Performance Psychology

Commissioning Editor: Claire Wilson
Development Editor: Catherine Jackson
Project Manager: Sukanthi Sukumar
Designer: Stewart Larking
Illustration Manager: Gillian Richards
Illustrator: Cactus

Performance Psychology

A Practitioner's Guide

Edited by

Dave Collins BEd MSc PhD CPsychol CSci FSMA AFBPsS FBASES
Director, Grey Matters Performance/Chair of Coaching and Performance, University of Central Lancashire, Lancashire, UK

Angela Button PhD MSc BA(Hons)
Research Fellow, University of Otago, Otago, New Zealand

Hugh Richards CPsychol
Director, Postgraduate Programmes in Performance Psychology, Institute for Sport, PE & Health Sciences, University of Edinburgh, Edinburgh, UK

Foreword by

Andy Robinson OBE
Scotland Head Coach, Scottish Rugby, Murrayfield Stadium, Edinburgh, UK

CHURCHILL LIVINGSTONE

ELSEVIER

Edinburgh London New York Oxford Philadelphia St Louis Sydney Toronto 2011

CHURCHILL
LIVINGSTONE
ELSEVIER

ISBN: 978-0-443-06734-1

British Library Cataloguing in Publication Data
A catalogue record for this book is available from the British Library

Library of Congress Cataloging in Publication Data
A catalog record for this book is available from the Library of Congress

Notice
Neither the Publisher nor the Editors assume any responsibility for any loss or injury and/or damage to persons or property arising out of or related to any use of the material contained in this book. It is the responsibility of the treating practitioner, relying on independent expertise and knowledge of the patient, to determine the best treatment and method of application for the patient.

The Publisher

Printed in China

Contents

Foreword

Getting it right mentally is crucial to performance. Now acknowledged by performers and coaches alike, performance psychology is an increasingly important feature of preparation. However, psychological aspects are not just something which is addressed immediately before the big game. Getting it right mentally is something that starts a lot earlier, often before the elite coach gets his or her hands on the performers. This book covers the whole 'mental preparation' process; from talent development, though setting up the right environment, to designing and deploying practice regimes. Oh yes, AND doing everything right in preparation for the specific event.

Reflecting this longer term perspective, this book offers exemplars for each stage of the process. Just as importantly, the four stage process is crucial to performance in many domains. The expert panel in this book serve to demonstrate how each stage is crucial for performance in the long term, across domains as varied as athletics, rugby, dance and extreme sports. If the principles work across this lot, they will work anywhere!

Andy Robinson, OBE
Scotland Head Coach

Acknowledgements

Over the years and in the different places and jobs that we have worked, many individuals have contributed to our understanding of psychology and its impact on performance. There are far too many to mention individually, but include colleagues, clients, collaborators, students, supervisors and supervisees. We are grateful for the opportunities this work has provided and for the insights that we have gained from you.

We would also like to acknowledge the contributions made to this book by the authors, photo providers and others who have helped to shape its content.

Dedications

Dave's Dedication
To HelsBels, Joe, Judy, Rosie, Ruby and Lily

Angela's Dedication
For my Familiy

Hugh's Dedication
To Elspeth and to my girls, Anya, Lucy and Bronwyn

List of Contributors

Andrew Abraham MSc
Principal Lecturer in Sports Coaching, Leeds Metropolitan University, Leeds, UK

Joseph Baker PhD
Associate Professor of Lifespan Health and Development, School of Kinesiology & Health Science, York University, Toronto, Canada

Veronica Burke BA(Hons) PGCE MA PhD
Programme Director – General Management Programmes, Cranfield University, School of Management, Bedford, UK

Angela Button PhD MSc BA(Hons)
Research Fellow, University of Otago, Dunedin, New Zealand

Chris Button BSc(Hons) PhD
Associate Professor, School of Physical Education, University of Otago, Dunedin, New Zealand

Claire Calmels PhD
Researcher, INSEP, Research Service, Paris

Dave Collins BEd MSc PhD CPsychol CSci FSMA AFBPsS FBASES
Director, Grey Matters Performance/Chair of Coaching and Performance, University of Central Lancashire, Lancashire, UK

Judy Collins BSc Psych CertCBT
Psychology Department, University of Leicester, Leicester, UK

Nicola J. Hodges BSc MSc PhD
Associate Professor, School of Human Kinetics, University of British Columbia, Canada

Paul Holmes PhD
Director, Institute for Performance Research, Manchester Metropolitan University, Crewe, Cheshire, UK

Patrick W. Howard BPharm MPS FINSIA
Chief Operations Officer, Cromwell, Brisbane, Australia

John Kiely HDip BSc(Hons) MSc
Senior Lecturer in Elite Performance, Institute of Coaching and Performance, University of Central Lancashire, Lancashire, UK; Strength and Conditioning Consultant, UK Athletics, Athletics House, Solihull, West Midlands, UK

Clare MacMahon PhD
Senior Lecturer, Motor Learning and Skilled Performance, Institute of Sport, Exercise and Active Living (ISEAL), Victoria University, Melbourne, Australia

Áine MacNamara PhD
Senior Lecturer in Elite Performance, Institute of Coaching and Performance, University of Central Lancashire, Lancashire, UK

Alan C. MacPherson PhD
Lecturer in Sport and Exercise Psychology, Institute of Sport, Physical Education & Health Sciences, University of Edinburgh, Edinburgh, UK

Amanda Martindale BSc(Hons) MSc CPsychol PhD
Lecturer in Sport and Performance Psychology, Physical Education, Sport and Leisure Studies, University of Edinburgh, Edinburgh, UK

Russell Martindale BSc MSc PhD
Lecturer in Sport Psychology and Coaching, Napier University, Edinburgh, UK

Duncan R.D. Mascarenhas PhD
Senior Lecturer in Sport and Exercise Psychology, Sport and Exercise Sciences, Glyndŵr University, Wrexham, UK

Rich Masters BA(Hons) MA DPhil
Professor and Assistant Director (Research), Institute of Human Performance, The University of Hong Kong, Hong Kong

Aidan Moran BA MA PhD
Professor of Cognitive Psychology, School of Psychology, University College, Dublin, Ireland

Patrick Mortimer BEd(Hons)
Private Consultant, Aubrey Performance, www.aubreyperformance.co.uk; formerly Performance Manager, Rugby Football League/Chelsea Football Club Academy, Cheshire, UK

Hugh Richards CPsychol
Director, Postgraduate Programmes in Performance Psychology, Institute for Sport, PE & Health Sciences, University of Edinburgh, Edinburgh, UK

Sheelagh Rodgers DClinPsychol MSC MBA BA(Hons)
Area Clinical Psychologist, NHS Highland, Inverness, UK

Nickolas C. Smith PhD CPsychol
Principal Lecturer, Sport and Exercise Psychology, Department of Sport and Exercise Science, Manchester Metropolitan University, Cheshire, UK

Britt Tajet-Foxell BSc MSc
Cognitive Behavioural Psychotherapist, The Royal Ballet, London, UK; Chartered Psychologist, Olympiatoppen, The Olympic High Performance Centre, Oslo, Norway

Joan N. Vickers EdD
Professor, Faculty of Kinesiology, University of Calgary, Alberta, Canada

Mark R. Wilson PhD
Senior Lecturer in Sport Psychology, School of Sport and Health Sciences, University of Exeter, Exeter, UK

Performance Panel

Steve Backley OBE
Retired Athlete and Olympian; Designated Partner, www.BackleyBlack.com

Kevin Bowring BEd
Head of Elite Coach Development, Rugby Football Union, Bristol, UK

Sara Matthews
Artistic Director, Central School of Ballet, London, UK

Ray Rowe BCU Level 5 Coach
Teacher, UK

Introduction
Performance psychology: developing a peak performance culture

Dave Collins

Grey Matters/UCLan

CHAPTER CONTENTS

> Times are bad. Children no longer obey their parents and everyone is writing a book.
>
> Cicero, c. 43 BC

So, on the basis that some things haven't changed much since Roman times, we decided to get together with some friends and colleagues and write one ourselves. Our motivation in producing this magnificent tome was simple; to attempt the provision of a comprehensive guide for mental aspects of physical performance.

What do we cover and why?

There are loads of texts on sport psychology, and an increasing number that look at the application of these techniques to other performance domains such as dance, music and/or business. To our minds, however, the vast majority make the error of concentrating on the 'traditional' methods of sport psychology, namely the mental skills and strategies taught to athletes, rather than considering every aspect of the performance environment. In simple terms, what we try to provide here is a guide to developing your own performance pathway, right from consideration of *preparation* (early identification/selection – if this is really advantageous), through *provision* (of support – structuring and managing your training and performance environment) through considerations of *practice* and the mental skills stuff to help you to ensure the best *performance*.

At the time of writing there seems to be an ever increasing number of subspecialisms in performance support. On a personal level, I would always rather work in an inclusive and inter/crossdiscipline fashion to ensure benefits from the component subjects and their interactions. As Gandalf says 'he that breaks a thing to find out what it is has left the path of wisdom' (p. 276). OK, that's a bit pretentious, but I do feel that treating coaching, skill acquisition and talent identification as separate concerns carries some risk. Consequently, you will find them all covered, and hopefully integrated, in this text.

Why might psychology be different from other support disciplines?

> Sport science is a multi-disciplinary field concerned with the understanding and enhancement of human sporting performance. Sport science can be thought of as a scientific process used to guide the practice of sport with the ultimate aim of improving sporting performance. It is about using the best available evidence at the right time, in the right environment, for the right individual to improve their performance.
>
> Bishop, 2008, p. 254

DOI: 10.1016/B978-0-443-06734-1.00026-2

Consider the ways in which support disciplines are embedded within performance support programmes. Physiotherapy, strength and conditioning and, more recently, nutrition are well accepted across almost all the physical domains. Even biomechanics and its more user-friendly subshoot, movement analysis (is there a difference?), is commonly accepted. Despite the obvious acceptance that performance has a massive mental component, however, psychologists and psychological principles have not received an equivalent level of attention.

At least two possible explanations occur to me. Firstly, perhaps mental characteristics aren't as easily operationalized. In this respect, it might be worth remembering the futility of only working on things you can measure. Performance isn't a Schrödinger's cat setting; try to measure it and it suffers. Neither, however, are we limited to a need for total objectivity all of the time. As such, intuition and thinking out of the box are always going to be part of the armoury when you are focused on innovation; on getting an edge over the competition (even when what you do isn't overtly competitive) as a central part of your role. In short, if you stay in your comfort zone as a scientist, quoting references all day, you are unlikely to be accepted into the performance environment, whatever it is. Without a consistent, 'no compromise' (a commonly stated, very uncommonly followed principle) focus on the end result, you may become guilty of self-satisfying academic activity at the genuine expense of the performance you are employed to enhance.

At the other end of the scale, however, psychologists might not get a look in because what they do is viewed as a bit fuzzy or fluffy-bunny for the hard world of performance. Certainly, when I hear a leading proponent of sport psychologist training state that performance is not important compared to performer wellbeing, I cringe! Perhaps psychologists need to acknowledge the stated needs of the client? If they want pushing, then we should help to push! And furthermore, this pushing should be across the disciplinary spectrum since virtually everything done has a mental component. Perhaps some performance psychologists don't know enough, or at least understand and apply enough, to make a notable contribution. Accordingly, ensuring the quality and hard-edged-ness of science in what you do is also vital. Without this quality, your input takes on a salesperson quality, with impact based more on powers of persuasion than demonstrable cause and effect.

So how do we cover it and why?

Reflecting these parallel considerations (comprehensive coverage, scientific rigour and performance focus) has been our concern throughout. We have selected authors whose approach characterizes the 'scientist–practitioner' model; high-quality, pertinent research and theoretical evidence underpinning practical and impactful advice. Chapters will say clearly what they suggest, what they don't agree with *and why*. This qualifier is important in a world where reputation ('Do you know how many medallists I've coached?'), politics ('Do you know that organization X or person Y appointed me?') or sport-specific connection ('Of course, when I was performing with...') often have a completely disproportionate influence, unless of course you stick to the 'no compromise' principles that such individuals so frequently espouse! As such, chapters will be technical, well referenced and academic in the best sense of the term.

To further ensure the real-life application, however, we are privileged to have secured the input of a performers' panel (hereafter referred to as the PP): a group of experts drawn from across the performance domains who have contributed to action summary chapters at the end of each section. The names, brief backgrounds and abbreviations used in this book are shown in Table A1 below.

Two more things to note and we can get started. Our attempt to cover physical environments is genuine but, to avoid the frequent use of multiple terms, please take 'performer' to mean all such species (athlete, player, dancer, etc.) and 'coach' to mean every variant of those who technically help and develop them (including teacher, instructor, sensei/sifu or grand wazir).

Enfin

I started with a quote....so here's another to finish.

> Many thanks for your book. I shall waste no time in reading it.
>
> Benjamin Franklin

I hope your experience is somewhat more positive than Ben's. Happy reading!

Table A1 The performer's panel membership – brief profiles

Name	Current role	Performance domain	Brief resumé
Steve Backley (SB)	Private consultant	Individual sports	• International athlete and former WR javelin • Triple Olympic/double world medallist • Four times European champion
Kevin Bowring (KB)	Head of elite coach development, Rugby Football Union (RFU)	Team sports	• First class and Barbarians rugby player • Coach of Wales 1995–98 • Winner of the SCUK 'Dyson' award
Sara Matthews (SM)	Director, Central School of Ballet	Dance	• Professional dancer with Ballet Rambert for 11 years • Teaches contemporary dance and also choreographs for Ballet Central • Teaches internationally, including recent trips to Cuba and Japan
Ray Rowe (RR)	Teacher	Extreme sports	• Paddled in two flat-water world championships, selected Olympian, Munich • First descents in Wales, First ascents Iran, First crossings in Alaska, Australia, Arctic Norway, etc. • First solo completion – Three Peaks

References

Bishop, D., 2008. An applied research model for the sport sciences. Sports Med. 38, 253–263.

Gandalf (1418 sr). Cited in Tolkein, J.R.R. (Ed.), 1968. The Lord of the Rings (single-volume paperback edition). George Allen & Unwin, London, p. 276.

Section 1

Preparation

Introduction: getting ready to perform

1

Dave Collins

Grey Matters/UCLan

Many texts concentrate on the mental skills necessary to perform at top level, and self-help books of variable quality and extremely variable theoretical provenance abound. What is less common, bar a few 'parenting your superstar' books from the US market, are resources that provide a critical consideration of what it takes to get there; that is, the challenges which need to be faced on the pathway to elite performance and the associated skills to overcome them. In parallel to this dearth, the majority of the literature about young performers has, at least until recently, been focused on the identification of talent rather than the best way to develop it (talent identification and development: TID).

To an extent, this focus is understandable, especially when one considers the predominance of 'hard science' approaches, largely physiological, in the history of performance enhancement. The predominance of periodization, the tightly controlled and well ordered planning for future success is one such approach (which may well be flawed – see Chapter 10), which has been a major influence on the ways we work with performers. These ideas receive 'support' with the clear success that has resulted from tightly controlled and achievement-focused performance systems in past (e.g. the eastern European, most notably Russia and East Germany) and present (e.g. Chinese) regimes. Add in the widely touted and 'clearly apparent' importance of genetic endowment and early identification, and placement in a highly pressured 'hot-house' environment becomes the obvious solution to the need for performance success, irrespective of domain. These approaches still abound across performance domains. Young children are selected for high-status training on the basis of anthropometry (e.g. ballet or rowing) and/or early performance accomplishment (e.g. tennis or athletics) and, until recently, no questions have been asked about the efficacy or even the ethics of this approach.

It is against this backdrop that this section proposes a psychologically based approach to talent; in fact, one more focused on development than identification (TID) because we believe this to be the most effective and efficient approach to the dual challenge of realizing potential while also promoting lifelong physical activity and an achievement orientation. In making this point, the authors are not combative but rather raise issues with previous approaches when considered against the aims and processes of TID schemes in a western society. As such, we do not deny that early selection and hot-housing will be effective in certain cultures (see Ch. 2). Just in passing, however, you might like to consider the points made about the role of genetics in Table 1.1. Of course, genetic endowment plays a role. I am about 120 kg on a good day. I won't make much of a dancer, while Angela (50 kg) won't succeed as a prop forward in rugby despite her Welsh Heritage! It's just that things are somewhat more complex than many genetics-based initiatives (e.g. the comparative length of your middle finger or testing all army recruits for the possession of an SAS gene) may suggest.

So, on with the content. The section gets an excellent base from Angela Button in Chapter 2. Angela's treatment of the issue is both comprehensive theoretically and practical in its guidelines and implications.

Nicola Hodges and Joseph Baker present a scholarly and thorough consideration of expertise in

DOI: 10.1016/B978-0-443-06734-1.00001-8

Table 1.1 Talent. . . .are you really born with it?

Question	Some observations	The point
What do geneticists think?	'If you gave me money and said, 'Build a football team', I'd be better off paying boys' clubs to give me first crack at their talented youngsters than spending it on genetic tests' (Hugh Montgomery – geneticist from University College London, quoted in Wilde 2003)	Genetics can't address enough of the variance (i.e. explain or measure enough of the causative factors)
How effective is 'genetic engineering'?	Only one in 10 turns out to be a thoroughbred. For example: • Snafee Dancer (sired by Northern Dancer) cost £13.1m but never raced • Red Rum was bred as a sprinter but won three Grand Nationals	The best organized genetic engineering system in the world is, at best, 10% efficient. Even when it works, attempts to breed 'Usain Bolt' can result in 'Paula Radcliffe'

Chapter 3. Optimum development of expertise is a big part of the pathway to excellence, so an understanding of how this may best be achieved is part of the core armoury for all those involved in talent development (TD).

In Chapter 4, Áine MacNamara presents some of the key implications of the theoretical coverage provided by Angela. Áine introduces the idea of psychological characteristics of developing excellence (PCDEs) as arguably the most important characteristics needed by a developing performer. The psychological bias is obvious (but look at the title of the book!) but is also justified by many of the arguments in the preceding chapters. This, we believe, is the best way to realize potential and develop talent.

Finally, Russell Martindale considers the design characteristics of optimum TD environments in Chapter 5. A triangulation of theory with perspectives from coaches and developing performers reveals a pleasingly consistent picture of what is needed. These practical parameters are supported through input from Paddy Mortimer, the second author, who, at the time of writing, was engaged in the evolution of the well supported and well led academy at Chelsea FC (a fairly good football club in London, in case you hadn't heard of them).

As the common feature in every section, the performance panel (PP) chapter concludes with some more practical considerations and guidelines for practitioners in the TD field.

Reference

Wilde, S., 2003. Runs in the family. Sunday Times 6 July. Available on line at: http://www.timesonline.co.uk/tol/sport/article1148435.ece (accessed 30.10.09).

Aims, principles and methodologies in talent identification and development

2

Angela Button

Dunedin, Otago, New Zealand

CHAPTER CONTENTS

Introduction

Talent identification (TI) has undoubtedly become big business. Across a range of different performance domains including sport, art, dance and education, researchers are continually attempting to find effective methods to identify the best performers for the future. These fields are united in many societies around the world by high levels of competition to achieve success against limited financial resources (Abbott et al 2005). In addition, research suggests that talented individuals need to experience 10 years of developmental opportunities before they excel in their chosen domain (Ericsson et al 1993, Starkes 2000). As such, implementing processes for recruiting and developing talented individuals before they are snatched up by other competitors has become a priority for many organizations (e.g. a business or a national governing body of sport). For example, in the mid-1990s, the English Football Association recognized that their talent development (TD) system was inadequate for serving the needs of young players (Holt 2002). Consequently, the TD system was restructured and all Premier League clubs were required to operate an elite development academy and all Football League clubs a centre of excellence aimed at recruiting and developing talented footballers from the age of 9 upwards. This increased popularity of academies and centres of excellence

DOI: 10.1016/B978-0-443-06734-1.00002-X

has occurred not only in sport but across other performance areas (e.g. dance, art and drama) as organizations increasingly recognize the importance of providing a coordinated and systematic approach to TD from early participation through to elite level.

The implementation of effective talent recruitment and development systems would appear to be a particular concern for those countries that don't have the luxury of selecting from a large population base. For example, within sport, Australia and the UK have to select from a relatively small population base compared to USA, Russia and Germany. Therefore, this chapter will initially consider current approaches for identifying the talented and reflect on their appropriateness for identifying the performer most likely to attain excellence within a domain. Based on this evaluation, and a recognition of what it takes to develop into a successful elite performer, general principles that need to underpin talent identification and development (TID) models are discussed. How coaches/trainers can adhere to the principles advocated when working with their performers is discussed further in Chapters 4 and 5, and exemplars/ideas for practice are covered in Chapter 6.

Traditional talent identification processes

Traditionally, TID resources (coaching expertise, access to facilities, funding, etc.) have been targeted at those youngsters who are judged to have performed the best during age group competitions or who stand out during trials or auditions (Abbott & Collins 2004). In addition, within sport, more systematic processes of identifying talent where the physical and physiological characteristics of youngsters (e.g. height, speed) are contrasted with an 'ideal' physique for a specific sport have been increasingly employed. Such processes were originally initiated (with some success) in the former Eastern Bloc countries in the 1960s and 1970s and continue to underpin the majority of systematic TI processes employed in sport today (for an overview of such processes, see Abbott & Collins 2004). The potential role of physique on the performance of athletes has been recognized by sport practitioners for decades. For example, physical education teachers commonly position players in teams on the basis of their physique (e.g. the tall student is steered towards basketball and the short student towards gymnastics). The music teacher may consider students' hand structure (e.g. length of fingers) when directing them towards a specific instrument (e.g. the piano). The dance teacher may look at the flexibility and body proportions of their pupils as an indication of those most likely to excel. The performance and physical make up of a young performer continue to be the dominant approaches for identifying the 'talented' (Abbott & Collins 2004). In fact, the increased interest in genetics appears to have further fuelled the interest in physique-based selection processes.

Of course, it may well be that, in environments/societies where psychological issues such as motivation can be discounted, these approaches offer an effective answer to the TID question. Under certain regimes, for example, all children are expected to commit themselves to the needs of the state. In others, poverty makes the pursuit of sporting success so attractive that almost everyone is highly committed to achievement, whatever the personal cost or challenge. Fortunately from a humanitarian point of view, such situations do not typify the majority of countries. Accordingly, and most simply, choice makes the individual perspective a crucial extra factor that must be catered for. In short, even if person A has the perfect build (or it at least seems that they will eventually have it) and motor ability for an activity, they may just not want to take part. Reflecting this tenable possibility, therefore, the remainder of this section (and indeed the book) considers things from the individual perspective, within an environment that does not 'demand' that people stay with whatever they are allocated to.

This caveat notwithstanding, however, the youth performance/anthropometric/genetic approach still exhibits significant weaknesses. It may be that even the old Eastern Bloc got some things wrong! In fact, the limitations of both performance- and physique-based approaches for identifying those individuals most likely to develop into successful senior competitors are increasingly being acknowledged by both researchers and practitioners (Abbott et al 2005). The following section will provide an overview of these major limitations.

Limitations of performance- and physique-based TI models

Using performance and/or physique as the main (or sole) criteria for selection ignores the fact that performance can be constrained by a range of factors, many of which can vary over time. For example, if an individual is excelling at a particular point in time, is this as a result of his/her talent or is it a result of his/her physical maturity in comparison with his/her peers? Consider a young rugby player who stands out due to his ability to score regularly. If the youngster is more physically mature than his peers, this success may be a result of an ability to overpower his opponents rather than as a result of possessing a 'rugby' talent. Such physical maturity biases are commonly apparent in age-group sport as considerable interindividual variation can occur in the processes of maturation and an early maturer may start puberty 5 years before a late-maturing peer (Boreham 2001). Therefore, the impact of this variation is that adolescents who excel at strength sports (e.g. rugby, weightlifting) tend to be 'early maturers' (Blanksby 1980, Bloomfield 1995, Shakespear 1980) while 'late maturers' tend to excel in coordination sports (e.g. rowing, gymnastics) (de Garay et al 1974, Moore et al 1998).

A detailed example of the impact of relative age in selection processes was emphasized recently in Belgian football. Helsen et al (2000) highlighted how, until 1997, the Belgian selection year started on 1 August and ended on 31 July. Youth players born between August and October (the early part of the selection year) were more likely to be identified as talented and eventually to become successful senior players. In contrast, players born later in the selection year tended to drop out of football as early as 12 years of age. However, the change in the start of selection in 1997 to the first of January has resulted in a shift in the birthdates of individuals being selected. Only individuals within the 16–18 age group did not experience this shift. This is probably because those players who were born in the first and second quarters of the year (January–July) were deselected before the age of 16, because of the old selection process. This finding highlights the problem with employing performance criteria for identifying talent, since those individuals born later in the selection year are likely to be later maturers. Of relevance, Malina et al (2000) found that, within Portugal, football appeared systematically to exclude late-maturing boys and favour average and early-maturing boys. Consequently, late maturers are likely to be eliminated during adolescence and will not have the opportunity to develop the required skills to be reselected into the sport once they have matured physically.

To illustrate how individual variation in timing and rate of biological maturation can have profound repercussions for the adolescent athlete, consider a selection policy that positively discriminates in favour of those individuals who are able to overpower their less mature competitors through size and strength, that is, on current performance. For a 'late maturer' to develop successfully along the athletic continuum, he/she would have to be technically superior just to 'hang in there' (Van der Walt 1988). Unfortunately however, evidence suggests that rather than 'hanging in there', players born later in the selection year tend to drop out of 'strength' sports as early as 12 years of age (Helsen et al 1998). Consequently, many late maturers are likely to be ignored during adolescence and will not have the opportunity to develop the required skills to be reselected into the sport once they have matured physically. Crucially however, those few late maturers who do persevere are often likely eventually to surpass the performance of the early maturers, who have not been required to develop optimum technical skills, nor even perhaps to develop and exhibit similarly high levels of work rate and determination. Additionally, once 'caught up' by these late developers, the early maturers often drop out; frustrated perhaps by their sudden inability to compete with these technically superior athletes and their lack of experience in working through difficulties (Abbott et al 2002). Therefore, adolescent performance, rather than reflecting the talent of an individual, may say more about the physical maturity of that individual. In consequence, TI models that select on the basis of either performance or physical variables alone (and these are unfortunately typically employed with prepubescent or pubescent children) are likely to identify adolescents who happen to have a physical advantage at the time of testing, as opposed to identifying the individuals with the most talent.

A second problem with physical and performance-based TI models is that they underplay potential. Since the focus of such models is on age-group success, the potential of an individual to develop into a successful senior player is typically overlooked. The vast majority of coaches/teachers are able to highlight individuals who showed early promise as youngsters but who failed to develop into successful adult performers. This failure to translate early 'potential' may be a result of a range of factors such as a lack of commitment, poor decision-making skills, short-term physical advantages or an inability to perform under pressure. In contrast, many performers have made it to the top of their chosen domain despite not showing promise as a junior. For example, within sport, a longitudinal study of elite German tennis players found no early predictors of tennis performance in early adulthood (Schneider 1993, see also Monsaas 1985). This research is supported by anecdotal evidence across a range of disciplines. One of many examples of individuals that have excelled in sport despite being discounted is Pietro Mennea. Mennea held the 200 m world record for 17 years from 1979–1996. As a youth he was given little hope of athletic achievement since it was believed that his slight physical frame was inappropriate for sprinting. Reflecting on his athletic background, Mennea stated, 'When I took up athletics almost all the coaches doubted that I could ever achieve any significant results. I always used that as a stimulus to prove them wrong and become a success. And I did' (Birri 2000). Apparently, dedication, application and technique development were the key factors in his outstanding success and enabled Pietro Mennea to overcome his physical 'shortcomings'.

Biographies of individuals who have excelled within arts and music also highlight the fact that early achievement is not a necessary prerequisite for adult excellence. For example, Sosniak (1985) studied 24 exceptionally able young professional pianists and found that there were few indicators of the musicians' potential when they were very young. Even after 6 years of relatively intensive training, confident predictions about the eventual success of the young musicians could only have occurred in a minority of cases. Sloboda (2005, p. 269) comments that 'the notion that very early achievement is the normal precursor of adult excellence finds very little support in the documented research literature. The child prodigy may be the exception rather than the norm.'

Consequently, the key problem is not so much in identifying the best performer at any one time or the youngster with the 'ideal' physical profile but rather identifying over time which factors may be limiting TD (Kunst & Florescu 1971, Simonton 1999). Therefore, while discrete performance variables may be helpful in signposting potential athletes during development, we should not be fooled into believing that they can distinguish future performers (Abbott et al 2005). If an individual does not currently display a desired attribute (e.g. effective decision making), this may be because an important factor (e.g. self-confidence) is absent or because it will not develop or emerge until later. The lack of a characteristic, such as mental focus, that may take several years to fully develop (Gould et al 2002) may hinder the identification of young and otherwise very talented athletes. In addition, as evidenced by the success of Pietro Mennea, 'shortcomings' in one area may be successfully compensated for by strengths in other areas.

Another important quality that is often ignored by discrete physical or performance measures is the ability of an athlete to adapt performance to suit different situations and environments. In golf, for example, the fairways on British Open courses are typically wider and the greens slower than on the US Open course. In tennis and cricket, players must also learn to adapt their game to various playing surfaces. Many examples exist of players who have failed to make the crucial adaptations required. For example, the USA tennis player Andy Roddick won the US open (hard court) in 2003 and was a finalist in 2006. He also reached the Wimbledon (grass court) finals in 2004, 2005 and 2009. However, Roddick has struggled to adapt his game to clay court surfaces and in the last 7 years has been eliminated four times from the first round of the French open. In golf, Phil Mickelson, who has achieved 31 PGA tour victories to date, has finished in the top 10 only once in 13 British Open appearances. In an interview with Christine Brennan (2006), Mickelson, reflecting on his past performances in the British Open, stated that:

> It wasn't until 2004 that I really understood the technique of hitting the ball properly into the wind, I was swinging hard, just like I normally do, and I wasn't able to get that low, penetrating shot. It just took me a lot longer to trust that 50–100 yards of roll that we get and took me a while to learn how to trust the little knockdown, little chip shots that travel a couple hundred yards because of the hard fairways.

In contrast, Tiger Woods adapted his US game quickly to meet the demands of the British Open, finishing third in 1998, his second full season as a professional, and winning the championship in 2000, 2005 and 2006. In fact, the subtle adaptation (or transfer) of coordination patterns is arguably what enables elite sports people such as Tiger Woods to maintain very high levels of performance consistency over the course of several playing seasons (Button et al 2006). The clear message is that the ability to adapt is a genuinely key feature of true elites but that this ability is unlikely to be identified by snapshot observations (e.g. single testing days) and/or single-environment TI events.

In summary, this section has highlighted how talent in any performance area is both multidimensional and non-linear. Therefore, traditional TI programmes that identify the 'talented' through summative scores on a limited range of physical and/or performance measures may lack sensitivity and predictive power and therefore may prematurely eliminate many potentially talented but late-maturing youngsters. Additionally, such models may lead to the demotivation of children, since early selection of an individual, due to his/her display of age-group excellence, may be closely followed by deselection once their peers 'catch up' and any early advantages are minimized or eliminated. Consequently, the following section argues that there is a need to combine TI and TD processes so that emphasis can be placed on the development of a range of key variables that underpin success rather than focusing on snapshots of a few unstable variables to identify the 'talented'.

Acknowledging the multidimensional and dynamic nature of talent within TID programmes

Despite the multidimensional and dynamic nature of talent highlighted in the previous section, TI processes across performance domains continue to rely on snapshots of a limited number of discrete variables (e.g. grouping/selecting athletes on height and weight; see Abbott & Collins 2004 for a review). Such processes reflect the belief that TI can be a distinct process that precedes effective TD. However, as highlighted above, long-term predictions cannot be made solely on the basis of a few physical or performance characteristics, at the very least because of their unstable and non-linear development over time. In addition, there are clear limitations to TI models where no consideration is given to many key performance determinants, because of their developmental, and therefore non-predictable, nature. For example, the real life examples presented in Box 2.1 and Box 2.2 highlight (a) performers who excelled in their chosen domain despite apparently displaying poor values on one or more 'key' performance variables during childhood and (b) performers who excelled as youngsters but did not or have yet to transfer this early success into senior competition. These examples reinforce the multidimensional nature of talent and how, through appropriate developmental opportunities, weaknesses in one area can either be overcome or compensated for by strength

Box 2.1

Examples of individuals who have excelled at the senior level despite a weak profile as a junior

Athletics: Linford Christie was involved in athletics as a youth. However, until the age of 16, this involvement lacked commitment. The turning point appears to have been in the summer of 1985 (aged 25) when his coach Ron Roddan and Andy Norman, the promotions officer for British athletics, sent letters to him saying, in effect, use your talent or leave athletics. That lit a fire, and the next year Christie lowered his 100 m best from 10.42 to 10.04 and went on to claim his first major title. In 1992, he became the Olympics 100 m title holder.

Ballet: At the age of 14, Ryan Nye was on track to play cornerback or linebacker one day for the Waterville Senior High School football team when he took up ballet. At 14 he was a late starter and had to reshape his body before he could master the many movements and the extraordinary extension demanded of a quality ballet dancer. However, by the age of 15, he was playing lead roles in the Bossov Ballet.

Football: Alan Ball was a 5 ft 6 in (1.68 m) English professional footballer who was the youngest member of England's 1966 World Cup winning team. However, as a teenager Alan Ball was rejected by both Wolverhampton and Bolton Wanderers football clubs. While on trial at Bolton, Bill Ridding, Bolton manager at the time, told Ball 'You'd make a good little jockey'. However, despite his lack of height, Ball gained 72 English caps and scored more than 180 league goals in a career spanning 22 years.

Box 2.2

Examples of individuals who have failed to excel at the senior level despite a strong profile as a junior

Athletics: Mark Lewis Francis burst on to the scene at an early age, setting UK age-group 100 m records at 14, 15, 16, 17 and 18 years of age, showing himself to be a brilliant prospect. At 19 years of age Lewis Francis ran an amazing time of 9.97 seconds and it was considered by many that a world record was inevitable. Yet he has consistently performed badly in championships and has actually become slower as he has moved into his twenties (9.97 remaining his personal best).

Football: Despite only losing on penalties in the Under-16 World Football Cup final in 1989, Scotland has failed to exploit this success as a basis for subsequent performance.

in other areas. Hence, the multidimensional and dynamic evolution of talent seems to suggest that the focus of TI processes in sport, and probably other performance domains, should shift from early identification towards developmental aspects. Therefore, before considering the best approaches for identifying and developing talent, this section considers how talent evolves over time.

The development process

Hopefully, in relating the concepts discussed in the previous sections to your own experiences, the multidimensional and dynamic nature of talent has been reinforced and the limitations of employing traditional approaches for identifying TI acknowledged. Clearly, in order to optimally target scarce TD resources, the complexity of talent needs to be recognized and catered for irrespective of the performance domain. As such, practitioners will need to acknowledge that (a) many of the key performance determinants in sport are not fixed and are not easily measurable but rather can be developed with the appropriate training opportunities (decision making, technique, etc.) and (b) eventual expertise will not require an individual only to develop a strong profile on the determinants of performance but also to develop those attributes that enable them to successfully negotiate the inevitable ups and downs they will encounter as they develop within their performance domain (perseverance, mental toughness, etc.). While many individuals working with developing performers may emphasis the development of these latter skills, current evidence suggests that they are not systematically being promoted across the development years of the performer. As such, the focus of this section will be on identifying some of the attributes that inhibit and facilitate athletes' ability to successfully develop in sport before a consideration is given to how TID systems can be refocused to ensure that appropriate emphasis is given to these key skills. While the primary focus of this section is on sport, the wider implications across performance domains should be apparent.

Successful development within a performance domain

As highlighted above, the pathway to success is rarely smooth. The progressive development of a world-class performer is a long-term process that research has suggested takes a minimum of 10 years or 10 000 hours (Ericsson & Charness 1994). The pathways to achieving excellence are characterized by sudden unpredictable jumps (or slumps) in development (i.e. are non-linear) and athletes pass through various stages of development as they progress from a novice to an expert in sport (Bloom 1985, Côté 1999, Durand-Bush & Salmela 2001), albeit at different times and for different durations. This non-linear TD is reflected in Figure 2.1, which tracks the 400 m freestyle performances of Australian swimmers Grant Hackett and Ian Thorpe since 1997 across five major championships.

Bloom's (1985) research in the USA explored the development of athletes, musicians and academics and considerably added to our understanding of the non-linear nature of expertise development. Furthering this work, Van Tassel-Baska (2001) highlights how a key component of Bloom's work was the focus on the evolution of talent as opposed to seeing talent as a phenomenon governed solely by genetic predispositions. Bloom (1985) highlighted three distinct stages of development in the athletic career (initiation, development and mastery) and stressed the influence of environment on the progress of individuals within each of these stages. For example, Bloom highlighted that champion tennis players benefited from being instructed by increasingly able coaches as they progressed. More recently, Côté (1999) presented the 'stages of sport participation' model, which looked at involvement in sport up to the age of 18 years and also identified the 'sampling', the 'specializing' and the 'investment' years:

> In general, the sampling years are characterized by a lower frequency of deliberate practice and a higher frequency of deliberate play; the specializing years are marked by more equal amounts of deliberate play and deliberate practice; and the investment years are characterized by a higher frequency of deliberate practice and a lower frequency of deliberate play
>
> Côté, 1999, p. 413

Côté also highlighted that there was likely to be a fourth stage of development typified by the maintenance and perfection of skills. This is consistent with work by Kreiner-Phillips & Orlick (1992) that highlighted the distinction between 'getting there' (producing a world-class performance) and 'staying there' (consistently producing world-class performances). The nature of these four stages of development is illustrated in Figure 2.2.

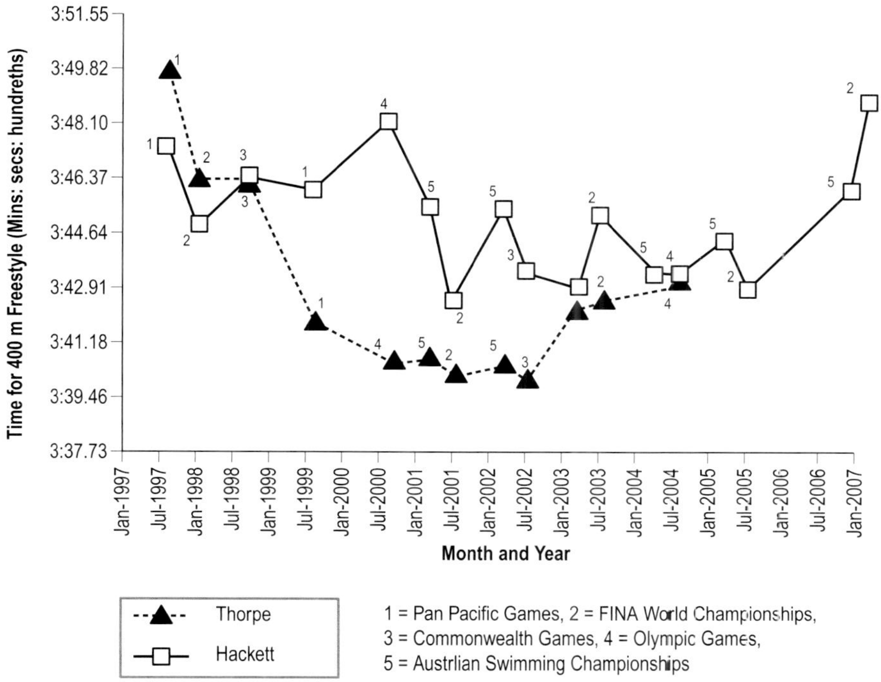

Fig. 2.1 • The non-linear 400 m freestyle performances of Australian swimmers Grant Hackett and Ian Thorpe since 1997 across five major championships.

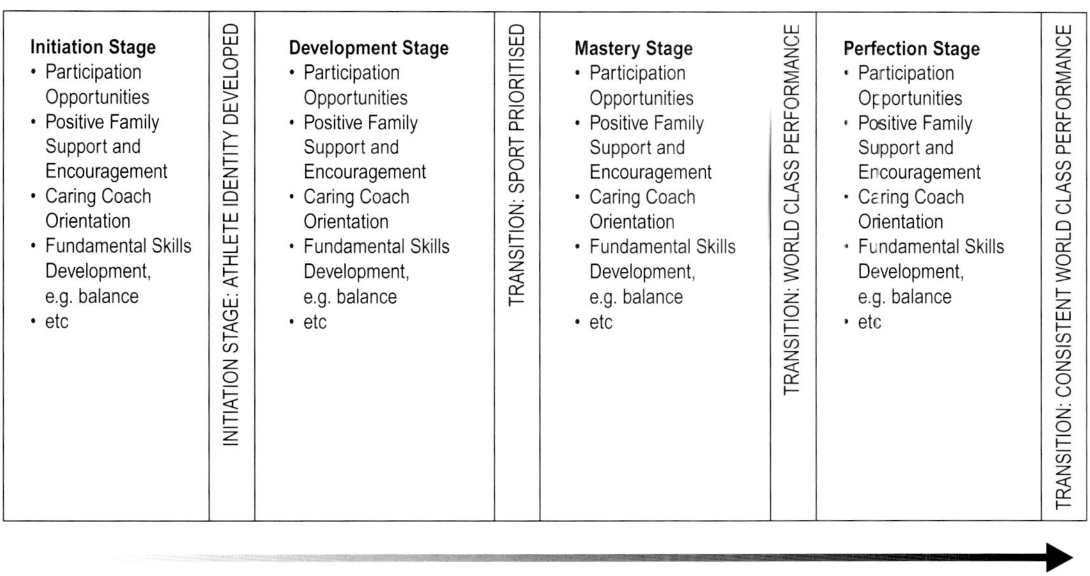

Fig. 2.2 • Stages of development that an elite performer is likely to progress through.

The existence of these stages suggests that the ability to achieve the changes required to successfully transfer between stages and to cope with the pressures within each stage will be crucial to the development of an athlete. Thus, an important question in understanding the characteristics of those that excel is 'Why are some individuals able to deal with and progress through the inevitable setbacks (e.g. injury, personal tragedy) they encounter during their development while the same setback may lead to other individuals dropping out of the sport altogether?' For example, speed skater Dan Jansen was favoured to win medals in both the 500 m and 1000 m races at the 1988 Olympic Games. However, his older sister died of leukaemia 7 hours before he raced in the 500 m event. Even though her death had been expected, Jansen was obviously shaken. Just 10 seconds into the race, he fell rounding a turn and was out of the competition. Three nights later, he fell again while on a winning pace in the 1000 m race. In the 1992 Olympics Jansen was once again favourite to win the 500 m and 1000 m events but finished a disappointing fourth in the 500 m race and 26th in the 1000 m race. However, despite these setbacks, Dan Jansen continued to strive towards achieving his dreams, and on entering the 1994 games was the only skater ever to have broken the 36 s mark for 500 m. Incredibly, Jansen once again fell during the 500 m race and finished in a disappointing eighth place. In the 1000 m race Jansen started fast and was on pace to beat the time of the current leader when he felt himself begin to lose his balance. Unlike in previous races, however, Jansen was able to regain focus and set a world record on his way to becoming the Olympic champion. Clearly, Jansen's perseverance in face of multiple setbacks enabled him to achieve his goals. Faced with similar hurdles and setbacks, many others may have become demotivated and have ended up withdrawing from competition before achieving their ambitions.

As well as overcoming setbacks, for individuals to fulfil their potential they must be able to initiate the changes required to make the transition from one stage of development to the next (e.g. increasing the hours of deliberate practice, changing coaches), then work effectively to achieve the transition and establish themselves at the next stage. The failure of many elite junior athletes to fulfil their potential will be apparent to many coaches. In 1979, Norm Osborne (then chairman of the Amateur Athletics Union Coaching Committee in Australia) and Dr John Boas (Australian jumps coach) discovered that, at the under-19 level, 90% of those who had won national junior titles and 75% of those who had won a medal had failed to make the transition to elite national or international level. While figures have improved today, 50% of athletes competing at the junior championships still fail to represent Australia at the senior level (Perera 2000). Within swimming, Malina (1997) highlights that it is not uncommon for a child to be successful in one age group only to be relegated to a low position in the ranking when s/he moves to the next age group. Fisher (1996) explained how a senior English Football Association coach traced back the England football teams for the World Cups of 1986 and 1990 to find that only one player, goalkeeper Peter Shilton, had played for England at youth level. Similarly, despite only losing on penalties in the U16 World Football Cup final in 1989, Scotland has failed to exploit this success as a basis for subsequent performance in the adult game (McCleish & Collins, 2002).

The crucial point is that, as performers encounter opportunities (e.g. opportunity to train with specialist coach), obstacles (e.g. an injury) and progressions (e.g. transition to the next stage of development), many aspects of their performance may become unstable and it is the ability of the developing athlete to cope with these unstable periods and to restabilize that is key to their continued development. The following section considers the skills that research suggests are crucial to this process.

Attributes likely to facilitate successful development

Research (e.g. Kreiner-Phillips & Orlick 1992, McDonald et al 1995, Morrone & Pintrich 1997, Schunk 1990) has demonstrated that the application of psychological behaviours such as being able to effectively evaluate performance, set realistic goals and self-reinforce are crucial to enable developing performers to cope with the unstable periods they will encounter as they progress within and across the four development stages (initiation, development, mastery and maintenance) highlighted by previous research. In effect, athletes use 'psychological behaviours' as transition mechanisms that can guide them into more effective, stable levels of performance and consequently these underpin the potential of an individual to become a successful and consistent elite performer (Abbott et al 2002). For example, the ability to produce consistently world-class performances is often viewed as the mark of a true champion. However, national standard athletes may struggle to progress to the world-class level if they do not possess the will to train to a sufficiently high intensity ('out of their comfort zone') or the mental skills to cope with 'off days' (handle failure) and deal with the associated instability in their performance. Interestingly, Kreiner-Phillips & Orlick (1992) found that, out of 17 athletes who had won major international titles in a range of sports, only seven continued to maintain their level of performance. The remaining athletes either experienced prolonged performance slumps ($n = 6$) or were never able to reproduce comparative performances ($n = 4$). Kreiner-Phillips and Orlick reported that only psychological factors were able to distinguish between consistent performers, those who experienced prolonged performance slumps and those who failed to reproduce comparative performances. Consequently, any TI processes should promote and monitor athletes on these key psychological behaviours.

A somewhat related issue is the ability of performers to successfully transfer across disciplines (e.g. from one sport to another, from one musical instrument to another). This 'discipline' transfer has been identified as an important experience of elite performers in British sport (Moore et al 1998) and music (Sloboda & Howe 1992), which aids the realization of top level performance. For example, Sloboda & Howe (1992) reported the background of 42 students at Chethams School of Music, Manchester, UK. Students at this school, aged 8–18, are selected nationally on the basis of musical audition and many students go on to professional careers as performing musicians. Sloboda and Howe found that only 45% of the students currently focused on the very first instrument they studied. In fact, for 10 of the musicians their principal instrument was often the third or even fourth instrument tried. Further, only two of the students had worked with just one instrument. Some interesting examples of performers transferring 'disciplines' are provided in Table 2.1.

The fact that so many examples exist of performers successfully changing disciplines (and specializing) late in their development and excelling despite not having accumulated the 10 000 hours of discipline-specific practice typically accepted as being required suggests that this transfer is facilitated by the skills they have developed in their original performance area. For example, Sloboda & Howe (1992), in their study of musicians, reported that 15 out of the 42 subjects began their musical careers on the recorder and concluded that classroom-based instruction on instruments such as recorders may be a useful stepping-stone to excellence on other instruments. Within sport and the performing arts many of the psychomotor skills (e.g. coordination, decision making) that contribute to success in one activity may also contribute to success in an alternate area. The television program 'Strictly Come Dancing'/ 'Dancing with the Stars', which requires famous people to learn how to dance, provides a good example of how athletes have successfully transferred the motor skills that underpin sport (e.g. coordination, balance) to a 'novel' activity. Examples of athletes that have successfully applied their dedication and agility to dance training include Colin Jackson (110 m hurdles), Denise Lewis (heptathlon), Darren Gough (cricket), Mark Ramprakash (cricket), Matt Dawson (Rugby Union), and Norm Hewitt (Rugby Union). Reflecting on how he managed to exploit his cricketing prowess when he was learning to dance, Ramprakash stated 'As a batsman, I do work a lot on technique, and always think about balance, my arms, where the feet go and how far they move' (Lane 2006).

Table 2.1 Examples of performers who have successfully transferred from one performance area to another

Name	Original sport	Current/ultimate Sport
Nigel Walker	100 m hurdling	Rugby Union
Iwan Thomas	BMX riding	400 m running
Eddie Eagan	Boxing	Bobsled
Ryan Nye	American football	Dancing
Marion Jones	Basketball	100 m sprinting
Arthur Milton	Football	Cricket

Therefore, given the generic nature of motor skills such as coordination and balance, it seems that children would benefit from involvement in a broad range of activities during the early stages of development. Unfortunately, the current trend of encouraging sport-specific involvement at an earlier age (e.g. mini-rugby) to ensure that the 'talented' get appropriate developmental opportunities is likely to prohibit the ability to transfer between disciplines and could further restrict the number of athletes who develop into successful senior international performers. The problem is that if children are not encouraged to experience and practise a range of different motor skills at a young age, this may prevent them from capitalizing on individual strengths or transferring these skills when specializing at later stages.

The broad activity background advocated above may also facilitate the ability of an athlete to adapt performance to suit different situations and environments, an ability that was identified earlier in this chapter as key for successful athletes. Bompa (2000) discusses the findings of two research projects by Nagorni (1978) and Harre (1982) that looked at the advantages and disadvantages of early and late specialization. Harre, from the former East Germany, conducted an experimental longitudinal study contrasting the impact of a traditional North American early specialization programme with an approach that developed sport-specific traits alongside generic skills. Nagorni, from the former USSR, carried out a descriptive longitudinal survey regarding youth developmental programmes. Their results yielded similar findings and highlighted the benefits of a multilateral training regimen in the early stages of development for promoting a strong, stable foundation for athletic success. For example, those individuals who had experienced a multilateral development programme early in the early stages of development increased their performance consistencies within competitions, while specialization led to inconsistencies. A range of recent research also supports diversified physical activity involvement during childhood (e.g. Baker et al 2003, Lidor & Lavyan 2002, Stevenson 1990).

Another feature that may be important in enabling successful performers to transfer their skills across different performance environments is the psychological behaviours discussed above (e.g. realistic performance evaluation, imagery, goal setting). For example, Mark Ramprakash highlighted how his sporting background has not only provided him with the balance and coordination required in dance but has also proved useful in preparing to compete under pressure: 'I try to get myself mentally in a frame of mind to perform, to have positive thoughts, to visualize myself going out there beforehand. It's trying to build confidence' (Lane, 2006). Research that has identified that the same psychological behaviours underpin success across a range of performance environments (e.g. surgery, athletics, music, dance) supports Ramprakash's experiences. For example, imagery has been found to be important for carrying out successful surgical operations (McDonald et al 1995), and for excelling as an athlete (Orlick 2000) and a musician (Talbot-Honeck & Orlick 1998). However, the surgeon, the athlete and the musician will clearly apply this psychological behaviour in a very context-specific way. Therefore, not only will TI processes that promote and monitor performers on key psychological behaviours help developing performers deal with the inevitable ups and downs they will experience as they develop within their specialist area, but these 'generic' skills will also facilitate athletes achieving their potential across different performance areas (e.g. academia, music).

To illustrate some of the TI issues that have been discussed so far, we can consider hypothetical data from three budding gymnasts (Collins, Button and Richards). We have measured three components of gymnastic performance that may help to distinguish which athlete is most talented. Looking at Figure 2.3, consider which of our gymnasts you think would have been identified by traditional TI models that select on the basis of physical or performance determinants? (Bear in mind that, in gymnastics, it is generally considered a disadvantage to be tall, as shorter people have a lower centre of gravity and can generate angular momentum quickly.) Time's up! It is probable that you chose Button, as he was the shortest gymnast of the three and did comparatively well on the other two components (commitment and agility). However, the concerns that have been raised in this chapter thus far also apply here. At present, the component that receives most emphasis is a physical factor (height), but the inclusion of psychobehavioural and psychomotor characteristics provide a more holistic description of talent. Still not simple, though! Even if you acknowledged this fact and added the contributions of the three components to provide a total score of talent, this still does not provide us with an understanding of the interaction of these factors over time. In Figure 2.4, each factor is monitored over time, depicting the changes in stability associated with each individual performer.

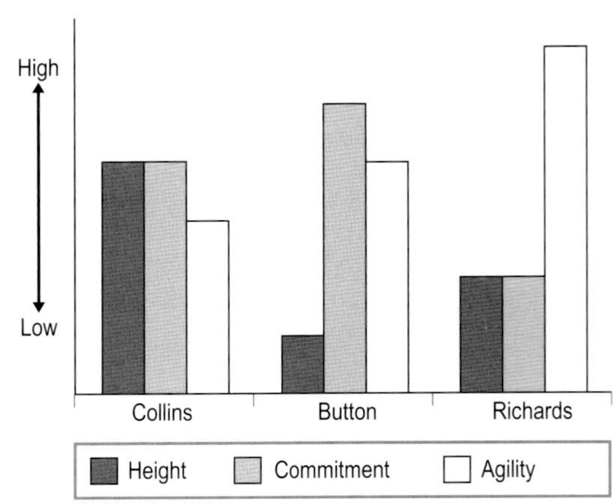

Fig. 2.3 • Hypothetical description of possible performance determinants amongst gymnasts: three possible components of talent measured for three different performers (height, agility and commitment).

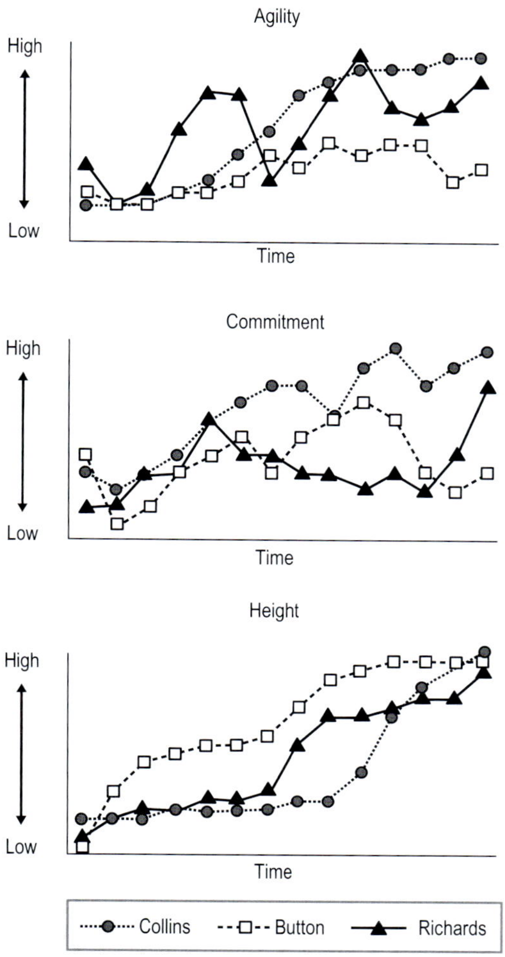

Fig. 2.4 • Changes in agility, commitment and height for each gymnast over time.

Also, rather than simply adding the mature values of each component, consider the multiplicative effect that each might have on talent and how the history of each factor will be of importance.

Which gymnast would you select now? It is possible that, instead of Button, you chose Collins, as his values for height, commitment, and agility were favourable at the final re-test. Alternatively, it might have been interesting to consider Richards; the lack of stability in his components may indicate the fact that he is progressing through a transitional period. Either way, the important message is that one-dimensional, discrete measures of performance related variables will be less effective than an approach that monitors and promotes athletes on a range of variables over time (Abbott et al 2005).

A real-life example recently emerged in the form of the Russian artistic gymnast Svetlana Khorkina, who was originally thought to be too tall to compete at the elite level and was advised to take up rhythmic gymnastics instead. However, Khorkina insisted on pursuing the sport she loved most and excelled despite her height disadvantage (she become a multiple world champion across various gymnastic disciplines). In fact, she turned her added stature to an advantage by producing slower and more graceful long, levered movements. This example highlights the limitations of basing selection on just a few discrete measures of 'ideal' performance, since performers may be able to overcome a physical weakness by emphasizing alternate strengths (e.g. grace, commitment, dedication, etc.).

Summary

Literature highlights how the traditional conception of talent is simplistic as it fails to account for the dynamic and multidimensional nature of talent (de Garay et al 1974, Jokl 1964, Tanner 1964, Tittel 1965). Irrespective of physical make-up, unless athletes actively interact with the environment and have the resilience to cope with the challenges and setbacks they encounter as they strive to develop, they will fail to excel (Holt & Dunn 2004). Accordingly, the previous section emphasized the need for a reconceptualization of sporting talent that can account more fully for its multidimensional and dynamic nature. In keeping with this principle, it was proposed that talent should be conceived as a construct that evolves as a result of active interactions between an individual and his/her environment, and that this evolution is facilitated through the application of psychological behaviours.

This emphasis on the development of sporting talent does not discount genetic influences but rather, aims to overcome the failure of traditional perspectives to recognize that sporting talent does not just require the tangibles (i.e. the physical attributes such as speed, size and strength), but also that an individual needs to actively engage with the environment to fully exploit them. For example, Michael Phelps, who won six gold and two bronze swimming medals at the Athens Olympics, would appear to have an ideal body shape for swimming – he is 6 ft 4 in (1.93 m) tall, has size 14 (48½) feet, a 6 ft 7 in (2 m) 'wingspan', and an extra-long torso. However, he is also reported to have an incredible work ethic – swimming on average 7 miles a day in practice, 365 days a year (Sokolove 2004). In short, many are the right shape, but few work hard enough to make sure they are chosen! To enable individuals to actively and appropriately engage with the environment, TID processes need to acknowledge and exploit both the role of psychobehavioural characteristics and the appropriateness of the training environment for enabling athletes to optimize their development (see Chapter 5).

Moving away from traditional TID approaches: the total picture

Clearly, the distinction between 'performance' and 'talent' is an important one but a difference that does not appear to have been grasped fully by organizations and personnel involved in the development of talent (e.g. national governing bodies of sport, funding agencies, coaches). Indeed, to achieve excellence at the world-class level, excellence at the junior levels may even have to be sacrificed, since the characteristics of individuals who will excel at the two levels may be different. In other words, the determinants of performance and the determinants of potential during adolescence are likely to be disparate. For example, a child may excel in age-group rugby because of his/her advanced physical maturity; however, (and often as a result of this early but 'effortless' success) s/he may not have the resilience to cope with the inevitable setbacks encountered as s/he strives to become a world-class performer. In short, traditional TI models have been based almost exclusively on the existence of current skills and ability (what may be termed a 'current performance' model), together with a less evident focus on 'innate' early indicators of talent (e.g. height, strength). Procedures need to evolve so that development coaches pay most attention to those factors that are likely to impact on the capacity of a young athlete to translate early potential into successful performances at the senior level, rather than those that aid their current achievement. This approach requires a shift away from the establishment of short-term initiatives that primarily emphasize quick results to justify public investment (Balyi & Hamilton 2000, Reid 2003). Consequently, this final section considers processes for practitioners (teachers, coaches, etc.) that will enable them to place a greater emphasis on the development of talent.

As highlighted across the preceding sections, the adoption of an approach that emphasizes the capacity of an athlete to develop would imply that considerable focus be placed on the promotion of key psychobehavioural characteristics. Psychobehavioural characteristics appear to significantly impact on the capacity of an individual to cope with 'unforeseen twists' and therefore to translate potential into successful performance at the senior level. However, while coaches typically recognize the crucial role of psychology in translating potential to talent, and many of the psychological behaviours may be being currently promoted by development coaches, our present evidence suggests that there is no coherent system in place (Morris 2000). This dichotomy between understanding and practice may reflect uncertainty regarding how psychological attributes can be optimally promoted alongside psychomotor skill development. For example, recent research by Kelling et al (2007) highlights that coaches perceive that imagery can be beneficial for athletes but they rarely advise athletes to employ it because they lack knowledge about imagery techniques and have little confidence in their ability to advise athletes on its use.

In addition, research that has looked at the perceived role of sport psychologists has emphasized that both athletes and coaches typically perceive sport psychology as a service that has the potential to benefit only problem or weak athletes (Ferraro & Rush 2000, Kremer & Marchant 2002, Pain & Harwood 2004, Partington & Orlick 1987). This problem-focused emphasis is in contrast to the approach being advocated within this chapter, where sport psychology is seen as a tool that should be exploited to optimize athletic development. Consequently, the establishment of explicit processes that enable coaches to provide athletes with opportunities to develop psychological behaviours alongside sport-specific skills is crucial if a coherent approach to TID is to be advanced within (and across) performance domains.

Transferable advantages for achievement in a range of performance domains

It is possible that many of the issues discussed in this chapter that relate to TID in sport and art transfer to other performance domains (e.g. business, education, surgery). Indeed, many of the psychological behaviours that are considered necessary for TD in sport (such as mental focus, goal setting and self-evaluation) are beginning to receive greater attention across a range of performance domains (Jones 2002, Loehr & Schwartz 2001). It is widely accepted that for an individual to excel within a performance area (e.g. sport, music, mathematics), 10 years of deliberate practice is required (Ericsson et al 1993, Simon & Chase 1973). A high level of motivation is clearly required to persevere over such long periods. Accordingly, the importance of self-motivation for high attainment has been highlighted by a number of researchers (e.g. Heller et al 1993, Ziegler & Raul 2000).

In repeated observations (initially by Meij 1992 and then by Meij et al 1995) it was found that individuals achieving excellence in academia exhibited, without exception, higher levels of competence motivation and were clearly and significantly more persistent and enthusiastic than less successful individuals. Thus, both the level and style of an individual's motivation will determine the frequency and persistence of his/her interactions with the relevant environment and thereby will influence his/her development. In this regard, Riksen-Walraven & Zevalkink (2000, p. 204–205) stated that 'given that the motivation of competence in a given field literally drives a person towards interactions that foster development, competence motivation can be considered as the primary *engine* of development'. This strong relationship between motivation and attainment has also been reported by Bloom (1985), Csikszentmihalyi et al (1997), Gottfried et al (1994) and Sosniak (1985) in the areas of sport, art, academia and music, respectively.

The clear and positive message is that current research highlights that the same psychobehaviours are consistently found to underpin achievement in different performance domains. Goal setting, self-awareness, performance arousal and arousal control are all advantageous qualities that will assist individuals in every walk of life. For example, being able to maintain focus and confidence in anxiety-provoking situations is a skill that is helpful in sport but is equally valuable when performing on stage, going for a job interview or carrying out a surgical procedure. In fact, many examples exist of retired athletes who have become successful business people: Fritz Hobbs (rowing to chief executive at a Wall Street investment bank), Wilt Chamberlain (basketball to successful coach, businessman, writer and even actor), John Eales (Rugby Union to successful business consultant), Greg Norman (golfer to successful entrepreneur).

The 'transferability' of psychological behaviours is particularly appealing when one considers the funding shortfalls and a range of often competing sectoral interests such as education, welfare and elite sports development apparent in today's society (Houlihan 2000). Consequently, such links should be actively promoted and exploited across achievement areas. In fact, actively promoting the transfer of psychobehaviours across achievement domains seems necessary, since individuals may need assistance in making the connections between sport demands and demands in other walks of life (Danish & Nellen 1997).

Developing motor competence and perceptual-cognitive skills alongside psychobehavioural skills

As psychobehaviours characterize the means by which an individual interacts with the environment and therefore the extent that they make the most of the opportunities that exist, this chapter has emphasized the need to place early emphasis on these key developmental attributes. Practitioners need to recognize the key role psychobehaviours can have in positively facilitating the interaction of individuals with their environment and enabling successful negotiation of the path to excellence (or fulfilling one's potential) (Freeman 2000). Of course, participation in physical pursuits such as sport and dance also requires individuals to perform a wide array of different motor movements. While many of these movements are complex, specialized skills (e.g. top slice in tennis, the spike in volleyball or the grand jeté in ballet), the majority of these specialized movements are underpinned by common skills (e.g. running, jumping, throwing). For instance, the ability to combine the movements of running, jumping, hopping, leaping and landing is of greater relevance to triple jumpers than each in isolation. These basic movements, which are common to a range of activities, are known as fundamental motor abilities (Gallahue & Ozmun 1998).

Research evidence suggests that early diversification in sport and physical activity facilitates this ability to match 'coordinative structures' with specific situations (Baker 2003) because of the existence of 'identical movement elements' between tasks (Schmidt & Wrisberg 2000). To put it simply, involvement in a range of activities requires fine adjustment to be made to coordinative structures and therefore encourages adaptability. For example, with appropriate developmental experiences, catching a ball by trapping with two hands can be adapted to carrying out a successful movement that requires the body to be oriented to enable the ball to be caught with one hand and to adapt to variations in ball trajectory. Such diversified activities facilitate adaptations required within a sport, a quality that was highlighted earlier in this chapter as key to attaining excellence within a performance environment (see Ch. 9).

As well as the physical movements required to excel within a performance arena, a considerable literature attests to the superior perceptual cognitive skills displayed by elite performers (e.g. athletes, pilots, surgeons) (Vickers 2007). For example, consistent differences emerge between skilled and less skilled players in their anticipation and decision-making skills (Williams et al 1999). Differences are thought to be a reflection of their superior knowledge developed through practice and instruction, as opposed to any pre-existing differences in visual hardware such as acuity, colour vision or depth perception. Because of the existence of identical perceptual elements (i.e. performance-related decisions) and common conceptual elements (i.e. strategies, guidelines, and rules regarding performance) between tasks (Schmidt & Wrisberg 2000), it has been suggested that diversification is likely to facilitate this learning process. For instance, field hockey and football both require participants to be aware of and interpret the actions of their opponents in order to be successful; therefore, these sports share this perceptual element. Gymnastics and diving share conceptual elements (e.g. similar rules), as do basketball and netball (e.g. similar strategies). Therefore, involvement in a range of sports and activities at younger ages is likely to facilitate the development of 'identical conceptual and perceptual elements' and, therefore, the ability of individuals to adapt their knowledge to different contexts (Baker et al 2003).

In summary, while limited research has directly compared the benefits of early versus late specialization within a performance area (due largely to the difficulty of carrying out controlled longitudinal research), initial research supports the benefit of early physical experiences of youngsters primarily being in diversified activities that promote a basic movement vocabulary (e.g. the ability to catch) and the ability to combine these into increasingly complex coordinative structures (e.g. the ability to run, catch and throw a ball). This concept parallels processes employed within language education where individuals are initially taught basic skills (i.e. words) before being required to employ these within increasingly complex phrases and sentences (i.e. grammar). Diversified physical practices should encourage individuals to adapt coordinative structures to various conceptual and perceptual demands. For several years, physical education specialists have utilized intuitively appealing but relatively atheoretical methods such as 'games for understanding' (Bunker & Thorpe 1982) and 'tactical games' (Griffin et al 1997) in an attempt to build children's generic capacity to understand, and thus get involved in, team games. Such approaches implicitly acknowledge the role of knowledge structures as essential components of preparation for effective play. Recent research has highlighted the mechanisms through which this 'declarative' knowledge (Anderson 1993) can be developed (e.g. Rovegno et al 2001) and the apparent generic benefits that accrue in a child's decision-making style. Once again, varied experiences offer the best medium to develop this declarative knowledge base, providing performers with the capacity to be more innovative and creative in their (eventually) selected area.

While the promotion of diversified physical activity could be met by an effective primary physical education programme, recent investigations suggest that current pedagogical processes are not providing children with the competencies (perceived and actual) required to successfully participate in physical activities (e.g. Currie et al 2004, Reuschlein & Vogel 1985, Ross et al 1985). Therefore, although this chapter has emphasized the need to develop psychobehavioural characteristics, a curriculum that enables the development of motor skills and perceptual-cognitive skills in tandem with these psychobehavioural characteristics is essential. As discussed in the next section, such a curriculum would not only facilitate performance excellence but also has the potential to contribute to an individual's personal, non-performance goals.

Contribution of psychobehavioural and psychomotor skills to non-performance environments

The psychobehavioural and motor competence skills discussed throughout this chapter not only underpin achievement across performance arenas (e.g. art, business) but also have the potential to contribute to the attainment of personal goals in non-performance environments (e.g. hobbies, parenting, healthy living) and are therefore also believed to be of lifelong value. In this regard, Miller & Kerr (2002) highlight how personal excellence, defined as 'the achievement of developmentally appropriate tasks across the lifespan and the acquisition of personal qualities that contribute to optimal health and wellbeing', can be successfully promoted alongside performance excellence. Bloom (1985) emphasized that, as a performer develops along the TD continuum, s/he will assume greater responsibility for his/her own development and behaviours (see Fig. 2.2). However, this ability to take personal responsibility is believed to be not only of value for achievement but also of lifelong value to all individuals' welfare (Miller & Kerr 2002). For example, with global concerns over an increasingly sedentary population, and more and more research establishing links between inactivity and health issues (e.g. heart disease, diabetes, high blood pressure, colon cancer) (US Department of Health and Human Services 1996), uptake of and adherence to lifelong physical activity is a crucial concern for many (e.g. health professionals, government). The same psychobehavioural skills that have been found to underpin successful development, such as the ability to set realistic goals, to plan and to take personal responsibility, are likely to significantly affect the long-term health behaviours of an individual (Summerfield 1995).

In addition, proficiency across a range of fundamental movement skills (e.g. catching and running) has been shown to be central to the physical competence of children (Rose 1994, Rose et al 1997), and are seen as the 'building blocks' for future successful participation in recreational activities (Armstrong 1990, Department of Education and Science 1991, Sports Council 1993). By contrast, a perceived lack of competence in fundamental motor skills has been reported to be a barrier to future participation in physical activities for both primary-school (Haubenstricker & Seefeldt 1986) and secondary-school children (Clough et al 1993). If competency (perceived and actual) is not achieved on these generic skills, an individual may avoid the physical settings required for him/her to adopt a healthy lifestyle (Seefeldt et al 1979). As Seefeldt et al (1979, p. 21) state: 'Children who possess inadequate motor skills are often relegated to a life of exclusion from organized and free play experiences of their peers, and subsequently, to a lifetime of inactivity because of their frustration in early movement behaviour.'

Other authors have also supported the wide-ranging implications of poor fundamental movement skills. Skinner & Piek (2001, p. 13), in considering the psychosocial implications of poor motor coordination, stated that their research had 'indicated that poor motor skills may have adverse social and emotional implications for children and adolescents. The difficulties experienced are not confined to the movement domain but may affect how children and adolescents view themselves physically, socially and scholastically'. For example, children with developmental coordination disorder ('clumsy children') can suffer from a range of psychosocial problems (Cummins et al 2005, Smyth & Anderson 2000). Consequently, fundamental movement skills are seen as essential precursors to both excellence in sport and successful participation in health-related activities throughout life. Accordingly, early involvement in a diversified range of activities that encourage children to develop competence (perceived and actual) across a range of psychomotor skills will not only provide the basis for successful participation in performance sport but should provide children with the confidence to choose to participate in physical activity and therefore adopt a physically healthy lifestyle (Bernstein 1967).

In summary, TD environments not only have the potential to optimize performance excellence (e.g. achievement in sport, academia, etc.) but, if appropriately structured, can be used as a vehicle for enhancing overall wellbeing (e.g. self-esteem) and personal excellence (e.g. acquisition of personal qualities that contribute to optimal health and wellbeing). Therefore, while personal excellence is typically only promoted outside the performance environment (in classrooms, counselling centres, etc.), TID programmes have the opportunity to adopt a philosophy that envisions performance and personal excellence as coexisting in the high-level performance setting, where the attributes being promoted contribute to the achievement and overall development of the individual (Miller & Kerr 2002). A positive feature of adopting a philosophy where personal excellence is promoted in tandem with performance excellence is the potential for addressing the current split between educational and sporting community over the ethics of performance sport. It is only once this split is addressed that the opportunity to provide coherent and systematic processes across the development of performers will truly exist.

Coherent and systematic processes across the development of performers

In order to adhere to the philosophies advocated within this chapter, it is important that long-term development (LTD) be consistently promoted across performer experiences. Of course, the coach/trainer may recognize the need for LTD but feel that the national governing body is judging/rewarding age group coaches on the success of age-group performers/teams. Such a process would encourage a focus on short-term success where performers are selected on the basis of age-group success and is likely to result in a 'yo-yo' effect as performers move in and out of squads as they mature and develop. At best, the lack of consistency evidenced within this yo-yo effect would hinder sporting experiences and coaching opportunities for many performers. At worst, many talented performers who do not achieve good results early on will be lost from the sport as they become demotivated and withdraw. In contrast, TID processes that focus on long-term aims would require individual attention to be given to equip developing performers with the skills that will help them get to, and then stay at, the top of their chosen event. Therefore, a coherent and unified focus on equipping performers with the attributes that have the potential to help them negotiate the complex pathway to success is essential. Consequently, it is recommended that governing organizations consider the extent that current education and rewards for coaches/trainers optimally promote the development of performers.

To develop a holistic approach to development, knowledge of attributes that typify the stages of development presented in Figure 2.2 (i.e. initiation, development, mastery and maintenance) could be used as a basis for rewarding coaches/trainers. Rather than rewarding those who develop successful age-group performers/teams, coaches who have worked with performers who successfully transfer from one stage of development to the next should be acknowledged (for example, the effectiveness of a coach working at grass roots level could be assessed by the number of his/her athletes who go on to make the transition from the initiation to the development stage). The provision of support dictated by the stage of development of a performer would encourage a coherent focus on long-term development rather than short-term ambitions (such as age-group success). In other words, focus will be on identifying the skills and support a performer requires to progress to the next stage of development and will help prevent an overemphasis on excelling at their current level. For example, three 13-year-old athletes in the initiation, development and mastery stages respectively would employ psychological behaviours in different ways (e.g. coach- or parent-led versus self-determined motivation). In addition, these three athletes are likely to have very different goals for their sport participation, e.g. enjoyment, skill development or performance mastery. Therefore, coaches need to recognize and acknowledge these differences and ensure that education and support provided to athletes are development/stage-specific rather than age-specific. This focus on providing appropriate developmental experiences as opposed to focusing on age-group performances, may be essential, as a successful transition from one stage of development to another (e.g. development to mastery) may require adjustments (in technique for example) that may negatively affect performance in the short term. As well as emphasizing LTD, this focus would also facilitate a more interdisciplinary approach to TD from early on in the development process (e.g. physical and mental considerations).

For an effective LTD programme to be established within any performance arena, effective collaboration among a range of organizations will be essential. For example, within sport, a range of organizations (schools, regional clubs, national sporting organizations, etc.) will have an input into the development of athletes. Similarly, within dance/music, school, academy and company/orchestra are examples of organizations that affect the development of potential dancers/musicians. Without a coherent and systematic development process across these organizations, mixed messages are likely and the criteria for measuring progress are likely to conflict. This collaboration is in itself a major challenge, as the current evidence suggests that organizations typically work in isolation even when addressing related issues (Kirk & Gorely 2000).

Why are so many continuing with the traditional approach?

Within sport, national organizations are increasingly recognizing the limitations with traditional TID approaches that only emphasize 'genetic' determinants of talent. For example, SportScotland, SPARC

(New Zealand), Sport England and Northern Ireland all recently rejected the Australian Talent Search approach where selection is based on children's profile across 10 standard anthropometric (e.g. height) physiological (e.g. speed) and performance (e.g. catch) attributes. For example, an individual who scores well on height, depending on the rest of his/her profile, may be guided towards participation in basketball. However, despite this shift in attitude, many sport-specific organizations from these same countries continue to employ one-dimensional and oversimplistic determinants of 'talent'. For instance, a recent report presented in New Zealand highlights that SPARC, the national body of sport, wishes to move away from relying on traditional TID approaches and advocates a greater emphasis on TD (Mahon 2004). Unfortunately, other organizations within New Zealand continue to pursue the Talent Search approach. For example, the Peter Snell Institute (PSI) aims to employ a systematic process for seeking out talented school-age athletes within New Zealand that demonstrate the capacity necessary to ultimately succeed at international level. Although PSI acknowledges that talent is a result of physical, physiological, psychological and skill attributes, it adopts the Talent Search approach and selection is based on children's profile on 'seven standard physical education tests'. Specifically, the approach aims to identify 'talented' athletes on the basis of the height, weight, arm span, vertical jump performance, seated basketball throw performance, 40 m sprint performance and shuttle run performance of children tested.

Within the UK, several government agencies and sport governing bodies continue to employ a TI system that selects the 'talented' on the basis of performance on a limited range of anthropometric and physical determinants. This approach continues despite the national sporting organizations for Wales, Scotland and England 'officially' rejecting the approach. Of course, certain sports (e.g. rowing, cycling and discus) have clear physiological and/or anthropometric demands and assessment of individuals on physiological and anthropometric components will be a useful, and sometime crucial indicator, of their potential to excel within these sports. For example, without adequate fast twitch fibres an individual will be unable to excel as a weight lifter or sprinter. However, it is important to recognize that many of the physiological and anthropometric attributes of an individual will remain unstable until the later stage of adolescence, making it more difficult to predict physical potential in younger subjects (Borms 1994). For example, since aerobic capacity is affected by body mass and maturity (Welsman & Armstrong 2000), performance on the multistage fitness test will not stabilize until after puberty. Similar problems exist with measuring the anaerobic capacity of adolescents, since the metabolic characteristics underpinning the relevant energy responses are also subject to growth influences. A final caution is that, even when physical assessment is being conducted with older (post-pubertal) athletes, it is important to recognize that, irrespective of physical make-up, unless an athlete actively interacts with the environment and has the resilience to cope with the challenges and setbacks s/he encounters within and between the various stages of development, s/he will fail to excel (Holt & Dunn 2004). In consequence, sporting talent needs to be reconceptualized so that TID processes account more fully for its multidimensional and dynamic nature.

The continued emphasis on one-dimensional models of TID across many sport and other performance areas may seem surprising. However, this mixed picture of current practices may reflect the practical complexities that result from a multidimensional and dynamic concept of talent and the absence of explicit alternative strategies. In contrast, the (apparent) ease of implementation of the traditional one-dimensional approach may make it an appealing option, especially for those organizations in the early stages of establishing systematic TI processes. In addition, the nature of funding strategies used to support developing performers may directly affect the focus of development programmes. For example, within sport, funding for athletes is typically based on age-group performance rather than potential to develop. Again, this encourages a focus on short-term success as opposed to the long-term development focus being advocated within this chapter.

Nevertheless, despite this somewhat disjointed picture, the evidence is that progress is slowly taking place at the policy level, where governing organizations are currently reconsidering their TID systems in accordance with a multidimensional and dynamic concept of talent. For example, SportScotland have recently emphasized how all future work will aim to embrace the multidimensional and dynamic concept of talent. This is in contrast to previous work that supported age-group performers without considering the potential of these youngsters to develop into successful athletes at the senior level. Chapter 4 aims to help transfer this philosophical shift into practice by providing practitioners with exemplar systems that enable them to adhere to the principles advocated by a multidimensional and dynamic model of TID.

Conclusion

It is important to re-emphasize that, while the principles presented within the final section of this chapter emphasize the role of psychology in actualizing one's potential, talent is a multidimensional concept and therefore multiple interactive and compensatory processes take place within and between a range of variables including physical, psychological, motor, sociological and environmental factors. Consequently, individuals should not be identified or deselected on any one component, since weaknesses in one area (e.g. height) may be compensated for by an advantage in another or a combination of other components (speed and commitment). Additionally, because of the evolutionary nature of talent, the need to continually monitor and develop all components that may influence the fulfilment of an individual's talent is an essential principle of the model proposed. This integration of TI and TD processes requires a shift from the current emphasis on selection and elimination, which is typically based on 'one-off' performance observations (e.g. scouting in football). Instead, selection processes should consider a child's progress and behaviour (e.g. commitment) during a development programme, as opposed to purely considering performance levels. A key question should be whether the individual successfully learns skills during the development phase and whether s/he shows a commitment to his/her development, especially when faced with adversity. Such a system should also help guide the support provided to the athlete at different stages of development. This is in contrast to an approach where selection is based on an individual's performance despite this being purely due to an early physical advantage.

While evidence exists that organizations are increasingly recognizing the need to adopt a multidimensional and dynamic approach to developing talent, this philosophical shift has yet to systematically occur in practice. Consequently, Chapter 4 aims to facilitate the ability of coaches to adhere to a multi-dimensional and dynamic concept of talent within their development programs.

References

Abbott, A., Collins, D., 2004. Eliminating the dichotomy between theory and practice in talent identification and development: considering the role of psychology. J. Sports Sci. 22, 395–408.

Abbott, A., Collins, D., Martindale, R., et al., 2002. Talent identification and development: an academic review. Report for SportScotland by the University of Edinburgh. SportScotland, Edinburgh.

Abbott, A., Button, C., Pepping, G.-J., et al., 2005. Unnatural selection: talent identification and development in sport. Nonlinear Dynamics Psychol. Life Sci. 9, 61–88.

Anderson, J.R., 1993. Rules of the mind. Erlbaum, Hillsdale, NJ.

Armstrong, N., 1990. New directions in physical education. Human Kinetics, Champaign, IL.

Baker, J., 2003. Early specialization in youth sport: a requirement for adult expertise? High Ability Studies 14, 85–94.

Baker, J., Côté, J., Abernethy, B., 2003. Learning from the experts: practice activities of expert decision-makers in sport. Res. Q. Exerc. Sport 74, 342–347.

Balyi, I., Hamilton, A., 2000. Key to success: long-term athlete development. Sports Coach Autumn. 30–32.

Bernstein, N.A., 1967. The co-ordination and regulation of movements. Pergamon Press, Oxford.

Birri, S., 2000. Pietro Mennea: Europe's fastest politician. Trans World Sport, program 703. Available on line at: http://www.trans-world-sport.com/includes/cobranded_nav/nav_tws/181000pietro.htm

Blanksby, B.B., 1980. Measures of talent identification in competitive swimming. Sports Coach 15 (4), 13–19.

Bloom, B.S., 1985. Developing talent in young people. Ballantine, New York.

Bloomfield, J., 1995. Talent identification and profiling. In: Bloomfield, J., Fricker, P.A., Fitch, K.D. (Eds.), Science and medicine in sport. Blackwell Science, Cambridge, pp. 206–221.

Bompa, T.O., 2000. Total training for young champions: proven conditioning programs for athletes ages 6 to 18. Human Kinetics, Champaign, IL.

Boreham, C., 2001. The physiology of exercise in children. In: Maffulli, N., Chan, K.M., Macdonald, R., et al. (Eds.), Sports medicine for specific ages and abilities. Churchill Livingstone, Edinburgh, pp. 65–72.

Borms, J., 1994. From theory to practice: talent identification and selection – the future for British Governing Bodies. BOA CAG Seminar, London.

Brennan, C., 2006. Parched British Open, unusual course provides mental test. USA Today. Available on line at: http://www.usatoday.com/sports/columnist/brennan/2006-07-19-british-open_x.htm (accessed 14.02.09).

Bunker, D.J., Thorpe, R.D., 1982. A model for the teaching of games in secondary schools. Bulletin of Physical Education 18 (1), 5–8.

Button, C., Davids, K., Schöllhorn, W., 2006. Co-ordination profiling of movement systems: a multi-disciplinary perspective. In: Davids, K., Bennett, S., Newell, K.M. (Eds.), Variability in the movement system: a multi-disciplinary perspective. Human Kinetics, Champaign, IL, pp. 133–152.

Clough, J., McCormack, C., Trail, R., 1993. A mapping of participation rates in junior sports. ACHPER National Journal 40 (2), 4–7.

Côté, J., 1999. The influence of the family in the development of talent in sports. Sport Psychologist 13, 395–417.

Csikszentmihalyi, M., Rathunde, K., Whalen, S., 1997. Talented teenagers: the roots of success and failure. Cambridge University Press, Cambridge.

Cummins, A., Piek, J.P., Dyck, M.J., 2005. Motor coordination, empathy and social behaviour in school-aged children. Dev. Med. Child Neurol. 47, 437–442.

Currie, C., Roberts, C., Morgan, A., et al., 2004. Young people's health in context. Health behaviour in school-aged children (HBSC) study: international report from the 2001/2002 survey. In: Health Policy for Children and Adolescents No. 4. World Health Organization Regional Office for Europe, Copenhagen.

Danish, S., Nellen, V.C., 1997. New roles for sport psychologists: teaching life skills through sport to at-risk youth. Quest 49, 100–113.

De Garay, A., Levine, L., Carter, J.E., 1974. Genetic and anthropological studies of Olympic athletes. Academic Press, New York.

Department of Education and Science, 1991. National curriculum physical education working party: interim report. Her Majesty's Stationery Office, London.

Durand-Bush, N., Salmela, J.H., 2001. The development of talent in sport. In: Singer, R.N., Hausenblas, H.A., Janelle, C. (Eds.), Handbook of sport psychology. John Wiley, New York, pp. 269–289.

Ericsson, K.A., Charness, N., 1994. Expert performance. Am. Psychol. 49, 725–747.

Ericsson, K.A., Krampe, R.T., Tesch-Romer, C., 1993. The role of deliberate practice in the acquisition of expert performance. Psychol. Rev. 100, 363–406.

Ferraro, T., Rush, S., 2000. Why athletes resist sport psychology. Athletic Insight 2 (3). Available on line at: http://www.athleticinsight.com/Vol2Iss3/Resistance.htm (accessed 14.02.09).

Fisher, R., 1996. Gifted children and young people in physical education and sport. In: Armstrong, N. (Ed.), New direction in physical education: change and innovation. Cassell Education, London, pp. 131–143.

Freeman, J., 2000. Teaching for talent: lessons from the research. In: van Lieshout, C.F.M., Heymans, P.G. (Eds.), Developing talent across the life span. Psychology Press, Hove, Sussex, pp. 231–248.

Gallahue, D.L., Ozmun, J.C., 1998. Understanding motor development, third ed. Brown & Benchmark, Dubuque, IA.

Gottfried, A.E., Fleming, J.S., Gottfried, A.W., 1994. Role of parental motivational practices in children's academic intrinsic motivation and achievement. J. Educ. Psychol. 86, 104–113.

Gould, D., Dieffenbach, K., Moffett, A., 2002. Psychological characteristics and their development in Olympic champions. Journal of Applied Sport Psychology 14, 172–204.

Griffin, L.A., Mitchell, S.A., Oslin, J.L., 1997. Teaching sport concepts and skills: a tactical game approach. Human Kinetics, Champaign, IL.

Harre, D., 1982. Principles of sports training: introduction to the theory and methods of training. Sportverlag, Berlin.

Haubenstricker, J., Seefeldt, V., 1986. Acquisition of motor skills during childhood. In: Seefeldt, V. (Ed.), Physical activity and well-being. American Alliance for Health, Physical Education, Recreation and Dance, Reston, VA, pp. 41–102.

Heller, K.A., Mönks, F.J., Passow, A.H. (Eds.), 1993. International handbook of research and development of giftedness and talent. Pergamon Press, Oxford.

Helsen, W.F., Starkes, J.L., Hodges, N.J., 1998. Team sports and the theory of deliberate practice. Journal of Sport and Exercise Psychology 20, 12–34.

Helsen, W.F., Hodges, N.J., Van Winckel, J., et al., 2000. The roles of talent, physical precocity and practice in the development of soccer expertise. J. Sports Sci. 18, 727–736.

Holt, N., 2002. A comparison of the soccer talent development systems in England and Canada. European Physical Education Review 8, 270–285.

Holt, N., Dunn, J., 2004. Toward a grounded theory of the psychosocial competencies and environmental conditions associated with soccer success. Journal of Applied Sport Psychology 16, 199–219.

Houlihan, B., 2000. Sporting excellence, schools and sports development: the politics of crowded policy spaces. European Physical Education Review 6, 171–193.

Jokl, E., 1964. Essay on medical sociology of sports. In: Thomas, C.L. (Ed.), Medical sociology and cultural anthropology of sport and physical education. Charles C. Thomas, Springfield, IL, pp. 65–71.

Jones, G., 2002. Performance excellence: a personal perspective on the link between sport and business. Journal of Applied Sport Psychology 14, 268–281.

Kelling, M.R., Short, S.E., Lindsay, R.-S., 2007. Imagine that...': how coaches advise their athletes to use imagery in practice settings. Journal of Sport and Exercise Psychology 29, 175–176.

Kirk, D., Gorely, T., 2000. Challenging thinking about the relationship between school physical education and sport performance. European Physical Education Review 6, 119–134.

Kreiner-Phillips, K., Orlick, T., 1992. Winning after winning: the psychology of ongoing excellence. Sport Psychologist 7, 31–48.

Kremer, P.J., Marchant, D.B., 2002. Reflections and considerations of providing sport psychology services with professional football players. In: Spinks, W. (Ed.), Science and football IV. Routledge, London, pp. 294–299.

Kunst, G., Florescu, C., 1971. The main factors for performance in wrestling. National Sports Council, Bucharest.

Lane, M., 2006. Why are cricketers such good dancers? BBC News Magazine 24 November. Available on line at: http://news.bbc.co.uk/2/hi/uk_news/magazine/6132706.stm (accessed 14.02.09).

Lidor, R., Lavyan, N., 2002. A retrospective picture of early sport experiences among elite and near-elite Israeli athletes: developmental and psychological perspectives. International Journal of Sport Psychology 33, 269–289.

Loehr, J., Schwartz, T., 2001. The making of a corporate athlete. Harv. Bus. Rev. 79, 120–128.

McCleish, S., Collins, D., 2002. Talent identification and development in Scottish soccer: where did we go wrong? Department of Physical Education, Sport and Leisure Studies, University of Edinburgh, Edinburgh.

McDonald, J., Orlick, T., Letts, M., 1995. Mental readiness in surgeons and its links to performance excellence in surgery. J. Pediatr. Orthop. 15, 691–697.

Mahon, T., 2004. Linking promise to the podium: talent identification and development (TID) in New Zealand. A Report to SPARC's Board from the TID Taskforce into potential. New Zealand Academy of Sport, Wellington. Available on line at: http://www.sparc.org.nz/Talent-Identification-and-Development (accessed 22.02.09).

Malina, R.M., 1997. Talent identification and selection in sport. Available on line at: http://road.uww.edu/road/jonesd/Coaching-463/Readiness for Sport/ (accessed 30.10.09).

Malina, R.M., Reyes, M.E.P., Eisenmann, J.C., et al., 2000. Height, mass and skeletal maturity of elite Portuguese soccer players aged 11–16 years. J. Sports Sci. 18, 685–693.

Meij, J.T., 1992. Sociale ondersteuning, gehechtheidskwaliteit en vroegkinderlijke competentie-ontwikkeling [Social support, attachment, and competence]. Doctoral dissertation, Catholic University, Nijmegen.

Meij, J.T., Riksen-Walraven, J.M.A., van Lieshout, C.F.M., 1995. Patterns of change and consistency in parental support as related to children's competence motivation. In: Koops, W., Hoeksma, J., van den Boom, D. (Eds.), Proceedings of 'Early mother–child interaction and attachment: old and new approaches'. North-Holland, Amsterdam.

Miller, P.S., Kerr, G., 2002. The athletic, academic and social experiences of intercollegiate student-athletes. Journal of Sport Behavior 25, 346–367.

Monsaas, J.A., 1985. Learning to be a world-class tennis player. In: Bloom, B.S. (Ed.), Developing talent in young people. Ballantine, New York, pp. 211–269.

Moore, P., Collins, D.J., Burwitz, L., et al., 1998. The development of talent study (DOTS). Sports Council, London.

Morris, T., 2000. Psychological characteristics and talent identification in soccer. J. Sports Sci. 18 (9), 715–726.

Morrone, A.S., Pintrich, P.R., 1997. Achievement motivation. In: Bear, G., Minke, K., Thomas, A. (Eds.), Children's needs II: psychological perspectives. National Association of School Psychologists, Washington, DC, pp. 387–395.

Nagorni, M.F., 1978. Facts and fiction regarding juniors' training. Fizkulturai Sport, Moscow.

Orlick, T., 2000. In pursuit of excellence, third ed. Human Kinetics, Champaign, IL.

Pain, M.A., Harwood, C.G., 2004. Knowledge and perceptions of sport psychology within English soccer. J. Sports Sci. 22, 813–826.

Partington, J., Orlick, T., 1987. The sport psychology consultant evaluation form. Sport Psychologist 1, 309–317.

Perera, S., 2000. Cricket with a plot: nationalism, cricket and diasporic identities. Journal of Australian Studies 26, 14–26.

Reid, P., 2003. More than a game? The role of sports governing bodies in the development of sport education programmes. European Physical Education Review 9, 309–317.

Reuschlein, P.L., Vogel, P.G., 1985. Motor performance and physical fitness status of regular and special education students. In: Clark, J.E., Humphrey, J.H. (Eds.), Motor development. Princeton, Pennington, NJ, pp. 147–165.

Riksen-Walraven, J.M., Zevalkink, J., 2000. Gifted infants: what kinds of support do they need? In: Van Lieshout, C.F.M., Heymans, P.G. (Eds.), Developing talent across the life span. Taylor & Francis, Philadelphia, PA, pp. 203–229.

Rose, B., 1994. The importance of gross motor coordination in the psycho-social lives of children. PhD thesis, University of Western Australia, Perth, Western Australia.

Rose, B., Larkin, D., Berger, B., 1997. Coordination and gender influences on the perceived competence of children. Adapted Physical Activity Quarterly 12, 210–221.

Ross, J.G., Dotson, C.O., Gilbert, G.G., et al., 1985. What are kids doing in physical education? Journal of Physical Education Recreation and Dance 56, 31–34.

Rovegno, I., Nevett, M., Babiarz, M., 2001. Learning and teaching invasion-game tactics in 4th grade: introductions and theoretical perspective. Journal of Teaching in Physical Education 21, 177–192.

Schmidt, R.A., Wrisberg, C.A., 2000. Motor learning and performance: a problem-based learning approach. Human Kinetics, Champaign, IL.

Schneider, W., 1993. Acquiring expertise: determinants of exceptional performance. In: Heller, K.A., Mönks, J., Passow, H. (Eds.), International handbook of research and development of giftedness and talent. Pergamon Press, Oxford, UK, pp. 311–324.

Schunk, D.H., 1990. Self concept and school achievement. In: Rogers, C., Kutnick, P. (Eds.), The social psychology of the primary school. Routledge, London, pp. 70–91.

Seefeldt, V., Haubenstricker, J., Reuschlein, S., 1979. Why physical education in elementary school curriculum? Ontario Physical Education and Health Education Association Journal 5 (1), 21–31.

Shakespear, P., 1980. Identification and selection of talent in rowing. Sports Coach 15 (4), 9–12.

Simon, H.A., Chase, W.G., 1973. Skill in chess. Am. Sci. 61, 393–403.

Simonton, D.K., 1999. Talent and its development: an emergenic and epigenetic model. Psychol. Rev. 106, 435–457.

Skinner, R., Piek, J., 2001. Psychosocial implications of poor motor control coordination in children and adolescents. Hum. Mov. Sci. 20, 73–94.

Sloboda, J., 2005. Exploring the musical mind: cognition, emotion, ability, function. Oxford University Press, Oxford.

Sloboda, J.A., Howe, M.J.A., 1992. Transitions in the early musical careers of able young musicians: choosing instruments and teachers. Journal of Research in Music Education 40, 283–294.

Smyth, M.M., Anderson, H.I., 2000. Coping with clumsiness in the school playground: social and physical play in children with coordination impairments. British Journal of Developmental Psychology 18, 389–413.

Sokolove, M., 2004. Built to swim. New York Times 8 August. Available on line at: http://www.nytimes.com/2004/08/08/magazine/built-to-swim.html. Accessed 30 October 2009.

Sosniak, L.A., 1985. Learning to be a concert pianist. In: Bloom, B.S. (Ed.), Developing talent in young people. Ballantine Books, New York, pp. 19–67.

Sports Council, 1993. Young people and sport: policy and frameworks for action. Sports Council, London.

Starkes, J.L., 2000. The road to expertise: is practice the only determinant? International Journal of Sport Psychology 31, 431–451.

Stevenson, C.L., 1990. The athletic career: some contingencies of sport specialization. Journal of Sport Behavior 13, 103–113.

Summerfield, L.M., 1995. National standards for school health education. Eric Digest. ERIC Clearinghouse on Teaching and Teacher Education, Washington, DC. (EDRS No. ED387483). Available on line at: http://eric.ed.gov/ERICDocs/data/ericdocs2sql/content_storage_01/0000019b/80/14/2f/d6.pdf (accessed 22.02.09).

Talbot-Honeck, C., Orlick, T., 1998. The essence of excellence: mental skills of top classical musicians. Journal of Excellence 1 (1), 66–81.

Tanner, J.M., 1964. The physique of the Olympic athlete. George Allen & Unwin, London.

Tittel, K., 1965. Zur Biotypologie und funktionellen Anatomie des Leistungssportlers. Nova Acta Leopoldina 30, 172.

US Department of Health and Human Services, 1996. Physical activity and health: a report of the surgeon general. Centers for Disease Control and Prevention, Atlanta, GA.

Van der Walt, T.S.P., 1988. Antropometriese tipering by topdeelnemers in verskillende Olimpiese sportsoort. [Anthropometrical typecasting amongst competitors in different Olympic events]. South African Journal for Research in Sport Physical Education and Recreation 11, 101–120.

Van Tassel-Baska, J., 2001. The talent development process; what we know and what we don't know. Gifted Education International 16, 20–28.

Vickers, J.N., 2007. Perception, cognition, decision training: the quiet eye in action. Human Kinetics, Champaign, IL.

Welsman, J.R., Armstrong, N., 2000. Longitudinal changes in submaximal oxygen uptake in 11- to 13-year-olds. J. Sports Sci. 18, 183–189.

Williams, M., Davids, K., Williams, J., 1999. Visual perception and action in sport. E & FN Spon, London.

Ziegler, R.S , Raul, T., 2000. Myth and reality: a review of empirical studies on giftedness. High Ability Studies 11, 113–136.

Expertise: the goal of performance development

3

Nicola J. Hodges* Joseph Baker†

*University of British Columbia, Vancouver, British Columbia, Canada
†York University, Toronto, Ontario, Canada

CHAPTER CONTENTS

Introduction

It has long been acknowledged that practice is an important ingredient in obtaining expertise in sports. However, there has been debate concerning the importance of this variable and whether practice is both a necessary and a sufficient ingredient. There has been a tendency for researchers, perhaps spurred on by practitioners, to devote their efforts to looking for predispositions or innate factors that serve to give the expert advantage. This has been at the expense of looking to the specifics of the practice environment. This changed significantly in the early to late 1990s when Ericsson et al (1993) presented evidence to show that a specific type of domain-relevant practice, so-called deliberate practice, was positively related to expertise level in musicians. In other words, the more skilled the musician, the more domain-relevant practice had been accumulated. Since this time there has been a significant collection of evidence in sports showing similar relations between practice and performance in domains as varied as soccer and field hockey (Helsen et al 1998), karate (Hodge & Deakin 1998), wrestling (Hodges & Starkes 1996) and triathlon events (Baker et al 2005, Hodges et al 2004).

Although there has been debate over this correlational-type research and hence our ability to imply cause and effect, the fact that methods were now available to measure practice quantity and quality resulted in some important and interesting questions in the field of skill development. People now wanted to know the critical ages for starting practice and whether practice could stave off declines in performance associated with age or even overcome performance differences as a function of sex (for recent reviews see Baker & Côté 2006, Hodges et al 2007, Ward et al 2004). In this chapter, we aim to provide the reader with an overview of this research, with specific emphasis placed on implications for best practice and 'talent development'. We will attempt to review studies where practice and performance relationships have been examined with the purpose of understanding which conditions best promote the chances of succeeding within a sporting domain, as well as maintaining a high level of performance in a domain beyond established peaks.

To guide our discussions and reviews, the chapter is divided into two general sections. In the first we examine research evidence in terms of three major

DOI: 10.1016/B978-0-443-06734-1.00003-1

constraints on practice outlined by Ericsson et al (1993): resources, motivation and effort. We also examine the concept of sport enjoyment in this section as it relates to the concept of motivation. In the second section we look at various practice behaviours as a function of the stage of development of the performer, whether this is as a child, during the adult and peak performance years or as an ageing performer (i.e. master athlete). There are obvious links between the two sections in terms of the various constraints and conditions that are likely to affect practice and performance at the different stages of skill development.

Constraints on practice

Ericsson and colleagues pointed to the critical influence of sheer quantity of time in deliberate practice. However, they acknowledged that the accumulation of this practice would be constrained by three categories of factors: resources, effort and motivation. In this first section we examine these constraints on practice in terms of relatively recent research findings in sport that identify the conditions most conducive to success. Although we will discuss these categories of constraints separately, it is clear there is significant interaction among them. This is particularly noticeable in terms of our discussions of effort and motivation, such that some of the issues and research evidence presented in these sections could fall into either category of constraint. Our aim in this first section is to raise awareness of certain conditions that are likely to affect the amount and quality of practice and to discuss conditions that appear optimal for the development of high-level performance skill. As will be clear in this discussion, some of these 'constraints' are within the individual's control and can be changed or accommodated to fit the individual. However, some of these factors will be out of the individual's control and might be relatively impervious to changes in the environment. Another consideration is the relative importance of these various factors in affecting skill development. As will hopefully be clear, the necessity of certain conditions for the development of considered elite performance levels is very much open to debate.

Resources

Access to essential resources appears to be a fundamental constraint on the ability to acquire high-quality, domain-specific practice. Baker and Horton (2004) suggested that this is an important secondary factor that moderates the influence of direct or primary factors such as training. Below we review some of the more prominent resource-related factors affecting skill development in sport.

Significant others (coaches and parents)

In many cases, coaches have complete control over an athlete's training and, not surprisingly, they can have a critical influence over the rate at which athletes progress. A key characteristic of expert coaches is meticulous planning and the ability to maximize training time (Voss et al 1983). Research consistently indicates that the structure and content of expert athletes' practice is superior to that of non-experts (see Baker et al 2003a, Starkes et al 2001 for reviews). Moreover, there is evidence that proper coaching is critical for promoting adaptations to more advanced levels of learning and development (Horton & Deakin 2008). In studies of coaching effectiveness it has been shown that effective and successful coaches give more correct and precise feedback to their players (e.g. More & Franks 1996, Rutt-Leas & Chi 1993) as well as engaging players in drills that most closely resemble actual game scenarios, both in terms of intensity and competitive realism (Deakin & Cobley 2003). Bloom (1985) has presented evidence that 'talented teenagers' are more likely to report having an influential coach or teacher in developing their skills, often requiring the child to travel significantly or even move to prosper from expert tuition. However, it is unclear whether the various characteristics of a good coach change in importance as a function of skill and hence engender expertise. As we will outline in the second section of this chapter, when learners advance in skill development, cognitive, physical and emotional needs change and the role of the coach will also need to change accordingly. There has been a clear trend in sport to employ successful players as coaches of highly prominent teams when they retire. Presumably this is fostered by the belief that the more successful the player the more likely it is that s/he or she will be a good coach. As far as we know, this premise (i.e. the relationship between skill performing and skill teaching/coaching) has not been examined in the coaching literature. It may well be that the successful player–coach has more of an inspirational than an informational role and that the latter characteristic is more important for skill development in the early years than the former.

It is common today for an aspiring athlete to have a team of coaches who specialize in particular aspects of trainings, such as fitness, sport psychology, choreography and match analysis. One of the main changes that occur as an athlete develops is this increased access to coaching resources and specialists (see Starkes et al 1996 and their discussion of coaches in national figure skating).

Researchers have also highlighted the important role that parents play in promoting the athletic development of their children (Bloom 1985, Côté 1999). For instance, Bloom (1985) found that parents were important resources in nurturing the development of a wide variety of skills in their children. Similar to coaches, the roles of parents shift as the athlete advances in skill development, moving from a source of financial support and leadership in early development to a source of emotional support during later stages of development (Côté et al 2003). In a recent study of youth soccer players who had been selected to train and play in affiliation with professional academies in England, over 80% of the elite players reported that their parent was the most influential person in their career. In contrast, for the subelite players questioned (i.e. those playing primarily in school leagues), only about 40% remarked on the significance of their parents in influencing their decision to play soccer (Ward et al 2007).

Developmental context (culture, size of birthplace and relative age)

The importance a nation or community places on a particular sport may also have a dramatic influence on an athlete's success. For example, the sport of ice hockey has become a fundamental component of the national identity in Canada and recent estimates indicate that Canada has three times more children playing ice hockey than Russia, Sweden, Finland, the Czech Republic and Slovakia combined (Robinson 1998). Given these factors, Canada's international success is not surprising. Other countries, such as Austria in skiing and Kenya in distance running, emphasize the association between culture and sporting success.

A factor that may be linked to culture and has recently been identified as a predictor of expert performance is the size of one's birthplace. Preliminary research has indicated that birthplace size affects one's likelihood of attaining elite level performance (Baker & Logan 2007, Côté et al 2006). Figure 3.1 provides an example of this effect using

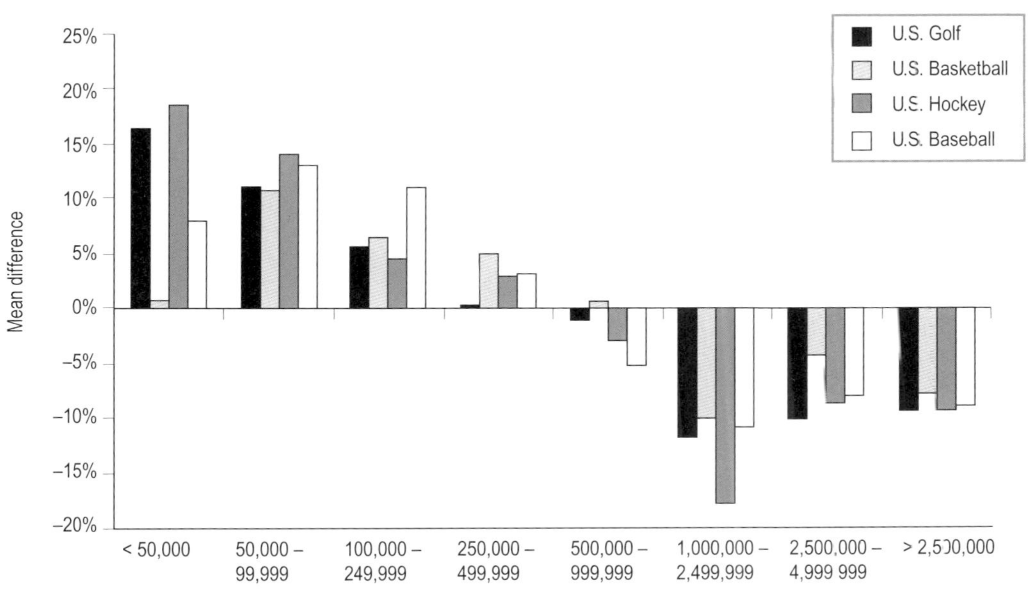

Fig. 3.1 • Birthplace effect in Canadian athletes from the National Hockey League (NHL). Columns above the line (0%) represent an over-representation relative to expected values while columns below the line represent an under-representation. Adapted from Côté et al 2006.

data modified from Côté et al (2006). In general, the research suggests an optimal environment size for promoting expertise development as geographical regions that are too small or too large result in a disadvantaged environment. While the mechanisms for this 'birthplace effect' are not known, it is likely that a range of factors, such as safety, sport opportunities, identification of 'talented' individuals and level of competition, play a role.

Relative age effect

Another factor related to the acquisition of expertise is the 'relative age effect' (see Musch & Grondin 2001 for a review of this concept). It is common in many sports to group participants by age in order to equalize evaluation and competition. However, research indicates that, during early development, older individuals in a given age cohort (i.e. that have a greater relative age) report higher levels of proficiency. This discrepancy has been found to have considerable influence on an athlete's chances of developing into an expert. To date, this effect has been reported in sports ranging from professional ice-hockey (Barnsley & Thompson 1988) and baseball (Barnsley et al 1991) to junior football (Barnsley et al 1992). The relative age effect seems to have manifested in the 1970s and was probably a result of sport development programmes that placed significant emphasis on talent identification and enhancement (Wattie et al 2007). One of the more serious consequences of the relative age effect is that a late-maturing individual born late in the selection year is doubly disadvantaged in terms of sport selection and being identified as 'talented' relative to his or her peers. One also has to consider other factors that covary with a higher relative age, e.g. more time to practice. However, the role of practice in this effect might not be quite as significant as the body size/strength advantage. A reversed relative age effect has been demonstrated in female gymnastics, whereby children born later in the selection year are more likely to succeed (Ste-Marie et al 2000). In gymnastics (and perhaps also in classical ballet), it is hypothesized that there are advantages associated with being a late-maturing individual in terms of maintaining a slight body frame and relatively homogenous body proportions. These characteristics are associated more with aesthetics than skill, although physical changes associated with the onset of puberty could have implications for balance and coordination.

Motivation, commitment and enjoyment

In view of the high quantity and quality of practice that is required to attain an expert level of sport performance, researchers have started to look at the factors that are likely to precipitate this dedication to practice (as detailed in the period of specialization discussed below). Many researchers, including Ericsson et al (1993), have remarked on the fact that if someone was interested in identifying talent and predicting expertise then they would be wise to select individuals who are the most motivated and committed to the sport and to practice. Despite this widespread agreement, there have been very few studies where these two factors, i.e. motivation or commitment and deliberate practice, have been considered and measured together.

Commitment and motivation have often been used interchangeably to examine interest in sports and to measure an individual's desire to practice and to excel. The general goal has been to identify the common factors that lead to continued sport involvement and high levels of performance within a domain. This has led people to examine the variables that best predict commitment and hence long-term involvement, as well as the motivation to succeed in a particular sport or activity.

Much of the work on sport commitment has been conducted by Scanlan and colleagues (Carpenter et al 1993, Carpenter & Scanlan 1998, Scanlan et al 1993) which has culminated in the Sport Commitment Model (Scanlan et al 1993). Sport commitment has generally been defined as 'the psychological state representing the desire or resolve to continue sport participation' (Scanlan et al 1993, p. 6). Notice that this definition does not relate to success, just participation, although obviously the latter is a necessity for the former. Original models of sport commitment were based on studies of social relationships in the home and workplace and hence factors were identified that were expected to be related to the strength of a relationship, such as the degree of personal investment, other alternatives and overall level of satisfaction (e.g. Kelley 1983, Rusbult 1980, Thibault & Kelley 1959). One major change between the non-sport models and subsequent sport models was the replacement of 'satisfaction' with the concept of sport enjoyment (Scanlan et al 1993). Weiss et al (2001) argued that sport enjoyment was the only factor to directly affect sport commitment and that other factors, such as other sport alternatives, exerted their influence through this concept of enjoyment (i.e. the mediational model of sport commitment). Although there has been support for both models, Augaitis (2005) recently showed that, for novice and intermediate level triathletes, sport enjoyment did not mediate the influence of other variables such as personal investment, involvement opportunities and involvement alternatives. Rather, these latter variables were all significant independent predictors of sport commitment. In subsequent analysis of this data, Augaitis et al (in preparation) examined the relationship between practice behaviours (current practice hours and accumulated practice hours) and commitment (based on a 5-point scale, see Scanlan et al 1993). Moderate positive correlations were observed for current and past practice estimates. Practice hours in the past year based on seasonal variations in practice (i.e. pre-race, race, off-season estimates) showed a moderate-sized correlation with commitment, r (134) = 0.42. Average number of hours/week training yielded a correlation of r (141) = 0.34. Commitment and accumulated practice showed a correlation of r (141) = 0.30. These data are illustrated in Figure 3.2. Although cause and effect statements are difficult to make from this type of research, it is tempting to speculate that these markers of commitment predict practice behaviours and hence performance. However, because commitment levels are most highly correlated with weekly and yearly practice, as opposed to practice across the athlete's career, there might be reason to suspect that commitment is only a transient measure of current levels of performance investment. In future research it will be important to track practice behaviours and sport commitment or other motivation-related variables concurrently to try to ascertain the direction of the relationship and whether commitment to the sport is the driving force behind engagement in practice. Although Augaitis et al looked at performance markers (i.e. triathlon times) in addition to practice variables and commitment, the relationship between practice behaviours and performance was not as strong as reported in previous studies (although this could be due to the lower skill level of the athletes in comparison to other studies as well as the difficulty in comparing times across supposedly similar triathlon events where there can be variability in distance, conditions and difficulty of the courses). The other important issue to consider is whether commitment to a sport is the same as commitment to practice and whether commitment to a specific sport is related in a more general way to a person's disposition to generally be more committed to people,

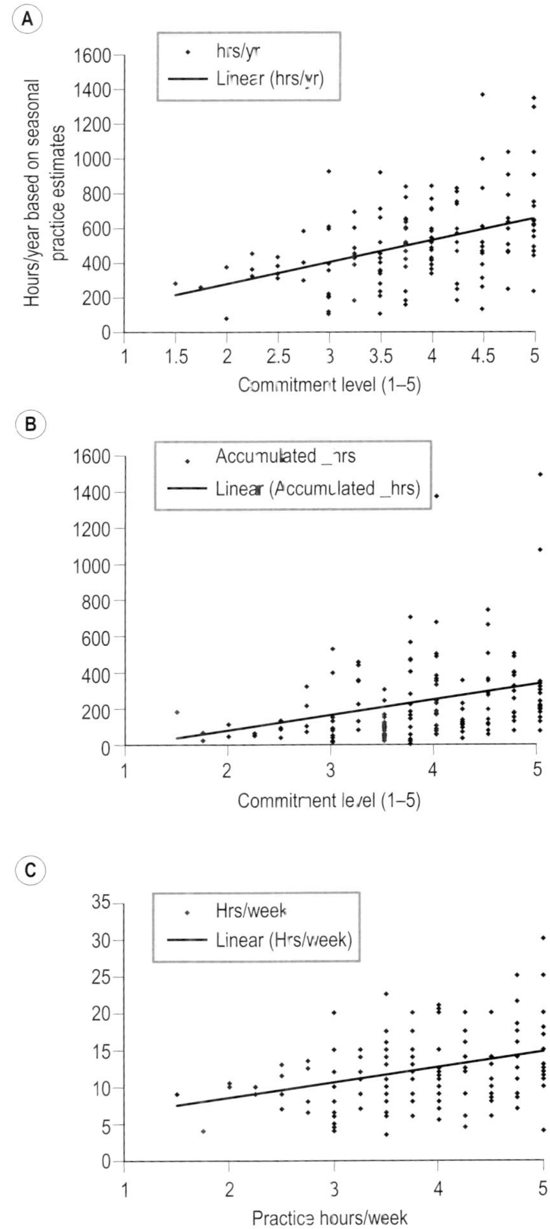

Fig. 3.2 • Scatter diagrams showing the relationship between reported levels of commitment and practice amounts for age-level triathletes (a) hours/year; (b) career accumulated hours; (c) hours/week in current season.

activities and things. Research is necessary to determine whether commitment can be fostered through participation in a specific sport or whether there are certain features of individuals which appear to predispose them to seriously engage in practice.

A number of researchers have asked general motivation questions across different classes of skill to try and ascertain the reasons for engagement in the sport and hence the desire to practice. There is evidence that perceptions of competence in a domain drive feelings of intrinsic motivation (e.g. Deci & Ryan 1985, Ryan & Deci 2000) and hence motivation is seen to be a result of practice and performance rather than necessarily predictive of performance. However, other factors have also been suggested to underlie motivation, including enjoyment of an activity and the desire to excel and meet challenges (e.g. Lens & Rand 2000). The general assumption has been that sport participation in general is enjoyable and that this enjoyment engenders further engagement (see, for example, Kowal & Fortier 1999).

In an examination of various practice activities and behaviours across elite and subelite youth soccer players between the ages of 8 and 17 years, Ward et al (2007) asked the players to give their reasons for involvement in soccer in order to get a better understanding of the motivating factors across the developmental continuum as a function of both age and skill level. Motivation factors were assessed using an adapted version of the Sport Commitment Questionnaire (Scanlan et al 1993). Perceived competence was also assessed (Harter 1981, 1982). Elite players reported being significantly more dedicated and competent than subelite players across all ages. Both skill groups rated soccer as highly enjoyable, with the elite level players giving slightly higher ratings than the subelite players. The elite players cited improvement in skill as the main reason for playing in the current year, irrespective of age, whereas enjoyment was cited as the most common reason for their subelite cohorts. Although it is difficult to make any clear predictions about the importance of motivation and self-perceived competence in predicting continued involvement and performance, we see a high correlation between skill level and these measures across the age continuum. Moreover, the elite players across the age continuum report a desire to improve their current skill level as a more important factor underlying engagement than enjoyment.

It is apparent from the above discussion that enjoyment features prominently in any discussion of motivation and commitment, although there does not appear to be a clear relationship between enjoyment, practice and performance. There has been some controversy in the sport domain when researchers have tried to examine Ericsson et al's (1993) original ideas about the concept of enjoyment and its unnecessary role in encouraging practice behaviours and hence in developing skill. This is primarily due to three factors. First, Ericsson et al (1993) have often been misreported as claiming that engagement in the actual activity (e.g. music or sport) is not enjoyable. More correctly, Ericsson et al claimed that engagement in 'deliberate practice' was not considered to be high in inherent enjoyment (see also Ericsson & Charness 1994). Second, this judgment of enjoyment was determined through relative comparisons with other activities that were deemed to be inherently enjoyable, such as socializing with friends or watching TV. Deliberate practice was perceived as more enjoyable than not enjoyable (on a scale of enjoyment), but this concept was not an important or necessary characteristic of practice. This led Ericsson and colleagues to argue that people engaged in deliberate practice primarily to improve or maintain performance, rather than for its inherent enjoyment value. Finally, Ericsson et al (1993) were very careful in their assessment of enjoyment using interview techniques and purposely asking people to differentiate enjoyment gained from participating and hence perceptions of the results of practice, what others have termed satisfaction, from enjoyment experienced during the practice session.

Although there have been a few studies where practice behaviours have still been rated as highly enjoyable, despite more controlled assessment of enjoyment, differences in the way practice has been assessed appear to be the primary reason for the majority of discrepancies in results across studies. Two recent studies have served to confirm this interpretation. Hodges et al (2004) asked competitive and recreational triathletes to keep diaries detailing their engagement in various types of physical activity each day. In addition to recording the time spent in these activities, the athletes rated each activity in terms of its relevance to improving performance, effort and concentration, enjoyment experienced during the activity and general feelings of satisfaction with the results of the activity once it was completed. There were three important findings. Ratings of enjoyment were not significantly correlated with ratings of relevance or effort, although the ratings were significantly higher than the overall mean. Second, general feelings of satisfaction were related to perceptions of relevance and effort. Third, when the athletes were asked to provide ratings in a questionnaire and these were compared to the diaries, a high correlation between enjoyment and relevance was observed. These data confirm the conclusions of Ericsson et al (1993) that deliberate practice activities (i.e. activities rated high in terms of relevance to improving performance and high in effort) might be perceived as enjoyable, especially when people are asked to generally rate their perceptions of various practice activities in a questionnaire, but that enjoyment is not a necessary condition for deliberate practice. Similar distinctions between enjoyment obtained from the process (i.e. actual participation) and enjoyment based upon appraisal of the outcome of each activity led Ward et al (2007) to reach similar conclusions about the role of enjoyment in practice. Young players, irrespective of skill class, typically gained enjoyment from actual participation in the activity but, as age increased, players tended to shift their emphasis toward appraising the outcome of the activity when rating training activities for enjoyment. Overall, it appears that perceptions of enjoyment are not necessary correlates of effective practice and arguably the development of skilled performance, but that motivation and commitment to practice might be partially mediated by enjoyment. As we discuss elsewhere, enjoyment in sports and activities in general might be fostered in the early years of sport participation but performance success and satisfaction are more important mediators of continued involvement at higher levels of performance skill.

Effort

One of the methods for ascertaining how enjoyable and effortful practice activities are as a function of skill level has been to perform an in-depth analysis of particular practice sessions. This approach is usually conducted through time–motion analysis whereby a skilled observer records the time spent in various practice activities reported to be the most relevant to improving performance.

There has been evidence that elite performers maximize their time at practice sessions by engaging in the most important practice activities as well as taking less time for rests. Deakin and colleagues (see Deakin & Cobley 2003, Starkes et al 1996) found that elite skaters spent approximately 20% more of their time practising jumps and 30% less time resting during on-ice practice than subelite skaters. Perhaps not surprisingly, these data show that the quality of practice for elite performers is superior to that of subelite performers, not just the amount. Whether the quality of the practice differentiates across skill levels at a young age and is predictive of later skill is yet to be tested. Ward et al (2007) examined how practice sessions were differentiated in youth soccer players between the ages of 8 and 17 years, although this analysis was based on self-report rather than the more objective time–motion analysis. Surprisingly, there was little difference between the groups as a function of skill level and no evidence that the more elite players were spending less time resting during their practice. The only activity to differentiate across the skill groups was time spent in strategic decision-making activities, with the elite players reporting more time training in this aspect of performance than their subelite counterparts (see also Rutt-Leas & Chi 1993).

A more refined analysis of practice has also been achieved through measurement of practice across a performance year, what has been referred to as periodization of practice. If athletes maintain a constant level of training throughout the season then it is to be assumed that the activity itself is the primary motivating variable. However, practice vacillates as a function of time of season, giving evidence that practice is designed to maximize performance rather than because of its inherent enjoyment. Practice periodization has been examined in the sport of triathlon where individuals engage in three events and hence the organization of practice is quite critical to overall performance in an event. Hodges and colleagues, as reported in Ward et al (2004), found that the stronger athletes were more likely to divide their practice sessions equally across the three events in comparison to the less competent athletes, who favoured the event they were best at. There are also data obtained from questionnaires and heart rate monitors that show that across the practice season the more highly skilled performers practice at a higher intensity than their less skilled counterparts (Baker et al 2005, Hodges et al 2007, Ward et al 2004).

In their original discussions of constraints on practice, Ericsson et al made the point that the amount of practice aspiring performers could devote to a specific domain would be limited by their ability to maintain concentration at high levels for extended periods of time. Effort (both physical and cognitive) would therefore be expected to interact with age, skill level (in that less effort would be expected for the same activity as skill level increases) and the performance domain/sport. Although there is evidence that skilled athletes appear to engage in more effortful practice (in terms of the type of practice and amount of rest within a practice session), there has not been any evidence that skilled athletes are able to overcome effort constraints on practice perhaps associated with eventual burnout. There is likely to be a link between commitment levels or intrinsic motivation and effort. It is probable that for young, developing athletes, effort to attend practice and engage effortfully during practice is highly facilitated by significant others such as the coach and parents (i.e. is externally mediated). Later in development, internal factors are likely to play a more important role in encouraging deliberate practice.

Athlete training across the stages of development

Developmental psychologists have produced several models delineating the stages or periods of human development and researchers in the field of expertise have done the same. In general, researchers have suggested that athletes, as they move from novice to expert, move through three or four qualitatively different stages that are related both to skill level and age (e.g. Bloom 1985, Côté & Fraser-Thomas 2007, Ericsson et al 1993). Below, we review three primary stages leading to the development of expertise and the type of training required to augment the acquisition of expertise. We have also included a fourth stage of development that is characteristic of skilled performance with advancing age. These various stages are illustrated in Figure 3.3.

In attempting to differentiate across the skill continuum with respect to various stages of development, we have assumed that these four stages can also be qualitatively described in some manner. The early years typically reflect the initial involvement of children in a sport, although the actual age of starting can vary considerably across domains. For example, wrestlers often begin early involvement around puberty whereas gymnasts or soccer players begin much earlier, sometimes around 4–5 years (see Starkes et al 1996). We would argue that this early stage of development and the amount of involvement is highly influenced by the primary caregiver. The second stage, what we have referred to as the intermediate stage of performance, is indicative of specialization within a sport. Again, there could be considerable variability in the age of specialization and it is unclear where the boundary exists between this specialization period and the attainment of expertise (stage 3). People's definition of expertise has been shown to vary widely in the research literature and hence it is somewhat problematic to discriminate these two stages. Typically, expertise is thought to reflect world-class performance and hence criteria such as professional status or international competition might be used to qualitatively define true expertise. University-level

Stage 4 – Masters Involvement

- Increased emphasis on endurance activities rather than sprint/power training
- Reduction in absolute time spent training

Stage 3 – Expertise

- World class performance
- Almost exclusive focus on deliberate practice
- Enjoyment, social engagement and recreation are secondary to performance improvement

Stage 2 – Intermediate Development

- Increase in specialization and investment in training
- Highly skilled coaches and high quality resources increasingly important

Stage 1 – Early Development

- Initial involvement in sports and physical activity
- Learning occurs at a rapid rate
- Focus on acquisition of general, fundamental skills

Fig. 3.3 • Stages of development for expert athletes.

athletics might be the highest level for some individuals, or involvement in professional youth academies, but arguably this skilled performance at a pre-adult age or at a relatively local level is not quite true expertise, although it is certainly indicative of a high level of skill. Some authors (e.g. Bloom 1985, Ericsson et al 1993) have separated the 'expertise' stage from a later 'maintenance' stage. Although it is true that there are probably differences in improving and maintaining performance, we do not deal with these stages separately in this chapter as they are difficult to distinguish empirically and no practice-related research with young athletes has been conducted to date that would necessitate this separation. The 'maintenance' stage could in some cases be viewed as a period that overlaps the 'expertise' stage and the 'masters' stage, which we detail below. However, not all masters athletes have necessarily achieved expertise in their youth. Our final stage, elite masters competition, is easier to define, although it appears to be sport-dependent. The entry age for participants in the World Masters Games, the largest multisport event in the world, is 30 years of age, but athletes can participate at this level at younger ages in some sports (e.g. swimming, gymnastics and figure skating). This stage is often underrecognized in models of athlete development.

Stage one: early years of sport involvement

Research typically indicates that future sports experts begin involvement in sports (either organized or unorganized) at around 5 years of age. However, there is some disagreement about what form training should take at this stage. The issue pertains to the extent to which children should 'specialize' their training and involvement during this period. Contention exists around this issue because of the negative consequences associated with a specialized approach. For instance, it has been linked to compromised physical, social and psychological development and may even be counterproductive to the development of expertise because of the possibility of decreased motivation and dropout (see Baker & Côté 2006 for a review). However, researchers advocating a specialized approach (e.g. Ericsson et al 1993) point to the robust relationship between time spent practising and proficiency (Newell & Rosenbloom 1981) as outlined elsewhere in this chapter. Accordingly, it is perceived to be necessary to start practising at an early age in order to accrue the necessary hours of practice needed to be identified as 'talented' and compete at the highest levels of the sport.

Regardless of which position proves ultimately correct, researchers from both camps generally agree that training in the early stages of athlete development differs significantly from training in the later stages. Typically during this period there is a focus on the acquisition of general, fundamental skills, either through focused, specific training, as advocated by the specialists (see Ward et al 2007) or through unorganized and unstructured general play, as advocated by the generalists (Côté et al 2007).

According to the research literature, learning occurs quickly and rapidly during this initial phase of development. Figure 3.4 presents one hypothesized profile of rates of learning over time, the power law of practice, which has been shown in skills ranging from learning to read upside-down text to rolling cigars. What the profile indicates is that the largest advances in learning (as measured by performance) occur during this period but that the magnitude of these learning advances gradually decreases over time. The rapid increases in learning/performance are probably due to general changes or restructuring in the biological and cognitive systems responsible for performance in the sport. For instance, at the onset of an aerobic training programme, general systemic changes in cardiovascular functioning (e.g. increases in heart size and blood volume) contribute to the rapid improvements in performance (Rowell 1986). However, training must readily adapt to continue providing appropriate training stimuli to the developing athlete. The primary objective of this early stage of development is to lay a foundation of general skill from which to build domain-specific

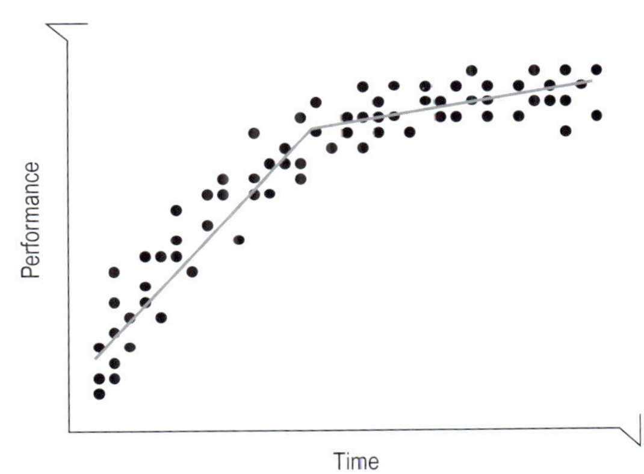

Fig. 3.4 • Hypothetical profile of performance over time indicating the power law of practice.

expertise in the future. It is highly probable that the 'seeds' of expertise are planted during the early phases of development; however, it is currently not clear how the early experiences of the expert are different from those of the non-expert. In their study of youth soccer players, Ward and Williams (2003) showed that, even as young as 9 years of age, measures of cognitive skill, such as recall of game-related scenarios and decision making (both accuracy and speed), differentiated across skill class. Players who had been selected to play in professional soccer clubs' youth academies showed advantages in these so-called 'software' measures of performance in comparison to schoolchildren, but tests of perceptual hardware (e.g. visual acuity, colour contrast perception) did not differentiate across skill. Subsequent evaluation of these age groups showed that, even as young as 9 years of age, the youth 'experts' had accrued approximately 700 more hours of individual practice than the school-level, subelite soccer players (Ward et al 2007). As remarked earlier, the elite players reported spending more time on tactical decisions during structured training, but it was difficult to make comparisons across age groups in this study because of the low number of subelite players who engaged in structured practice at a young age.

'Sampling' a variety of related sports may play an important role in expertise development via transfer of skills between related activities. For instance, Abernethy et al (2005) found that the ability to recognize specific offensive and defensive patterns of play was transferable across similar sports. However, there are some data to suggest that, if transfer of skill occurs in the development of expertise, it is confined to this early phase of development. In a review of cross-training effects, Loy et al (1995), concluded that transfer of training effects occurs primarily during the early stages of development when individuals are at lower levels of fitness and that as individuals become more skilled the value of transfer diminishes. Baker et al (2003b) investigated expert decision makers from the sports of basketball, netball and field hockey and reported that participation in other relevant activities during the early phases of development augmented the physical and cognitive skills necessary in their primary sport (see also Baker et al 2005). Although more work remains to be done on this interesting and important topic, these results suggest that the relationships among structured and unstructured training and play versus practice are dynamic and probably dependent on several factors, including age and skill level.

Stage two – intermediate phase of athlete development

The intermediate phase of athlete development covers much undiscovered territory. Côté and his colleagues (e.g. Côté & Hay 2002) consider this period a 'transition' from the unstructured involvement of childhood, when participation takes the form of various sporting activities performed in a play-like manner, to the structured, specialized involvement of the high-performance adult performer. Developmental investigations of this period indicate that it is a time when there is an increasing investment in adult-like training (i.e. 'deliberate' practice), coupled with a gradual reduction in participation in other activities. Training becomes much more specialized during this period.

Examinations of training profiles generally indicate that this is the period where experts begin to distance themselves from their non-expert counterparts. Before this time, there is usually very little, at least in their training profiles, to distinguish the expert from the non-expert. In this intermediate stage, experts increase their focus on high-quality, sport-specific training, such that the total accumulated hours of practice is drastically different from the non-expert. For instance, a recent study of Ironman-level triathletes (Baker et al 2005) showed that experts had amassed nearly twice as many hours of training as their peers at an intermediate level of skill and three times as much training as peers at a low level of skill. Similar results have been noted in a range of studies, in sports ranging from field hockey (Helsen et al 1998) to basketball (Baker et al 2003b), and from gymnastics (Law et al 2007) to darts (Duffy et al 2004). In their developmental study of youth soccer players, Ward et al (2007) showed that during this intermediate stage there was a decrease in the amount of soccer engaged in just for fun (i.e. play-related), coupled with a concurrent increase in the amount of structured team practice. This was true for both skill groups. Based on retrospective estimates of practice, Helsen et al (1998) also showed a reported reduction in the amount of individual practice in exchange for structured team practice with increasing age among semi-professional soccer players in Belgium.

Stage three – expertise

The highest stage of expertise development is characterized by the demonstration of world-class performance. At this level, there are considerable cognitive, psychological, physiological and biomechanical differences between experts and their less-skilled counterparts. A great deal of research has been conducted examining the training environments of expert performers. Typically, this research indicates that experts spend the vast majority of their time in deliberate, high quality practice, under the supervision of professional expert coaches and with access to superior training resources (e.g. facilities, sports scientists). General rules of expertise development suggest that a minimum of 10-years or 10 000 hours of involvement in a domain are required to achieve this stage of performance (Ericsson et al 1993, Simon & Chase 1973); however, others point out that these guidelines are quite crude and probably not applicable to all areas of human performance (Baker & Horton 2004).

Usually there is no consistent involvement in other sports during this period, although recreational involvement in physical activity during the 'off-season' can be common. Baker et al (2003b) found that expert decision makers from Australian national teams regularly spent time in the off-season competing in recreational sports such as golf and tennis. In sum, this period is demarcated by a very systematic approach to training that is exclusively intended to improve (and maintain) performance. Enjoyment, social engagement and recreation are secondary concerns.

What seems clear is that the development of expertise requires a balance between the type of training stress required for optimal skill development and the psychosocial and physical limitations of the developing person. For instance, some researchers suggest that a primary focus on adult-like training during early development exceeds the capabilities of young performers; in other words, their system is not 'ready' for this type of training. Athlete development may be best characterized as a period of continued adaptation to training constraints as we have detailed above. These training constraints must be continuously modified to promote maximal adaptation over time. Interestingly, there is evidence that the amount of time that can be devoted to deliberate practice is limited even at the highest levels. For example, in a comparison of musicians and athletes across various domains, Starkes et al (1996) found that the amount of training time per week for the highest-achieving athletes within a domain was reported to be on average 25 hours per week and this was relatively consistent across domains. If this number reflects a limit in practice amount, based on the various constraints detailed in the previous section, there are a number of reasons why multi-sport athletes, compared to their single-sport counterparts (e.g. swimmers or runners) would be expected to circumvent these limits. First, they are not as dependent on resources to practice, compared to swimmers, for example, who require a pool to train. Triathletes are able to run or cycle if access to a pool is not forthcoming. Second, triathletes are likely to be able to overcome constraints on effort. Muscle fatigue is typically specific to certain muscle groups, such as the deltoids and triceps in swimming. If the triathlete has muscle fatigue in the arms s/he is still able to run and cycle and should be more resistant to injury. Finally, triathletes are likely to be able to circumvent some of the motivational constraints. They are less likely to suffer from boredom and burnout from participating in only one activity as opposed to three. Despite these predictions, Hodges et al (2004) failed to find evidence that triathletes were engaging in more hours of sport-specific practice than elite swimmers, as illustrated in Figure 3.5. The elite triathletes (see Fig. 3.5a) reported about 18 hours per week in the three sport-specific activities combined (swim, cycle and run), in comparison to approximately 24 hours per week for the international swimmers (and 18 hours for the junior–national level swimmers) spent just on swimming practice (see Fig. 3.5b). This consistency in practice amounts across domains at the highest level of skill attests to the fact that practice should be acquired in a distributed manner across many years, as there is little evidence that the constraints on practice time can be circumvented in order to 'catch up' by doing more in advancing years.

Stage four – masters involvement

In outlining stages of development in sport involvement across a person's career, it is important not to ignore performance beyond what is assumed to be peak levels of physical fitness. The choice of an athlete to retire from international competition is often stimulated by performance declines that appear to be age-related, both as a result of factors that are intrinsic (such as injury or a decline in fitness) and extrinsic to the athlete (e.g. family, career). There are also cases of people who only begin participation in a sport/activity at a later age and only enter into older-adult or what is called 'master level'

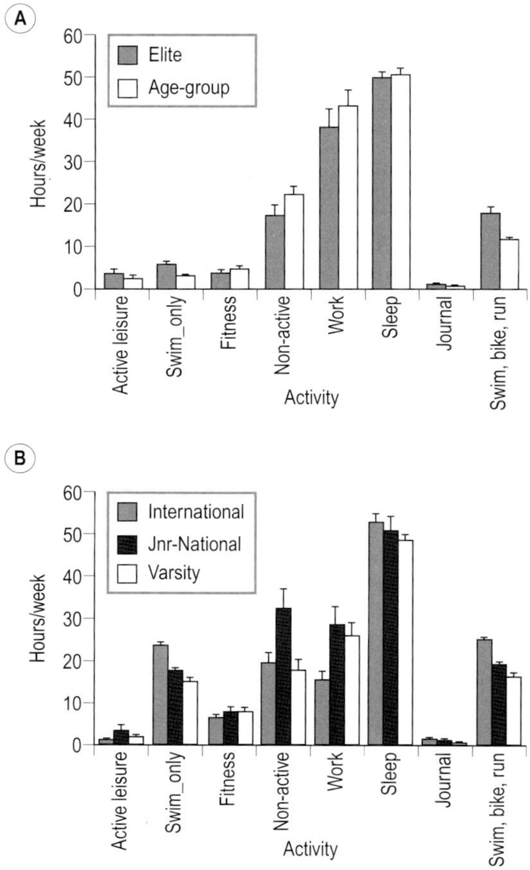

Fig. 3.5 • Average reported hours per week in various everyday (non-active = non-active leisure time) and sport-specific activities for triathletes (a) and swimmers (b).

competition. Across the world, high-level competition beyond the traditional age norms is observed (usually above 35 years of age with no upper limit). For example, in track and field, the World Association of Masters Athletics (WMA) hosts competitions for athletes around the world who continue to compete at a high level and who maintain training beyond what would be considered merely recreational hours.

How individuals are able to maintain performance beyond peak years and continue to compete at a high level of competition is an important question from both a theoretical and an applied standpoint. Researchers have attempted to study how performance and ageing are related in order to understand the process of ageing and features that are particularly susceptible to decline (such as aerobic or anaerobic fitness). Through mainly correlational analyses and cross-sectional comparisons of different age groups of performers in sport, it has been possible to quantify the age–performance relationship in a variety of domains. For example, it is relatively well established that many performance-related variables change linearly with age until approximately 60 years of age, after which the rate of change accelerates and becomes more quadratic in nature (Salthouse 1992, Stones & Kozma 1981). It has been shown that these declines are more noticeable in endurance-related activities, such as long distance running or swimming, than anaerobic activities, such as sprints (e.g. Weir et al 2002). Further, the top-achieving athletes in these older age groups were also shown to change the types of activity they engaged in to compensate for performance decline, such as decreasing the amount of time spent in power and technique training and increasing the amount of time working on cardiac/respiratory function. Starkes et al (2004) have suggested that maintenance of performance after the peak years might be achieved through a changing skill set. For example, declines in perceptual–motor abilities, such as speed, might not be noticeable if coupled with improvements in cognitive–perceptual abilities, such as better decision making and anticipation. Therefore, it is important to look carefully at the types of skill that constitute skilled performance, and hence interpretations of ageing decline in performance need to take account of the various facets that make up skilled performance. When declines are not observed, this does not mean that the ageing process has not started to take its toll but that perhaps the skills and the type of practice have changed to compensate for declines in other areas. A recent study of the careers of PGA golfers supports this conclusion. Baker et al (2007) examined the component skills of golf performance and found that some skills decreased more rapidly than others (e.g. driving distance versus putting, respectively) but that golfers were able to maintain a remarkable level of performance overall (i.e. a decline of less than 0.15% per year after peak performance).

The declines that have typically been documented in the sport literature as a function of age have usually been based upon cross-sectional comparisons of different age groups. There is, however, evidence that comparisons of different groups of people as a function of age portray quite a negative picture of the ageing process in comparison to analysis of ageing and performance within the same individual (i.e. longitudinal data, see Baker et al 2007, Starkes et al

1999, Stones & Kozma 1981, Weir et al 2002). In some cases, the declines appear to be almost twice as steep as in longitudinal data. This effect is expected to be related to changes or consistency in factors external to the individual that have an impact on the maintenance of practice. For example, a person who continues involvement in a domain beyond the peak years is likely to maintain their practice amounts at a similar level and hence any declines are more likely to be a result of intrinsic, rather than extrinsic factors. There has been evidence to support this conclusion in music (Ericsson & Krampe 1996) as well as case study data collected from long-distance runners. Starkes et al (2003; see also Young & Starkes 2005) showed that when practice amount was maintained over a 30-year period for one athlete (i.e. between 26 and 56 years of age), although performance had slowed in this time, the amount of slowing was considerably less than that predicted by estimates based on cross-sectional data (i.e. world, age-related grading). Ericsson and Krampe (1996) have proposed a 'selective maintenance' account of ageing. This was based on findings among ageing pianists showing that performance declines were restricted to general activities and skills such as simple reaction time. Skills specific to playing the piano were not subject to such declines if practice was maintained with advancing years. This was especially true if practice was maintained between the ages of 50 and 60 years. One of the highly positive results of the recent sport-related research is that performance improvements have been observed later in life as a result of increased training. Starkes et al (2003) present a case of an athlete who achieved his best performance in the mile at 41 years of age (achieving a level of performance that would rank him among the top 10% in the world for his age).

Summary, conclusions and implications for coaches and athletes

In this chapter we have outlined various conditions that are likely to engender best practice and facilitate the need to devote many hours of domain-relevant deliberate practice. Ericsson et al (1993) considered these conditions 'constraints' on practice. In this review we argue that these factors should be considered as stepping stones on the expertise journey, certainly providing important career boosts, such as being born at the right time, in the right place and maturing physically at an optimal time. However, these conditions alone would not be considered either necessary or sufficient for the attainment and maintenance of a high level of skill (Figure 3.6). At the current time it is still unclear how critical motivation and commitment are as factors necessary to promote practice and engender skill development. We do not know whether motivation to practise and succeed is a stable trait characteristic of certain individuals and hence whether lacking the motivation phenotype is a constraint on skill development. It might be that motivation is task- and sport-dependent, emerging out of success in a sport and feelings of competence and therefore limited to a particular domain. In this latter view, motivation per se is not a limiting factor but could perhaps be nurtured and developed through careful mentoring. Indeed, it might be that the early enjoyment fostered through play and diversification in sports could be the catalyst for motivation to grow and hence the investment of the necessary quality and quantity of practice.

It should be clear from this review that there is still some debate as to whether early practice experiences should be specific or general in nature and how these experiences impact on later sport involvement. It might be the case that many athletes are unnecessarily dropping out of sports because of pressure to specialize at an early age and that the ones who succeed are better suited to focused, domain-specific, specialized practice. Although

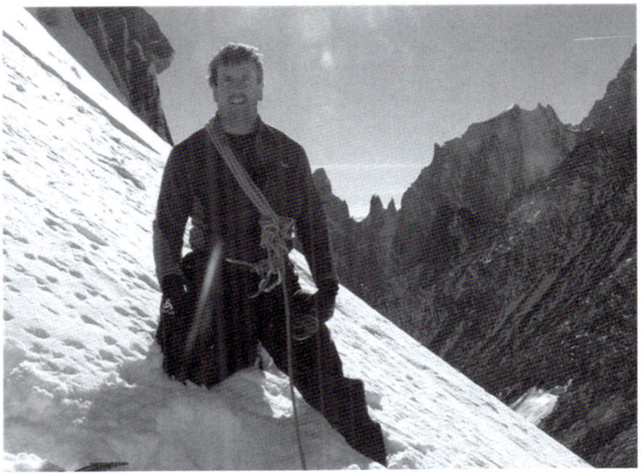

Fig. 3.6 • Peak performance! Mountaineering is often low expertise but high physical loading. Even here, however, there are skills which must be mastered if safety is to be maintained. Photo with thanks to Katherine Flynn. © Katherine Flynn.

there is some evidence that early experiences in sports in general may have some performance benefits in specific domains later in development, research evidence is still lacking. There is a need for researchers to examine more carefully the types of skill and ability that are likely to transfer across domains in order to make predictions as to how early diversification and sampling of various sports might facilitate later specialization and success in one domain.

Additional research is needed to develop our understanding of the factors promoting the transition from the more general sports experiences of early life, emphasizing enjoyment and play-like involvement, and the more structured, intense involvement representative of adult training. Moreover, we know very little about the training and development of elite older athletes and these performers may provide us with vital information regarding skill maintenance with advancing age.

References

Abernethy, B., Baker, J., Côté, J., 2005. Transfer of pattern recall skills as a contributor to the development of sport expertise. Applied Cognitive Psychology 19, 705–718.

Augaitis, L., 2005. The sport commitment model: commitment and outcome behaviours of age-group triathletes, MA thesis, University of British Columbia, Vancouver, BC.

Baker, J., Côté, J., 2006. Shifting training requirements during athlete development: the relationship among deliberate practice, deliberate play and other sport involvement in the acquisition of sport expertise. In: Hackfort, D., Tanenbaum, G. (Eds.), Essential processes for attaining peak performance. Meyer & Meyer, Aachen, pp. 93–110.

Baker, J., Horton, S., 2004. A review of primary and secondary influences on sport expertise. High Ability Studies 15, 211–228.

Baker, J., Logan, A.J., 2007. Developmental contexts and sporting success: birthdate and birthplace effects in NHL draftees 2000–2005. Br. J. Sports Med. 41, 515–517.

Baker, J., Horton, S., Robertson-Wilson, J., et al., 2003a. Nurturing sport expertise: factors influencing the development of the elite athlete. Journal of Sports Science and Medicine 2, 1–9.

Baker, J., Côté, J., Abernethy, B., 2003b. Sport specific training, deliberate practice and the development of expertise in team ball sports. Journal of Applied Sport Psychology 15, 12–25.

Baker, J., Côté, J., Deakin, J., 2005. Expertise in ultra-endurance triathletes: early sport involvement, training structure and the theory of deliberate practice. Journal of Applied Sport Psychology 17, 64–78.

Baker, J., Horton, S., Pearce, W., et al., 2007. Maintenance of skilled performance with age: a descriptive examination of professional golfers. J. Aging Phys. Act. 15, 299–316.

Barnsley, R.H., Thompson, A.H., 1988. Birthdate and success in minor hockey: the key to the NHL. Canadian Journal of Behavioural Science 20, 167–176.

Barnsley, R.H., Thompson, A.H., Steblelsky, G., 1991. Born to play ball: relative age effect in major league baseball. Sociology of Sport Journal 8, 146–151.

Barnsley, R.H., Thompson, A.H., Legault, P., 1992. Family planning: football style. The relative age effect in football. International Review for the Sociology of Sport 27, 77–87.

Bloom, B., 1985. Developing talent in young people. Ballantine Books, New York.

Carpenter, P.J., Scanlan, T.K., 1998. Changes over time in the determinants of sport commitment. Pediatric Exercise Science 10, 356–365.

Carpenter, P.J., Scanlan, T.K., Simons, J.P., et al., 1993. A test of the sport commitment model using structural equation modeling. Journal of Sport and Exercise Psychology 15, 119–133.

Côté, J., 1999. The influence of the family in the development of talent in sport. Sport Psychologist 13, 395–417.

Côté, J., Fraser-Thomas, J., 2007. Youth involvement in sport. In: Crocker, P.R.E. (Ed.), Sport psychology: a Canadian perspective. Pearson, Toronto, ON, pp. 266–294.

Côté, J., Hay, J., 2002. Children's involvement in sport: a developmental perspective. In: Silva, J.M., Stevens, D. (Eds.), Psychological foundations in sport. Merrill, Boston, MA, pp. 484–502.

Côté, J., Baker, J., Abernethy, B., 2003. From play to practice: a developmental framework for the acquisition of expertise in team sports. In: Starkes, J.L., Ericsson, K.A. (Eds.), Expert performance in sports: advances in research on sport expertise. Human Kinetics, Champaign, IL, pp. 89–114.

Côté, J., MacDonald, D., Baker, J., et al., 2006. When 'where' is more important than 'when': birthplace and birthdate effects on the achievement of sporting expertise. J. Sports Sci. 24, 1065–1073.

Côté, J., Baker, J., Abernethy, B., 2007. Play and practice in the development of sport expertise. In: Tenenbaum, G., Eklund, R.C. (Eds.), Handbook of sport psychology. John Wiley, New York, pp. 184–202.

Deakin, J.M., Cobley, S., 2003. A search for deliberate practice: an examination of the practice environments in figure skating and volleyball. In: Starkes, J.L., Ericsson, K.A. (Eds.), Expert performance in sports: advances in research on sport expertise. Human Kinetics, Champaign, IL, pp. 115–135.

Deci, E.L., Ryan, R.M., 1985. Intrinsic motivation and self-determination in human behaviour. Plenum Press, New York.

Duffy, L.J., Baruch, B., Ericsson, K.A., 2004. Dart performance as a function of facets of practice amongst professional and amateur men and women players. International Journal of Sport Psychology 35, 232–245.

Ericsson, K.A., Charness, N., 1994. Expert Performance: its structure and acquisition. Am. Psychol. 49, 725–747.

Ericsson, K.A., Krampe, R.T., 1996. Maintaining excellence: deliberate practice and elite performance in young and older pianists. J. Exp. Psychol. 125, 331–359.

Ericsson, K.A., Krampe, R.T., Tesch-Römer, C., 1993. The role of deliberate practice in the acquisition of expert performance. Psychol. Rev. 100, 363–406.

Harter, S., 1981. A new self-report scale of intrinsic versus extrinsic orientation in the classroom: motivational and informational components. Dev. Psychol. 17, 300–312.

Harter, S., 1982. The perceived competence scale for children. Child. Dev. 53, 87–97.

Helsen, W.F., Starkes, J.L., Hodges, N.J., 1998. Team sports and the theory of deliberate practice. Journal of Sport and Exercise Psychology 20, 12–34.

Hodge, T., Deakin, J.M., 1998. Deliberate practice and expertise in martial arts: the role of context in motor recall. Journal of Sport and Exercise Psychology 20, 260–327.

Hodges, N.J., Starkes, J.L., 1996. Wrestling with the nature of expertise: a sport specific test of Ericsson, Krampe and Tesch-Römer's (1993) theory of deliberate practice. International Journal of Sport Psychology 27, 400–424.

Hodges, N.J., Kerr, T., Starkes, J.L., et al., 2004. Predicting performance from deliberate practice hours for triathletes and swimmers: what, when and where is practice important? J. Exp. Psychol. Appl. 10, 219–237.

Hodges, N.J., Huys, R., Starkes, J.L., 2007. A methodological review and evaluation of research of expert performance in sport. In: Tenenbaum, G., Eklund, R.C. (Eds.), Handbook of sport psychology, third ed. John Wiley, New York, pp. 161–183.

Horton, S., Deakin, J., 2008. Expert coaches in action. In: Farrow, D., Baker, J., MacMahon, C. (Eds.), Developing sports skill: researchers and coaches put theory into practice. Routledge, Abingdon, Oxfordshire, pp. 75–85.

Kelley, H.H., 1983. Love and commitment. In: Kelley, H.H., Berscheid, E., Christensen, A. et al., Close relationships. WH Freeman, New York, pp. 265–314.

Kowal, J., Fortier, M.S., 1999. Motivational determinants of flow: contributions from self determination theory. J. Soc. Psychol. 139, 355–368.

Law, M.P., Côté, J., Ericsson, K.A., 2007. Characteristics of expert development in rhythmic gymnastics: a retrospective study. International Journal of Sport and Exercise Psychology 5, 82–103.

Lens, W., Rand, P., 2000. Motivation and cognition: their role in the development of giftedness. In: Heller, K.A., Monks, F.J., Sternberg, R.J., et al. (Eds.), International handbook of giftedness and talent. second ed. Elsevier, Amsterdam, pp. 193–202.

Loy, S.F., Hoffmann, J.J., Holland, G.J., 1995. Benefits and practical use of cross training in sports. Sports Med. 19, 1–8.

More, K.G., Franks, I.M., 1996. Analysis and modification of verbal coaching behaviour: the usefulness of a data-driven intervention strategy. J. Sports Sci. 14, 523–543.

Musch, J., Grondin, S., 2001. Unequal competition as an impediment to personal development: a review of the relative age effect in sport. Developmental Review 21, 147–167.

Newell, A., Rosenbloom, P.S., 1981. Mechanisms of skill acquisition and the law of practice. In: Anderson, J.R. (Eds.), Cognitive skills and their acquisition. Lawrence Erlbaum Associates, Hillsdale, NJ, pp. 1–55.

Robinson, L., 1998. Crossing the line: violence and sexual assault in Canada's national sport. McClelland & Stewart, Toronto, ON.

Rowell, L.B., 1986. Human circulation: regulation during physical stress. Oxford University Press, New York.

Rusbult, C.E., 1980. Commitment and satisfaction in romantic associations: a test of the investment model. J. Exp. Soc. Psychol. 16, 172–186.

Rutt-Leas, R., Chi, M.T.H., 1993. Analyzing diagnostic expertise of competitive swimming coaches. In: Starkes, J.L., Allard, F. (Eds.), Cognitive issues in motor expertise. Elsevier, Amsterdam, pp. 75–94.

Ryan, R.M., Deci, E.L., 2000. Self-determination theory and the facilitation of intrinsic motivation, social development, and well being. Am. Psychol. 55, 68–78.

Salthouse, T.A., 1992. Mechanisms of age-cognition relations in adulthood. Lawrence Erlbaum Associates, Hillsdale, NJ.

Scanlan, T.K., Carpenter, P.J., Schmidt, G.W., et al., 1993. An introduction to the sport commitment model. Journal of Sport and Exercise Psychology 15, 1–15.

Simon, H.A., Chase, W., 1973. Skill in chess. Am. Sci. 61, 394–403.

Starkes, J.L., Deakin, J.M., Allard, F., et al., 1996. Deliberate practice in sports: what is it anyway? In: Ericsson, K.A. (Ed.), The road to excellence: the acquisition of expert performance in the arts and sciences, sports, and games. Lawrence Erlbaum, Mahwah, NJ, pp. 81–106.

Starkes, J.L., Weir, P.L., Singh, P., et al., 1999. Aging and the retention of sport expertise. International Journal of Sport Psychology 30, 283–301.

Starkes, J.L., Helsen, W., Jack, R., 2001. Expert performance in sport and dance. In: Singer, R.N., Hausenblas, H.A., Janelle, C.M. (Eds.), Handbook of sport psychology. second ed. John Wiley, New York, pp. 174–201.

Starkes, J.L., Weir, P.L., Young, B.W., 2003. Retaining expertise: what does it take for older expert athletes to continue to excel? In: Starkes, J.L., Ericsson, K.A. (Eds.), Expert performance in sports: advances in research on sport expertise. Human Kinetics, Champaign, IL, pp. 251–272.

Starkes, J.L., Cullen, J., MacMahon, C., 2004. A model of skill acquisition and retention of perceptual-motor performance. In: Williams, A.M., Hodges, N.J. (Eds.), Skill acquisition in sport: research, theory and practice. Routledge, London, pp. 259–281.

Ste-Marie, D.M., Starkes, J., Cronin, A., et al., 2000. The relative age effect: A 'flip-flop' phenomenon in gymnasts. Proceedings of the Canadian Society for Psychomotor Learning & Sport Psychology Conference. Waterloo, Canada.

Stones, M.J., Kozma, A., 1981. Adult age trends in athletic performances. Exp. Aging Res. 7, 269–280.

Thibault, J.W., Kelley, H.H., 1959. The social psychology of groups. John Wiley, New York.

Voss, J., Green, T., Penner, B., 1983. Problem solving in social sciences. In: Bower, G. (Ed.), The psychology of learning and motivation: advances in research theory17, Academic Press, New York, pp. 165–213.

Ward, P., Hodges, N.J., Williams, A.M., et al., 2004. Deliberate practice and expert performance: defining the path to excellence. In: Williams, A.M., Hodges, N.J. (Eds.), Skill acquisition in sport: research, theory and practice. Routledge, London, pp. 231–258.

Ward, P., Hodges, N.J., Williams, A.M., et al., 2007. The road to excellence in soccer: a developmental look at deliberate practice. High Ability Studies 18, 119–153.

Ward, P., Williams, A.M., 2003. Perceptual and cognitive skill development in soccer: the multidimensional nature of expert performance. Journal of Sport and Exercise Psychology 23, 93–111.

Wattie, N., Baker, J., Cobley, S., et al., 2007. A historical examination of relative age effects in Canadian hockey players. International Journal of Sport Psychology 38, 178–186.

Weir, P.L., Kerr, T., Hodges, N.J., et al., 2002. Master swimmers: how are they different from younger elite swimmers? An examination of practice and performance patterns. J. Aging Phys. Act. 10, 41–63.

Weiss, M.R., Kimmel, L.A., Smith, A.L., 2001. Determinants of sport commitment among junior tennis players: enjoyment as a mediating variable. Pediatric Exercise Science 13, 131–144.

Young, B.W., Starkes, J.L., 2005. Career-span analyses of track performance: longitudinal data present a more optimistic view of age-related performance decline. Exp. Aging Res. 31, 69–90.

Psychological characteristics of developing excellence

4

Áine MacNamara

University of Central Lancashire, Lancashire, UK

CHAPTER CONTENTS

Introduction

Talent is often oversimplified as the ability to perform at an elite level but little consideration is generally given to the factors that contribute to the ability to achieve this superior performance. For instance, even if an athlete has the physical attributes to succeed in sport, their potential to develop is also dependent on other determinants of success such as commitment, motivation and the availability of developmental resources. In fact, talent is increasingly, and more correctly, viewed as a dynamic and multidimensional concept with a parallel awareness of an array of factors (e.g. physical, technical, psychological) that contribute to the realization of potential (Ceci et al 2003, see Ch. 2). This understanding is especially important, as the pathway to excellence is usually complex and the aspiring elite must optimize development opportunities (e.g. first-time appearances at a new level of competition), adapt to setbacks (e.g. injury) and effectively negotiate transitions (e.g. selection on to teams) encountered along the way if they are to realize their potential. Without the mental skills and psychological behaviours to successfully deal with these developments, talent may well end up as unfulfilled potential.

Accordingly, this chapter is concerned with ensuring that young performers have the best chance of becoming successful by equipping them with the psychological skills identified as prerequisites for learning and development. To guide this discussion, the chapter is divided into two sections. The first section outlines the philosophy underpinning the use of psychological characteristics of developing excellence (PCDEs) in the development of talent, while the second section examines the behaviours associated with PCDEs and how these can be developed, deployed and refined within talent identification and development (TID) processes.

DOI: 10.1016/B978-0-443-06734-1.00004-3

The philosophy underpinning the use of psychological characteristics of developing excellence

While some physical and physiological variables are clearly advantageous in sport (e.g. height in basketball), the ability to perform at the top level is also governed by the athlete's capacity to engage with the performance environment and successfully cope with a range of challenges. For those already at the top, there is an abundance of literature highlighting the central role that mental skills and psychological factors play in elite performance (e.g. Ericsson & Charness 1994, Durand-Bush & Salmela 2002). For instance, an array of psychological success factors (e.g. high level of commitment, long- and short-term goals, imagery, focus, pre- and in-competition planning) has been found to distinguish successful performers from their less successful counterparts (Orlick & Partington 1988). Supporting these findings, Gould and his colleagues observed that successful Olympic athletes were more committed and focused, and engaged in more extensive mental preparation than less successful performers (Gould et al 1999). Less successful athletes were not as effective in their planning and experienced problems related to focus and commitment. Further support for this contention comes from Durand-Bush & Salmela's work (2002) with Olympic and world champions. They identified self-confidence and motivation as salient personal characteristics of elite athletes. Not only were these athletes confident about their ability to succeed, they were also motivated to invest considerable time and effort into training in order to be the best they could be. In addition, these elite athletes employed imagery and self-talk both to prepare for competition and to remain focused during high-level performances. Thomas & Thomas (1999) found that successful athletes not only utilized a variety of psychological skills during competition but also used a wider range of mental skills during training (e.g. goal setting, imagery, self talk, emotional control, relaxation) than athletes of a lower standard. Reflecting this, Kane (1986, p. 191) stated that 'The ultimate factors accounting for achievement are likely to be the unique personal and behavioural dispositions which the individual brings to the actual performance'.

Undoubtedly, psychological skills play a critical role at elite levels but they also play a pivotal role in helping athletes get to the top of their sporting domain (Gould et al 2002, Orlick & Partington 1988, Williams & Krane 2001). Recognizing this, modern TID approaches are beginning to stress the initial possession, then subsequent development of such psychological behaviours (Abbott & Collins 2004). These psychological characteristics of developing excellence (PCDEs; Abbott & Collins 2004) can encompass both trait characteristics (the tendency to...) and state-deployed skills (the ability to...when...), and have been shown to play a crucial role in the development of potential and the realization of elite performance. In sum, PCDEs underpin effective development in a number of ways. For instance, focus, distraction control and quality practice facilitate the acquisition of skills, while goal setting and realistic performance evaluations help athletes get the most out of each coaching session. PCDEs also allow athletes to stay on the pathway to excellence by enabling them to invest the requisite time to practise and stay committed to the development process, especially when peers may be engaged in more enjoyable activities. These PCDEs are outlined in Box 4.1.

Critically, current research suggests that the same psychological skills that underpin successful development in sport (Box 4.1) also support development in many other performance domains, from music to business to dance (Ericsson 1996, Jones 2002, MacNamara et al 2006, Orlick & Partington 1988). Consequently, TID processes that promote PCDEs not only encourage and facilitate children to achieve their potential in their current performance domain

Box 4.1

Psychological characteristics of developing excellence

- Commitment
- Focus and distraction control
- Imagery
- Realistic performance evaluations
- Quality practice
- Goal setting
- Coping with pressure
- Planning and organizational skills
- Self awareness

See Orlick & Partington 1988

but also allow for the 'cross-fertilization' of talent into other domains at later stages of development (Moore et al 1998). As significant are the long-term health benefits of promoting and developing PCDEs in children. The PCDEs that underpin development in achievement domains also seem to be the same psychological characteristics that promote a physically active lifestyle (Brustad 1993, Sallis et al 2000). Thus, these psychological factors influence an individual's capacity to be physically active and underpin the competence to make appropriate health and exercise choices; a significant benefit given the growing physical inactivity levels of youth and the health risks associated with this inactivity (Boreham & Riddoch 2001). In short, from both performance and educational perspectives, there appears to be substantial benefit from the systematic development and facilitated deployment of these skills.

Defining behaviours associated with PCDEs in achievement domains

Incorporating PCDEs into TID processes encourages developing athletes to behave like champions. However, it is important to understand exactly what that behaviour entails and what athletes should be doing to demonstrate these 'champion behaviours'.

PCDEs must be defined as clear and observable behaviours. By doing so, the performer will be able to understand exactly what behaviour is expected of them, and coaches/teachers can effectively monitor and reinforce appropriate actions. Let us take one PCDE, 'commitment', to illustrate this point. If different coaches were asked to explain what being committed meant to them, they would be likely to arrive at a host of different answers. Examples of responses could vary, from 'an athlete who would never miss practice' to 'an athlete who engages in lots of independent training' to 'someone who never gives up'. Therefore, it is important to break down each PCDE into observable and objectively defined behaviours that can be easily assessed, measured and reinforced. By doing so, coaches, parents or even the performers themselves can monitor and reinforce desired behaviours. In sum, if we are intent on promoting certain behaviours in young athletes, all concerned must understand what behaviours are important for their particular activity and consistently model and/or reinforce them. Reflecting this focus, it is critical that the psychological behaviours are defined in a manner that is meaningful to both the individual performer and the context in which they perform.

Recognizing this, the application of PCDEs also appears to be, at least partly, domain-specific. Simply put, the behavioural component of the PCDE may look different across different performance domains, or perhaps even within performance domains, depending on the individual's specific challenges (e.g. event, playing position or musical instrument). Again, let us take commitment as an example. A young musician might be able to demonstrate their commitment by engaging in independent practice, and arriving for their music lessons prepared and ready to learn. On the other hand, a young rugby player might show his commitment by tackling hard in a match or taking part in extra training sessions. While both behaviours are characteristic of the same PCDE – commitment – the performers are behaving in different ways that, by and large, are dictated by the activity they are involved in. Even within performance domains there may be differences in how psychological behaviours are manifested. For instance, a front-row forward in rugby may use effective and controllable imagery to psych themselves up for the first scrum of the game by imaging the feeling of a big hit and the aggression associated with that action. On the other hand, effective and controllable imagery for the place kicker may involve them mentally rehearsing a successful kick at goal prior to the physical execution of the actual kick. The main consideration here is that each PCDE must be operationalized with the specific needs of the individual in mind.

Finally, the application of PCDEs must cater for the particular emphasis placed on the individual by, for example, the coach/instructor, the current focus of the development process or the target for that session. It is also important to recognize that young performers will interpret PCDEs differently from adult performers (Abbott & Collins, 2004). Thus, when attempting to define and operationalize PCDEs, it is important to recognize how the stage of development as well as the mental maturity of the individual performer will impact on their ability to apply the desired behaviour. For example, although the ability to set appropriate goals is important throughout development, it is applied differently depending on the age and maturation levels of the performer. In the early years, it may be appropriate for a young athlete to follow simple coach- or teacher-led goals. However, as the athlete gets older more complex and self-driven goal setting may be put in place. As such, each of the PCDEs identified in

Box 4.1 must be defined in relation to the specific needs of the performer, taking account of their level of growth and maturation (Abbott & Collins 2004) and recognizing that these needs will vary both across and within performance domains.

Negotiating the challenges of the pathway to excellence

The developmental pathway is unlikely to be smooth and the aspiring elite performer must negotiate an array of challenges and opportunities if they are to reach the top of their chosen domain. For example, research exploring the development of expertise has shown that athletes pass through various stages of development as they progress from novice to elite (sampling, specialization and investment; Côté 1999, Durand-Bush & Salmela 2002), and that the requirements of individuals will change as they progress through these stages (see Ch. 3). Given the changing requirements encountered along the pathway to excellence, it may well be that different behaviours are required at different stages, for different activities, or even idiosyncratically for different individuals. With this in mind, it is important to understand the challenges that performers face at different stages of development and equip them with the PCDEs that will optimize their ability to cope with difficult periods of development. In fact, the successful negotiation of the pathway to excellence is governed by the phase- and indeed incident-specific application of certain PCDEs.

Furthermore, the degree to which specific PCDEs must be applied and reinforced is complicated by differences between activity-related developmental pathways. For instance, early success in sprinting may be achieved with little effort or even deliberate practice if the athlete possesses natural ability and a superior physique to their peers. In contrast, the same early success is unlikely to be evident in team sports such as rugby or hockey if the athlete hasn't yet developed the necessary technical and tactical skills to engage successfully with that sport. As an even more extreme case, a young musician or dancer must engage in highly technical and demanding practice before they can even begin to perform. Given that different performance environments require different levels of deliberate practice at different stages of development, it may be that there are activity-related differences in the set of behaviours required. Illustrating this, MacNamara and colleagues (2006) found that young classical musicians employed a range of PCDEs (e.g. commitment, imagery, focus and distraction control) from very early stages of development in order to cope with the performance and training requirements of that domain. In fact, because of the substantial demands placed on young musicians so early in their careers, these performers already possessed, developed and then deployed a range of PCDEs comparable to the psychological characteristics employed by elite performers (Gould et al 2002). Conversely, the world-class sprinters interviewed for the same study, although very successful in their junior careers, did not display similar 'champion behaviours' until they had to make the transition into adult levels of competition. It was only then that these sprinters started to prioritize their sport and make considerable sacrifices for training and preparation.

Transitions: a special challenge?

Unfortunately, the challenges of each stage of development can seem slight when compared to the pressures of achieving crucial transitions between these stages (Tebbenham 1998). For instance, the transition to what Côté (1999)) termed the 'specialization years', with its associated need for deliberate practice and greater performance demands, is essential for further development. Tebbenham (1998) noted that successfully negotiating these transitions might be even more significant than coping with the challenges of the stages themselves. In fact, Abbott and colleagues (2005) suggest that the ability of developing athletes to cope with these unstable periods is the key to the successful transition from one stage to the next. In essence, they propose that developing athletes use PCDEs as transition mechanisms to guide them into subsequent stable and effective levels of performance. Again, similar findings are found in other achievement domains (e.g. music). MacNamara and colleagues (2006), among others (Burt & Mills 2006, Pitts 2002), identified two key transitions in the career of aspiring classical musicians: the entry to full-time music education and entry to the music profession. They found that developing musicians used a variety of psychological behaviours to cope with the challenges of these transitions. For instance, the musicians noted that tertiary music education demanded considerable autonomous learning and practice. In order to cope with these demands, the performers used goal setting to plan their practice schedule, as well as imagery to augment their physical practice.

Furthermore, while performers must de facto progress through these macro stages of development (Côté 1999), they will also encounter many micro-and meso-stages of developmental transition (e.g. injury, selection on to teams, technique change; Ollis et al 2005). While these micro-stages are generally of shorter duration, they are of no less importance and must be overcome effectively to maintain progress. Consequently, equipping performers with the necessary PCDEs and promoting their timely deployment is crucial if they are to remain on the pathway to excellence. Critically, given that many of these transitions (e.g. injury) are unexpected, TID programmes should systematically develop and promote key PCDEs throughout development so performers are able to cope with these challenges if and when they arise.

Reinforcing and encouraging targeted behaviours

Once key PCDEs have been identified, it is important to understand how they can be promoted and reinforced in training and competition. People strive to behave in ways that are likely to produce reinforcement, and therefore the effects of other people's action (e.g. the rewards and punishments they provide) have an important influence on how an individual behaves. Operant conditioning suggests that these consequences can modify the occurrence and form of desired behaviours, and suggests an interrelationship between antecedents, behaviour and consequences (ABC; Martin & Pear 2003). Simply, this ABC approach suggests that if antecedent stimuli are present, and/or consequences are controlled to systematically reinforce certain actions, then an individual will increasingly engage in certain behaviours. Attention to the antecedents, or setting conditions, makes the incidence of certain behaviour more likely. In a somewhat similar fashion, if behaviour results in a positive reinforcement it increases the likelihood of that behaviour occurring again in the future. For example, a requisite of effective development is the ability to engage in quality independent practice. If coaches wish to encourage their athlete to engage in this behaviour, they must offer a consistent and supportive environment (the antecedents) and consistently reinforce the athlete when they engage in independent practice (the consequences). Over time, this behaviour will become accepted and internalized by the athlete, especially when justification is also offered as part of a broader educational process. Eventually, the behaviours occur spontaneously and unconsciously, and the learner will experience a sense of discomfort if alternative behaviour is forced upon them. 'Good manners' are another example of this; most of us feel a wave of irritation if someone jumps a queue or fails to hold the door open. These behaviours, systematically encouraged by our parents and reinforced with approval, become ingrained and subsequently occur as a matter of course. Clever coaching can do the same, resulting in an athlete who 'automatically' demonstrates the elite behaviours described earlier to the benefit of their performance.

Reflecting this ABC approach, it is important to recognize how the systematic application of reinforcement can promote desired behaviours (and indeed eliminate undesirable ones) in talent development environments (Gould & Weinberg 2007). Behaviour modification (Donahue et al 1980) refers to attempts to structure the environment, or setting conditions, through the systematic use of reinforcement. Evidence in the literature has shown that these reinforcement techniques can effectively modify a range of behaviours. For example, Galvan & Ward (1998) employed behaviour modification techniques to reduce inappropriate on-court behaviours (e.g. verbal abuse, racquet abuse) in tennis players. A baseline measure of inappropriate behaviours was taken and publicly displayed in the locker room. Each tennis player was individually informed of their inappropriate behaviours and given strategies to reduce these behaviours. In addition, coaches positively reinforced the players for engaging in appropriate on-court behaviours. By the end of the competitive season there was a significant reduction in inappropriate behaviours, suggesting that behaviour modification can eliminate detrimental and promote desirable behaviours.

A number of guidelines can increase the effectiveness of these behaviour modification techniques. Firstly, as previously suggested, it is important to target and define the behaviours that need to be addressed. It is essential to limit this focus to only a couple of behaviours, otherwise both the athlete and coach can get overwhelmed by attempting to change too much too quickly. Furthermore if a limited number of behaviours are targeted, it becomes easier to reinforce these effectively and consistently. Secondly, coaches, teachers and significant others must provide feedback and reinforcement that clearly indicates the individual's progress towards achieving the desired behaviours. This feedback, provided within a supportive environment, not only increases motivation but, as explained previously with the ABC model, increases the likelihood of the desired behaviour occurring again in the future. Finally, athletes must have a clear understanding of what behaviour is required and coaches must clearly state the outcomes of performing, or not performing, these targeted behaviours. For example, a music teacher can positively reinforce a young musician's committed behaviour by offering praise and attributing quick progress to their preparation. Conversely, as a consequence of being unprepared for lessons, the teacher may withdraw the student from a recital or performance. In this manner, consequences are controlled to systematically reinforce desired actions. In sum, the coach/teacher must clarify what behaviours are expected and what the consequences are of engaging or not engaging in those behaviours. It is important to keep these principles in mind as we now consider how coaching practices encourage athletes to develop and deploy PCDEs.

Table 4.1 Exemplar commitment behaviours associated with judo

Behaviours being promoted	Coach system	Coach behaviour
Keeps going in training	Clear objectives, expectations are published in advance of each session	Adherence to plan (start and finish time, content)
Addresses weaknesses and shows progress	Fortnightly one-to-one goal setting and progress meetings	Encourage athlete involvement Process goals Provide specific goal-orientated behaviours

Adapted from Abbott et al 2007

Table 4.2 Exemplar commitment behaviours associated with curling

Behaviours being promoted	Coach system	Coach behaviour
Practise away from the team	Fortnightly team goal-setting session (individual and team goals)	Public and private recognition of goals and improvement
Supports others' efforts	'Buddy' system of support and feedback on individual goals	Knowledge of and active input to 'buddy systems' (who, goals, feedback style liked)

Adapted from Abbott et al 2007

Coaching practices that encourage the application of psychological behaviours

Recognizing the importance of both antecedents and consequences for modifying behaviour, it is imperative for coaches to consider how both their own actions, and the system within which they work, promote desired (and, unfortunately, dysfunctional) behaviours. This section will discuss how a combination of coach behaviours and coach systems can effectively promote the PCDEs underpinning effective development.

As already stated, different achievement domains require athletes to behave in different ways. Tables 4.1 and 4.2 illustrate how exemplar commitment behaviours can vary across two different sports – judo and curling. Coaches must carefully consider their interactions with the athlete if these specific behaviours are going to be promoted, strengthened and thus likely to reoccur. For example, a judo player (Table 4.1) can behave in a committed manner by addressing weaknesses and showing progress in training. The coach can reinforce these actions through 'coach behaviours' such as providing goal-orientated feedback based on the athlete's performance and their progression in relation to their goals. As such, the coach is systematically reinforcing the desired behaviour (the athlete addresses weaknesses and shows progress) by controlling consequences (e.g. providing goal-orientated feedback). It is also important to consider how the coach system can increase the likelihood of the desired behaviour occurring. This system may take the form of regular goal setting and progress meetings between the coach and athlete. Thus, the combination of these coach behaviours and coach systems should encourage the athlete to address weaknesses and show progress. If these practices are continually adhered to, the athlete will accept and internalize these behaviours to the point where they occur as a matter of course, to the benefit of the judo player's performance.

Of course, it is imperative that the relationship between setting conditions, athlete behaviour and coach behaviour is consistent over time and across situations. Lack of consistency leads to a confused athlete who feels a 'lack of control' over the environment and good habits are unlikely to result. For example, if a curling coach (Table 4.2) wants their athletes to engage in individual practice away from the team, then the coach's behaviour must positively reinforce this desired behaviour by, for instance, both public and private recognition of goals and improvements. However, if the coach does not reinforce individual goals, or fails to design coach systems to guide this behaviour (e.g. regular goal setting meetings) it is unlikely that the curler will carry out independent practice independently. Thus, coach behaviours and coach systems are only effective when they work in combination with each other and clearly outline to the athlete what behaviour is expected.

Additionally, it is important that all those involved in the coach system (e.g. coaches, managers, national governing bodies, parents) 'sing from the same hymn sheet' and systematically promote targeted behaviours. Athletes can easily get confused if they are receiving mixed messages from different agents within the development process and are unlikely to develop the targeted behaviours as a result. An important consideration is that coach action has two important components; how the coach behaves and the system they use. Just like athlete behaviours, these are observable and open to a similar ABC approach (Martin & Pear 2003), with the coach 'supervisor', mentor or meta-coach playing a central role in setting antecedents for, and reinforcing, effective (and, unfortunately, ineffective) coach behaviours. For example, if coaches are reinforced for being successful in competitive games at young ages they are likely to make short-term decisions that lead to this immediate success, regardless of the long-term development implications. This early success is unlikely to be a predictor of mature adult performance (surely the goal of effective TID processes), and young athletes may burn out because of over-training and inappropriate expectations. From a developmental perspective, coaches who work with this agenda also fail to promote the key transitional skills (e.g. PCDEs) needed to convert early 'promise' into world-class achievement. One only has to look at the number of 'world-class' juniors who have failed to make the transition to senior sport and have either dropped out of the sport completely or compete at lower levels than would be expected. For example, only 20% of teenage soccer players recruited to professional teams are still contracted to these teams beyond their teens (Simmons & Smith 2004). Likewise, only three players from the Irish under-19 team that won the under-19 Rugby World Cup in 1998 went on to represent Ireland at senior level. One approach to overcome the difficulties in converting underage promise to senior success is to incorporate PCDEs into TID processes and systematically promote these as part of development process. Furthermore, by advocating TID models that monitor and develop all the components that influence the fulfilment of potential we are shifting the emphasis away from an early identification of talent based on some predetermined 'X' factor towards a consideration of progress and behaviour during development. As a consequence, the efficiency of TID models is increased by neither excluding 'potential' through inappropriate early identification procedures nor ignoring crucial talent development variables that contribute towards the fulfilment of potential (see Ch. 1 for a thorough review of TID challenges).

The key message here is that PCDEs play a key role in helping athletes negotiate the pathway to excellence. In order to help aspiring elites behave like champions, it is important to understand how to encourage and promote these behaviours in full cognisance of the needs of individual performers. The next section overviews each PCDE (Box 4.1) and offers exemplar structures for promoting the psychological behaviours that underpin successful development.

Commitment

It is clear that no matter how physically talented an athlete might be, unless they have the commitment to stay with the development process, especially in times of adversity, they will never realize their potential. Firstly, it is important to understand how athletes behave in a committed manner. Some of the behaviours associated with commitment are presented in Box 4.2.

Of course, different achievement domains will prioritize different behaviours. Such variation would

Box 4.2

Commitment behaviours

- Arrives early to training
- Keeps going hard in practice
- Trains independently away from the rest of the team
- Shows a consistent effort and good preparation
- Works hard at their own level
- Understands and is responsible for both training and rest where appropriate
- Is resilient when faced with obstacles and setbacks during development

Adapted from Abbott et al 2007

not be surprising given that the challenges that must be overcome on the pathway to excellence are, to say the least, diverse (Baker et al 2003; see also Ch. 3). It is critical that coaches evaluate what is appropriate for their particular athletes at their individual level of participation and in their particular context. For instance, 5 hours of practice a week would be indicative of high levels of commitment for a 12-year-old rugby player but would not be for a swimmer of the same age or a senior rugby player. Thus, PCDEs must be defined and operationalized in relation to the particular emphasis placed on that individual by, for example, their specific performance domain, their current stage of development, or indeed the particular target for that session.

The example shown in Table 4.3 demonstrates how a coach has identified that a committed athlete *works hard at his or her own level*. We will now consider how to systematically promote and subsequently reinforce this behaviour. A coach could promote and reinforce this behaviour by giving the athlete individualized feedback based on their own performance. Since the coach is trying to encourage the athlete to work hard at their own level of performance, this feedback must be related to the specific individual and situation, based on previously agreed goals. Over time, this positive reinforcement leads to the targeted behaviours becoming ingrained in the athlete, who then begins to behave in this manner independently. Furthermore, in order to encourage the athlete 'to work hard at their own level' the coach has identified a coach system that takes the form of regular meetings to review progress and provide feedback. These antecedents encourage athletes to engage in the targeted behaviour by providing a supportive and consistent environment that facilitates their deployment. Reflecting the ABC model previously presented, it is important that coach behaviours and coach systems work in combination with each other if this approach is to be effective. For example, if the coach gives feedback to the athlete unrelated to previous goals, or in comparison to others, they would not be encouraging the athlete to 'work hard at their own level'. In fact, this coach behaviour would defeat the purpose of holding regular meetings to set goals and review progress, and might even encourage the athlete to evaluate performances relative to others. Thus, the relationship between coach systems and coach behaviours must be clear and consistent over time and reinforced in as many ways as possible (e.g. meetings, talks, training).

It is also important to consider how a coach/teacher can develop this PCDE in specific contexts. The second example, presented in Table 4.4, suggests that developing performers (especially at later stages of development) show their commitment by *engaging in independent practice*. For instance, young musicians or dancers must engage in a great deal of independent quality practice throughout their career. It is important to understand what combination of coach behaviours and coach systems can

Table 4.3 Examples of coach systems and behaviours for promoting the application of commitment behaviours within training in sport

Behaviours being promoted	Coach system	Coach behaviour
During training, the athlete works hard at their own level	1. Regular meetings are held to review progress 2. Regular meetings are held to set goals for training	1. The coach gives individual goal-orientated feedback 2. The coach gives feedback relative to individual goals

Adapted from Abbott et al 2007

Table 4.4 Examples of coach systems and behaviours for promoting the application of commitment behaviours within music or dance education

Behaviours being promoted	Coach system	Coach behaviour
The performer engages in independent training and practice	1. Guidelines are given about what and how much to practise 2. The content of subsequent lessons is discussed in a de-brief session at the end of every lesson	1. The teacher questions the performer about their practice 2. The teacher reinforces the role of independent practice 3. The teacher praises performers who spend time engaging in independent practice

Adapted from Abbott et al 2007

encourage the learner to practise independently. For example, the teacher could hold a post-lesson debrief that clearly outlines the content of subsequent sessions. Accordingly, this debrief guides the musician's independent practice by outlining key areas that could be attended to. This system, and the guidance the teacher provides, also ensures that the independent practice is of the requisite quality and content to make it worthwhile. The teacher can also promote this behaviour by providing positive reinforcement to pupils who engage in independent practice. The teacher should also engage with, and question, the young musician during these meetings about the extra practice that they are doing. By attributing quick progress to this extra practice, the teacher can also help the musician recognize the benefits of their efforts. Thus antecedents (e.g. post-lesson debriefs) are put in place that promote desired behaviours (e.g. engaging in independent practice), and consequences (e.g. positive reinforcement) are controlled to increase the likelihood of that behaviour occurring again in the future.

The need for realism is an important caveat when encouraging commitment. Without care, many will fall into the negative spiral of 'more is better', with increasing guilt (a negative example of internalized behaviour and self reinforcement!) the consequence unless an increasingly punishing schedule is kept to. In time, this usually results in some kind of burnout, and another high-potential individual is lost to the activity. Thus, the sensible coach or teacher will ensure that the learner's targets and self-reinforcement are realistic to the particular setting. Important concepts of quality training, effective recuperation and peaking will be lost unless the learner is convinced (and accepts and internalizes) that often 'less is more'.

It is important to remember all these principles as we consider the other PCDEs, since similar concerns and methods exist whatever the targeted behaviour. Coaches must be aware that the behavioural component of the PCDEs may look different depending on the specific challenges faced by individual performers (e.g. performance domain, playing position) at different stages of development. With this in mind, the following sections provide examples of how a coach could develop and reinforce PCDEs across these different contexts.

Focus and distraction control

Like elites, developing performers must compete and train in environments full of distractions such as noise, spectators and other competitors. If athletes are going to perform optimally, and train to their maximum, they must be able to block out such distractions and focus on the cues relevant to their performance (Fig. 4.1). In fact, the ability to focus and not be distracted by erroneous cues not only facilitates good performances but also allows athletes to learn effectively and develop at a faster rate. There are a number of clear and observable behaviours that are indicative of focus and distraction control across performance domains (Box 4.3). Again, it is likely that performers in different domains will behave in different manners, but this list gives generic examples of the types of behaviour that enable athletes to stay focused and avoid distraction.

Table 4.5 presents an example of a rugby coach who has identified the importance of his athletes being able *to block out distractions in competitive settings*. While this ability is important at all levels of participation, it is particularly salient when athletes

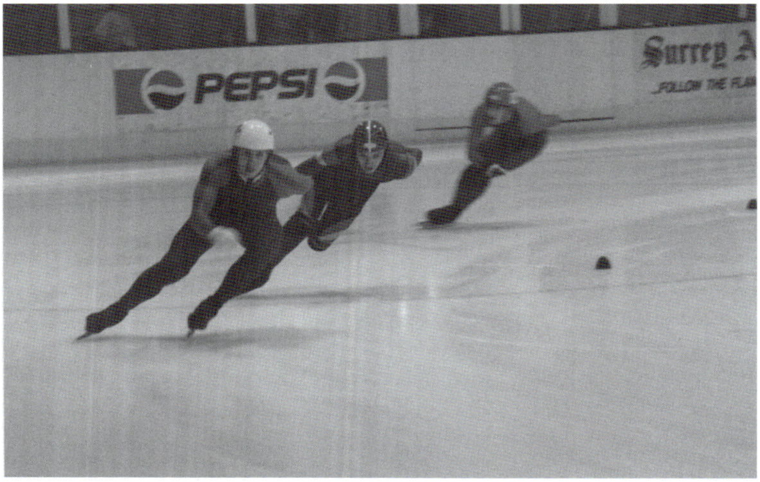

Fig. 4.1 • Focus is a key characteristic of elite and developing performers. Olympic and World medallist Nicky Gooch competes at the Short Track National Championships (Thanks to Alan Luke for the photo)

Box 4.3

Focus and distraction control behaviours

- Remains focused under distraction
- Stays calm under pressure
- Blocks out distractions
- Displays a consistent pre-performance routine
- Maintains a focus on appropriate cues during competition
- Shows an understanding of when distraction is likely

Adapted from Abbott et al 2007

begin to compete in novel environments where such distractions are plentiful (e.g. first-time appearances at major competitions). A combination of coach behaviours and coach systems can again help the coach promote and encourage this behaviour. For example, if the coach emphasizes and reinforces the importance of focusing on task-relevant cues, the athlete is likely to engage in that behaviour in their eagerness to get positive reinforcement. In addition, the coach has identified a system that also facilitates the development and promotion of this behaviour. In order to prepare athletes to block out the inevitable distractions of competition (e.g. noise, crowd presence, opponents), similar conditions can be simulated in high-resource practice settings. Using this simulation training, the athlete can learn to block out distractions in a very supportive setting in preparation for the competitive environment. Another coach system that could promote the ability to focus on relevant cues would be the development of mental skills such as thought stopping or cue words through team meetings or workshops. Essentially, this encompasses equipping athletes with a toolkit of mental skills on which they can draw to block out the distractions that interfere with their performance. Again, what is important here is that

Table 4.5 Examples of coach systems and behaviours for promoting the application of focus and distraction control for first time appearances at major competitions

Behaviours being promoted	Coach system	Coach behaviour
The performer is able to block out distractions during first-time appearances at major competitions	1. Simulate match situations in high resource settings 2. Allow athletes to develop a range of mental skills to help them cope with distractions in their environment 3. Allow athletes time to practise these skills	1. Discuss potential distractions with the athlete and plan for these effectively 2. Emphasize that to perform optimally you need to focus on relevant cues

Adapted from Abbott et al 2007

all three aspects – athlete behaviour, coach behaviour and the coach system – work coherently together with the coach reinforcing appropriate behaviour and providing appropriate setting conditions that support the development and deployment of these behaviours. It is important to remember that there may be many coach systems and coach behaviours that contribute to the effective promotion of a set of behaviours. This recognizes the activity-specific and context-specific (e.g. developmental level) factors discussed in the first section. As such, PCDEs must be defined, and coach behaviours and systems developed with the needs of each performer in mind.

Box 4.4

Effective and controllable imagery behaviours

- Using imagery to rehearse new skills
- Using imagery to cope with difficult situations and negative emotions
- Using imagery to mentally prepare for games or competitive situations
- Using imagery to simulate novel environments

Adapted from Abbott et al 2007

Effective and controllable imagery

The effects of imagery are broad ranging, including improvements in performance (Taylor & Shaw 2002), enhanced confidence (Callow et al 2001) and decreases in anxiety (Long & van Stavel 1995). In fact, imagery has been called the Swiss army knife of mental skills – it can help almost anything! Imagery allows an athlete to practise skills perfectly even when they are injured and unable to physically train. Not only is imagery effective for learning skills (Martin et al 1999) but it also allows athletes to deal with difficult situations and mentally prepare for big occasions that they might not necessarily have previous experience of (Munroe et al 2000). Some of the athlete behaviours that demonstrate effective and controllable imagery are outlined in Box 4.4.

The example in Table 4.6 shows how a coach has identified that a high jumper can use imagery effectively *to deal with difficult situations* such as failing to clear the opening height in a competition. There is no doubt that we often experience negative emotions and thoughts when we perform, especially when under pressure or in competitive settings. Cognitive thoughts such as 'I am not good enough', as well as somatic manifestations of these emotions (e.g. butterflies in the stomach), are common in the run up to and during performance. Such emotions and thoughts are inevitable, and in fact attempts to suppress them are futile (Wegner 1994). However, even though the athlete can't suppress these negative thoughts, they can effectively deal with them by employing a range of psychological skills. For example, combination of coach behaviours and systems can encourage the high jumper in this situation to use imagery to cope with failing to clear the opening height in competition (Table 4.6). There are a number of coach behaviours that can promote this skill. For instance, the coach can reinforce this application of imagery by helping the athlete include realistic coping in their imagery scripts. The athlete should include feelings of nervousness and anxiety in their image to reflect the emotions that are associated with performing in high-pressure situations. However, the athlete should image himself or herself overcoming these feelings and clearing the height at the next attempt. The coach system could take the form of regular meetings between athlete and coach to discuss the feelings and emotions associated with performance and how to effectively cope with these. Again, it is essential to remember that coach systems

Table 4.6 Examples of coach systems and behaviours for promoting the application of imagery for coping with difficult situations

Behaviours being promoted	Coach system	Coach behaviour
The high jumper uses imagery to cope with failing to clear the opening height at the first attempt	1. Regular meetings are held between the coach and athlete to discuss feelings and emotions associated with performance	1. The coach encourages the athlete to use realistic coping in their imagery 2. The coach reinforces the role of imagery in preparation for performance

Adapted from Abbott et al 2007

and coach behaviours are effective as a combination. For instance, the coach system in this example (regular meetings) is rendered meaningless unless the coach gives the athlete the opportunity to use imagery in preparation for competition. As such, it is critical that the relationship between coach behaviours and coach systems is consistent and coherent to ensure that each PCDE is effectively promoted.

Realistic performance evaluations

The ability to realistically evaluate one's own performance has been identified as a discriminating factor between elites and subelites (Gould et al 1992, Orlick & Partington 1988). This ability is also seen as a crucial determinant of development. In fact, McCall and colleagues (1992) found that underachievers in an academic context (defined as children who performed below their expected capabilities) had unrealistic standards and subsequently low persistence in that domain. These ideas reflect our earlier concerns about keeping expectations realistic to the performer's current level. Performers must understand that world-class performances or personal-best performances cannot be produced in every event. The ability to make realistic evaluations of performance is crucial if athletes are to remain motivated in pursuit of excellence despite poor performances or slumps in progress. In fact, the ability to realistically evaluate performance and attribute success and failure appropriately also enables athletes to identify areas that need improvement, and in turn to design strategies to improve those areas. Observable behaviours associated with the ability to make realistic performance evaluations are outlined in Box 4.5.

The coach in the example in Table 4.7 has identified that athletes who can make realistic performance evaluations are able to *evaluate performance regardless of win/loss outcome*. Sometimes an athlete might perform to the best of their capabilities but not win a competition because of the quality of the opposition. In a similar fashion, an athlete might perform quite poorly in relation to their potential but still win because the opposition was relatively weak. The coach can encourage the athlete to 'evaluate performance regardless of win/loss outcome' by emphasizing the process of the performance. Coaches (or indeed significant others) can encourage athletes to evaluate performances regardless of outcome by providing 'process-oriented feedback' that is informative and related to each individual's goals. For example, a 100 m sprinter should not only be encouraged to consider their outcome performance (e.g. where they were placed in the race) but should also receive feedback and reinforcement about particular elements of the race (e.g. start, each phase of the run). These consequences (e.g. feedback and reinforcement) in turn promote the athlete's own ability to make realistic evaluations of performance. Once again, these coach behaviours are only effective when implemented in combination with appropriate coach systems. For example, an appropriate coach system could take the form of post-match reviews that act as a forum for discussing and understanding performance outcomes.

Box 4.5

Realistic performance evaluation behaviours

- The ability to analyse what you do well and what you don't
- The ability to realistically evaluate performance regardless of win/loss outcome
- The ability to attribute success and failure appropriately

Adapted from Abbott et al 2007

Table 4.7 Examples of coach systems and behaviours for promoting the application of realistic performance evaluations for reviewing performances in sport

Behaviours being promoted	Coach system	Coach behaviour
An athlete who can realistically evaluate performance regardless of win or loss	1. Process-oriented feedback 2. Feedback related to roles/goals 3. Encourage athlete involvement	1. Individual meetings every 3 weeks 2. Post-match review

Adapted from Abbott et al 2007

Quality practice

Ericsson's environmental approach to talent development suggests that it takes 10 years of deliberate practice to progress from novice to elite in any domain (Ericsson et al 1993). Deliberate practice is difficult, effortful and not inherently enjoyable but is necessary to develop the requisite skills that effectively aid an athlete's development. However, it is the quality and not necessarily the quantity of practice that is most salient (Côté et al 2007). In fact, if an individual is to maximize their experiences in training and practice they must be aware of the purpose of the activities that they are involved in. Some observable behaviours associated with quality practice are outlined in Box 4.6.

Let us consider an example from the performing arts. The ballet teacher in Table 4.8 has identified that her pupils engage in quality practice when they *have the ability to maximize understanding in training*. In order for her to encourage her pupils to maximize this understanding, she has developed a system where the concepts and aims of the class are discussed prior to the start of the class. By putting appropriate systems in place, pupils are primed to understand the purpose of the lesson and the activities they will be involved in. In combination with this system, the teacher can reinforce quality practice by giving clear explanations to each pupil as well as checking this understanding through questioning and probing techniques. This teacher behaviour, in combination with an effective coach system, should promote the desired behaviour by giving each pupil a clear and coherent message about what behaviour is expected and consistently reinforcing appropriate practice.

Goal setting

The ability to set realistic yet challenging goals and adhere to such targets is one of the key psychological behaviours associated with elite performers. In fact, goal setting is also an essential part of becoming elite as goals give direction and purpose to both training and competition. Effective goal setting strategies improve the athlete's ability to focus their attention and motivation on key elements of their performance. Setting appropriate goals also motivates athletes to train hard, especially when training may be arduous and difficult. Some of the behaviours associated with effective goal setting are outlined in Box 4.7.

Box 4.6

Quality practice behaviours

- The ability to maximize understanding in training
- Showing an understanding of why they are doing what they are doing
- The ability to evaluate their (and their team-mates') progress in training
- Asking questions to clarify understanding and purpose of training

Adapted from Abbott et al 2007

Box 4.7

Goal setting behaviours

- The ability to independently set goals
- The ability to set goals for both training and competition
- The ability to independently reinforce achievements
- The ability to set short, medium and long-term goals
- The ability to set appropriate goals

Adapted from Abbott et al 2007

Table 4.8 Examples of coach systems and behaviours for promoting the application of quality practice in ballet or music

Behaviours being promoted	Coach system	Coach behaviour
The ballet dancer maximizes their understanding in training	1. Pre-lesson meetings are organized to clarify the aims and concepts of the lesson	1. The teacher clearly explains the different activities and their purpose 2. The teacher checks understanding through questioning and probing techniques

Adapted from Abbott et al 2007

Table 4.9 Examples of coach systems and behaviours for promoting the application of goal setting in training and competition

Behaviours being promoted	Coach system	Coach behaviour
The athlete sets goals for training and competition	1. Regular meetings are held to monitor progress and re-evaluate goals 2. A written log of goals and progress is recorded	1. The coach provides feedback relative to individual goals 2. The coach monitors progress relative to individual goals

Adapted from Abbott et al 2007

How can a coach encourage their athletes to engage in effective goal setting? For example, the coach might identify that it is important for his athletes *to set goals for both training and competition* (Table 4.9). In order to promote this behaviour the coach should be aware of each individual's goals and provide feedback to individuals relative to their progress towards these targets. The coach should also monitor, and positively reinforce, the progress that is made in relation to individual goals. Furthermore, appropriate coach systems should be put in place to increase the likelihood of the athlete engaging in the desired behaviour; for instance, regular meetings should be held between the coach and athlete to review progress and set goals for both training and competition. Athletes can also be encouraged to maintain a written log that records their goals and their progress. This system also encourages the athlete to be part of the goal setting process by giving them the responsibility for maintaining records and evaluating progress. The ability to take responsibility for one's own learning and development is a hallmark of successful development (Bloom 1985, Zimmerman 2000). Critically, these coach systems and coach behaviours are designed to work together to promote the ability of the athlete to set goals.

It should now be becoming obvious that similar methods (e.g. coach systems and coach behaviours) can be employed to encourage a range of different behaviours. In fact, it may well be that a single coach system or coach behaviour can promote a number of desired athlete behaviours. The example highlighted in the previous paragraph is a perfect illustration. Not only did these coach behaviours and coach systems encourage the athlete to set goals for training and competition, they also encouraged the athlete to take responsibility for their own learning. This approach is actually beneficial as it simplifies the coaching process and increases the probability of each system and behaviour being effectively implemented.

Coping with pressure

There is no doubt that the ability to perform at elite levels is, at least partly, dependent on an athlete's ability to cope with the psychological pressures of competing. In fact, the ability to cope effectively with the performance environment and to regulate arousal has been long associated with high levels of performance (Landers & Boutcher 1998). It seems likely that performers at all stages of development need similar coping skills to deal effectively with the challenges that they face. For instance, athletes must cope with the pressures of increased deliberate practice during the specialization years (Côté 1999), as well as the pressures of competing in highly competitive environments if they are to successfully develop in sport. Some coping behaviours that performers use to manage the pressures of their involvement in achievement domains are outlined in Box 4.8.

The ability to *show confident behaviour and thrive under pressure* is characteristic of those athletes who can cope with the pressure of competition (Table 4.10). This is very important as, by its very nature, sport takes place in a cauldron of pressure and expectation. To succeed, athletes must not only cope with this pressure but must also learn to use it

Box 4.8

Coping with pressure behaviours

- Respond positively to training and competitive situations
- Show confidence to thrive under pressure
- Confident to do their best in competitive situations
- React appropriately to mistakes and criticism

Adapted from Abbott et al 2007

Table 4.10 Examples of coach systems and behaviours for promoting the application of coping behaviours in competitive events

Behaviour being promoted	Coach system	Coach behaviour
The athlete shows confident behaviour and thrives under pressure in competitive settings	1. Use video to reinforce confident behaviours 2. Simulate high-pressure situations in training	1. The coach helps the athlete identify confident behaviours and reinforces these 2. The coach reinforces confident behaviours

Adapted from Abbott et al 2007

to their advantage and thrive on it (Jones & Swain 1995). The example below is particularly relevant to athletes who are competing at competitive and evaluative events (e.g. championship finals) where they may have only one chance to perform to the best of their ability. Coach behaviours and coach systems must prepare the athlete for these highly pressurized situations by promoting the behaviours needed to thrive. An example of how this can be encouraged through coach behaviour is as follows. The coach can identify confident behaviours and body language and encourage the athlete to display these behaviours, especially perhaps when opponents might not be displaying the same behaviours (Prapavessis et al 2004). The coach system could encompass the simulation of high-pressure situations to encourage athletes to display appropriate confident behaviours in these settings in preparation for competition. In this manner, both coach systems and coach behaviour are working in cooperation to ensure that this essential transitional and developmental skill is promoted.

Planning and organization

As athletes develop in sport a variety of factors (e.g. training, competition, rest, work and study commitments) compete for their time and attention, and thus these athletes must learn to balance commitments from both within and outwith their sporting domain. If athletes are to maintain a steady progress, they must plan and organize their lifestyle in line with their training and competition demands. Furthermore, as athletes get older the responsibility for their progress and development moves from significant others such as parents and coaches to themselves (Bloom 1985, Côté 1999). This is especially important in performance domains (e.g. music, endurance events) where a performer must engage in large amounts of deliberate practice outside the supervision of coaches or teachers. Recognizing this, athletes must develop the skills (e.g. self-regulating their own practice schedules) that will enable them to independently progress along the pathway to excellence when the nature of support changes. In fact, not only do planning and organizational skills help athletes maintain development and progress, but they are also the same skills that ensure that they can perform to the best of their ability on important occasions. Box 4.9 outlines some of the behaviours associated with effective planning and organization.

The example shown in Table 4.11 suggests that coaches may want young athletes to demonstrate effective planning and organizational behaviours by *arriving in plenty of time for training and matches*. The coach can promote this behaviour by setting a good example and always arriving for training early and prepared. Modelling – the process where a person learns behaviour by observing others – is a very effective means of changing behaviour (Bandura 1986). Orlick and McCaffrey (1991) highlighted the importance of a well-chosen model for modifying behaviour and suggest that teachers, parents, peers and even other performers can all promote targeted behaviours through their own actions. An effective

Box 4.9

Effective planning and organizational skills behaviours

- Arrive early for training and matches
- Be appropriately prepared for training and matches
- The ability to balance lifestyle commitments
- The ability to prioritize different activities
- The ability to plan effectively for competition

Adapted from Abbott et al 2007

Table 4.11 Examples of coach systems and behaviours for promoting the application of planning and organization behaviours at early stages of development

Behaviours being promoted	Coach system	Coach behaviour
The athlete arrives in time for training and matches	1. Publish a timetable of training session 2. Adhere to the arranged schedule 3. Always start and finish sessions on time	1. Positively reinforce athletes who arrive in time for sessions 2. The coach should set a good example and always be on time

Adapted from Abbott et al 2007

coach system in this case could be the publication of a timetable of events in order that the athlete understands what is expected of them and what is occurring throughout the course of a session. Recognizing the importance of modelling (Bandura 1986), the coach must also adhere to this schedule and start and finish sessions at the established times. If the coach offers this supportive environment and consistently reinforces and models the desired behaviours, the athlete will in turn accept and internalize these to the point where they will automatically engage in these planning and organizational behaviours.

Conclusion

Rose (1995) proposed that people have dispositions and not destinies. Therefore, individuals must make the most of their dispositional tendencies if they are to realize their potential. As such, we propose that promoting the behaviours associated with PCDEs in young athletes is an effective way to develop talent as it recognizes the individual needs of the athlete as well as the demands inherent in their domain (Abbott et al 2007). In fact, this approach supports the research that recognizes that psychological characteristics play a critical role throughout development and not just when the performer achieves elite status.

Furthermore, while the importance of psychological skills at elite levels of performance is already well established in the literature (e.g. Callow et al 2001, Durand-Bush & Salmela 2002, Gould et al 2002), the approach outlined in this chapter recognizes the importance of formally reinforcing these psychobehavioural skills throughout development. In this manner, aspiring elites are equipped with all the skills necessary to make the most of the opportunities that present themselves during development (Abbott & Collins 2004, Bailey & Morley 2006). What is also important to remember is that all the PCDEs are interrelated and as such have both a direct and an indirect effect on each other. Consequently, it is critical that TID processes incorporate all PCDEs in an integrated and balanced manner to increase the likelihood of young performers staying on the pathway to excellence and realizing their potential.

References

Abbott, A., Collins, D., 2004. Eliminating the dichotomy between theory and practice in talent identification and development: considering the role of psychology. J. Sports Sci. 22, 395–408.

Abbott, A., Button, C., Pepping, G.J., et al., 2005. Unnatural selection: talent identification and development in sport. Nonlinear Dynamics Psychol. Life Sci. 9, 61–88.

Abbott, A., Collins, D., Sowerby, K., et al., 2007. Developing the potential of young people in sport. SportScotland, Edinburgh.

Bailey, R., Morley, D., 2006. Towards a model of talent development in physical education. Sport, Education and Society 11, 211–230.

Baker, J., Cote, J., Abernethy, B., 2003. Sport-specific practice and the development of expert decision-making in team ball sports. Journal of Applied Sport Psychology 15, 12–25.

Bandura, A., 1986. Social foundations of thought and action: a social cognitive theory. Prentice-Hall, Englewood Cliffs, NJ.

Bloom, B.S., 1985. Developing talent in young people. Ballantine Books, New York.

Boreham, C., Riddoch, C., 2001. The physical activity, fitness and health of children. J. Sports Sci. 19, 915–929.

Brustad, R.J., 1993. Who will go out and play? Parental and psychological influences on children's attraction to physical activity. Pediatric Exercise Science 5, 210–223.

Burt, R., Mills, J., 2006. Taking the plunge: the hopes and fears of students as they begin music college. British Journal of Music Education 23, 51–73.

Callow, N., Hardy, L., Hall, C., 2001. The effects of a motivational general-mastery imagery intervention on the sport confidence of high-level badminton players. Res. Q. Exerc. Sport 72, 389–400.

Ceci, S.J., Barnett, S.M., Kanaya, T., 2003. Developing childhood proclivities into adult competencies: the overlooked multiplier effect. In: Sternberg, R.J., Grigorenko, E.L. (Eds.), The psychology of abilities, competencies, and expertise. Cambridge University Press, Cambridge, England, pp. 126–158.

Côté, J., 1999. The influence of the family in the development of talent in sports. Sport Psychologist 13, 395–417.

Côté, J., Baker, J., Abernethy, B., 2007. Play and practice in the development of sport expertise. In: Tenenbaum, G., Eklund, R.C. (Eds.), Handbook of sport psychology. third ed Wiley, New Jersey, pp. 184–202.

Donahue, J.A., Gillis, J.H., King, K., 1980. Behavior modification in sport and physical education. Journal of Sports Psychology 2, 311–328.

Durand-Bush, N., Salmela, J.H., 2002. The development and maintenance of expert athletic performance: perceptions of world and Olympic champions. Journal of Applied Sport Psychology 14, 154–171.

Ericsson, K.A., 1996. The road to expert performance: empirical evidence from the arts and sciences sports and games. Lawrence Erlbaum, Mahwah, NJ.

Ericsson, K.A., Charness, N., 1994. Expert performance: its structure and acquisition. Am. Psychol. 49, 725–747.

Ericsson, K.A., Krampe, R.T., Tesch-Romer, C., 1993. The role of deliberate practice in the acquisition of expert performance. Psychol. Rev. 100, 363–406.

Galvan, Z.J., Ward, P., 1998. Effects of public posting on inappropriate on-court behaviors by collegiate tennis players. Sport Psychologist 12, 419–426.

Gould, D., Weinberg, R., 2007. Foundations of sport and exercise psychology, fourth ed Human Kinetics, Champaign, IL.

Gould, D., Eklund, R.C., Jackson, S., 1992. 1988 US Olympic wrestling excellence: mental preparation, pre-competitive cognition, and affect. Sport Psychologist 6, 358–382.

Gould, D., Damarjian, N., Medbery, R., 1999. An examination of mental skills training in junior tennis coaches. Sport Psychologist 13, 127–143.

Gould, D., Dieffenbach, K., Moffett, A., 2002. Psychological characteristics and their development in Olympic champions. Journal of Applied Sport Psychology 14, 172–204.

Jones, G., 2002. Performance excellence: a personal perspective on the link between sport and business. Journal of Applied Sport Psychology 14, 268–281.

Jones, G., Swain, A.B.J., 1995. Predispositions to experience debilitative and facilitative anxiety in elite and non-elite performers. Sport Psychologist 99, 201–211.

Kane, J.E., 1986. Giftedness in sport. In: Gleeson, G. (Ed.), The growing child in competitive sport. Hodder & Stoughton, London.

Landers, D.M., Boutcher, S.H., 1998. Arousal-performance relationships. In: Williams, J.M. (Ed.), Applied sport psychology: personal growth to peak performance. Mayfield Publishing, Mountain View, CA.

Long, B.C., Van-Stavel, R., 1995. Effects of exercise training on anxiety: a meta-analysis. Journal of Applied Sport Psychology 7, 167–189.

McCall, R.B., Beach, S.R., Lau, S., 2000. The nature and correlates of underachievement among elementary schoolchildren in Hong Kong. Child Dev. 71, 785–801.

MacNamara, Á., Holmes, P., Collins, D., 2006. The pathway to excellence: the role of psychological characteristics in negotiating the challenges of musical development. British Journal of Music Education 23, 285–302.

Martin, G., Pear, J., 2003. Behavior modification: what it is and how to do it, seventh ed Prentice Hall, Englewood Cliffs, NJ.

Martin, K., Moritz, S., Hall, C., 1999. Imagery use in sport: a literature review and applied model. Sport Psychologist 13, 245–268.

Moore, P., Collins, D.J., Burwitz, L., et al., 1998. The development of talent study (DOTS), English Sports Council, London.

Munroe, K., Giacobbi, P., Hall, C., et al., 2000. The 4 W'S of imagery use: where, when, why and what. Sport Psychologist 14, 119–137.

Ollis, S., MacPherson, A., Collins, D., 2005. Expertise and talent development in rugby refereeing: an ethnographic enquiry. J. Sports Sci. 24, 309–322.

Orlick, T., McCaffrey, N., 1991. Mental training with children for sport and life. Sport Psychologist 5, 322–334.

Orlick, T., Partington, J., 1988. Mental links to excellence. Sport Psychologist 2, 105–130.

Pitts, S.E., 2002. Changing tunes: musical experience and self-perception amongst school and university music students. Musicae Scientiae 6, 73–92.

Prapavessis, N., Grove, R., Eklund, R., 2004. Self-presentational issues in competition and sport. Journal of Applied Sport Psychology 16, 19–40.

Rose, R., 1995. Genes and human behaviour. Annu. Rev. Psychol. 46, 625–654.

Sallis, J.F., Prochaska, J.J., Taylor, W.C., 2000. A review of correlates of physical activity of children and adolescents. Med. Sci. Sports Exerc. 32, 963–975.

Simmons, C., Smith, S., 2004. Thinking inside the box. Inside Knowledge 7, 8–10.

Taylor, J.A., Shaw, D.F., 2002. The effects of outcome imagery on golf-putting performance. J. Sports Sci. 20, 607–613.

Tebbenham, D., 1998. The nature of talent development and the importance of athletic transition in UK Sport. MSc thesis, Manchester Metropolitan University, Alsager, Manchester.

Thomas, K.T., Thomas, J.R., 1999. What squirrels in the trees predict about expert athletes. International Journal of Sport Psychology 30, 221–234.

Wegner, D., 1994. Ironic processes of mental control. Psychol. Rev. 101, 34–52.

Williams, J.M., Krane, V., 2001. Psychological characteristics of peak performance. In: Williams, J.M. (Ed.), Applied sport psychology: personal growth to peak performance. fourth ed Mayfield Publishing, Mountain View, CA, pp. 162–178.

Zimmerman, B.J., 2000. Attaining self-regulation: a social cognitive perspective. In: Boekaerts, M., Pintrich, P.R., Zeidner, M. (Eds.), Handbook of self-regulation. Academic Press, San Diego, CA, pp. 13–39.

Talent development environments: key considerations for effective practice

5

Russell Martindale* Patrick Mortimer†

*School of Life, Sport and Social Science, Edinburgh Napier University, Edinburgh, UK;
†Aubrey Performance (formerly Chelsea Football Club Academy, Heswall, Cheshire, UK)

CHAPTER CONTENTS

Introduction

The ultimate achievement for any coach or organization interested in high level performance is to nurture people effectively, enabling them to realize their full potential and succeed at world-class level. In this type of excellence orientated environment, the identification and development of talent are both an integral and intertwined part of a successful process (Abbott et al 2002, Bloom 1985, Martindale et al 2005). This is reflected in the amount of resource that is often directed at talent identification and development (TID) programmes. Some organizations plough significant financial resources into buying in ready-made stars to ensure success; however, this type of practice is unlikely to develop truly sustainable success over the long term or benefit international teams where home grown talent is a necessity (Douglas & Martindale 2008). It is no surprise that many of the most successful organizations have worked this out and, accordingly, openly value and prioritize resource in this area. The aim of this chapter is to outline some of the key issues in talent development and suggest a focus for the requirements of effective talent development environments (TDEs). The next section will outline some key facts regarding talent and highlight some potential pitfalls. The sections

DOI: 10.1016/B978-0-443-06734-1.00005-5

following on from this will focus on two key issues: first, the characteristics of effective practice for young children with regards to building the foundations for future progression and second, the requirements of effective TDEs at a level where athletes are considered to have potential and are actively pursuing long-term excellence (Bloom 1985).

Operationalizing a long-term focus – potential pitfalls

Almost every single sporting organization will have a documented vision and mission statement relating to the aim of becoming and/or remaining successful on the elite world-class stage, where identifying and developing young talent to that senior level is high on the agenda. For example, the UK's high-performance sports agency, UK Sport has a stated mission of 'working in partnership to lead sport in the UK to world-class success'. The programmes that they fund through sports governing bodies are implemented through three levels called world-class podium, world-class development, and world-class talent, to help support and structure this process. Research shows that this type of long-term vision is essential for success at a senior level (Bailey & Morley 2006, Bloom 1985, Ericsson et al 1993, Howe et al 1998). However, the subtleties of understanding the nature and requirements of development within a long-term agenda are often overlooked, and the external pressures of what typically constitutes perceived effectiveness, particularly at developmental stages (e.g. winning at age-group level) can take over.

Age-group success is not well correlated with world-class success

Eventual world-class success does not require someone to have been a 'successful' age grouper within the same domain (Abbott et al 2005, Bloom 1985, Martindale et al 2007, Moore et al 1998). Unfortunately, this perception is not often recognized within sports and many people, coaches, parents and youngsters alike, perceive there to be a strong link between the two. However, there is significant evidence to highlight this as a myth. For example, Bloom (1985) carried out a retrospective study on 120 elite 'performers' within a variety of domains, which included sport, whose elite status was defined as top 25 in the world. He found that fewer than 10% of those adults showed a level of performance at the age of 11 and 12 good enough to signal to their parents and coaches that they had the potential to reach the heights of achievement that they eventually did. Bloom concluded that:

> being good in one phase of the learning may not have a high relation to being good at a later phase, even though both phases are in the same talent field... without the purposeful step by step talent development process, it is unlikely that even the individuals we studied (world top 25) would have reached the high levels of talent development reported.
>
> (Bloom 1985, p. 532–534)

Furthermore, it is worth considering that, if 90% of eventual world top 25 performers do not necessarily shine supreme at young ages, what chance is there of identifying a more broad range of future sport professionals, and distinguishing them from other enthusiastic young sportspeople by watching their early performances? Indeed, the peak age of many top sportsmen and women is not always particularly early (although there are variations between sports). For example, Helsen et al (1998) found that international hockey players, on average, do not peak until their late twenties, highlighting that there is not necessarily any rush to produce. This becomes far more pertinent when you consider that early specialization and emphasis on 'age-group winning' is also often associated with early dropout and wasted talent, ideas that are explored through this section (Baker et al 2003, Gould et al 1982, Valeriote & Hansen 1986). Of course, although there are problems with an overemphasis on winning and being the best at developmental stages, it is important not to ignore good performers at young ages, and certainly not 'good performances'. For example, 'precociousness in a talent field is not to be dismissed, it can only be realistically viewed as an early stage in talent development. There are many years of increasingly difficult stages of talent development before mature and complex talent will be fully attained' (Bloom 1985, p. 538). Indeed, Bloom (1985) also highlights the benefits of being recognized as having potential and the role of perceived competence and self-belief in the pursuit of excellence. However, this doesn't necessarily have to come from winning or high-level age-group representation; it often comes most powerfully from coaches and an understanding of the requirements of long-term development.

To make such a shift in our philosophy of youth sport, it is necessary to reward good development

Box 5.1

Two examples of how coach practice is often focused toward winning not development

How to get a prestigious coaching job – gain recognition for high achievement

United States Olympic Committee (2002) – 'Top Coaches of the Year' are publicly recognized for quality coaching through demonstration of winning percentages, without any reference to the coach's ability to help individual athletes progress through the system to senior level, as measured for example by the eventual progression and success of the athletes coached. Unfortunately in our view this provides reinforcement and clear direction to aspiring coaches that winning percentages are required to demonstrate good-quality coaching.

When you get a prestigious job – what is your remit?

In 1989, having led 2–0 at half time, Scotland lost the final of the U16 FIFA World Cup to Saudi Arabia 5–4 on penalties, after being clawed back to 2–2. With such a great result, the future was looking bright for Scottish and Saudi football. Unfortunately, almost none of these 15- and 16-year-olds progressed to an international senior level, with the exception of Paul Dickov. Indeed, the World Cup winners, Saudi Arabia, have never been a top footballing nation at senior level. However, Craig Brown, Scotland's U16 manager at the time, went on to manage Scotland's senior team between 1993 and 2001. While this tournament provided an opportunity for these young players to showcase their skill, there appeared to be no explicit developmental agenda behind player selection or the tournament itself, casting some doubt on the rationale behind such a tournament at U16 level from a player development perspective.

coaching where it occurs. Unfortunately, as the two examples in Box 5.1 highlight, rewards and the agenda of age-group coaching often focus around winning.

Physical maturity can enhance perceptions of 'talent'

In a system that makes it a necessity for young developing athletes (and coaches) to win and be one of the best in order to gain opportunities, it is inevitable that many youngsters with future potential will be missed and left behind, leaving any future developments to chance. In this regard, evidence suggests that it could be almost impossible to 'catch up' if deselected (Csikszentmihalyi & Robinson 1986, Krampe & Ericsson 1996, Starkes et al 1996), resulting in early deselection meaning permanent deselection, with a subsequent reduction in talent base and quality at the top. This is of particular concern when you consider that many of those who 'perform' better or win at early ages do so because of physical maturity biases, as opposed to 'talent' or 'potential' (Côté et al 2006; see Ch. 2). When there is an overriding focus on winning, this is particularly problematic (Baxter-Jones & Helms 1996, Helsen et al 2000, Richardson & Stratton 1999). Interestingly, research has shown that 'eventual' world champions are often brought up in environments where close support networks make efforts to de-emphasize the importance of 'success' through developmental periods (Gould et al 2002).

Without such an informed and supportive environment, initial selection may result in a subsequent self-fulfilling process of selection, training, quality interaction and improvement for those initially involved and perceived to have more potential because of their ability to outperform others (Dweck 1986, Solomon et al 1996). However, this extra help is likely to be the reason for improved standards, not the athletes' level of potential. For example, Ward & Williams (2003) concluded that the higher skill levels of 'elite' soccer players as young as 8 are likely to be as a result of the 200 additional hours of expert coaching they have received as opposed to any genetic superiority. Crucially, Abbott et al (2002) highlight that this initial bias can impact through the rest of the system. For example, in sports such as rugby or football, a higher proportion of 'older' players (i.e. relative to others in their year group) are represented at senior level, while many of those born late in the selection year tend to drop out early (Helsen et al 1998). With the reverse being true in gymnastic-type sports, these situations provide classic examples of creating a 'self-narrowed' talent base (Barnsley et al 1992). Given that age-group selection systems are potentially important sources of perceived competence and opportunity, careful consideration must be given to the aims and rationale of their design (Bloom 1985, Deci & Ryan 1985, Solomon et al 1996).

Performance versus potential – the effects of training

Without question you can have young players who are excellent performers but who will never become experts as adults. It is clear that our TID systems need to recognize the differences between the attributes that characterize someone with 'potential' to be an expert adult and those that characterize someone who can 'perform' at age group better than others at a particular moment in time (Abbott & Collins 2002, Bailey & Morley 2006, Bartmus et al 1987, Bloom 1985, Regnier & Salmela 1987). This is important, as much of the expertise and skills associated with high level performance can be improved and developed dramatically through training (Bailey & Morley 2006, Csikszentmihalyi et al 1993, Ericsson & Lehmann 1996, Helsen et al 1998, Howe et al 1998, Starkes 2000). In fact, because weaknesses can be improved easily over time and 'natural ability' can hide itself until explicitly developed, early training can mask those with true potential, especially if large discrepancies exist between children's opportunities at early ages (Ericsson 2003). When you consider the huge changes and progression that are required over a career, high ability can often not be apparent until later, again masking our ability to identify talent at development stages and reinforcing the need to keep larger pools of performers on the books (Bartmus et al 1987, Bloom 1985, Howe et al 1998, Simonton 1999). Furthermore, certain skills and knowledge important for future performance often do not become fully developed or do not impact explicitly on performance until later, even though they may be trained and show improvement at early ages (Abernethy & Russell 1987, Tenenbaum et al 2000). For example, important memory skills can take up to 10 years to develop fully, but rarely show themselves before 16 (French & McPherson 1999). Therefore, training that benefits long-term preparation may often not be as 'observably successful' in terms of short-term performance gains as intense sport- or competition-specific practice. This is important because it is sometimes difficult for coaches to accept the benefits of or the need to repeat and persevere with 'apparently unsuccessful' or mistake-ridden drill and practice (Côté & Hay 2002). However, if the focus is to develop individuals into successful senior performers then clear agendas must be put in place.

Is early 'success' poor preparation for 'the big time'?

While the evidence suggests that early selection based only on performance leads to many with potential not getting the necessary opportunities, ironically, those who are selected early may also be at a disadvantage if strong guidance is not available. While they will improve initially, early achievers may be prone to premature dropout through unnecessary competitive pressure (Gould et al 1982, Moore et al 1998, Ommundsen et al 2006). Furthermore, those selected may miss crucial (long-term) development experiences (Côté & Hay 2002) by focusing too much on performance as opposed to learning (Ericsson 2003). Thus, while many will 'win' at junior levels by relying on physical attributes or tactics that work at that age, they may fail to develop the skills required for later progression and end up ill-prepared to make the important next step (Moore et al 1998, Stafford 2005). Indeed, those who do perceive 'outperforming' others and 'age-group selection' as the only indication of future potential may have a torrid roller-coaster ride, trying to impress different coaches at different times and battling to maintain 'performance' levels year in, year out. This is particularly problematic when you consider that different determinants of performance have been shown to characterize success through the age groups (Regnier & Salmela 1987). For example, hard running and physical maturity may be key to rugby success at the age of 12 but, as athletes get older and size and strength factors balance out, mental factors such as decision-making and anticipation become more important for success (Abbott & Easson 2002). Of course, certain skills are important for performance at many different ages (8–18 years old), such as certain perceptual and cognitive skills (Ward & Williams 2003), so it would be appropriate to identify what is key for future progression and success and systematically develop these skills in as many youngsters as possible from early stages.

It is clear that, in order to provide youngsters with the best chance of realizing their potential in the longer term, TDEs must focus on providing foundations for future success. In other words, they must develop habits and skills that will be effective for that individual at later stages (even if this might not optimize chances of 'success' now), and enhance a youngster's ability to learn, develop and progress successfully into the future. Ideally, such programmes will reconceptualize 'winning', and pay careful attention to the rationale behind identification and selection policies to help stress appropriate development, while avoiding common mistakes such as overemphasis on factors associated solely with age-specific success. However, we need to be careful. Factors such as competition, winning, the will to win, and learning how to win and perform under pressure are not bad things to promote and they can be easily achieved by targeting certain competitions as having a 'developmental' or 'win' agenda. In fact, they are a necessity and a certain event, challenging competition, performance success or disappointment can be the very thing that triggers an athlete into a higher developmental level (Bloom 1985, Martindale et al 2005, 2007). However, there is a right time and place for these things and a developmental focus needs to remain at the forefront of policy and coach decision making in our TID programmes. Recognition of the differences between 'performance' and 'potential' and the provision of clear expectations, roles and understanding within each level of development will provide a coherent base that will promote long-term development throughout a sporting system. This is particularly pertinent when we consider the research that looks at what types of experiences provide a good foundation for future success at early stages. This is where we look next.

Setting up the foundations for world-class success

Given that we know it takes many years of dedicated and deliberate practice to become good (Ericsson et al 1993), it might seem sensible to adopt early identification and specialization policies because the earlier a youngster starts, the sooner large quantities of practice can be achieved (Côté & Hay 2002, De Knop et al 1996, Ericsson et al 1993, Ewing & Seedfeldt 1996, Hedstrom & Gould 2004, Hill & Hansen 1988, Soberlak and Côté 2003). However, 'what a learner does, how he or she does it, and how things change as the years pass, are certainly more important variables than the absolute amount of time spent doing an activity' (Sosniak 1985, p. 409). The simplistic view of 'start specializing early' fails to account for many developmental, motivational and psychosocial factors that lead to the necessary capability and dedication required for the achievement of excellence while avoiding the potentially negative consequences of dropout and burnout (Baker & Côté 2006, Wiersma 2000). This quantity versus quality argument is explored in more depth in Chapter 3. The key to addressing this apparent dilemma is to consider what is done when; in other words, what is the optimum makeup of the magic 10 000 hours of practice at each level of development.

In line with the arguments above, while early specialization and large amounts of hours of sport-specific practice may produce 'better' athletes initially, this has not shown to be the most beneficial foundation for future success. Evidence suggests an advantage for those who specialized later (approximately 13–17 years old) and engaged in more diverse deliberate play before committing to one sport (Côté 1999) as well as participating in a greater variety of different sporting activities (Baker et al 2003). Such individuals develop more successfully into elite-level sport, shown by a reduction in the amount of deliberate practice subsequently required to become 'elite' (i.e. national team selection) and remain at this 'elite' level (Baker et al 2005, Côté et al 2003, Côté & Hay 2002, Durand-Bush & Salmela, 2002). For example, Baker et al (2003) found that (eventual) experts participated in more extracurricular activities than non-experts between the ages of 5 and 12, before starting to specialize. To illustrate this, Bloom (1985) highlighted that only four out of 18 elite tennis players specialized solely in tennis in the early years. However, even after the age of 17, when these experts had entered more advanced development years, they still remained involved in up to three activities for relaxation and cross-training purposes. Furthermore, Côté (1999) highlighted the nature of these different stages. Between the ages of approximately 6 and 12 there was a high frequency and variety of deliberate play (e.g. inherent fun, process-oriented, not monitored) and low levels of deliberate practice (e.g. purposeful improvements, outcome-oriented, monitored), with the opposite being true through later investment stages (16+), when specialization in one or two main activities appeared to be paramount. Indeed, it is during the later years that a huge amount of deliberate and structured activity appears to characterize and lead to world-class success, but not before. Of course, special consideration needs to be given to those sports that compete at an early age, such as gymnastics, but even here many of the same considerations hold true.

Varied participation and less pressured experiences enable youngsters to experiment with movement skills and develop many fundamental and transferable skills that are functionally significant for later development (Baker et al 2003, Beamer et al 1999, Côté et al 2006, Ericsson 1998). These skills underpin the development and adaptability of more complex sport-specific skills (technical, tactical, physical and mental) required in more specialized contexts (Beamer et al 1999, Jess & Collins 2003, Soberlak & Côté 2003). However, these basics are not innate qualities and do need to be developed systematically (Gallahue 1982), perhaps ideally in addition to varied sports participation as well as through it. Although it is much more useful for these skills to be taught from an early age (Moore et al 1998), if the skills are not already in place then their development needs to be prioritized and incorporated as part of sport-specific training. Indeed, flowing coordination and quality fundamental movement are often cited as one aspect that characterizes someone with potential (Abbott et al 2002).

Importantly, these early experiences also appear to generate the level of intrinsic motivation and emotional attachment required to commit later down the line to the large amount of deliberate practice that is needed to become an expert and deal with the 'performance lifestyle' without losing motivation (Abernethy et al 2002, Deci & Ryan 1985, Gould et al 1996). This makes sense because early specialization and highly structured training is likely to take away feelings of choice and ownership while prioritizing external motives, which are key factors associated with a reduction in intrinsic motivation (Deci & Ryan 1985, Lepper & Greene 1975), which is known to lead to dropout and burnout. Bloom (1985, p. 141) illustrated this:

> the early years were the crucial years, even more crucial than those that follow, because it is in this period that our subjects became interested and caught up in the sport of swimming. In time that interest became self motivating. Had there been no excitement during the early years, and no sense that the young swimmer was very successful, there would never have been a middle or later period.

Not only are important physical and mental attributes developed in these times, as many as 40% of eventual elite British athletes switched sports comparatively late (approximately 14) from a completely different sport in which they were successful age-groupers (Moore et al 1998). This highlights another reason why transferable and adaptable skills are essential components of early development experiences, regardless of the possible 'side effect' of less winning at early ages (Moore et al 1998). Given this 'likelihood' of direction change, extending choice by keeping 'more doors open' for young people as they develop provides a significant advantage to all TID programmes (Côté et al 2003). Willing sporting governing bodies could benefit each other enormously by keeping transfer links alive and promoting generic skills within their specific sports for both talent development and physical activity promotion.

In short, there are good reasons for developing youngsters towards the 'long haul' in physical activity. Not only are the young participants equipped for lifelong physical activity participation (Jess & Collins, 2003), they are also able to select which activity offers them the best pathway to fulfilment of their personal aims. One example of well structured collaboration is the British Judo and Leicester Tigers Rugby initiative, which is built within Leicester's 2005 programme, the 'Tiger Pathway'. The development of judo skills is funded by the rugby club and is unashamedly targeted at eventual high performance in that sport. The joint approach helps young players to keep their options open while developing skills necessary for success in these, and other, sports. How many less formal but equally effective relationships could be built between, say, athletics and team games clubs? Play soccer in the winter, sprint in the summer and learn the key skills of competition from both? These ideas are explored in more depth in Chapter 6.

Implementing an effective talent development environment

Building a holistic skills package

The need for the development of fundamental skills and an intrinsic love for sport and activity has been highlighted. The skills and physical attributes that are important at later stages of development are a sport-specific concern. Studying the senior game and predicting any likely trends is very important in understanding what may be most usefully developed now. However, while it may be easy to identify effective habits, it may take time to teach them well, especially where poor habits, such as overdribbling in hockey or raw power in rugby, are often rewarded with success at younger ages. This tactic will quickly lose its effectiveness at higher levels, however, when skills such as decision making under pressure and fast, accurate passing become key. Unfortunately, many young players may give up at this stage, demotivated by the sudden drop in performance standard previously achieved by a well conditioned but now limiting skill (Blanksby 1980) and the realization that other previously less successful peers are coming through. For example, skills developed at a younger age by a physically underdeveloped rugby player to help them survive and avoid contact situations may become the very skills that make them shine when they catch up physically.

Research highlights that it would be sensible to incorporate a wide variety of cognitive, perceptual and motor skills into training programmes (Janelle & Hillman 2003), as many such 'teachable' factors are important in distinguishing the best performers at later stages (Helsen & Starkes 1999, Simonton 1999, Ward & Williams 2003, Williams & Reilly 2000: for a fuller review of this objective evidence of factors associated with the development of performance, see Starkes & Ericsson 2003, Williams & Hodges 2004). For example, only an integration of anthropometric, physical, psychological and sport-specific factors could distinguish senior footballers at elite and subelite levels (Reilly et al 2000), and many researchers have highlighted the diversity of necessary skills (Abbott & Collins 2004, Bailey & Morley 2006, Durand-Bush & Salmela 2002, Elferink-Gemser et al 2004; Falk et al 2004, Helsen & Starkes 1999, Williams 2000, Williams & Reilly 2000) and domain-specific knowledge bases (Ericsson & Charness 1994), which need to be used as development and assessment tools for elite players. As the hockey example highlighted, it is often only the integration of skills such as decision making and passing that is effective at later stages. Therefore it is extremely important that habits and skills are formed in an interdisciplinary and integrated manner in order for them to be truly useful and transferable (Durand-Bush & Salmela 2002). Indeed, the importance of interdisciplinary work is well documented within sport science research (Burwitz et al 1994). In conclusion, it is crucial that sports have a very clear and holistic developmental 'curriculum'. This would cover technical, tactical, physical and mental development as a minimum, whereby it would be possible to identify and develop progression for any youngster of any ability within a programme (see the Five Rings model presented in Ch. 6).

The psychology of long-term development requires special attention

There are three clear strands to the importance of psychology in long-term development (Jones et al 2002): first, its role in learning and development, second, its role in performance and third, its usefulness in lifestyle management. Getting all the skills and attributes that are required for world-class success into place takes a lot of time, effort and learning. Consequently, it is easy to miss the fact that underpinning this effective development are important psychological skills and attributes such as dedication, commitment, motivation, desire, 'coachability', confidence, planning, reviewing and goal setting (Bloom 1985, Ericsson et al 1993, Gould et al 2002, Talbot-Honeck & Orlick 1998). It would appear obvious that motivation is absolutely paramount to successful development at all levels and that, if we are to improve, develop and succeed over time we must have the desire to do so. Indeed, Ericsson (2003, p. 63) argues that 'most amateurs do not improve their performance only because they have reached (in their minds) an acceptable level'. Furthermore, learning autonomy is an important aspect of successful development and is underpinned by strategies such as taking active control over the thinking processes involved in learning (i e. adopting a metacognitive overview), planning, monitoring, self-evaluation and a mixture of attitudes, such as curiosity, persistence and confidence (Freeman 1995). Therefore, it is all these mental skills that would help characterize someone with potential and provide a focus for development.

In terms of performance, it is clear to see that mental skills are very important for success at the highest level. We all know examples of top-level sports men and women who were on the verge of winning a major tournament only to crumble when most under pressure or when approaching the winning line. This 'mental toughness' and the associated psychological skills have long been identified as factors that discriminate between the very good and the very best. In other words, they are often the dividing line between winning and losing on the day, particularly when skills and physical attributes are very similar (Gould et al 1993, Kane 1986, McCaffrey & Orlick 1989, Orlick et al 1978, Orlick & Partington 1988, Silva et al 1985, Talbot-Honeck & Orlick 1998). These mental skills are also the same factors that discriminate between those who are able to win at the highest level and then remain at the top of their game and those who either win sporadically or end up as 'one-off wonders' (Durand-Bush & Salmela 2002, Kreiner-Phillips & Orlick 1993).

The third important role of psychology within talent development, but perhaps the least acknowledged, is being able to deal with the lifestyle issues that surround sport development (Bloom 1985). Young athletes must be able to handle their performance lifestyle and manage this with other aspects of their lives, such as family, work, social life (partying, growing up, relationships) and education. It is clear that athletes must be motivated to put in the many hours of deliberate practice required to excel in any field (Bloom 1985, Ericsson et al 1993) and to be able to keep progressing through a host of ups and downs, for example, selection, deselection, injuries, dealing with relationship stress (Bloom 1985, Sinclair & Orlick 1993). Not only can it be a 'very hard and boring slog', many sacrifices need to be made, particularly at a young age when friends are going out enjoying themselves (Bloom 1985, Rowley 1992). Therefore, psychological skills and mental resilience and their development are a necessary and specific requirement.

Although a definitive set of mental skills has yet to be agreed, research from a number of fields of study consistently identifies similar factors (Bloom 1985, Gould et al 2002, Orlick & Partington 1988, MacNamara et al 2006, 2008). Notably, however, while there are important psychological states such as confidence, mental toughness, anxiety and motivation, it is the application of mental skills by an athlete that underpins them. Key skills such as effective and controllable imagery, focus and distraction control, realistic performance evaluation and attributions, commitment and role clarity, planning and organization, perceptions of pressure, goal setting and self-reinforcement, and quality practice are teachable and need to be used in an integrated way within the sporting context. A special mention needs to be given to the importance of athlete responsibility. While this construct is somewhat related to psychological skills and motivation, it is something that consistently crops up separately as crucial to elite development (Bloom 1985, Bull et al 2005, Van Rossum 2001). Once an athlete starts to take development in sport seriously, as characterized by Bloom's (1985) developmental and mastery stages of progression, a commitment needs to be given to an increase in dedication, sacrifice, discipline and quality (i.e. the constituent parts of athlete responsibility). As more and more is demanded and required to keep progressing, an ever-increasing level of independence, responsibility and autonomy over learning, performing and decision making becomes crucial to further success and development (Bee & Mitchell 1984, Hellstedt 1995, Knowles et al 1998, Schmidt & Wrisberg 2000). Indeed, a very high level of intrinsic motivation must be in place and nurtured for this to be an effective process. For example, this can be promoted by providing opportunities for ownership over development and clear feedback on mastery, ability and process requirements for further success (Deci & Ryan 1985). Furthermore, athletes need to be challenged and supported appropriately to help them develop the required self-responsibility, awareness and understanding (Csikszentmihalyi et al 1993, Martindale et al 2007; Box 5.2). Importantly, coaches must find a way of promoting the development of these facets of someone's personality and ability within the coaching environment (Martindale et al 2007).

However, it would appear that this may be a difficult trade off for coaches. For example, telling athletes the answer will produce fast, but perhaps more superficial results, while challenging them and allowing them the time and experience to work it out for themselves takes more time, and much more effort, but is more likely to produce the long-term change required (Martindale et al 2007). It is easy to 'take the athletes to the water' too many times, and of course coaches are very willing to give advice, especially if they have been through the whole thing themselves and have coached other athletes. But it is dangerous to point out too many of the pitfalls because it blocks the development of responsibility and that pre-empts the learning curve that is crucial for development (Martindale et al 2007).

Box 5.2

Extracts from expert developmental coaches

I'd challenge the athlete to find their way of doing what I know they've got to do. So, that's part of the challenging culture. It's not good either, giving too much away, but more and more, the athlete will take responsibility of his or her own actions the better. That's the best way to learn.

Individual sport coach

I (the coach) would ask them to explain why they made the decision and then i say to them 'well what were your other options?' And they've gotta understand why, because if they understand why they will then try and change their habit. So that is an important stage.

Team sport coach

Ownership and self-awareness, I just feel players who are directed all the time lack self-awareness and don't develop, you know, become robotic, whereas if he can get an understanding the way to design drills, the why you do them, to have a clear model of the skills that they're trying to work on... if you can get that sort understanding then you've got players who can self-coach and they can go out any time and do the drills.

Team sport coach

Source: Martindale et al 2007, p. 196

Balancing act

The ability to organize and balance one's lifestyle is also extremely important within a TD environment. Research indicates that stress is a cumulative process and comes from a variety of physical and psychological factors (Silva 1990). Therefore, being able to balance one's life stresses and 'recover' physically and emotionally is extremely important in staying injury-free, motivated, and developing and performing well (Durand-Bush & Salmela 2002, Salmela & Moraes 2003). For example, this can be achieved through the use of good nutrition and hydration strategies, cool down, stretching, time out, social support, periodization programmes or additional activities. Finally, one must consider the stress that retirement can cause to athletes, especially if it is enforced through injury (Sinclair & Orlick 1993). Such a transition has been shown to be smoother and more beneficial to future development and wellbeing if there are clear goals and skills that can be utilized after an athletic career is over. Notably, a high proportion of parents of high-achieving athletes highlighted the importance of continuing education through development stages (Côté & Hay 2002). Therefore, as part of a healthy training and performance career, education, vocational training, life experience and/or personal development must play an ongoing role in preparation and as part of recovery and relaxation away from the sport. However, as aspirations, beliefs and hope are crucial for future success (Holt & Dunn 2004, Solomon et al 1996), it is important that the need for a balanced development for a future 'in case of failure' should not take away the dreams of success for young people. Of course other activities, be it sporting, educational or vocational, can be very effective for emotional recovery, avoidance of burnout and general wellbeing, although, given the cumulative nature of stress, this needs to be weighed up on an individual basis. For example, for the first year in which a young rugby player turns professional, the additional physical and mental pressure of training and competing may demand a full focus until the required physical and emotional adaptations are acquired.

Setting the right ethos: 'demanding' change and development through the environment

While it is apparent that there needs to be a strong sense of holistic development within any TDE, psychological development underpins the development and effective use of a range of skills and attributes. The way in which these key psychological attributes are developed needs careful consideration (Durand-Bush & Salmela 2002, Gould et al 2002, Martindale et al 2007) and it is clear that a 'professional ethos' is required to promote the attainment of excellence (Bloom 1985). This 'professional ethos' incorporates certain attitudes and relationships as well as a clear and deliberate application in training and competition. However, while there is a lot of research highlighting ways in which psychological attributes can be taught successfully (Greenspan & Feltz 1989, Hanton & Jones 1999), crucially, they are often developed because the environment (e.g. peer pressure, support or coaching style) 'demands' it, but are not necessarily explicitly taught. For example, confidence can grow through successful experiences but without a specific psychological intervention (Bloom 1985, Csikszentmihalyi et al 1993, Salmela 1996). Indeed, Durand-Bush & Salmela (2002) highlight that often even sport psychology practitioners incorrectly assume that mental skill training has to be structured and involve specialized performance enhancement techniques to be effective. Having said this, explicit planning for setting up the TDE to encourage psychology growth and development is crucial (Bull et al 2005, Côté et al 2006, Gould et al 2002, Martindale et al 2007). The impact of such an 'informal environment' is seen clearly in the strong family environments that produce balanced young men and women as opposed to the youngsters who are unable to adhere to elite sport development social guidelines.

This is supported by research by Gould et al showing that the nature of psychological development in Olympic champions incorporated environmental influences such as the sports process itself as well as individual development, in addition to more explicit education through sport personnel. Research within cricket has highlighted foreign competition and training as an important source of psychological development, as well as experiences of setbacks and being 'asked to earn success' (Bull et al 2005). Furthermore, Durand-Bush & Salmela (2002) highlighted that an ethos derived through coaches, team mates, support staff and other athletes is an important influence and driver of the required psychological development. In fact, a strong sense of cultural value for the talent domain and the behaviours associated with excellence development helps promote clarity and reinforce commitment to what is required (Csikszentmihalyi et al 1993, Gould et al 2002). Interestingly, research in group processes

(Carron et al 2005) also highlights the powerful impact that the environment can have on shaping individual behaviour within a group, particularly when it is done through informal and formal group norms. Informal, emerging roles and norms within a group and the communication of clear expectations (again either formally or informally) can exert a very powerful pressure on attitudes, beliefs and behaviour. This can provide a number of essential benefits for long-term development, including a strong work ethic, clear long-term goals, adoption of mentally tough attitudes and behaviours, routine, life management and recovery behaviour. However, the environmental influence on psychological development is clearly something that is best developed through design rather than left to chance. Therefore, individuals needs need to be assessed and then the environment changed accordingly to encourage change, perhaps alongside more explicit help, communication and support (Box 5.3).

Research also highlights the importance of effective role models and the powerful effects observing and interacting with role models can have on people's behaviour and attitudes (Bandura & McDonald 1963), particularly if the role model is considered to be high-status. Of course, different people at different times can be more influential than others, or at least equally influential. As mentioned earlier, this includes a wide range of individuals from coaches, teachers, schools, peers and successful adults (Côté 1999, Csikszentmihalyi et al 1993, Durand-Bush & Salmela 2002, Gould et al 2002). Hence, the utilization of a variety of positive role models at different levels is required to maximize the impact on the development and choices of any youngster (Abernethy et al 2002, Brustad 1993), particularly, if the athletes mix across levels and ages (Côté et al 2006, Pancoe 1999, Veenman 1995). Therefore, it is important to try to utilize as many role models as possible throughout the development environment and, given the key role of parents in this process of support and building support, special efforts to disseminate knowledge and understanding, as well as including them in the development process, are key. Of course, the ethos that an athlete is involved with is not always beneficial for long-term development. For example, university education would seem to be beneficial for an athlete, by providing holistic development, preparation for retirement and 'balance' while they are within a professional or full-time sport set up. However, in certain circumstances this may be counterproductive. Universities are renowned for being associated with late nights, drinking and poor eating habits. If the pressures on athletes take them away from the lifestyle that will enable long-term sport development then serious consideration needs to be given to the nature of how it must be set up and managed.

Box 5.3

Examples of using individual assessment, environmental challenge, support and review to facilitate player development

Transition to the top

Developing the 'mental resilience' required at a high standard of rugby may involve giving young players (who are deemed physically and emotionally ready) the opportunity to compete in that environment, under pressure. Indeed, setting up the training environment and mixing younger players with higher-level (elite) players can help this transition, as can providing competitive second team fixtures. In other words, purposeful, carefully chosen challenges can help develop the required confidence and mental skills required to make the step up. Fundamental to this process is subsequent review and support, which will help to ensure positive development and progression from such experiences. This sort of challenge can help close the 'gap' that exists between levels by showing athletes first-hand, clear comparison expectations and requirements and also that they are not as far away as they perhaps at first perceived.

Mental toughness: one-on-one physicality

Young rugby players may have talent but lack the 'confidence or toughness' in one-on-one physical battles, for example at the breakdown. By incorporating 'another sport' (in this specific case judo) into the training regime of players, personal demands are made of them that develop a range of benefits back to the rugby field, not least strength, flexibility and agility as well as the required 'confidence' in one-to-one physical battles and mental toughness to battle on.

The key message is to identify specific areas for psychological development and provide experience and support that will develop it 'in action'. This sort of challenging and supportive culture was highlighted by Csikszentmihalyi et al (1993) as crucial for talent development.

Source: P. Mortimer, personal communication, 2007

Understanding the nature of the development years

It is convenient to use staged approaches to talent development, not least because on a practical level we have progressive, often age-related stages in our school system and sport pathways. In addition, research has produced a complementary stage model (Bloom 1985, Côté & Hay 2002, Durand-Bush & Salmela 2002, Ericsson et al 1993, Van Rossum 2001). However, while it is important to have a good understanding and definition of what is required at different developmental 'stages', research highlights that the developmental process is individual, dynamic and unpredictable (Abbott et al 2005, Bloom 1985, Simonton 1999), where individuals often pursue completely different 'paths' to world-class status. Simonton's (1999) work on the development of talent highlighted it as multidimensional, whereby a number of factors can contribute to the existence of talent within any domain. In addition, these various factors are likely to develop at different rates in different individuals. Therefore, 'infancy, adolescence and even adulthood will see the latent components undergoing various transformations' (Simonton 1999, p. 442). In other words, talent will develop and change over time in both adaptive and maladaptive ways, depending on the interaction between certain innate and environmental factors. It is a combination of clearcut and more subtle personal transitions that triggers or hinders development (Abbott et al 2005, MacNamara et al 2006, Simonton 1999). For example, on a more generalized level, we know that physical development and performance factors are unstable because of factors such as maturation and training effects (Abbott & Collins 2002, Ward & Williams 2003). Consequently, we can provide support and opportunities to those who, while being identified as 'having potential', may not be performing to a high level because of maturation (e.g. growth spurts) or training effects (e.g. heavy strength and conditioning requirements). On a more subtle level, a competition experience, for example competing against but being beaten by a high-class athlete, may provide a realization of what is required at the top level. This, in turn, may mentally narrow the gap between themselves and the best, triggering an athlete to the next level of development because of increased confidence and belief in their ability. This example can obviously be 'transferred' down to any level of ability.

The implications of such a dynamic process are that systems must be 'flexible' enough to allow for such variations and provide for the realization that there may not be set stages that any one individual may progress through. Indeed, improvements and peaks may follow troughs and fallow periods and vice versa (Moore et al 1998) and, as long as we understand why and we are taking steps to facilitate future development, this is not a problem. General templates may help organize our programmes and help us understand the priority at any particular moment in time or stage of development for a particular individual, but prescriptive packages and plans must be avoided. The players who appear to be doing the best at younger ages may well be passed 3 years later by someone who has been doggedly training away, perhaps catching up physically through late maturation, having started or transferred to the sport late, having missed early training opportunities or even just that it has taken time for the individual to develop the required skills. Ultimately, the message is clear. It is important not to write anybody off too early because things can change dramatically over a short time, particularly through the adolescent years.

Providing structures that cater for developmental variation

The structure of our sports systems and competitions can help allow for this non-linear developmental variation. For example, while we know quality physical education and extracurricular clubs in schools can provide a good foundation for future development for all, a good club structure can provide a wide range of opportunities for a variety of junior and senior athletes at different standards, helping to keep large numbers of youngsters and adults involved in sport. This could be done by providing a number of teams throughout the club system, e.g. U12s, U14s, U16s, U18s, Seniors, with a number of teams at each stage, so someone could play for the seniors' fourth team or U14s seconds. This will facilitate players at any standard to take part and move in and out of better or worse standards as their development and motivation allows, without loss of resources or opportunity. In minority sports, efforts need to be made to set up multiple and sustainable opportunities to bring like-minded individuals together. Coherent coach education and philosophy could minimize this still further. This can help avoid any negative impact on youngsters through premature and overly selective age-group teams, whereby perhaps out of 50 or 60 young, enthusiastic 13-year-olds who could all one day be great players, 40 or 50 are 'told implicitly' that they are not good enough by the selection of a lucky (or physically mature, or more practised) few to the county U14 squad (Martindale et al 2007). Of course, this may be particularly problematic when players are selected for the sole purpose of 'winning' the county tournament. At a more 'elite' level, examples of systems that can provide high-quality training environments for a wider range of youngsters with potential might include a number of regional excellence centres/development squads with flexible age ranges. Under this approach, selection is based more holistically on standards, general athletic ability, development and commitment, rather than just selecting a squad of players centrally at each age group on the basis of performance. The management of such a process might allow longer 'probation periods' for talent to develop over time, with clear goals where deemed appropriate and retaining the benefits of interacting with role models and resource. If players are 'dropped', then it would be sensible to provide clear feedback and advice to the athlete and their coach about the required developments for re-entry at a later time.

Indeed, depending on the sport – if there is no professional club system for example – it may be necessary to develop national centres of excellence in order to bring together like-minded and talented athletes with the coaching, role models and resources required to step up to a world-class level. It is important to point out that national centres would sensibly have a clear and explicit link to 'world-class performance and world-class performers' as opposed to an overemphasis on national age-group success. Furthermore, there is evidence to suggest that keeping young athletes within structured age-group bands is not as effective as development with a mixture of age-groups/standards (e.g. academy players/first teamers or 15-year-olds/adults) (Côté et al 2006), particularly if this allows interaction, such as training, playing, watching day-to-day activities, with elite level performers at an appropriate level (Martindale et al 2007). Therefore, the greater the integration and interaction between 'levels' the better. Furthermore, these types of system help to build a structure where the 'gaps' between levels of ability are decreased and clear expectations are reinforced, through which good practice and TI can be disseminated, particularly, for example, if coaches in regional centres are linked in some way to local clubs and schools.

Building the pathways and managing the networks

It is fair to say that in different regions of the country you will find a different sporting infrastructure and different opportunities, in terms of breadth and quality. For example, there may be four top-flight professional sports clubs and academies in a certain city but none in the whole of another county. There may be a strong tradition of county sport in certain sports and not others, there may be some strong school or club systems that attract and develop sporting talent effectively, or not. Therefore, there is no one single template for the most effective 'sporting structure'. For a sport, a country, a county or a professional club, it is important to clearly identify, develop and be part of pathways that allow young sportspeople to develop and be monitored and identified over time (Abbott et al 2005) and get the necessary quality competition and training required (Durand-Bush & Salmela 2002), while providing opportunities for keeping people involved (Simonton 1999), and for late developers to emerge and be picked up (Moore et al 1998), and providing clarity and understanding about the required standards, expectations and opportunities that exist for those aspiring to become top-level performers (Martindale et al 2005). Indeed, such pathway structures and communication among the network of people involved also provide opportunities to disseminate good practice, which in itself will help to provide wider and better-quality opportunities.

Providing quality and managing quantity

Given that high-quality and challenging competition experiences, as opposed to high-quantity (Van Aken 2005), become a very important development tool once developmental and mastery stages are reached (Bloom 1985, Côté & Hay 2002, Durand-Bush & Salmela 2002), it would be sensible to give special consideration to the development of a system that can cater for such needs. One crucial aspect of the development of young athletes into world-class competitors is to enable them to get the quality of competition that will challenge them to learn, develop and utilize the skills and confidence required to make the step up to the top level. This is a critical part of any sporting structure and needs to be designed and managed carefully. Indeed, competing at too low a level too often will not demand quality play and the types of on-field behaviour (e.g. skills, tactics, physicality, psychology) necessary for progression. This is likely to breed bad habits that will be ineffective at a higher level, due, for example, to the ease in which points can be scored by that particular talented individual.

As a common consequence, players may even resort to more 'fanciful' play in order to be recognized. It can also be the case that a youngster is unable to distinguish one game from the next and a long adult season may therefore not be effective for development. The addition of breaks allows for regeneration, review and feedback, during which global lessons/themes can be drawn out, then practised and then tested, adding to the quality of the competition experience. Playing week after week in a 7-day cycle may not allow this to occur.

Another problem that young talented individuals face is a demand on their time and ability. It could be possible for any one individual to play for a school, county, regional, national age group and professional sport academy team in any one season, possibly in more than one sport too. The case for the dangers of overplaying young people has been made many times over the years (Gould et al 1996) and is an aspect of development that requires management, with a priority focus by all involved on the development of the individual youngster, not the teams they 'play' for. Indeed, priorities for the youngster (e.g. long-term development, health, athlete choice and aspirations) must be clearly identified, discussed and communicated to the youngster themselves, parents, schools, clubs, select teams, etc. While the sole responsibility for this is not always clear, it would seem sensible to include parents and the person most responsible for the youngster and their sporting aspirations. This is where communication among the people and clubs/schools/squads in the 'pathway' is crucial, and, indeed, having and developing good working relationships between all those involved is highly beneficial. This is perhaps more important and relevant the more in demand or talented the youngster is. These communication channels and relationships across a 'pathway network' can lead to a more effective network of TI (through dissemination and understanding of what potential 'looks like') and help bring youngsters to the attention of those who have the talent selection remit. The coherent development of this talent can then be helped through dissemination of knowledge and coaching, for example inviting coaches to watch and be involved with coaching 'higher level' athletes, leaflets, websites, discussion forums, formal and informal meetings/interaction. However, it must be recognized that what is best for the development of the individual athlete must remain the priority.

Focusing on individuals: walking the walk, not just talking the talk

Because of the dynamic, individualized nature of development and given that 'no uniform *sport* performance ability exists: Indeed, deficiencies in one area of performance can be compensated for by a high level in others' (Bartmus et al 1987, p. 415), it is clear that individual needs must be recognized and prioritized (Russell 1989). Therefore, it is imperative that youngsters are treated as individuals, and their needs are individually met as often as possible (Van Tassel-Baska 2001). In order to achieve programme individualization, coaches should conduct a series of activities and actions. These should include regular goal setting, purposeful feedback and personal review, in conjunction with informal and formal opportunities to communicate. Time spent getting to know the youngsters through these steps ensures effective individualized needs analyses and development (Côté & Fraser-Thomas 2007, Durand-Bush & Salmela 2002, Ericsson et al 1993, MacPhail & Kirk 2006, Martindale et al 2007, Wiersma 2000). While it is recognized that individualizing practice is a big coaching commitment, the effectiveness of such teaching and educational approaches is well documented (Yesseldyke & Christenson 1987). Recent work has shown that the eventual development of high-level talent can depend on the extent to which coaches commit to individualized attention (Bloom 1985, Csikszentmihalyi et al 1993, Gould et al 2002). The individualized nature of many behavioural change interventions supports the importance of individualized practice, especially when combined with clear reinforcement links to performance and development goals (Siedentop 1978). Furthermore, informal methods of communication and interaction have been identified as crucial and provide a number of advantages. For example, an expert development coach (hockey) interviewed by Martindale et al (2007, p. 197) highlights this clearly:

> I ring them occasionally, sit down and have a beer, have a coffee, particularly with two or three of the more senior players in the side. Have a check, you know how you think things are going; this and that and the other. And then you run into others at various other times and places and that's an opportunity to have a quiet word with them more. And obviously you stop people pre and post training, pre post match times. I believe to be honest with you that rather than a lot of formal situations that informal is best . . . That's what makes the whole team stick together, that communication. . . . It's just a

chat and it's a non-threatening environment. They'll tell you loads of things. Then you can get to know the players that bit better and know what makes them tick.

Such informal processes would need to be combined with a raft of formalized systems for individualized assessment and development, but ultimately the nature of the coach–athlete relationship is crucial for success (Box 5.4).

Provision of quality support networks

We have seen the need for individualized attention, due to the nature of development and differences in individuals themselves. While there is a significant role for coaches to help develop and support athletes through, there is also responsibility on the athletes themselves to work hard to overcome any barriers and be successful. This consideration notwithstanding, and given the time it takes to become an expert and the vast number of people and institutions involved in this process (Gould et al 2002), the likelihood is high that different people become more or less significant and important in development (Bloom 1985). Indeed, it is likely that different people will be more useful for helping an athlete through different problems and challenges, ranging from coaches to fellow athletes, friends and parents, to name a few. In this regard, UK research highlights the need to investigate and acknowledge the nature of sport-specific problem periods and set up a variety of support networks, education and training over the long term if more of our talented athletes are to be successful (Moore et al 1998, Rowley 1992). It appears that a wide variety of formal and informal, sport- and individual-specific support networks are crucial to the progression of many younger athletes in order to help prepare them for and support them through key transitions (Csikszentmihalyi et al 1993, Durand-Bush & Salmela 2002, Holt & Dunn 2004, MacNamara et al 2006, Morgan & Giacobbi 2006, Rees & Hardy 2000, Wylleman et al 2004). Social support has been found to be associated with effective TD and performance, with particular emphasis put on different types of support (Rees et al 1999). These include emotional support, esteem support, informational support and tangible support. Similarly, individual coping mechanisms are often used alongside other coping strategies, and their uses occur and can change depending on the circumstances (Rees & Hardy 2000). These can also occur at any time, within or outside any well defined transition, hence resourcing, widespread education and communication become all the more important.

Box 5.4

Examples of the nature of processes (formal and informal) that facilitate an individualized player development focus

We use a combination of methods to ensure an individualized approach: we are lucky enough to have a number of support people and coaches and every 6 weeks we do case study reviews, in which we sit down and discuss each player, their progress, their problems and work out what we need to do as a team to best develop them further. On top of that we do individual performance profiling and goal setting, where we assess a range of important features of their development and set stepping stones to reach goals. Also, the players review games of themselves and set their own weekly goals; this would also be done every so often with a coach or even one of the first teamers, to check and add value. In fact, we are lucky enough to have day-to-day contact with the lads and each other (as support staff), which allows us the opportunity to talk about players at any time. Equally, they can pop in and see us any time. This helps keep the process ticking over nicely and helps build relationships. Anything that can be done to understand the players better and provide an individualized approach adds value.

The importance of disseminating knowledge to parents and community

Outside influences, such as parents, communities and schools, are crucial but often not considered a priority. However, the scale of influence and dissemination of knowledge would sensibly extend down to those most able to affect the structure of the very early years of upbringing. Evidence of this is highlighted by Côté et al (2006), who have shown that it is initial community environments (e.g. parents, families, friends, teachers and coaches) that inadvertently foster and prepare youngsters for elite-level sport development by encouraging features such as intrinsic motivation, enjoyment, self-efficacy, problem solving, early success and recognition. They also provide social support, integration with older children and lots of varied, unstructured play and practice in a less competitive atmosphere. Even at later stages the necessary practical and financial support and development of a variety of support networks are often parent-led (Bloom 1985, Durand-Bush & Salmela 2002). There is evidence to highlight that key individuals in the athletes' socialization network need to be systematically educated and involved appropriately to foster desirable characteristics (Brustad 1993, Côté & Fraser-Thomas 2007, Gould et al 2002, Ommundsen et al 2006, Wolfenden & Holt 2005). Educational sessions are an obvious method of informing those important influences, but involving parents and others more directly could also be key. Evidence suggests that, even at elite level, the more interest and encouragement that is given by parents, the more likely it is that youngsters will stay involved (Weiss & Hayashi 1995). In fact, such support may be crucial; for example, it was found that in England around 40% of elite athletes aged 25 and under were still financially dependent on parents (Moore et al 1998). The reciprocal socialization effects of sport involvement (Weiss & Hyashi 1995) may also be useful for fostering extremely effective support networks, particularly if parents are given appropriate opportunities to contribute positively.

The need to develop and maintain effective communication

It would seem that there must be ample opportunity for effective communication patterns, not only between parents and coaches but also among university, work and other involved and important parties (Côté & Fraser-Thomas 2007, Gould et al 2002, MacPhail & Kirk 2006, Wiersma 2000). Indeed, this is where any problems or conflicts can be solved in the interests of the athlete and not in the interests of those with most power. Organizational psychology highlights that effective organizations explicitly promote clear expectations and open communication systems to allow provision for any conflicts that may arise (Bemowski 1996). The more opportunities for relationships to be built with those people and institutions involved with the development of young people the better. This has a number of added benefits. First, communication and strong relationships can allow for the management of the playing programme for a youngster, which is particularly problematic when they are highly talented and sought after by a number of different teams and sports. Secondly, the development of these relationships can help disseminate good practice and understanding, particularly to people who have a significant influence on a young person, most often the parents. For example, if the parents are the ones feeding the athlete, then it is crucial they understand about the right things to buy and cook. Furthermore, if the development of responsibility is key to an athlete, it is of limited value to promote this in the coaching environment if, at home, the youngster gets waited on hand and foot, with no demand for responsibility. Finally, if an athlete drops out of a 'select squad', back into the club system, then it is crucial that they have the opportunity for quality training and competition and that the 'new' coach understands what is best for the youngster; both factors that dissemination of best practice, communication and working relationships can help with.

There are many ways to encourage communication, knowledge sharing and working relationships: examples include formal education days or workshops; informal contact such as talking to parents at training or competitions; large education initiatives; practical coaching education; websites; booklets; providing events and occasions where athletes and role models can interact; actively encouraging positive involvement of influential people (e.g. parents); providing informal opportunities for coaches, support staff, parents, etc. to get together to allow crossover of information and ideas (perhaps by organizing a barbecue); phoning and speaking to other coaches who are involved with the same individuals; fortnightly meetings; a beer or coffee after work... the list goes on.

Conclusion

It is clear that long-term aims must be implemented consistently through the system to allow coaches, athletes, parents, schools, sports clubs, etc. to promote individual development effectively. The understanding of what leads to success at a world-class level is crucial. This has been explored at an early foundation level (fundamental movement skills and motivation), leading into an 'excellence environment level', highlighting the need to introduce clear expectations and direction, integration of 'levels' and role models, a wide variety of skills through quality

Key features	Key methods
Long Term Aims and Methods	• Develop a Long Term Vision, Purpose and Identity
Wide Ranging Coherent Messages and Support	• Provide Coherent Philosophies, Aims and Methods at a Variety of Levels (e.g. Parents, Coach Content, Practice and Reward Systems, Selection, Funding, Competition Structure, NGBs) • Educate Parents, Schools, Peers, Coaches and Important Others (and encourage positive contributions!) • Utilize Role Models at a Variety of Levels • Set Up a Variety of Support Networks Over the Long Term (e.g. Peer, Coach, Sport Staff, Family) • Provide Forums for Open and Honest Communication Patterns, Formal and Informal Coach/Athlete Interactions at a Variety of Levels
Emphasize Appropriate Development NOT Early Success	• Re-Conceptualize 'Winning' as Success at Developmental Stages • Provide Clear Expectations, Roles, and Meaning Within the 'Big Picture' at Every Level • Provide 'Stage Specific' Integrated Experiences and Teaching With Explicit Links to Performance Fundamental Physical and Sport Specific Skills (Technical, Tactical, Mental, Physical, Perceptual) Fundamental Mental Skills (Learning and Development; Life; Performance Related) Balance • Encourage Increasing Responsibility and Autonomy in Learning/Development • Develop Intrinsic Motivation and Personal Commitment to Process • Promote Personal Relevance, Athlete Understanding and Knowledge
Individualized and Ongoing Development	• Provide Accessible Opportunities and Fundamentals to as Many Youngsters as Possible • Provide Flexible Systems to Allow for Performance and Physical Development Variation • Identify, Prepare for, and Support Individuals Through Key Transitions • Provide Individualized Programmes and Regular Individual Goal Setting and Review Processes

Integrated, Holistic and Systematic

Fig. 5.1 • A summary of the key features of effective talent development environments.

training and quality competition, with particular consideration for the underpinning psychology. This requires the appreciation of the individualized, often unpredictable 'journey' to the top. With this understanding, a sporting structure can be put in place which will provide clear expectations and enable more effective movement between 'levels', and management of athletes within a more clear, multifaceted pathway(s). Indeed, where a player-centred approach genuinely exists, the treatment of youngsters as individuals is crucial, as is the development of an active and integrated network of support that can help guide athletes consistently to realize their potential. Figure 5.1 provides an overview of the key features of effective TDEs and summarizes the key messages presented throughout this chapter.

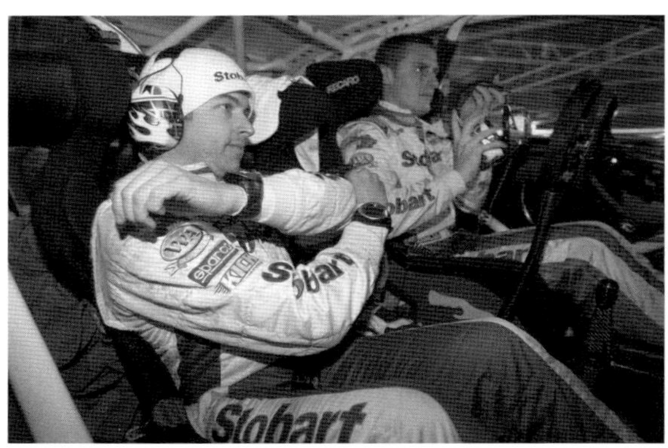

Working in an Academy set up. Rally Elite members Matt Wilson and Scott Martin getting ready to leave service for another batch of competitive stages. © Stobart Motorsport. With thanks to the Royal Automobile Motor Sport Association.

References

Abbott, A., Collins, D., 2002. A theoretical and empirical analysis of a 'state of the art' talent identification model. High Ability Studies 13, 157–178.

Abbott, A., Collins, D., 2004. Eliminating the dichotomy between theory and practice in talent identification and development: considering the role of psychology. J. Sports Sci. 22, 395–408.

Abbott, A., Easson, B., 2002. The mental profile. In: Hale, B., Collins, D. (Eds.), Rugby tough. Human Kinetics, Champaign, IL, pp. 17–33.

Abbott, A., Collins, D., Martindale, R., et al., 2002. Talent identification and development: an academic review. SportScotland, Edinburgh.

Abbott, A., Button, C., Pepping, G., et al., 2005. Unnatural selection: talent identification and development in sport. Nonlinear Dynamics Psychol. Life Sci. 9, 61–88.

Abernethy, B., Côté, J., Baker, J., 2002. Expert decision making in team sports. Technical report. Australian Institute of Sport, Canberra, ACT.

Abernethy, B., Russell, D., 1987. Expert-novice differences in an applied selective attention task. Journal of Sport Psychology 9, 326–345.

Bailey, R., Morley, D., 2006. Towards a model of talent development in physical education. Sport Education and Society 11, 211–230.

Baker, J., Côté, J., 2006. Shifting training requirements during athlete development: the relationship among deliberate practice, deliberate play and other sport involvement in the acquisition of sport expertise. In: Hackfort, D., Tenenbaum, G. (Eds.), Essential processes for attaining peak performance. Meyer & Meyer, Aachen, pp. 93–110.

Baker, J., Côté, J., Abernethy, B., 2003. Learning from the experts: practice activities of expert decision makers in sport. Res. Q. Exerc. Sport 74, 342–347.

Baker, J., Côté, J., Deakin, J., 2005. Expertise in ultra-endurance triathletes early sport involvement, training structure and the theory of deliberate practice. Journal of Applied Sport Psychology 17, 64–78.

Bandura, A., McDonald, F., 1963. The influence of social reinforcement and the behaviour of models in shaping children's moral judgements. J. Abnorm. Soc. Psychol. 67, 274–281.

Barnsley, R., Thompson, A., Legault, P., 1992. Family planning football style. The relative age effect in football. International Review for the Sociology of Sport 27, 77–88.

Bartmus, U., Neumann, E., De Marées, H., 1987. The talent problem in sports. Int. J. Sports Med. 8, 415–416.

Baxter-Jones, A., Helms, P., 1996. Effects of training at a young age: a review of the training of young athletes (TOYA) study. Pediatric Exercise Science 8, 310–327.

Beamer, M., Cote, J., Ericsson, K., 1999. A comparison between international and provincial level gymnasts in their pursuit of sport expertise. Paper presented at the 10th Annual European Congress of Sport Psychology, July 7–12. Prague, FEPSAC.

Bee, H., Mitchell, S., 1984. The developing person: a life-span approach. Harper & Row, New York.

Bemowski, K., 1996. Leaders on leadership. Quality Progress 29, 43–45.

Blanksby, B., 1980. Measures of talent identification in competitive swimming. Sports Coach 15 (4), 13–19.

Bloom, B., 1985. Developing talent in young people. Ballantine, New York.

Brustad, R., 1993. Youth in sport: psychological considerations. In: Singer, R.N., Murphey, M., Tennant, L.K. (Eds.), Handbook of research on sport psychology. Macmillan, New York, pp. 190–313.

Bull, S., Shambrook, C., James, W., et al., 2005. Towards an understanding of mental toughness in elite English cricketers. Journal of Applied Sport Psychology 17, 209–227.

Burwitz, L., Moore, P., Wilkinson, D., 1994. Future directions for performance-related sports science research: an interdisciplinary approach. J. Sports Sci. 12, 93–109.

Carron, A., Hausenblas, H., Eys, M., 2005. Group dynamics in sport. Fitness Information Technology, Morgantown, WV.

Côté, J., 1999. The influence of the family in the development of talent in sport. Sport Psychologist 13, 395–417.

Côté, J., Hay, J., 2002. Children's involvement in sport: A developmental perspective. In: Silva, J.M., Stevens, D. (Eds.), Psychological foundations of sport. Merrill, Boston, MA, pp. 484–502.

Côté, J., Baker, J., Abernethy, B., 2003. From play to practice: A developmental framework for the acquisition of expertise in team sport. In Starkes, J., Ericsson, K.A. (Eds.), Recent advances in research on sport expertise. Human Kinetics, Champaign, IL, pp. 89–114.

Côté, J., MacDonald, D., Baker, J., et al., 2006. When 'where' is more important than 'when': Birthplace and birthdate effects on the achievement of sporting expertise. J. Sports Sci. 24, 1065–1073.

Côté, J., Fraser-Thomas, J., 2007. Youth involvement in sport. In: Crocker, P. R.E. (Ed.), Introduction to sport psychology: a Canadian perspective. Pearson Prentice Hall, Toronto, Ontario, pp. 266–294.

Csikszentmihalyi, M., Rathunde, K., Whalen, S. 1993. Talented teenagers: the roots of success and failure. Cambridge University Press, New York.

Csikszentmihalyi, M., Robinson, R., 1986. Culture, time, and the development of talent. In: Sternberg, R.J. Davidson, J.E. (Eds.), Conceptions of giftedness. Cambridge University Press, New York, pp. 264–284.

Deci, E., Ryan, R. 1985. intrinsic motivation and self-determination in human behaviour. Plenum Press, New York.

De Knop, P., Engström, L., Skirstad, B., 1996. Worldwide trends in youth sport. Human Kinetics, Champaign, IL.

Douglas, C., Martindale, R., 2008. Player development review for PRL. PB Performance, UK.

Durand-Bush, N., Salmela, J., 2002. The development and maintenance of expert athletic performance: perceptions of world and Olympic champions. Journal of Applied Sport Psychology 14, 154–171.

Dweck, C., 1986. Motivational processes affecting learning. Am. Psychol. 41, 1040–1048.

Elferink-Gemser, M., Visscher, C., Lemmink, K., et al., 2004. Relation between multidimensional performance characteristics and level of performance in talented youth field hockey players. J. Sports Sci. 22, 1053–1063.

Ericsson, K., 1998. The scientific study of expert levels of performance: general implications for optimal learning and creativity. High Ability Studies 9, 75–100.

Ericsson, K., 2003. Development of elite performance and deliberate practice: an update from the perspective of the expert performance approach. In: Starkes, J.L., Ericsson, K.A. (Eds.), Expert performance in sports. Human Kinetics, Champaign, IL, pp. 49–83.

Ericsson, K., Charness, N., 1994. Expert performance: its structure and acquisition. Am. Psychol. 49, 725–747.

Ericsson, K., Lehmann, A., 1996. Expert and exceptional performance: evidence of maximal adaptation to task constraints. Annu. Rev. Psychol. 47, 273–305.

Ericsson, K., Krampe, R., Tesch-Romer, C., 1993. The role of deliberate practice in the acquisition of expert performance. Psychol. Rev. 100, 363–406.

Ewing, M., Seefeldt, V., 1996. Patterns of participation and attrition in American agency sponsored youth sports. In: Smoll, F.L., Smith, R.E. (Eds.), Children and youth in sport: a biopsychosocial perspective. Brown & Benchmark, Dubuque, IA, pp. 31–45.

Falk, B., Lidor, R., Lander, Y., et al., 2004. Talent identification and early development of elite water-polo players: a 2-year follow-up study. J. Sports Sci. 22, 347–355.

Freeman, J., 1995. Towards a policy for actualising talent. In: Freeman, J., Span, P., Wagner, H. (Eds.), Actualizing talent: a lifelong challenge. Cassell, London, pp. 174–192.

French, K., McPherson, S., 1999. Adaptations in response selection processes used during sport competition with increasing age and expertise. International Journal of Sport Psychology 30, 173–193.

Gallahue, D., 1982. Fundamental movement experiences for children. Wiley, New York.

Gould, D., Feltz, D., Horn, T., et al., 1982. Reasons for attrition in competitive youth swimming. Journal of Sport Behavior 5, 155–165.

Gould, D., Udry, E., Tuffey, S., et al., 1996. Burnout in competitive junior tennis players: I. A quantitative psychological assessment. The Sport Psychologist 10, 322–340.

Gould, D., Eklund, R., Jackson, S., 1993. Coping strategies by U.S. Olympic wrestlers. Res. Q. Exerc. Sport 64, 83–93.

Gould, D., Dieffenbach, K., Moffett, A., 2002. Psychological characteristics and their development in Olympic champions. Journal of Applied Sport Psychology 14, 172–204.

Greenspan, M., Feltz, D., 1989. Psychological interventions with athletes in competitive situations: a review. Sport Psychologist 3, 219–236.

Hanton, S., Jones, G., 1999. The acquisition and development of cognitive skills and strategies: Making the butterflies fly in formation. Sport Psychologist 13, 1–21.

Hedstrom, R., Gould, D., 2004. Research in youth sports: critical issues status. Institute for the study of youth sports. Michigan State University, East Lansing, MI.

Hellstedt, J., 1995. Invisible players: a family systems model. In: Murphy, S. M. (Ed.), Sport psychology interventions. Human Kinetics, Champaign, IL, pp. 117–146.

Helsen, W., Starkes, J., 1999. A multidimensional approach to skilled perception and performance in sport. Applied Cognitive Psychology 13, 1–27.

Helsen, W., Starkes, J., Van Wincel, J., 1998. The influence of relative age on success and drop out in male soccer players. Am. J. Hum. Biol. 10, 791–798.

Helsen, W., Hodges, N., Van Winckel, J., et al., 2000. The roles of talent, physical precocity and practice in the development of soccer expertise. J. Sports Sci. 18, 727–736.

Hill, G., Hansen, G., 1988. Specialization in high school sports – the pros and cons. Journal of Physical Education, Recreation and Dance 59, 76–79.

Holt, N., Dunn, J., 2004. Toward a grounded theory of the psychosocial competencies and environmental conditions associated with soccer success. Journal of Applied Sport Psychology 16, 199–219.

Howe, M., Davidson, J., Sloboda, J., 1998. Innate talents: reality or myth? Behav. Brain Sci. 21, 399–442.

Janelle, C., Hillman, C., 2003. Expert performance in sport: current perspectives and critical issues. In: Starkes, J.L., Ericsson, K.A. (Eds.), Expert performance in sports. Human Kinetics, Champaign, IL, pp. 19–48.

Jess, M., Collins, D., 2003. Primary physical education in Scotland: the future in the making. Physical Education and Sport Pedagogy 8, 103–118.

Jones, J., Hanton, S., Connaughton, D., 2002. What is this thing called mental toughness? An investigation of elite performers. Journal of Applied Sport Psychology 14, 205–218.

Kane, J., 1986. Giftedness in sport. In: Gleeson, G. (Ed.), The growing child in competitive sport. Hodder & Stoughton, London, pp. 184–204.

Knowles, M., Holton, E., Swanson, R., 1998. The adult learner. Gulf Publishing, Houston, TX.

Krampe, R., Ericsson, A., 1996. Maintaining excellence: deliberate practice and elite performance in young and older pianists. J. Exp. Psychol. Gen. 125, 331–339.

Kreiner-Phillips, K., Orlick, T., 1993. Winning after winning: the psychology of ongoing excellence. The Sport Psychologist 7, 31–48.

Lepper, M., Greene, D., 1975. Turning play into work: effects of adult surveillance and extrinsic rewards on children's intrinsic motivation. J. Pers. Soc. Psychol. 31, 479–486.

McCaffrey, N., Orlick, T., 1989. Mental factors related to excellence among top professional golfers. International Journal of Sport Psychology 20, 256–278.

MacNamara, A., Holmes, P., Collins, D., 2006. The pathway to excellence: the role of psychological characteristics in negotiating the challenges of musical development. British Journal of Music Education 23, 285–302.

MacNamara, A., Holmes, P., Collins, D., 2008. Negotiating transitions in musical development: the role of psychological characteristics of developing excellence. Psychology of Music 36, 335–352.

MacPhail, A., Kirk, D., 2006. Young people's socialization into sport: experiencing the specializing phase. Leisure Studies 25, 57–74.

Martindale, R., Collins, D., Abraham, A., 2007. Effective talent development: the elite coach perspective in UK sport. Journal of Applied Sport Psychology 19, 187–206.

Martindale, R., Collins, D., Daubney, J., 2005. Talent development: a guide for practice and research within sport. Quest 57, 353–375.

Moore, P., Collins, D., Burwitz, L., 1998. The development of sporting talent 1997: an examination of the current practices for talent development in English sport. English Sports Council, London.

Morgan, T., Giacobbi, P., 2006. Toward two grounded theories of the talent development and social support process of highly successful collegiate athletes. Sport Psychologist 20, 295–313.

Ommundsen, Y., Roberts, G., Lemyre, P., et al., 2006. Parental and coach support or pressure on psychosocial outcomes of pediatric athletes in soccer. Clin. J. Sport Med. 16, 522–526.

Orlick, T., Hansen, H., Reed, A., et al., 1978. Psychological attributes and on-ice indicators of high calibre hockey players. In: Terrauds, J., Gros, H.J. (Eds.), Science in skiing, skating and hockey. International Congress of Sports Sciences, Edmonton, Alberta, pp. 151–157.

Orlick, T., Partington, J., 1988. Mental links to excellence. Sport Psychologist 2, 105–130.

Pancoe, M., 1999. Multiage education. BA thesis. Alfred University Honors Program, New York.

Rees, T., Hardy, L., 2000. An investigation of the social support experiences of high level sports performers. Sport Psychologist 14, 327–347.

Rees, T., Ingledew, D., Hardy, L., 1999. Social support dimensions and components of performance in tennis. J. Sports Sci. 17, 421–429.

Regnier, G., Salmela, J., 1987. Predictors of success in Canadian male gymnasts. In: Petiot, B., Salmela, J.H., Hoshizaki, T.B. (Eds.), World identification systems for gymnastic talent. Sport Psyche Editions, Montreal, Québec, pp. 143–150.

Reilly, T., Williams, A., Nevill, A., et al., 2000. A multidisciplinary approach to talent identification in soccer. J. Sports Sci. 18, 695–702.

Richardson, D., Stratton, G., 1999. Preliminary investigation into the seasonal birth distribution of England World Cup campaign players. J. Sports Sci. 17, 821–822.

Rowley, S., 1992. Training of young athletes study (TOYA): TOYA and lifestyle. Sports Council, London.

Russell, K., 1989. Athletic talent: from detection to perfection. Science Periodical on Research and Technology in Sport 9, 1–6.

Salmela, J., 1996. Great job coach: getting the edge from proven winners. Potentium, Ottawa, Ontario.

Salmela, J., Moraes, L., 2003. Development of expertise: The role of coaching, families, and cultural contexts. In: Starkes, J.L., Ericsson, K.A. (Eds.), Expert performance in sports. Human Kinetics, Champaign, IL, pp. 275–294.

Schmidt, R., Wrisberg, C., 2000. Motor learning and performance, second ed. Human Kinetics, Champaign, IL.

Siedentop, D., 1978. Management of practice behavior. In: Staub, W.G. (Ed.), Sport psychology: an analysis of athlete behaviour. Mouvement Publications, Ithaca, NY, pp. 42–48.

Silva, J., 1990. An analysis of training stress syndrome in competitive athletics. Journal of Applied Sport Psychology 2, 5–20.

Silva, J., Shultz, B., Haslam, R., et al., 1985. Discriminating characteristics of contestants at the United States Olympic wrestling trials. International Journal of Sport Psychology 16, 79–102.

Simonton, D., 1999. Talent and its development: an emergenic and epigenetic model. Psychol. Rev. 106, 435–457.

Sinclair, D., Orlick, T., 1993. Positive transitions from high performance sport. Sport Psychologist 7, 138–150.

Soberlak, P., Côté, J., 2003. The developmental activities of elite ice hockey players. Journal of Applied Sport Psychology 15, 41–49.

Solomon, G., Striegel, D., Eliot, J., et al., 1996. The self fulfilling prophecy in college basketball: implications for effective coaching. Journal of Applied Sport Psychology 8, 44–59.

Sosniak, L., 1985. Learning to be a concert pianist. In: Bloom, B.S. (Ed.), Developing talent in young people. Ballantine Books, New York, pp. 19–67

Stafford, I., 2005. Coaching for long-term athlete development: to improve participation and performance in sport. Coachwise, Leeds.

Starkes, J., 2000. The road to expertise: is practice the only determinant? International Journal of Sport Psychology 31, 431–451.

Starkes, J., Ericsson, K., 2003. Expert Performance in Sports. Human Kinetics, Champaign, IL.

Starkes, J., Deakin, J., Allard, F., et al., 1996. Deliberate practice in sports: what is it anyway? In: Ericsson, K. (Ed.), The road to excellence: the acquisition of expert performance in the arts and sciences, sports and games. Lawrence Erlbaum Associates, Mahwah, NJ, pp. 81–106.

Talbot-Honeck, C., Orlick, T., 1998. The essence of excellence: mental skills of top classical musicians. Journal of Excellence 1, 66–81.

Tenenbaum, G., Sar-El, L., Bar-Eli, M., 2000. Anticipation of ball locations in low and high skilled performers: a developmental perspective. Psychology of Sport and Exercise 1, 117–128.

United States Olympic Committee, 2002. Amber Drury-Pinto named water polo's National Coach of the Year for USOC Coach Recognition Program. Available on line at:http://www.fansonly.com/printable/schools/cal/sports/w-wpolo/spec-rel/091902aaa.html (accessed 05.02.09).

Valeriote, T., Hansen, L., 1986. Youth sport in Canada. In: Weiss, M.R., Gould, D. (Eds.), Sport for children and youths. Human Kinetics, Champaign, IL.

Van Aken, I. 2005. Minutes of the ITF coaches' commission meeting, Paris, June. ITF, London.

Van Rossum, J., 2001. Talented in dance: the Bloom stage model revisited in the personal histories of dance students. High Ability Studies 12, 181–197.

Van Tassel-Baska, J., 2001. The talent development process: what we know and what we don't know. Gifted Education International 16, 20–28.

Veenman, S., 1995. Cognitive and noncognitive effects of multigrade and multi-age classes: a best-evidence synthesis. Review of Educational Research 65, 319–381.

Ward, P., Williams, A., 2003. Perceptual and cognitive skill development in soccer: the multidimensional nature of expert performance. Journal of Sport and Exercise Psychology 25, 93–111.

Weiss, M., Hayashi, C., 1995. All in the family: parent-child influences in competitive youth gymnastics. Pediatric Exercise Science 7, 36–48.

Wiersma, L., 2000. Risks and benefits of youth sport specialization: perspectives and recommendations. Pediatric Exercise Science 12, 13–22.

Williams, A., 2000. Perceptual skill in soccer: implications for talent identification and development. J. Sports Sci. 18, 737–750.

Williams, A., Hodges, N., 2004. Skill acquisition in sport: research, theory, and practice. Routledge, London.

Williams, A., Reilly, T., 2000. Talent identification and development. J. Sports Sci. 18, 657–667.

Wolfenden, L., Holt, N., 2005. Talent development in elite junior tennis: perceptions of players, parents, and coaches. Journal of Applied Sport Psychology 17, 108–126.

Wylleman, D., Alfermann, D., Lavallee, D., 2004. Career transitions in sport. European Perspectives Psychology of Sport and Exercise 5, 7–20.

Yesseldyke, J., Christenson, S., 1987. Evaluating students' instructional environments. Remedial and Special Education 8 (3), 17–24.

Implications and applications: views from the performer's panel

6

Dave Collins

Grey Matters/UCLan

CHAPTER CONTENTS

Unsurprisingly perhaps, the messages that emerge for talent development (TD) are very consistent. After all, as a glance at the reference list will show, most of the authors have worked together on several projects, so they are all familiar and in agreement with the general messages sent. However, this agreement is not based on friendship but rather on a critical review of the empirical evidence and through clear and justified analysis. On this basis, the agreed position on TD offers a clear way forward, even though there are some important issues that need consideration.

Key practical issues

The first, and possibly most challenging factor, is how well, if at all, talent can genuinely be identified at an early stage. Early performance and anthropometrics are pretty much dismissed as sole talent identification (TI) tools by every author in this section. Physique and maturity are identified as two confounds that make early TI very questionable. For example, consider age-group success in team sports, where players are selected as the best available rather than for their long-term prospects. In rugby, KB points out the problems of selecting props (typically a late-maturing position) for younger age-group teams; in fact, players selected as the best for this role at under 16 will rarely make it to senior success *in that position* (the italicized qualification is important – more on this in the 'What should you do' block). Similar challenges exist for other team games, especially in positions where size is important (e.g. goalkeeper in netball, forward guard in basketball).

The performers panel (PP) also highlighted the problems with performance as the tool. Selection of dancers at 15/16 (just before they enter 'academy'-style training), for example, will consider many more factors than current performance, despite the fact that these performers have usually already completed 5 or 6 years of training. SM describes the way selection must 'look through' the performance, and incorporate physical profiling together with fundamental movement/rhythm skills, to ensure that the process doesn't just choose the 'well drilled' or children of parents who can afford sound teaching.

The confounding factors of previous experience and relative maturity are further complicated by the application of different criteria for different ages. Some track and field athletics events are different at younger ages, for example, because of the relative size of the implements (e.g. lighter shot and lower hurdles). Of course, some age (and size) differentiation

DOI: 10.1016/B978-0-443-06734-1.00006-7

is essential but these modifications must be proportionate. Designing age-appropriate variations on adult sports, games and physical pursuits carries some subtle complexities. Consequently, where it exists (also in any implement sports, such as tennis, for example) the impact of differentially sized equipment coacts with maturation to make things even more confused. Consider two 11-year-old soccer players, one physically advanced and one comparatively immature, playing with a 'smaller than the adult game' size 4 ball. The mechanics of play will be different for both, but for one the ball is small, light and easy to kick while for the other it is large, heavy and cumbersome. Of course, individual skills would best be taught using 'size appropriate' equipment, especially as the aim should be eventual (i.e. adult) performance. Consequently, any football academy worth the name will have a stock of balls, size 1 through 5, to allow each player to be suitably challenged. When people play as a team, however, there is no way round this (you can't individualize with a ball per player!), and the differential size issue certainly adds to the complications of picking out who is talented and developing skills through common practices. These difficulties notwithstanding, the bottom line is clear. Performance at younger ages does not automatically demonstrate potential, so selection should be avoided or, if really necessary, must use a broader range of measures to test genuine potential *and* the capacity to get there. SM's points on dance were agreed across the PP:

> We see dancers with everything going for them physically but who really lack the drive to push themselves to practise consistently and with the amount of effort required to achieve elite level. Occasionally this can be as a result of low confidence or self-esteem which can be addressed through improved appropriate support but sometimes the young dancer simply doesn't enjoy hard physical work. The 'perfect' physique may even get themselves into a corps de ballet of a major company, but without real intrinsic drive and motivation and associated confidence levels they are highly unlikely to progress to soloist or principal level.

Another of the identified issues relates to 'fun': keeping things low key at the start of the involvement process is seen by many as important for attracting and keeping talented youngsters in the programme. All members of the PP commented on what 'fun' might mean (see our consideration of life balance in the next block). Of course, no one is suggesting a highly regimented and strict work ethic from day 1, but it is worth noting that talented youngsters, especially ambitious ones, get a lot of fun out of achievement, learning skills, challenging themselves and being part of an enthusiastic, high-effort environment. SB made an excellent point here about the 'sacrifice' that many perceive is essentially made by young performers. If success is what you want, and the work is taking you there, this isn't a sacrifice. RR describes the hours of practice, watching others and talking through moves that characterizes young 'crag rats' at the climbing wall; similar behaviours typify youngsters' addiction to many physical crazes such as skateboarding, bladeing, etc. SM explores the intrinsic satisfaction of getting better through her experiences as, and of, young dancers:

> As a trainee dancer I had no time to watch TV or do much in the way of social activity but achieving new physical skills and, more importantly, being cast in major roles by professional choreographers as a student dancer and subsequently studying and being successful in those roles gave enormous feelings of positivity and pleasure. There becomes a need for physical and artistic expression within the individual; the feeling of performance itself is addictive to the elite performer, the luxury of existing within the moment, being at your most honest. Who needs fun?!

So... be careful when researchers and well meaning experts cite 'fun' as the biggest motivating factor for youngsters and stress how important it is for recruiting and retaining them in the early stages. In extreme sports, RR stressed the need for an adequate and appropriate skill base, which often requires some pretty committed practice to acquire. Without the ability to avoid/get out of excessive danger, most extreme sports can get uncomfortably and uncontrollably extreme, far too quickly! The need for a careful blend is obvious. However, the bottom line here is that, so long as the environment is positive and supportive/rewarding of effort, quite young performers will commit and display a work ethic that transcends the play-police, badge-awarding environment so common in mini-sport and dance environments. While we are on the topic of badges, RR was 'not enthusiastic'!

> We built a coaching scheme where people's goal setting was based on moving up the coaching ladder. One often wondered if they'd heard of the sport.

Badge schemes can be a way to motivate and retain, but don't seem to be so successful in developing performers (or even participants) for the long haul. So if your goal as a coach is development for excellence and/or lifelong involvement, think carefully about the badge/award culture.

Finally, you must consider when young performers should specialize, and how much of this specialized work is really necessary. The authors are all in agreement with maintaining a breadth of activity for quite a long way though the development pathway – the PP agreed with this idea. As a general rule, the ages of 16 and 18 seem to be reasonable change points for cutting breadth and increasing depth, especially since the extra breadth will enable performers to catch up and surpass their earlier-specializing colleagues in short order.

This seems to be at odds, however, with the advice on practice volume, particularly the ideas presented on deliberate practice in Chapter 3. Not necessarily: the point is that, while young aspirant-elite performers need to be accumulating skills (clocking up the 10 000 hours), these don't have to be sport-specific. In fact, recent investigations, albeit retrospective, have suggested that elite performers (Australian Rules football – Berry et al 2008) can reach the top with substantially fewer than the 10 000 total (as low as 5000), and with a significant percentage of the total accumulated time in general play rather than specific and deliberate practice. There is lots of essential preparation work for any specific activity, which is often best accomplished in a generic or other-activity setting. In fact, if you have a budding genius on your hands, challenging her/him through a variety of activities is often the best development (breadth of movement vocabulary) and a good way to maintain interest and avoid burnout (see Ch. 5).

The real answer to the specialism question is defined, in the words of the PP, as 'it depends on the quality and long-termism of the coach'. In short, there are a number of factors that should be considered when making the decision to cut other activities or increase training volume. Simple guidelines like the 10 000 hours rule are much touted but often misinterpreted as well. From a performance perspective (and that is adult/senior performance), holding off on high-volume, single-activity commitments until 16 seems to offer more in the long run and staves off staleness/burnout issues at the crucial life transition age of 18. Volume of practice must be completed eventually, however. Even the Berry et al (2008) study showed that longer amounts of deliberate practice as a youngster were associated with better decision making in mature players.

Things to think about

Reflecting on the key issues raised in the previous block, designing the optimum environment requires some careful thought. Chapters 4 and 5 offer some excellent applied ideas for mental skill development, which has been well justified as essential for the successful evolution towards world class success. In this regard, it is worth considering the extent to which such development is a central and 'embedded' part of the learning environment. Often, when such 'life-skills' are taught in isolation, there is poor transfer and application to the task in hand. For example, consider the impact of healthy eating guidelines and life-skill planning lessons in schools; most coaches will acknowledge little or no transfer from these to young performers' habits in other facets of life. Accordingly, effective development coaches in any environment will make sure that they have the tools to teach mental skills in a sport/activity-specific way. Regular visits from your (hopefully) friendly local performance psychologist or providing a few self-help books just won't hack it! Developing and deploying the mental skills of excellence (including/incorporating PCDEs – see Ch. 4) must be taught and applied to current and future challenges in the particular performance domain; in fact, using coaches and older performers (ideally close in age to the target group) to exemplify or 'model' various techniques is an excellent way to ensure acceptance and application of the requisite skills. Indeed, if executed with sufficient 'cunning', the young performers end up almost coaching and encouraging each other on the skills and their use.

It is worth noting, however, that genuine 'budding elites' may often arrive possessing many of these important skills already. In fact, 'genuine' prodigies (i.e. those with potential to actually make it rather than just be successful at age-group level) may have already learnt how to compete, and know that they want this success, by the age of 12. They then spend the next few years looking for 'a sport that made sense' or 'the ticket to the party . . . . what would take me there' (both quotes from SB). The same ideas ring true across other performance domains: really talented youngsters may often move from one domain to another in search of 'the best vehicle for their talents' (quote from RR – an individual with prodigious and annoying levels of talent in many different extreme sports). The point here is that special individuals are . . . well, special! It is unfortunate that so many errors seem to be made around so rare a commodity. For example, how many talented youngsters are turned off an activity, maybe even all activity, for life by overexploitation and overwork at the hands of an often well meaning coach/teacher (see comments on 'life balance'). As the other side of this coin, how many infant world-class performers are spoilt by overpraise, overexposure and underwork?

The panel all talked about the need for 'reality' when dealing with precocious talent. The mentor role is often crucial here for keeping the aspirant elite on track, maintaining focus on the long game of adult performance rather than the quick hits of success and acclaim today. Two important points should be made about mentor recruitment, however: first, the need to avoid role conflicts. It should be recognized that the teacher/coach role and mentor role fulfil quite different functions and it is not necessary, indeed it can be very hard, for one person to do both. Furthermore a parent should not automatically act as a mentor. Parents already have an important relationship with the performer and attempting to simultaneously act as mentor means that inevitably one of these relationships will be compromised in the service of the other. In fact, it is usually better and less claustrophobic if two or three distinct individuals are involved, so long as their messages are coherent (see Ch. 5). Secondly, the mentor role is not necessarily best taken by a high-achieving ex-performer. Quite apart from what might be described as the 'Flashheart syndrome' – 'that's enough about me, now let's talk about me' (*Blackadder Goes Forth*), the role model can often more effectively model (exemplify and encourage) positive behaviours when closer in age and experience (e.g. a current performer, two or three stages ahead). Alternatively, when more distant in both age and experience (e.g. a parent-like figure, offering a realistic perspective on the often self-inflicted intensity of the performance environment), the mentor can act as an independent sounding board and source of wisdom. As ever, working relationships between two individuals require a complementary match to be found in line with their respective characteristics and preferences, so it is not possible to provide a definitive profile of a mentor, just as a definitive profile of a talented performer does not exist. What is clear, however, is that this role must be filled effectively as an important part of growing your superstar.

A further consideration relates to the developing performer's own values and self-schemata – literally, how they view themselves and the ways in which they reward themselves for various achievements. For example, consider one weekend for the 18-year-old javelin thrower SB. On the Saturday, in a British League Match (national) he threw 62 m and won by 30 m. Because of his 'prodigy' status, he then threw in a Grand Prix (international) on the Sunday, achieving second with a chuck of 75 m. It is worth considering which environment 'worked' for SB, which one he was most pleased with, and what this said about his potential for world-class competition in the future. Crucially, the extra distance 'generated' by the higher-pressure Grand Prix setting was an important learning point for SB – 'much more for no extra effort'. He used this insight, and his positive feelings around high-pressure competition, for the rest of his career.

For the well adjusted developing elite, common psychobabble sayings such as 'second is the first loser' are treated with the disdain they deserve, and effective progress towards elite status will involve a recognition that winning isn't the only thing at this level. Similar messages were suggested in the other performance environments. Resilience, be it physical (KB in team sports), mental (RR on taking the extreme sport challenges 'head on'), or emotional (coping with the inevitable roadblocks and checks to progress), was another essential characteristic to aim for. RR offered the quote from Confucius that could have been written for climbers everywhere: 'Our greatest glory is not in never falling, but in rising every time we fall'.

Keeping the high flier 'grounded' and taking personal responsibility for their progress (or lack thereof) was seen as another important cornerstone of effective TD. Even the genius prodigy will need firm handling at times, and all panel members were able to name some now high-profile performers who were cut from programmes, otherwise sanctioned and 'lured back from the dark side' of distraction, be it wine, (wo)men or song!

Finally, the PP made reference to what I will provocatively entitle 'the life balance myth' One of the protests raised against overinvolvement in an activity is that the young performer must maintain a life balance. In fact, all these terms, and the protests that result are completely relative. The point is that one person's balance is another's death knell; in simple terms, most enthusiasts, whether elite or not, are usually quite happy with lifestyles that others would view as harmful and dysfunctional. There are many examples of how the pathway to elite performance is viewed as unbalanced, but consider one common myth associated with deliberate practice. As well argued in Chapter 3, practice quantity/quality is important but this, in turn, depends on resources, effort and motivation. That is why other chapters make so much of developing the young performers' mental skills to ensure a positive attitude towards training. But is this training really so arduous? Note that, contrary to common perception, Ericsson did not say that deliberate practice was not enjoyable... just less enjoyable than other leisure activities such as TV. In simple terms, people engage in deliberate practice for later gains, be those next week or in 10 years' time. And therein lies the balance: namely, how the individual feels about and is affected by her/his involvement in the performance domain against all the other challenges of life. Good TID systems cater for, evaluate and work through this important perception, ensuring that each developing performer has, and can deploy, the necessary skills to self-monitor and adjust as pressures come and go. By this means we can ensure that each individual feels balanced and well adjusted, even if his/her training load and involvement seem superhuman (or even inhuman) to the uninformed/uninitiated observer. Reprising earlier points, note that the (self-perceived) balanced developing elite may make up this commitment with several activities or one; a busy lifestyle is likely to be a consistent feature, however.

So what should you do?

As I've said already, the chapters in this section are full of little nuggets of advice, together with some good applications and techniques. What might be missing is a way to synthesize all the information into guiding principles that can be applied to your own approach to structuring an effective talent development environment (TDE). So, here goes ....

Provide a comprehensive programme

The first step is to ensure your TDE meets the comprehensive needs of the developing performers. There are several ways to structure this. The way I approached this with Athletics is presented in Figure 6.1. Termed the 'Five Rings model', this aims to ensure an emphasis on all the key components.

The best way to consider this model is to look at the factors that cause derailment (dropping off the pathway) or limit performance in those performers who have achieved the top end. To offer an example, Table 6.1 presents some common issues from athletics. You might like to consider which combination of components from the Five Rings model (or, more accurately, lack thereof!) may underlie success/failure in each one, and consider how similar this situation is to your own performance domain.

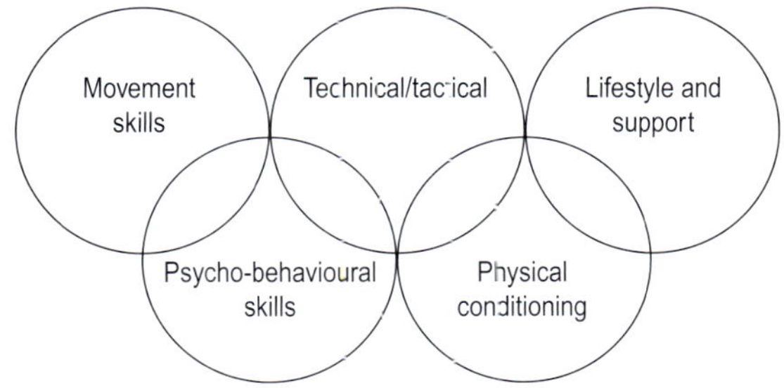

Fig. 6.1 • The 'Five Rings' skills package.

Once you have completed your 'audit' on derailers and limiters, you need to ensure that the necessary skills are in place and practised before the time when the issue would kick in (see Chs 2 and 4). Once again, an example may help. Many performance domains suffer with a substantial dropout during the transition from school to university (see Ch 4 for more discussion on this). Reasons for this often relate to interactions between poor mental skills (see Ch. 5), a lack of preparation for the newly autonomous lifestyle (can they cook, for example, or at least wait for an appropriate 'ping' from the microwave?) and an insufficient training base to cope with the changes (of coach, of workload, of approach) that usually occur.

Sensible TDEs, and well organized TDers, will address these possible limitations proactively, usually through a combination of formal and informal educational activity, peer and role model mentoring, discussion and planning involving domain-related significant others, and early liaisons with the new setup. For sport governing bodies or other performance organizations, it should be clear who is responsible for ensuring that all this takes place and accountable for excessive loss of talent! In this regard, there is a clear need for academy structures that aim to eliminate any roadblocks to progress while easing the pathway to avoid dropouts. As KB observed, academies are a process not a building. If you are part of a performance-focused organization, designing and deploying your own bespoke model should be of central importance. You could do a lot worse than the Five Rings model, if only as a starting point.

Table 6.1 Common derailers/limiters (and possible solutions) in track and field athletics: solutions draw on combinations of factors from the Five Rings

Observed behaviour	Caused by/shown by	Solutions may include . . .
Early promise 'collapses' under pressure	Self confidence damage 'hamstrings' athlete, preventing realization of full potential Lack of clear work ethic makes 'last 1%' gains even harder to achieve. As a result, confidence goes even lower	Specific work on confidence, using positive gains demonstrated by regular review 'Process' focus, stressing small but steady gains in component factors (e.g. strength, new technique, etc.)
Athletes can perform, but are extremely 'delicate'	High injury rates Need for a 'careful hand', meaning that training is often less than optimum Over-reliance on therapy. Consequent limitations on training and confidence	Early screening for weaknesses, then constant and monitored emphasis on improvement Emphasis on personal control – coach and performer, with specialist input (e.g. S & C, physio, Pilates, etc.)
High(ish) rise – quick fall	Excellent youth performances but leaves the sport. Always struggling to realize what they have 'obviously' got 'Could have been a contender' syndrome in athlete and coach, who moan about what 'might have been if *they*. . .'	Long term individualized developmental agenda De-emphasize today's success. Use a personalized set of targets against what each performer should achieve Realistic aspirations for coach, performer *and* parents
Fantastic physical potential but. . .!	Can't learn, won't learn Excuse City – always a reason why things haven't happened	Stress development in all components Realistic performance evaluations AND consequent action plans
They just don't quite make/have 'it'	Persistent (semi) finalist 'Lovely person. . .!' Shy and retiring 'cos that's a good place to be	Work on support and reward systems (e.g. family) Realistic aspirations What *do* they want to achieve? Is that OK with you?

Whatever system you end up with, it needs to be multilayered, with entry, exit and (a crucial but rare one, this) re-entry opportunities well established and understood. Significantly, these same criteria apply whether you are running a local talent group, a regional academy or centre, or a national programme. As Chapter 2 shows, the path to possible elite status is a long and winding one. The long-termism that we suggest is essential but will mean that some may 'come and go' from the process, unless you have limitless resources to keep the numbers in your special squad growing. As already highlighted, some individuals may be perfect for specific roles, or best suited to age-group challenges, but fall away when demands change. Quite apart from the human issues of discouragement, kids who drop out or who are dropped will often bounce back unless the system fails to cater for efficient and smooth re-entry to the programme/domain, or builds walls when they leave sufficient to discourage them from ever trying again.

Similar considerations apply to those of very high potential, the youngsters who seem to have it all. When dealing with precocious high-potentials, TDEs have to teach and develop/deploy the skills to prevent premature stardom, which in turn leads to variants of the usually terminal 'too-much-too-young' disease. As media attention becomes all-pervading and 24 hours a day, even low-key activities will be scanned regularly for news- or noteworthy items. As stressed throughout all the chapters in this section, keeping the genuine prodigies on track and grounded is a hard challenge, and messages may sometimes have to be fairly direct. *Suspending your Superstar* is not a bestselling book yet, but a development coach or teacher with the skills to know when to cut will be more effective than one who throws attention and emotional resource at a youngster who will eventually fail because they haven't the personal wherewithal to stand alone. All the PP members stressed the need for this hard but fair interpersonal style, which is at its most crucial when dealing with high-skilled and high-status potential. This message, in its many variations, is emphasized in the next two guidelines.

Provide a clear and consistent message

The need for the 'Five Rings' characteristics, or at least the mental skills component, should be clear from the ideas presented in the chapters within this section. In terms of actually realizing this, there are probably three key considerations. The first is to ensure that messages are clearly sent by using feedback systems that engage the developing performer and his/her significant others in conversation about progress and areas for attention. Chapter 24 will offer a useful tool (specifically Fig. 24.1) for this purpose. Briefly for the moment, the Athlete Performance Potential Template (APPT) is presented to performer and coach/teacher for completion. Discussion on the scores they award themselves, even more crucially the reasons why, helps to ensure a common and clear understanding of what the individual's ideal TDE will look like.

The second is to ensure consistency by engaging with all parties who are likely to have influence on the developee. Clearly, this will involve the parents, teachers and any other coaches/teachers involved. Less obvious, however, is the need to consider what messages the young performer is getting from his/her own peers. We all understand how important other people's thoughts are, especially in adolescence, which is the most common age range for aspirant elites in established TDEs. Accordingly, coaches or teachers in TDEs should constantly explore the conceptions and structures employed by developees and their significant others, using discussions, role models, videos and individual performer plans to monitor (and, if necessary, refine). Not only does this offer an essential check, it also encourages the development of declarative knowledge (the why knowledge – see Ch. 15), which helps the developee to understand, and therefore eventually further enhance, the development process.

The third key consideration is to 'never assume', and to use a variety of methods to check that the developee is completely au fait with what is expected of them, their current status and exactly where they need to go. A lack of conciseness and clarity is going to result in some very sad and bitter people later on, especially when the youngster is 'cut' from the group because of lack of progress. The approaches presented in the previous two paragraphs offer some means for 'check and balance'. To meet this particular need, however, it is essential to monitor – and adjust as necessary – the views held by the developees and their supporters. More value-added benefits here as well: the monitoring and feedback checks ensure that each individual has a realistic expectation of where they can get and knows where they are and what they need to do. Additionally and very positively, they generate an atmosphere of honesty, helping to ensure that all concerned believe what they are told and mutually encourage each other towards the genuine message.

Work on the 'feel and traditions' of your TDE

The detailed characteristics of the optimum TDE are covered in Chapter 5. However, the really effective 'talent factory' will go beyond these important but mechanistic procedures, establishing a social microcosm that all will remember with affection, pride and respect. This doesn't mean that the TDE is soft and fluffy, far from it, in fact. I am ex-military, and look back with these feelings on my basic training. No, I don't recommend that it be a boot camp either, although I do stress that some will fail to make it through any really worthwhile process (see Ch. 9 on 'peak performance organizations' and 'inspirational members')!

What I am suggesting is a supportive but pushy environment; a place where success and failure are personally referenced; a place where each individual is pushed to explore and extend her/his limits. The high-performing TDE will exude work ethic and enthusiasm; members will be competitive but collaborative, pleased when peers do well, dissatisfied when they don't themselves or when others let the side down. The environment will encourage high-quality work, interspersed with some 'team building' fun challenges. Anything that builds the right social setting will contribute to performance – it doesn't have to be domain-specific, just timely (best to avoid white-water rafting or 50 km bike rides 2 months before an Olympics, for example.... Yes, it did happen!). When inspecting your TDE, remember that quality practice is one of the key PCDEs; as SB points out: 'I was never a long trainer but I was a very intense trainer'.

If you think this sounds unrealistically idyllic, please think again. First of all, this sort of relationship is the norm in genuine elite environments. SB spent a lot of time working with Jan Zelezney, the world record holder in the javelin who was his nemesis at

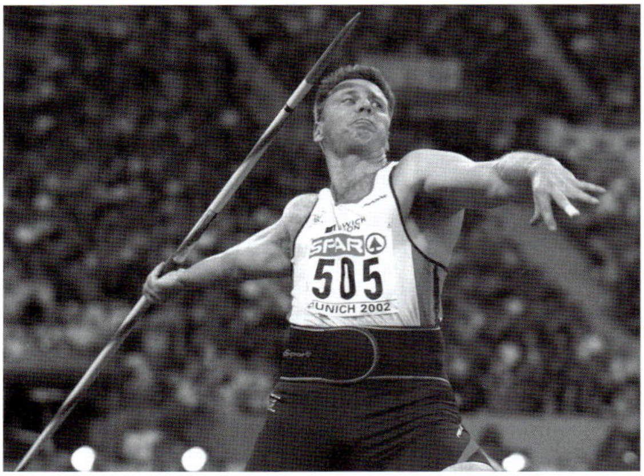

Performance Panel member Steve Backley winning his fourth European Gold at the 2002 Championships. © Mark Shearman Sports Photography. Reprinted with kind permission.

two Olympics (although Steve did beat him at the Europeans!). Rugby provides the recent example of two very high-profile and rather 'determined' characters who made a mutual non-aggression pact to help each other look good in practice and matches. This worked so well that these two previously antagonistic players both succeeded; in fact, one bought the other an expensive watch as a vote of thanks when he was selected to the England side. Even in the 'ego-rich' area of sprinting, top performers will often spend time together for mutual benefit; a combination of enhanced physical challenge, novel training ideas and a refreshing change from the norm all serve to rejuvenate both parties. The point is that elites often need the stimulus challenge of working with other elites, and developing elites should be no different.

Secondly, and as already described, development is enhanced by teaching others. Looking at your peers, considering their weaknesses and helping them address these benefits you as well. Finally, the push for collaboration helps to reinforce the fact that the important performance is yet to come. As already discussed, situations with real challenge inevitably entail exposure to the experience of failure but these moments in the development stage should be focused on the needs of the individual and represent critical learning experiences designed for performer-specific purposes.

This position is in stark contrast to those who condemn performance situations with the potential for failure as harmful for children: failure isn't negative, but an individual's issues or those imbued by significant others often make it so. In fact, learning to experience failure and setbacks well (to make use of the experience for overall development through realistic evaluations of good and bad points) is an essential step for all developers. For example, if a young dancer cannot cope with being 'upstaged' by other performers or performances, s/he will lack the ability to fully benefit from the interpersonal challenge that is inevitably part of any thriving school or company experience. In short, you shouldn't like failing but you shouldn't hate it so much that your self-beating is terminal!

Focus on the quality, not the quantity

This parameter is pretty central to the whole process but could be reworded in several ways to reflect its different components, all of which can influence (either positively or negatively) the impact and eventual outcome of the TD process. The problem you face is the apparently straightforward and definite advice so beloved of coaches but so very rarely correct! So simple guidance like the 10 000 hours rule or the need to fully exploit age-related windows of opportunity (see Balyi's Long term Athlete Development model (Balyi & Hamilton 2003)) are seductively clear and simple, leading many to accept and apply them enthusiastically but uncritically.

This 'trap' is avoided by careful consideration of the equally clear but slightly less simple guidelines that should emerge from careful study of this section. So the imperative for getting the right coach/teacher can be met by using the information in the preceding chapters to provide a checklist as to the best approach. Or how about 'Don't specialize too early'; by far the biggest factors in getting youngsters to specialize too soon relate to keeping them focused solely on that performance, making the teacher or coach look good and satisfying ego needs for success, be they the performer's, the organization's or even the parents'. Another pertinent aphorism might be 'Don't fall for the critical windows trap'. There is very little, if any, evidence for the existence of the critical windows for aspects of physical or mental development (Bailey et al 2009).

As KB points out, developing a young (in his case) rugby player is best achieved by developing an individual with a broad range of talents, the capacity and mental skill for hard work and the adaptability to change role, position or even sport as opportunities arise and full maturity is reached.

And finally... acknowledge and exploit the 'educational' benefits

Win–win situations are rare in life and, to date at any rate, many have seen a high commitment to a performance domain as likely to limit other aspects of life. Possibly the best news to emerge from this section is that this need not be so. Firstly, the physical skills developed in good academy environments can equip the developee for a successful life in many other physical domains. If your setup is well designed (see my earlier comments) you can often benefit from well trained transfers from other systems.

Secondly, and most pertinently, the skills described in this section, especially the psychobehavioural skills, are those that beget excellence whatever the performance domain. In short, graduation from an effective academy-style process built on these principles will equip the developee for life, providing skills that enable them to succeed wherever they choose to focus their endeavours. This idea of physical activity as 'character building' is seen as a myth by some. However, there is little doubt that the mental approach for success transfers well from arena to arena; consider Sebastian Coe (running to politics), Fran Cotton (rugby to the clothing business), Deborah Bull (dance to media), Gary Lineker (football to media via crisp sales) and Chris Bonnington (mountaineering to media). If your TDE is focused on developing these same skills (and this whole section offers evidence that it should), it is going to make an enormous contribution to all your performers, even if they don't make it in your own particular domain.

Finally, these same reasons make it a lot easier (and more morally acceptable) to encourage parents to support their children in committing to the development process. The point here is that, when done properly, the TD process is genuinely educational in the broadest sense. As such, commitment to your programme becomes a logical step, rather than a risk or dream chasing exercise. As an added benefit, you might consider emphasizing the developmental message within the performance environment (as highlighted by the examples in the previous paragraph), rather than possibly watering down or de-emphasizing the performance focus while paying lip service to the 'life-development' agenda.

Timing and make up of broader 'educational' activities also deserve deliberation. Consider once more the classic academy environment, where youngsters mad keen to make it are 'force fed' education. The motive is completely laudable: most won't make it and need something to turn to after football/dance/rugby (insert name of challenging environment here). How much do these individuals really benefit from this dual focus, however? Some alternative to the constant performance focus helps but, if this performance focus is genuinely developmental for the whole person as highlighted throughout this section, many of these educational resources (which are usually compromised in any case) can be kept and awarded as a 'parachute payment' once it becomes clear that their dream of the premiership/major company, etc. is unlikely to be realized. This sort of demob exit strategy works well in the military, meaning that resources are provided when individuals are both emotionally ready and optimally motivated to make use of them. It is doable and acceptable to parents so long as the performance environment can be shown to be making a demonstrable difference to the aspirant performer; which is, of course, exactly what it should be doing!

Conclusion

I hope that these perspectives and experiences from the panel help to contextualize the advice in the previous chapters. Even if, as a practitioner, you find some of the theory to be hard going, it repays the effort spent working thorough the arguments and evidence. There are always plenty of 'new miracle' techniques emerging in performance, especially in this hot-topic area of TD. A thorough understanding of the underpinning principles, coupled with regular selective dives into the research, will help to ensure that your TDE stays in world-class shape.

In similar fashion, researchers and academics in performance psychology must acknowledge the applied nature of this area. Regular consideration of the 'so whats?' of research findings will help to keep work relevant and genuinely useful to the field it is designed (or should be designed!) to inform.

References

Bailey, R., Collins, D., Ford, P., et al., 2009. Participant development in sport: an academic review. Report commissioned by Sports Coach UK, Leeds.

Balyi, I., Hamilton, A., 2003. Long-term athlete development update: trainability in childhood and adolescence. Faster Higher Stronger 20 (July), 6–8.

Berry, J., Abernethy, B., Cote, J., 2008. The contribution of structured activity and deliberate play to the development of expert perceptual and decision-making skill. Journal of Sport and Exercise Psychology 30, 685–708.

Section 2

Provision (of support)

Introduction: organizational issues in providing support

7

Dave Collins
Grey Matters/UCLan

The contents of this next section are crucial for the design and implementation of an effective performance support system. Given this importance, it is very surprising that, to date at any rate, these considerations have received very little consideration in performance psychology texts. All the more surprising since the quality assurance of support structures, unfortunately almost always on a unidisciplinary basis, is an obvious concern or even raison d'être for most professional associations such as the BASES or AAASP in sport, or BPS and APA in mainstream psychology (see Conclusion for a more thorough consideration).

In simple terms, it seems as if everyone acknowledges the need for support from an increasing number of specialist disciplines. It is also clear that performance organizations and/or funders recognize the importance of systems and structures in the achievement of excellence. However, very few authors (or planners or assessors) have employed the tools from cogent domains to examine the processes that underpin this support. Accordingly, that was the starting point when we considered the design of this book and this section: namely, to provide some critical consideration and guidance for how performance psychology (and related disciplines) may be most efficaciously employed to enhance performance.

In Chapter 8, Veronica Burke provides an overview of key concepts from the pertinent disciplines of organizational psychology and management. Students of sport psychology will spot much resonance in her work; concepts such as cohesion, role clarity and team identity are embedded with modern business thinking. Crucially, however, the different directions necessitated by the study of management provide a more performance-focused consideration. As such, the chapter provides a 'checklist' for the development of an effective organizational structure.

This theme is continued by Alan MacPherson in Chapter 9, where a wide range of considerations essential to effective group work are examined. The chapter is built around a series of exemplars drawn from the experiences of second author Pat Howard, who has enjoyed a prestigious career at the forefront of management in professional sport. Despite its rugby football flavour, the chapter offers a lens for critical examination of the team/large squad/company collective, which is the main structure in professional team and group activities. The overarching 'take-home message' lies with the initiation and maintenance of a performance culture in a team setting, a topic to which we return in the PP chapter at the end of the section.

In Chapter 10, John Kiely takes a big departure from his roots as a strength and conditioning specialist as he examines the considerations that should underpin the planning and deployment of a performance enhancement system. In many sports, this process is seen as highly scientific; built on the concept of periodization which is, for many practitioners and consumers, almost a science in itself. As John demonstrates, while there is 'some truth in the rumour', many of the sacred tenets of periodization are sacred cows! In fact, the science of prediction in performance, as with most other

DOI: 10.1016/B978-0-443-06734-1.00007-9

complex systems, is incredibly difficult. As such, the 'if... then... ' statements that are often taken as fact need very careful and critical application if the aims of 'peaking' are to be realized. The chapter demonstrates the importance of ongoing evaluation and refinement, almost an 'action research' approach, when working towards peak performance.

Finally, the PP chapter considers the implications and applications of these ideas when designing and managing your performance environment.

Organizing for excellence

8

Veronica Burke

Cranfield University, School of Management, Cranfield, Bedford, UK

CHAPTER CONTENTS

Introduction: the changing organizational environment

A substantial body of existing work in performance psychology has focused on aspects of mental skills training for individual performers such as controlling anxiety (Berger et al 2001), goal setting (Weinberg et al 2000), imagery (Hall 2001), concentration (Jackson & Csikszentmihalyi 1999), motivation (Smith 2001) and self-efficacy (McAuley & Blissmer 2002). However, it is essential for those working as performance practitioners (be they performers, performance managers, coaches, teachers or psychologists) to have a clear understanding of the support and pressure individuals may experience as a result of the organizational environment in which performance is developed, enhanced and maximized. Knowledge of this environment can help augment individual contribution and optimize performance while avoiding unnecessary disruptions and detrimental pressure that organizational structure might inadvertently exert. There are several dimensions of the organizational environment that are relevant in this regard. These are discussed in the following sections.

Conditions in the contemporary work environment have forced organizations to confront a 'flatter' organizational landscape, characterized by different political, economic and cultural variables (Friedman 2006). Government policies, changes to regulations and funding arrangements can all be influenced by global events and subsequent changes in priorities. The World-Wide Web has increased the sense of competitiveness for performance organizations while at the same time providing new ways of sharing knowledge and work to enable organizations to change and meet the competition. For example, performance practitioners can access information on the latest methodologies, research findings and professional expertise at the touch of a button. This way of working has also heralded a rise in part-time and flexible work patterns, including remote and virtual working, as employees increasingly comprise a vast, global pool of specialists. The impact of technological changes and abundant global communication has resulted in new ways in which people work together, where teams and individuals work flexibly without needing to be in the same place or work on tasks at the same time. This flexibility increases the capacity to collaborate with external partners and draw on a range of specialists for key areas of work. E-mail, search engines and sophisticated software

DOI: 10.1016/B978-0-443-06734-1.00008-0

enable intellectual capital to be delivered from anywhere – distributed and redesigned in a way that allows for new freedom in ways of working – especially work that requires brains as well as physical interaction.

Performers and performance practitioners frequently need to operate effectively in this new context. Rapid change and restructuring are commonplace, bringing with them uncertainty and fierce competition to achieve and then maintain the 'edge'. Whatever domain of the performance management environment people are working in, however, they can no longer afford to be parochial in their thinking. They must take account of changes in the wider environment likely to impact upon their work, such as new performance methods or techniques, leading edge research or pockets of expertise that may inform their practice.

What do these environmental changes mean for performance organizations such as professional sports teams, dance companies or institutes and governing bodies charged with developing elite performers? Given that organizations are essentially constituted of individuals, it is through the mechanism of individual contribution that organizational performance is optimized. It is therefore critical that the performance management team create an enabling context for performance – whether this is through supporting athletes, motivating coaches, developing performance managers or leading strategic change. At the local level, performance personnel are required to operate in dynamic settings in which organizational structures have become flatter and less hierarchical, where the lines of authority have become blurred and people move around (and out) of the organization in response to role changes or restructuring. At a practical level, there are fewer and less well defined stages in the decision-making chain as specialist knowledge can be accessed easily and directly and e-mail communication can dispense with some of the need for face-to-face meetings, speeding up the process.

The top-down 'rational' approach to organizational structure is not adequate in this new context and, in order to respond appropriately to these changes, managers, performers and support staff must develop strategies that fit the new realities. Management no longer represents the exclusive control of resource and information. Individuals have choices about where they focus their attention, how they behave and with whom they want to work. Increasingly, important decisions are arrived at through informal means via loosely configured networks of individuals, focused around common aims, coalitions or activities as the decision-making capability is dispersed more evenly throughout the organization. This context has heralded a change in the function of management, while these new circumstances have meant that performance practitioners must find ways to add value amidst uncertainty, scarce resources, competition and conflicting interests. Performance managers must look after their teams, compete for resources and manage the political dimension in order to achieve their objectives. In this new context, individual competence has become a crucial element in facilitating effective organizational performance. Table 8.1 represents these management changes, with associated examples.

Given these changes to the management role, the function of strategy becomes pivotal in ensuring organizational success. This means that the organization management and leadership group must have both a clear (as was always the case) and shared (a more recent imperative) understanding of where the organization is going – whether they are owners of an extreme sport team, the board of a football club or the executive group of a dance company. However, the task of setting strategy is one of the most complex tasks facing any management team.

Table 8.1 Changes to management function with associated exemplar implications

Management function	Example
Management no longer control resources	Responsibility for education, training and development budget given to staff member directly responsible for meeting goals to deploy in most effective way
Management no longer control information	With the Internet a team member can identify and contact directly key personnel in other areas of the organization without needing advice or input from a manager
Individuals choose what they do	An athlete and coach may select where and when to complete warm weather training or which events to enter to prepare for major event
Individuals choose with whom they do it	An injured performer harnesses the best national or international medical and rehabilitation expertise for advice, diagnosis and intervention

Pertinent management constructs for performance organizations

Strategy

Whatever area of performance development an organization is concerned with – whether dance, sport, adventure, or education – there must be a clear strategy. 'Some view of where and how the firm is trying to compete gives confidence to managers from the top downwards. It assists managers in making resourcing decisions, and it can instil a sense of purpose' (Bowman 1998, p. 1).

Strategy includes the aims, objectives and models of working that are central to the performance management setup. In short, strategy is about setting the long-term direction of the organization in order to achieve maximum success through the deployment of resources with the aim of fulfilling stakeholder expectations (Johnson et al 2005). In effect, this translates into the need for a shared understanding among key stakeholders, be they performers, managers, coaches, performance directors or support staff, about what they are trying collectively to achieve and where they want to go. Achieving this level of agreement is complex because the starting point is often an uncertain future. Much is written about mission statements and visionary leadership but perhaps a more usable notion is the one of 'being on purpose' (Pedlar et al 2004, p. 119). This idea is consistent with the notion that strategy making is a process that involves organizational members working together with a shared purpose that embodies core values. Everyone in the organization should know what the major goal is for the next 3 years and the underlying principles and values governing how they want to operate to achieve this. For the board of a sport governing body for example, this would mean working out the long-term objectives for development of the sport, such as improved number of medals or world rankings. In turn, this might require a multifaceted approach such as increased quantity and quality of domestic competition, more coaches taking qualifications at higher levels, targeting resources more specifically, based on refined criteria, reducing inefficiencies and greater retention of participants in transition from junior to senior levels. A clear goal provides focus for specifying clear priorities for performance management and establishes a number of tasks that the organization can monitor, and measure its progress towards achieving. The clear vision or raison d'être generated by strategy is to ensure the long-term survival of the organization, not about short-term, quick-fix approaches, and therefore frequently combines and balances both current performance and future development related activities.

However difficult strategy making may be, it is not an option but a requirement Without a clearly expressed, well understood and consistently executed strategy, an organization risks letting day-to-day short-term operational issues take up time at the expense of ensuring that priority tasks are completed, goals are met and the organization delivers successfully. Not only is strategy an essential requirement for performance organizations, it must also be developed and perceived to be developed by individuals at all levels. It is misguided to imply that strategy is the preserve of those at the top of the organization. Using this logic, the job of strategy is only for a few senior people: 'Our senior management used to be very hands-on and involved in everything. Then we had an inspection in which they were told they weren't sufficiently strategic. Since then we haven't set eyes on any of them' (Pedlar et al 2004, p. 120).

It is highly unlikely that the selected strategy can be achieved if the strategy is only known to a few. In order for the strategy to be collectively understood, the people responsible for initiating strategy formulation must develop ways of involving stakeholders in the process, of creating an engaging, long-term vision for the future and crucially, translating this into relevant activity to ensure the ongoing success of the organization.

Strategy making can be translated at three different levels – corporate, business and operational (Bowman 1998). Corporate strategy is made within large organizations (e.g. Sport England) where there are several autonomous operational departments or business units. An important consideration at this level is the rationale for grouping particular units together, as the organization of these must inform the way in which the units are managed from corporate headquarters. This process also determines the role of the corporate centre in the management of the units. In sum, there must be a logic for the grouping of units together, however they are configured.

The next level of strategy is at the individual business level. This would apply, for example, to organizations such as the CCPR, Outward Bound, UK

Athletics or the Royal Academy of Dance, which, although they have important stakeholders to manage, are not part of a corporate umbrella. The key question at the business level (and by business I refer to the core activities of the organization, whether these are concerned with physical education, dance or adventure sport) is how to remain successful. By implication, this requires a fundamental review of the rationale for the business unit. Key questions at this level include: Where do we want to excel? How should we do this and what is required for us to perform in the long term? What competencies do we need to realize this ambition and how should we organize our activities? In the light of these questions, the fundamental consideration is concerned with where we are now versus where we want to be (Bowman 1998).

Finally, operational strategy has a focus at the functional level. Most performance organizations have a specialized structure whereby people work in a subset of the overall tasks, for example elite performance, support services, education or grass roots development. Operational strategy is therefore concerned with the organization and direction of these functional areas. It would seem obvious that the business level strategy should be aligned with and inform the development of the operational strategy. However, in practice this is not always the case. One of the dangers is that each functional area can interpret the business strategy in a way that suits itself. This is not uncommon and may be done unintentionally as organizational members make sense of the strategic direction in the light of their own preferences and agendas. The three levels of strategy making are summarized in Table 8.2.

Making good-quality strategy is related to leadership capability, as there will inevitably be tensions between what might be desired and what is realistically achievable. The process of arriving at answers to these fundamental questions is driven by the values, beliefs and attitudes of those who are making strategy – usually those holding leadership positions – but should also explicitly involve the perspectives of those positioned vertically through the organization. Inevitably, strategy making is a messy process involving negotiation and management of competing interests and aspirations. Managing this political dimension is an important part of leadership function and will be discussed in more detail later.

Bowman (1998, p. 9) provides a useful framework for understanding how strategy is debated in organizations. He suggests three zones of debate:

Table 8.2 Strategy development within an organization

Level	Example	Nature of strategy	Key consideration
Corporate	Sport England	Direction of strategic business units by corporate headquarters	Must have logical rationale for grouping units
Business	CCPR UK Athletics	Review of rationale for business units	How to remain successful (against a clear statement of what success actually is)
Operational	Marketing function of a fitness franchise	Organization of functional areas	Linking the operational units together so they are aligned with the business strategy

1. The Zone of Comfortable Debate (ZOCD)
2. The Zone of Uncomfortable Debate (ZOUD)
3. The Intuitive Core.

In the Zone of Comfortable Debate, the main issues are avoided. Discussions are characterized by a comfortable feel about proceedings. The dialogue stays within acceptable boundaries and is not likely to have any real implications for individuals. Ambitious suggestions may be made in the safe knowledge that nothing is likely to happen anyway. In the ZOCD, there may be a focus on complaining about competitors, talking about irrelevant issues (e.g. car parking) or moaning about the status quo – in effect, rearranging the deckchairs on the Titanic! In order to get to the heart of strategy making, it is necessary to get into the Zone of Uncomfortable Debate.

The ZOUD is characterized by a heightened awareness and interest in real and relevant core issues. Unfortunately, a typical response is an attempt to diffuse the tension by prompting a slide back into the ZOCD. It is therefore up to those involved to keep the discussion in the ZOUD amidst attempts to throw the debate off track, animosity between individuals and the presence of dominant individuals intent on discrediting others' contributions in order to secure strategic decisions in support of their own agenda. Dealing with these issues is (or at least should be) an expected, routine experience for strategy makers (Butcher & Clarke 2001).

The final level of debate relates to the Intuitive Core. This refers to the collective assumptions and values held by the team and taken for granted. The more the team share common experiences, the less likely it is that these assumptions and beliefs will be brought into the open. Unless they are, it will be difficult for people to conceive of a different future for the organization. By getting into the ZOUD, the team are more likely to question these assumptions and be critical of the intuitive 'filter' through which they see the world.

At the individual level, strategy making requires people with a mindset or work orientation that enables them to see the bigger picture, who can envisage an ambitious but realistic future and who can be critical about the past, present and future. They also need to be able to help people get into the ZOUD and challenge assumptions previously held as fundamental to the organization This debate must happen among the strategy makers themselves and time has to be set aside from routine meetings for this to happen. This process could usefully utilize the contribution of skilled performance psychology practitioners to stimulate perspective taking, challenge key assumptions and debate the status quo. These specialists may also be a good source of independent external advice. The quality of the strategy will depend fundamentally on the value of the ideas and commitment to these by senior managers. Effective strategic management also requires that strategy makers work in partnership with all organizational members to secure commitment to the actions required for successful implementation.

Organizational structures

The structure that any organization takes must fit with the strategy that has been developed. An explicit and coherent link between the strategic direction and the organizational structure will optimize individual contribution and improve organizational performance. An appropriate structure enables key activities to be planned, directed and monitored (Mullins 2002). There are many factors to be considered to determine the most appropriate configuration, such as tasks and responsibilities, work roles and relationships, and channels of communication. The primary function of such structure is the division of work among organizational members and the synchronization of their activities.

In the last 50 years, the dominant 'top-down' hierarchical structure associated with the command and control style of working has been fundamentally challenged (Stewart 1999). This model was characterized by a few individuals at the top who held control and many more at the bottom, with several layers of bureaucracy in between. In this model, communication was assumed to be a linear process with authority for decision making resting with those at the appropriate hierarchical level. The increased use of team approaches, an emphasis on individual accountability, outsourcing of specialist services, and involvement of people in strategy have resulted in design efforts to loosen the bureaucracy and speed up decision making (Birchall 2001). The traditional notion of hierarchy has become obsolete in this new environment (Butcher 2001). The 'flatter' landscape, characterized by global web-based ways of sharing knowledge and work, and self-organizing, collaborative communities, has forced organizations to adapt to more flexible ways of working (Friedman 2006). The conditions of this landscape require organizations to make rapid decisions and respond flexibly to changing conditions. It is certainly not uncommon for performance practitioners to experience some form of organizational restructuring as teams, project groups and departments are streamlined to fit changing priorities. New coaching techniques, moves to change legislation, media pressure, increased funding demands and the need to justify performance to key stakeholders are just some of the conditions that require a response from the organization and it is essential that the structure supports this.

Accordingly, new organizational structures have emerged that seek to balance the vertical and functional work units with task forces that work across the organization. In many of these emergent forms, the hierarchy is flattened, much of the work is carried out in project teams and people frequently work remotely. Specialists are often employed as consultants to respond to specific needs or issues. The matrix structure is one notable example which combines two different types of structure – functional and project-based – such that people report to two bosses rather than one (Buchanan & Huczynski 2004, p. 481). Hence there is a dual rather than a single reporting line, which occurs because, in a matrix, one type of structure has been

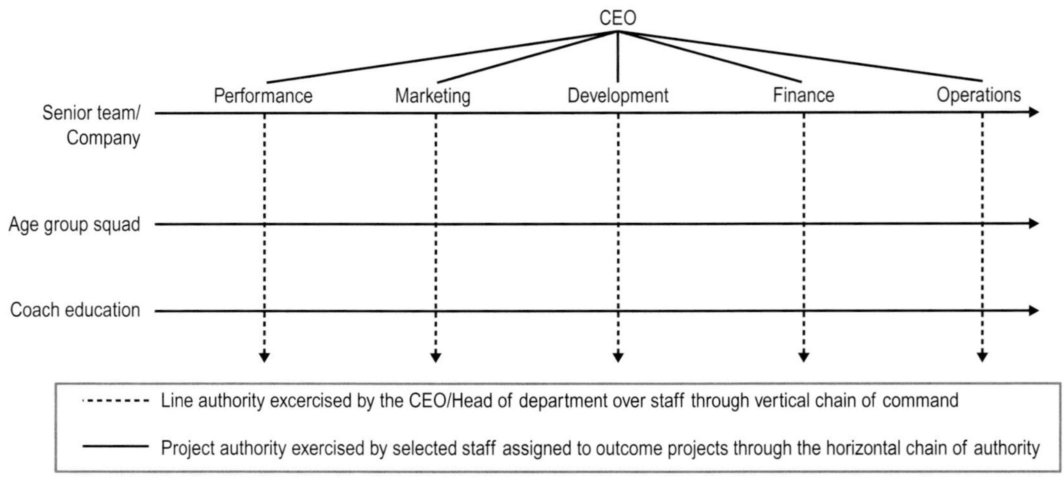

Fig. 8.1 • A hypothetical matrix structure in a sports national governing body.

superimposed upon another (Fig. 8.1). In performance management terms, this type of design can be seen where individuals report to one boss for the functional aspects of the role – e.g. finance, coaching, performance, research or events – and to another for a particular project or product such as a performance review programme or specialist coaching function. In athletics, for example, a javelin thrower may report to the senior performance manager for the functional dimension and a senior throws coach for the product. In educational institutions such as the Royal Academy of Dance, the reporting line may be to the head of department for the functional aspects of the role, e.g. ballet, and to the Director for a particular programme of study, e.g. a certificate or diploma for the product. Both bosses may also report to the same person, such as a performance director or dean of faculty, who coordinates the activities of both.

This sounds very attractive, and many performance organizations see themselves as already in, or moving towards, this system. The matrix design may be chosen under the following circumstances (Mullins 2005, p. 618):

- The organization has to have more than one critical orientation, i.e. functional and project-based. Hence the work of the organization is delivered through formal reporting lines as well as via functional teams that deliver specific projects or services.
- There is a requirement to concurrently process large amounts of information. This could involve, for example, coordinating the efforts of a variety of internal and external stakeholders in the management of a performer. Under these circumstances, the performance management function requires the creation of groupings based on project teams and the matrix design satisfies this need.
- There should be a need to share resources, which may involve the coordination of external support staff or professional services such as physiotherapists or psychologists. Thus it is necessary for members of staff from a variety of departments or functional areas to be assigned to a team for the duration of a defined project.

Matrix structures offer the advantage of flexibility in decision making, streamlining of resources and opportunities for staff development. However, they require people to work across functions in a more complex structure. Hence there may be problems in defining the extent of the project manager's influence over staff and of gaining the support of functional managers for particular projects. It has been suggested that an underlying difficulty with the matrix design is that divided loyalties and role conflict may arise as people report to more than one boss (Bartlett & Ghoshal 1990). However, this is a moot point since, arguably, role conflict, communication difficulties and lack of accountability are problems that beset most organizations at one time or another – whatever their structural configuration. Essentially, the emergence of new organizational structures requires leaders to deploy a high level of functional expertise alongside the capability to create an enabling context for performance at all organizational levels (Senior 2002). Leaders who are able to

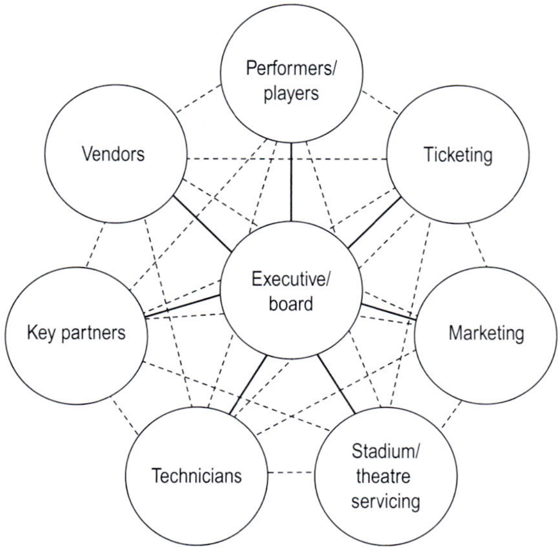

Fig. 8.2 • A hypothetical managed network structure in a professional club or company.

effectively deploy this capability are likely to add value to the organization, wherever they sit in the formal hierarchy.

An alternative to the matrix structure is the 'managed network' (Pettigrew & Fenton 2000), a loosely coupled organizational structure consisting of several interacting units with a central core unit that sets strategic direction and manages performance (Fig. 8.2). In this design, knowledge is shared among networks of organizational members and this informal structure gives rise to communication that is non-linear – people come together and disband as the work dictates. Like any network, it relies on responsible self-organization rather than tidy ordering of responsibilities and is more about organizing than organization (Pedlar et al 2004, p. 246).

The dilemma with this model is what to retain in the core. Networks may prove to be an attractive possibility for performance management organizations because of the flexibility they provide in service delivery. However, they pose a considerable challenge to those who prefer to operate in the command and control mode. Hastings (1993) cites a useful set of principles for operating in the managed network using the example of W.L. Gore & Associates, the makers of GoreTex. In this company, all units are small (150 people maximum), everyone is an associate and people choose their own work tasks subject to peer feedback and discipline. Associates is governed by four key principles, identified in Box 8.1.

Box 8.1

Principles governing behaviour in a managed network

- Work to principles of fairness in all transactions
- Encourage development of employees
- Honour business and personal commitments
- Consult with colleagues about all major business decisions

Source: Adapted from Hastings 1993, p. 15–16.

A central idea in the managed network is to create ways of working that add value to all who are associated with the organization, be they performers, funding body personnel or consultants. In performance management terms, this kind of structure may be appropriate for organizations where teams come together to provide services to the performer on an ad hoc basis. Examples include selection panels, ethics committees or performance testing events. In reality, although networks are apparently loose and fluid forms, they are always managed to an extent (Pedlar et al 2004). Under these circumstances, the challenge for performance practitioners lies in how to maximize the advantages of the network design while at the same time retaining the minimum requirements for organizational control. Making this design work depends a great deal upon the quality of relationships between people, as responsibility is devolved to the members across the structure and everyone has a role in organizing their contribution.

In determining and designing organizational structure, performance practitioners need to consider the formal and technological requirements of the work, the underlying principles of possible structures (e.g. matrix or network) and social factors such as the needs of the members. This last factor is critical in order to encourage commitment to participate in the selected structure and ensure the basis for optimal organizational performance.

Role clarity

Roles are a feature of every organization – even when the organization represents a set of specialists, as is the case in many performance environments. Roles are represented in the organizational hierarchy and the structure is specified through the spectrum of roles that the stakeholders are expected to play

(Buchanan & Huczynski 2004). This spectrum is likely to include roles associated with leadership, management and operations – although the precise configuration will vary according to the structure. People's roles are usually ranked by status; hence individuals occupying managerial roles are likely to be accorded more status than those at operational levels. Roles can be defined as the expected behaviours of the person occupying a particular position in the organization, such as Performance Director for example. Thus the roles of coach, mentor or performance manager may be associated with certain behavioural expectations. If roles are clearly delineated and there is a good 'degree of fit' between specified responsibilities, accountability and expectations, then it is more likely that role holders will be able to deploy the behaviours required of them.

Performance in a role is often the result of factors besides individual ability. Ostensibly, every individual accepting a role within an organization enters into an unwritten micro-contract with the organization that is beyond the capacity of any formal legal contract to capture. This is because of the detail and time-specificity that would make it impossible to contract formally. Thus, for the individual accepting a role, factors such as increased opportunity to travel or a new set of responsibilities or opportunities to undertake activities that might be considered to aid promotion may all be considered as part of the micro-contract for accepting a role. Working to a new philosophy, clearly stated by the executive but at odds with what has gone before, is another example of unwritten but 'should be' explicit contractual expectation.

Other individuals in the organization also hold their own, detailed view of what the role might include and these views may vary, be illogical or be based on poor knowledge of exactly what is involved. Nevertheless, if there is a mismatch between the role holder's expectations and those of other powerful people in the organization, this can lead to frustrations that are manifest through interpersonal difficulties (Slack 1997). Prouty (1988) describes how, when he was appointed as Director of the United States Cycling Federation, he was seen to be assuming responsibilities previously undertaken by board members, which resulted in attempts to have him fired. Hence, the extent to which key stakeholders accept the individual in the role, and are clear what the role is, is an important dimension in successful role performance.

Even when roles have been clearly defined, the problem of 'compliance versus commitment' is a common issue. How often have performance managers been heard to complain that they believed they had secured agreement to a particular course of action only to find that this had not been achieved? Because they had discussed what needed to be done and had apparently clarified responsibilities, the assumption was that progress would be made. In this scenario, compliance has been achieved but commitment is another matter. It may of course be some time before the situation is noticed and the delay can have a significant impact upon performance. Hence, although the formal structures indicate what people in the organization are supposed to be doing (e.g. via formal and apparently clearly understood job descriptions or role specifications), there may be a lack of clarity about, or commitment to, who does what in organizational terms. Efforts to surface assumptions and document changes to achieve agreement may help to surface unspoken agendas but this is a complex managerial problem. A useful starting point is to consider the personal and organizational agendas of individuals. People who understand their own and others' motives are likely to recognize that, in today's organizations, the neat alignment of individual and organizational agendas is not realistic. Rather, they understand that organizations are forums of self-interest and that it is necessary to recognize and work through these motives to deliver a worthwhile organizational contribution. Such managers take personal responsibility for specific projects, even when they run counter to the status quo (Butcher & Clarke, 2008, p. 112). In other words, they are prepared to challenge the current organizational situation, surface unspoken agendas and recognize the difficulties of achieving agreement because they are motivated to find new ways to deliver value to the business – even when this activity apparently falls outside the remit of 'formal' management work.

While it would be difficult to argue against the importance of role clarity in performance management contexts, achieving this aim can prove problematic. The process requires clarification of roles in relation to the overall strategy via a mechanism that 'unpacks' the behaviours associated with individual and team responsibilities and allows for them to be measured against appropriate criteria. However, engagement in this process by all involved is crucial and it is with this agenda that performance managers must connect. Above all, it is worth remembering that, whatever the formal role structure, it is frequently the informal (political) networks that prove to be significant in driving change. No matter what level they are working at, performance practitioners have the opportunity to exert influence, whether this is on an individual basis or by working with others to identify thought leaders who are able to initiate change by acting as 'cultural architects' (see Ch. 24 for more on this idea). This process tends to happen through the forging of strong relationships between organizational members – often outside, or even in spite of, the formal communication mechanisms. Hence, whatever their designated roles, performance practitioners are likely to be more influential if they work through formal and informal networks to make progress on the strategic agenda.

Leadership

Effective leadership is necessary at every organizational level in performance environments. Leadership is not a role preserved for the powerful few at the top, and title or position is no guarantee of leadership power. Effective, comprehensive leadership requires personal capabilities that cannot be reduced to a set of skills or a simple 'toolbox' of leadership behaviours. Leadership is not management, although, in practice, performance managers are likely to do both to varying degrees. Leadership is a deliberate process that involves creating direction for the organization by influencing those who work within it irrespective of their position (Butcher 2007). Leaders create strategic direction, implement changes to realize organizational potential and work through relationships to inspire others to action. They also employ an external perspective – the ability to enquire into, evaluate and generate usable knowledge from outside the organization boundaries to inform and strengthen their strategic influence. Once direction has been defined, management deals with the operational issues, systems of control and measurement and plans to achieve organizational stability (Pedlar et al 2004). Accordingly, performance practitioners must achieve a balance between leadership and management activity in order to deliver results against key strategic and operational objectives.

The relative balance between leadership and management activity is an important one. The changing work environment has decentralized accountability and individual contribution has become the vital currency. To help establish the essential balance between leadership and management action it is important to filter and prioritize work activities. One system for achieving this is a matrix proposed by Covey (2004, p. 151) that categorizes time spend into four quadrants related to two dimensions – importance and urgency.

If a project is important *and* urgent, it is likely to be deadline-driven, a crisis that has arisen or a short-term tactical problem. If it is important and not urgent, this may constitute strategic activity, relationship building or problem prevention. Projects that are urgent and not important may consist of pressing matters, some meetings, calls or reports or e-mail correspondence. Finally, activity that resides in the not important and not urgent category could be viewed as self-indulgent and may include attending to time wasters, indulging in irrelevant and enjoyable pursuits, or trivial work.

While such a model is useful to prompt thinking about the relative balance of short- and long-term activity, time management is not the real concern. It is managing ourselves that represents the core of the problem. Hence, the starting point is not to plan more activity in the hope that this will solve the problem. Rather, the focus needs to be on where the time is currently spent in relation to the four quadrants, as leadership credibility is earned through activity that resides in the first quadrants. Effective leaders are focused not on problems but on opportunities. While they need to be able to respond to crises, genuine leadership effectiveness will be achieved by attending to the important but not urgent activities that build capacity (Drucker 2004). This requires a fundamental shift away from the rather unsophisticated methods of time planning and working practices towards developing relationships and achieving results (Covey 2004). Leadership can therefore be seen as a mindset – a way of thinking about personal contribution – and crucially as a particular orientation that enables people to optimize organizational capability.

So what does this mindset look like in behavioural terms? Firstly, leaders must attend to what is strategically important. A future orientation is essential and this core characteristic is sometimes referred to as vision. The critical point about vision is that it represents a realistic, credible and promising future for the organization in ways that improve the current situation (Bennis & Nanus 1985, p. 89). The vision, or purpose, must be owned by those who will be implementing it, so the leadership role involves creating ways to engage people in building desirable pictures for the future. Leadership is essentially an activity rather than a position and it is leadership, rather than management activity, that represents core capability. Management is about achieving the smooth running of the organization via a focus on operations, planning and control. Leadership activity attends to organizationally crucial endeavours in order to deliver strategic value. Leaders must therefore work through their network of relationships to engage others to become involved in change to achieve the strategy and protect the long-term future of the organization (Butcher, 2007). In performance management settings, a clear strategic agenda, strong relationships across the organization and the ability to inspire others to action are crucial elements of leadership contribution.

Leadership action requires individuals to recognize the agendas of competing and mutual interest groups and use diplomacy – the process through which these interests are negotiated and reconciled – to achieve their goals. Politics exist in every organization and claims that leaders can be effective without being politically astute are naive. Working with and through constructive diplomacy (albeit this is a contradiction in terms for many people) is a mainstay of effective leadership (Butcher & Clarke 2001). If performance practitioners are going to be successful as individual change agents, they will need to operate diplomatically in ways that are outside the mainstream of 'official' managerial activity – via networking and building coalitions, for example – not all of which can be conducted in public.

In order to use diplomacy effectively in performance management settings, leaders must not only be politically astute but be aware of, seek and use power appropriately. Power can be seen as 'the ability to do, or to act, to get work done, to make things happen' (Pedlar et al 2004, p. 30). Power can be used constructively to drive action and involve others. It is also viewed by some as dangerous and a thing to be avoided. Yet lack of power is a problem too, leading to helplessness and boredom. Using power to beneficial effect while avoiding its destructive potential is complex. Seeking and using power for long-term organizational benefit lies at the heart of leadership and the motives underlying this are critical. Justifiable motives – in other words, those that are organizationally defensible – lie at the core of responsible political activity and leadership influence. 'A deserving and just cause in the service of others is a much easier motive to identify with than one of self-seeking ambition' (Butcher & Clarke 2001, p. 68). So long as the cause is principled – and in the best interests of those in the organization – the dialogue between leaders and their teams only sharpens the quality of decision making (Butcher & Clarke 1999). It is often easier to see what needs to be done than to make it happen. Responsible use of power to prompt and support positive change and action is one of the key challenges of leadership.

One of the most popular accounts of the sources of individual power comes from French & Raven's (1959) five part typology. This is presented in Table 8.3. Based on their work, certain sources of power have been seen to derive from *leadership position* while others are concerned more with *the leader*

Table 8.3 The five part typology of personal power

Position power	Role power	• The significance placed by others on your role and the status it accords • Linked to the organizational hierarchy and authority
	Coercive power	• Use of punishment to force compliance • Examples include withdrawal of promotion or privileges, disapproval, control of resources or exclusion from key networks
	Reward power	• Capacity to reward the compliant. Rewards include pay, conditions, recognition or allocation of desirable work
Personal power	Expert power	• Personal credibility and the value placed on competence in a given area; it may also be derived from specialist knowledge
	Referent power	• Respect and esteem in which you are held by others. Socially attractive people want to associate with you, 'to be in your gang'
	Connection power	• Based on networks and social competence • Not in French & Raven's original list

Source: after French & Raven, 1959

as a person and are linked to individual factors of status (Pedlar et al 2004, p. 68).

It would be difficult to ignore the importance of position power such as a performance manager. However, amidst the flattening of hierarchies and the emergence of new organizational forms, effective leadership requires personal power. An individual who is appointed to a managing role does not automatically become a powerful leader. The sources of personal power are of most significance as they relate to the core function of leadership, which is about influencing others to do things they might not otherwise agree to do in pursuit of long-term organizational interests. Although connection power is a later addition to French & Raven's power typology, it has become increasingly important in a world where informal means of influence are critical to leadership efficacy. Power is a relative concept – the amount of power a leader possesses in any given situation is dependent upon that of others. Leaders are only powerful because we allow them to influence us. This is why personal power is so important in leadership terms. If a performer is not persuaded by the strength of a coach or manager's argument, then s/he will have little power with, or over, the performer.

One of the most important roles of a leader in performance management terms is to act as a change agent by challenging the way things are done in order to get strategic issues on the agenda. This process can be initiated by people anywhere in the organization and runs contrary to the idea that leadership is the preserve of the chosen few formally designated in senior positions. Change is the common differentiator between management and leadership but, despite the popularity of top-down rational change initiatives, evidence of success is unconvincing (Pedlar et al 2004). In the new world of virtual working, remote partnerships, cross-functional teams and disparate networks, there is considerable flux and those who think they are in control may be very much mistaken. The depiction of change as a smooth linear process driven by the top is no longer adequate to explain how change happens.

> Study after study reveals employees from the top to the bottom of companies who have become frustrated, stressed, and disempowered by processes of organizational change that are designed to unleash their potential, not diminish it. Despite this evidence, 'thought leaders' on the new economy still promulgate the notion that vision and corporate higher purpose provide the essential point of stability and motivational framework, thereby enabling employees to commit their hearts and minds to an organization. Above all what this ignores is the self-interest and partisan mentality that is not only inherent in organizations, but if seen as destructive, becomes just that. Unwavering adherence to the principles of rationality, then, is eventually self defeating.
>
> Butcher & Clarke 2001, p. 11–12

Given these issues, a different approach to organizational change is required that acknowledges the management of self interest as central to success (Butcher & Clarke 1999, p. 11). In this model, working with constructive diplomacy is central to bringing about change. Recruiting others to share in decisions, inspiring commitment to take the next step and reading the motives of others are the new leadership priorities. Balancing self-interests against organizational motives is critical to leadership success. The best interests of the organization must dominate, otherwise 'destructive politics' will prevail and blatant self-interest will become the key driver. This approach necessitates strong relationships across, up and through the organization. With these relationships, leaders can act as change agents to initiate 'bottom-up' change, characterized by local initiatives that, through the power of strong relationships, build an inclusive approach that is altogether more authentic.

It is interesting to note that recruitment routes to performance management seem to have hitherto placed insufficient emphasis on the leadership dimension. All too often, leaders are appointed from within, or rise up through the ranks to earn their status, without sufficient scrutiny of their leadership capability. In football, for example, it is commonplace to appoint ex-players and coaches to leadership positions. A failure to recognize and select on the basis of the essential leadership skills is somewhat surprising given the intensity of relationships in performance settings but, more realistically, it reinforces the lack of sophistication in some aspects of current provision (Lyle 2002). Performance organizations need leaders who have the appropriate mindset coupled with behaviours that allow them to effect change. However, a lack of provision for leadership development may mean that a) these capabilities are not actively sought at recruitment and/or b) those currently occupying leadership positions do not possess these aptitudes and hence there appears to be no problem. In other words, they don't miss what they haven't got.

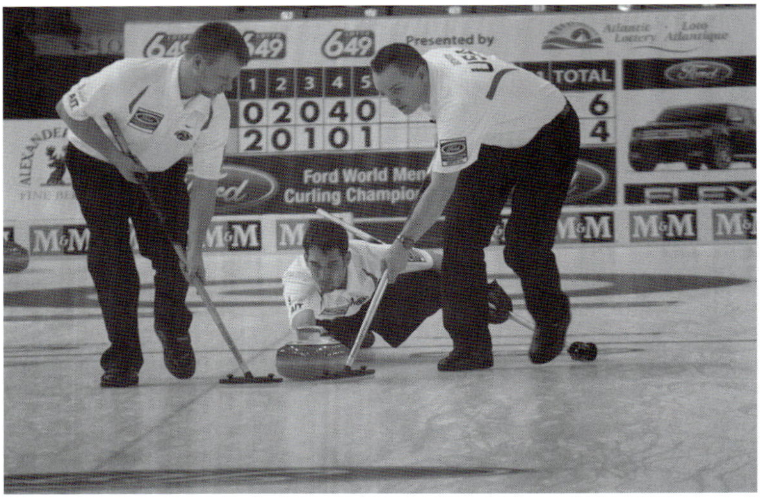

Fig. 8.3 • Teamwork in action. © Leslie Ingram-Brown. Reprinted with kind permission.

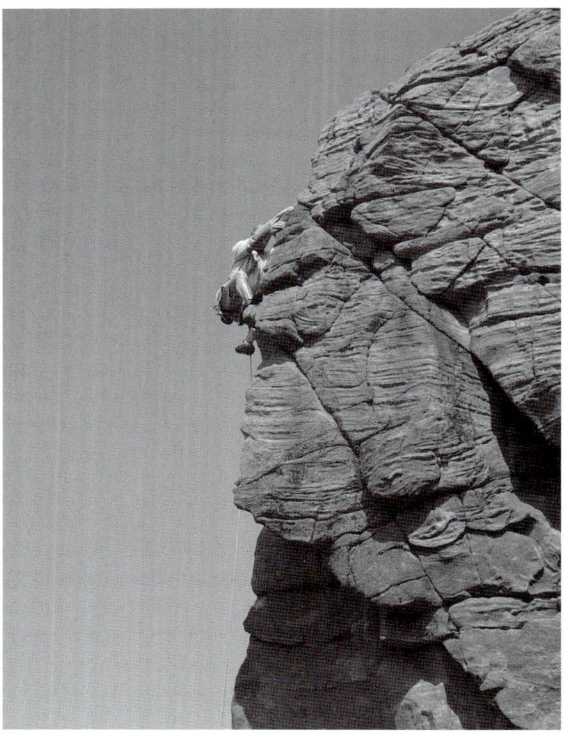

Fig. 8.4 • The outdoors is increasingly used as a 'training ground' for performers to learn key management skills.

Arguably, the positions of coach, mentor and performance manager could legitimately be cast as leadership roles, particularly in the domain of high-performance organizations. Nonetheless, there have been some notable attempts to address this 'gap' in provision, for example in sport performance, by using the principles of coaching and team building as mechanisms for management education (Figs 8.3 and 8.4) (Lyle 1997, Whitaker 1999). Unfortunately, much of this has been one way – business assuming it can learn from the 'urgent environment' exemplified by sport, while sport knows that what it does is clearly 'world class'! Crucially, however, insufficient attention to the requisite leadership capabilities coupled with lack of a coherent framework for development has meant that, in many performance settings, good practice has largely been the result of trial and error.

Pertinent psychological constructs for performance organizations

Emotional intelligence

Having a sound knowledge of the constituents of leadership is insufficient if it is not matched with the personal capability to take effective action. A growing body of evidence suggests that successful leaders possess a high degree of what has come to be known as 'emotional intelligence' (EI). EI has been defined as 'the ability to monitor one's own and others' feelings and emotion, to discriminate among them and to use this information to guide one's thinking and actions' (Salovey & Mayer 1990, p. 189). Being emotionally intelligent involves tuning into emotions, understanding the emotions in ourselves and others, and taking appropriate action based on this information. EI has been linked to outstanding accomplishments in a number of performance environments including sport (Lane & Lowther 2005), business (Zeider et al 2004) and academia (Parker et al 2004). Indeed, several writers have suggested that EI is a better indicator of career success than other tools (Goleman 1995, Lipsett 2006, Spencer & Spencer 1993). This is not to suggest that intelligence and cognitive skills such as strategic thinking are immaterial. Rather, they function as threshold or entry-level requirements for leadership roles. An individual may be well trained, bright and knowledgeable but these attributes may be of negligible importance if they are not matched by EI capabilities. Successful leaders are not at the mercy of out-of-control emotions. Notably, however, mastery of our own emotional state is not enough. Emotionally intelligent leaders are able to extend this expertise outwards and their empathy in dealing with others enables them to be influential (Eaton & Johnson 2001).

The four dimensions of EI involve perceiving emotion, using emotions to facilitate thought, understanding emotions and managing emotions (Salovey & Mayer 1990). The fundamental starting point for perceiving emotions is self-awareness. Individuals who are self-aware are neither overly self-critical nor especially hopeful – they are honest with themselves about their strengths and development areas. The decisions of self-aware people are often consistent with their values and they recognize how their emotions affect what they are doing. If people lack this competence, they are vulnerable to being sidetracked by emotions that are out of control. It is not difficult to find stories of technically competent managers who could not handle stress, or scientifically able coaches who did everything well except get along with people. Self-awareness is invaluable in many aspects of performance practitioner work. It helps individuals to maximize individual contribution, manage unruly feelings, maintain motivation and tune into the concerns of others around them in order to build good work-related social relationships. From this awareness develops another – a picture of how our feelings affect others. Being able to accurately perceive the emotions in the face or voice of others provides an important foundation for a more advanced understanding of how to use emotions to optimal effect.

The second element of the EI ability model relates to the capacity of emotions to enter into and guide our thinking. In other words, a capacity for self regulation – which is like an ongoing inner conversation – helps us manage our feelings. People engaged in such a conversation still feel upset and have bad moods but they find ways to channel their emotions in ways that are productive. This dimension can also help people to suspend judgement about certain events and think more carefully before acting (Goleman 1998a). The third branch of the EI model involves understanding emotions. So, for example, an athlete gaining selection for national squad may not necessarily feel happy with the decision if they have been waiting for some time for recognition and if they feel they may have been overlooked previously. They may feel satisfied and relieved but still bear some resentment (shown as hostility or anger), especially if they are expected to express gratitude for something they feel they have earned. High EI enables a person working with the athlete (manager, coach, psychologist) to more accurately determine and predict how and why they might feel this way in the context. This is important information to guide effective interactions and is much more based on 'why they feel it' than merely on recognizing that they do! If the athlete in this example also has high EI, the ability to understand why they feel this way may help them to explain effectively to others the reason and this is likely to be more acceptable (and hugely more beneficial for long-term relations) than if they simply demonstrate anger or hostility. In sum, this area of competence involves understanding what emotions mean, coupled with the capacity to reason about these meanings. Individuals who are able to do this well can realistically appraise setbacks, recognize good feedback and acknowledge their own emotional shortcomings. Finally, managing emotions in oneself and others is crucial to promoting personal and social goals. People who are able to use this ability well are adept at using their emotional radar to sense how others are reacting while mindfully fine-tuning their own response to push the interaction in the right direction.

Emotional intelligence is particularly pertinent to leadership because leadership involves recognizing others' emotional states, invoking emotions in others, managing these emotions accordingly and motivating by creating shared emotional experiences (Humphrey 2002). EI is a key factor in an individual's ability to be socially effective (George 2000) and enables smoother interactions with work teams, better conflict management and building of collaborative networks. Used well, these capabilities enable individuals to monitor how people are feeling and take appropriate action. Individuals are inspired by dreams, not plans, and experiences in the workplace generate both positive and negative feelings that are likely to motivate people to act. Put succinctly, leadership is not about deciding what tasks people should complete and how they should go about these. Rather, it is about intervening in the emotions of organizational life in order to enable others to act (Turnbull et al 2005, p. 300).

The current interest in EI has raised the question of whether it is possible to develop these competencies. A growing body of research on behavioural change suggests that it is possible to help people of any age to become more emotionally intelligent but an important starting point is to recognize a crucial distinction between emotional and cognitive learning (Goleman 1998b). Consider the example of a performance manager whose career was hindered because he was shy, introverted and too absorbed in the technical aspects of the role. Through cognitive learning, he may come to understand that it would be better for him to consult more, build relationships and connect better with the people around him. But just knowing these things would not enable him to take action. In order to develop this ability, a different type of learning is needed. Emotional capacities such as resilience and empathy differ from cognitive abilities in a number of ways; not least because they draw on different parts of the brain. Cognitive abilities are primarily based in the neocortex while the emotional centres are run from the amygdala via a circuitry that connects to the prefrontal lobes – the brain's executive centre. Effective learning for EI has to re-tune these circuits. Fundamentally, emotional learning involves breaking old habits of thought, feeling and action. Consequently, in order to develop EI capability, development provision must assist the learner to engage emotionally with the need to enhance their EI. In other words, they need to feel strongly that they want to change some aspect of their behaviour. Once emotional engagement is achieved, it is necessary to secure commitment to action – i.e. to trying out new ways of being – such as learning to approach people positively instead of avoiding them, listening better, giving feedback skilfully or communicating well in conflict situations. Unhelpful habits are usually developed from early life experiences and, for the learner, the process of developing new emotional responses often means a long and sometimes difficult journey involving much practice. Motivational factors may also interfere with this process. For some, the prospect of needing to develop greater EI is a bitter pill to swallow. A coach who is told, for instance, that they should learn more about a particular training technique is likely to be less upset or defensive than if he is told that he should control his temper and listen more to his athletes. Helping people to learn emotionally may therefore create resistance to change and has to be a carefully crafted process involving motivation, effort, support and sustained practice.

Conflict management

Individuals who are strong on EI may find this useful in dealing effectively with the inevitable differences that surface between people in organizations. Conflict defined as 'a form of interaction between parties that differ in interests, perceptions or preferences' (Brown 1979, p. 378) is extremely common in performance management settings and has an important role to play in development of a peak performance culture. Pressure to meet performance targets, lack of resources, management and power struggles may give rise to conflict and, accordingly, managers are often called upon to act constructively to resolve these difficulties and optimize the positive benefits.

In performance management environments, conflict may have many consequences: political bargaining, tacit compliance, absenteeism, employment of external figures to act as arbiters or moves to replace particular managers with others. Many of these conflicts occur on an individual as well as a collective basis and arise out of different conditions. Some conflicts are stimulated by the organizational environment as a result of changing structures or roles. Internal restructuring or changes in management responsibilities can cause conflict to escalate and it may also arise as a result of unequal reward systems, unfair treatment or a particular leadership style. A less hierarchical structure, a results orientation and increased emphasis on individual contribution have changed the performance environment and placed new demands on individuals. Responses to these factors are likely to vary considerably and render conflict levels susceptible to change as a result of diverse goals, work preferences and attitudinal differences. Although conflict may be classified as *interorganizational* (i.e. between organizations) the focus of this section is *intraorganizational* conflict (i.e. within an organization), which can be further categorized as intergroup, interpersonal and intrapersonal.

Intergroup conflict occurs between two or more units or groups within an organization. In performance management settings, it is not surprising that the needs, values and working practices of groups are frequently at odds and, although they are part of the same organization, their interests pull them in different directions. Conflict between groups can promote distrust and negative stereotyping, increased emphasis on differences and decreased communication. These effects can create a negative cycle whereby defensive aggression by one group makes the other group suspicious and promotes counteraggression, causing the conflict to escalate. An opposite scenario, in which trust, cooperation and positive stereotypes are generated, may also create a cycle of increasing collaboration between the groups (Deutsch 1973). There seems to be a link between cooperative situations and group formation, as those who believe their goals to be cooperative (rather than competitive) have been found to express their opinions openly, exchange information and ideas, explore each other's perspectives and work for mutually acceptable solutions (Tjosvold & Chia 1989). Effective management and positive employment of intragroup conflict are essential components of a performance team. For applied practitioners, these goals can be achieved by adopting a problem-solving approach when differences arise. By highlighting common aims, objectives or approaches, it is possible to build trust among colleagues, leading to a more open working environment where differences are actively aired in pursuit of better-quality decisions.

Interpersonal conflict refers to conflict between two or more organizational members. In performance environments, the education, information technology and administration functions may all be part of the same organization, but on occasion their interests may clash. Individuals have different aspirations and goals and it is inevitable that there will be some conflict as they strive to achieve them. It has been suggested that a degree of interpersonal conflict is likely to be healthy as people feel comfortable to express different opinions or points of view – whether their interests are compatible or not – and conflict may even be essential for organizational growth and development. This is not to suggest that conflict should be deliberately introduced into every meeting and debate. Indeed, the negative effects of too much conflict are well documented – ingrained hostility, inferior decisions and lack of commitment to much-needed change. Rather, the implication is that a lot of energy is wasted denying the existence of conflict when it could be used to constructively explore and resolve differences.

Finally, *intrapersonal conflict* is experienced by individuals when they feel pushed or pulled in opposite directions over a particular issue – in other words, the alternatives are both attractive, or both unattractive (Roloff 1987). This type of conflict occurs when a person is required to perform roles or tasks that do not match their expertise, interests, goals or values and may result in behaviour that appears to be inconsistent, hesitant or indecisive (Rahim 1992).

In performance management terms, conflict is of significance for one reason in particular – its influence on performance and productivity (Lyle 2002, p. 68). As long ago as 1976, a study by the American Management Association found that mid- and top-level managers spent approximately 20% of their time dealing with conflict (Thomas & Schmidt 1976). Indeed, given the new organizational forms that have since emerged, one could reasonably expect that the propensity for conflict in performance management settings would increase as new demands are made on people to be personally accountable amidst an environment of scarce resources and conflicting interests. (Slack 1997, p. 194). The negative effects associated with too much conflict, including decreased communication between conflicting parties, escalation of aggression and negative stereotyping, which contribute to a deterioration of working relationships, have received considerable attention (Baron 1989, Van de Vliert & Kabanoff 1990). The idea that too little conflict is dysfunctional has received less coverage (Davidson 1990) but, nonetheless, a lack of conflict can mean that groups take decisions that fail to take account of vital pieces of information or that little attention is paid to problem areas, resulting in organizational apathy or complacency.

The effectiveness of group performance can also be adversely affected by 'groupthink', which has been described as 'a deterioration of mental efficiency, reality testing and moral judgement that results from in-group pressures' (Mullins 2005, p. 570). Groupthink is characterized by the group accepting decisions without due consideration of either the consequences or the viability of alternatives. The phenomenon of groupthink involves the group believing they are invulnerable, rationalizing disagreeable information, creating negative stereotypes of opponents and putting pressure on individual members to conform. This helps to create an illusion of harmony and a false sense of unity, which supports poor decisions. Leaders who dislike conflict may inadvertently create ideal conditions for groupthink to emerge (Hambrick 2001). What this amounts to is that some conflict is desirable, if not essential for optimal performance.

Moderate levels of conflict are widely acknowledged to be associated with informed problem solving and constructive decision-making processes that take account of diverse perspectives. The contemporary view of conflict is that no organizational configuration or managerial strategy could, or indeed should, eliminate conflict altogether. Consequently, conflict is regarded as an important stimulus for change and some level of conflict, though not excessive, has been shown to increase organizational productivity (Feather 1990). As the capacity for conflict to influence performance has been acknowledged, this issue of conflict management has become important and the process of conflict handling is now considered to be a key managerial function (De Dreu 1997).

In performance management contexts, conflict can arise where there is a clash of roles – such as between a coach's value system and the expectations of the organization – albeit this is more likely in some settings than others. The propensity for conflict appears to be related to the reward system and the perceived pressures generated by individual accountability and outcome measurement (Lyle 2002, p. 71). Performance directors may also experience role conflict as they seek to work with the execution of the coaching process and the management of the performance system within which it takes place. It is not surprising that the task of regulating conflict levels often falls to those in management or leadership roles and this process involves ensuring that conflict levels facilitate constructive decision making but do not escalate so much that communication breaks down. One of the inherent difficulties is that an optimal level is likely to vary depending upon the situation, the people involved and the conflict issue. Some performance environments are characterized by high levels of interpersonal difference, while others appear to be relatively harmonious. In order to allow appropriate levels of difference to emerge, a degree of sensitivity is required on behalf of those dealing with conflict, as some people are more comfortable than others with expressed differences. An important factor in mediating the approach is the degree to which the conflict is contributing to better decision making and organizational productivity. In practical terms, skilled conflict handling involves 'turning up' or 'turning down' the amount of conflict so that differences are sufficiently aired and taken account of in decision-making processes. Consequently, performance managers may find themselves called upon to increase cooperation between opposing parties, promote a problem-solving approach in order to resolve interpersonal difficulties and develop a creative process whereby people can explore their options for resolving the conflict (Millson 1987).

It has been suggested that third parties (e.g. counsellors, managers or psychologists) who are called upon to deal with conflict need four kinds of skills (Deutsch 1994). The first relates to establishing a good working relationship with the conflicting parties in order to promote an atmosphere of trust, open communication and responsiveness. The second set of skills is concerned with creating a constructive, problem solving approach on behalf of those involved. Thirdly there are skills to do with developing a creative decision making process that facilitates a realistic assessment of potential courses of action. Finally, it is helpful for third parties to have information about the issues around which the conflict is centred. Skilled performance in this case would require the third party to adopt an enquiring approach to highlight core issues, suspending judgement until the relevant differences have been aired and implementing a productive process whereby people can explore their options for dealing with the situation. For those contemplating how to resolve a conflict, the Thomas & Kilmann Management of Differences instrument (Thomas & Kilmann 1974) offers five conflict-handling styles, mediated by two basic dimensions – assertiveness (i.e. the extent to which an individual tries to satisfy their own concerns) and cooperativeness (i.e. the extent to which an individual attempts to satisfy the other's concerns).

- **Competing** is both assertive and uncooperative and this style is characterized by trying to 'win' at the other person's expense. It is appropriate when quick, decisive action is necessary, or when the issue is vital and backing down is not an option.
- **Accommodating** is the opposite of competing and is unassertive and cooperative. When an individual is accommodating, they neglect their concerns in order to satisfy those of the other party. This style is useful where the issue is more important to the other party than to you, when you are outmatched and losing, or when consideration of a better position is necessary.

- **Avoiding** is both unassertive and cooperative. This style does not address the conflict and may take the form of sidestepping, ignoring or withdrawal. Avoiding is appropriate when the issue is trivial, where you have no opportunity to satisfy your needs or where deferral gives more time for vital consideration.
- **Collaborating** is the opposite of avoiding and is both assertive and cooperative. When collaborating, individuals actively work with others to achieve a mutually acceptable solution. This style is appropriate when the other party is willing to collaborate, where an integrative solution is necessary or the concerns of both parties are too important to be compromised.
- **Compromising** is at the midpoint for assertiveness and cooperativeness. The objective is to find a mutually acceptable solution that satisfies all parties. This might mean splitting the difference, engaging concessions or seeking the middle ground. This style is useful to achieve temporary settlements of outstanding issues or where goals are moderately important but not worth the disruption involved in using more assertive styles.

Most people have a preference for up to three of these styles and given that all are appropriate in particular situations, it is worth considering how to deploy non-preferred styles so that less usual behaviour may be adopted when the circumstances demand. That being said, over- or underuse of a particular response may indicate an organizational environment that requires the high or low use of that style.

No manager is a novice when they start learning about conflict handling. They have all been observers or participants in conflicts from childhood and these experiences are likely to result in preconceptions, preferences and ways of behaving that are deeply ingrained before any exposure to systematic training. In common with EI, skilled conflict handling involves learning in the emotional domain and, as people tend to vary in the degree to which they are emotionally aware, experience alone may not be a good indicator of competence in this area. Once again, this type of learning requires commitment to change, effort and repeated practice. Bespoke training provision should seek to incorporate these design elements in order to assist practitioners to act quickly to maximize the positive contribution of conflict in performance management settings.

Social identification

A potential source of conflict in performance management settings concerns the perceived degree of 'fit' between different social identities within a particular team or group. Hence, an understanding of the process of social identification is useful in the context of leadership in performance management, as people's behaviour is likely to reflect the extent to which they identify themselves as members of particular groups – both within and outside the organization. Indeed, in many situations there is often an explicit focus on the sense of belonging to the group – to be a part of the team. Groups in many contexts apply different devices to encourage members to strengthen their identity with them because of the many benefits that this confers upon the group's overall performance.

Social identification concerns how the individual perceives themselves in terms of group membership, and is defined by Tajfel (1972, p. 31) as 'the individual's knowledge that he/she belongs to certain social groups together with some emotional and value significance to him/her of the group membership'. Accordingly, a member of a team with a high level of social identification would not only acknowledge that they were a part of the team but would value that sense of belonging. Recognizing oneself as part of a particular group may have a number of effects including value placed on group membership (e.g. being a member of a particular team is important to me), emotional consequences (e.g. pride in the team's achievements) and impact on self-esteem through ascribed membership of a high-status group.

The positive impacts of a feeling of group identification upon behaviour have long been known. As early as the 1920s, Mayo (1924) suggested that, by allowing workers to develop their own social groups, staff turnover declined and productivity increased. This was supported some years later, by a study undertaken by Roethlisberger & Dickinson (1939), which suggested that, by enhancing workers' sense of social belonging, productivity and quality consequently increased. These findings have subsequently been replicated in a variety of contexts and settings in organizations. However, placing a positive value on group membership also requires a point of comparison such as another group or team. This comparison group must be judged as less valuable than the member's own group, which has the effect of raising the esteem of the member's group and their own self esteem. If comparisons are not positive, then there is no perceived value in being a group member and individuals will either leave the group or, worse still, continue to belong but become demotivated. In a similar fashion, if comparisons on salient features produce an apparently unfavourable result, i. e. 'that team is more skilful than us', this may result in a reappraisal until the chosen feature produces a favourable result to self esteem, even if detrimental to performance, e.g. 'We may be the worst team in the league, but we're the most aggressive'. Though not so overtly obvious in dance(!), such social comparisons and subsequent adjustment underpin many of the problems that keep a team down. In other words, once meaningful comparisons are no longer possible on the basis of directly 'performance-pertinent' characteristics, the move to establish an alternative source of 'pride' can serve to keep the team in a slump. This situation is often only remedied when an extreme step (e.g. change of manager/coach) imposes/demands a new comparator.

In performance management organizations, it is necessary for leaders to take account of the social identity of the group and, accordingly, analysis of the leaders' role cannot be separated from consideration of the group or organization of which they are a part (Haslam 2001, p. 66). Categorizing ourselves and others according to social groups appears to be a fundamental human characteristic. Because of two basic needs: to differentiate ourselves from others and a fundamental need for belonging, people expose themselves to the control of others (Buchanan & Huczynski 2004, p. 356). Members of the group are more likely to offer control to leaders whose attitudes and values are consistent with the group and also to leaders who seek to motivate and build a sense of belonging through team membership. It has been suggested that the potential of leaders to create a sense of shared identity among a given team or work group is an important determinant in the likelihood that their attempts to promote and sustain particular work-related behaviours will be successful (Reicher & Hopkins 1996). Furthermore, the extent to which leadership is accepted by the group may also be contingent upon the degree to which the members tend to either focus on the identity they share with the leader or consider the ways in which the leader is distinct from them (Ellemers et al 2004, p. 467). In this way, leaders' concerns are intimately bound up with the shared concerns of group members and, if the group is to function as more than an aggregate of individuals, its leaders must represent the concerns of the collective as a whole rather than their personal interests or those of a power elite (Haslam 2001).

For a variety of reasons, leaders are not always able to behave in ways that are consistent with the wishes of their group members. However, social identity effects mean that team members should generally be more inclined to have a positive view about the motives and intentions of leaders when they perceive them as 'in-group' rather than 'out-group' (Duck & Fielding 1999). One of the consequences of this is that leadership behaviour that deviates from the norm may be 'explained away' – for example, by attributing negative attitudes to external pressures – when the leader is perceived to be part of the in-group (Haslam et al 1998). People are also likely to understand behaviour that confirms previous expectations (i.e. positive in the case of in-group leaders and negative for out-group leaders) as more reflective of the true motives and reflections of their leaders (Hewstone 1990). Such in-group biases may constitute an important mechanism that acts to increase the propensity for leadership influence when the leader is perceived as in-group and decreases it when the leader is perceived as out-group.

Being acknowledged as in-group is an important step for a leader to wield effective control and to help minimize the negative impact when the leader has to take decisions unfavourable to the group membership. So leaders must identify the social identity of the group – i.e. the values and significance placed on membership, lead on the basis of this identity and guide groups from within (Reicher et al 2007). Furthermore, leaders are able to optimize their influence when they not only appear to belong to the group but also embody characteristics that make the group distinct from others. Leaders who separate themselves from the group by holding different social identities from it are likely to be less influential than those who represent the group's identity and lead from within. Under these circumstances, loyalty to an in-group leader is likely to emerge more unconditionally (Ellemers et al 2004) and this may increase the likelihood that the leader and their team will develop a positive relationship (Hogg & Martin 2003). The image of Nelson Mandela celebrating the 1995 Rugby World Cup success of South Africa in a replica shirt of the captain François Pienaar has often been cited as an iconic image for that country as it moved out of the apartheid era. The decision by Mandela to personally celebrate the victory so joyously may well have had the effect of aligning himself positively with the white rugby-playing/supporting community in South Africa – a group with which he had hitherto had few, if any, connections. Wearing the country's (indeed the captain's) shirt on an occasion when the country was explicitly opposed by other countries completed the key social identity tasks of minimizing within-group differences and maximizing between-group differences when the outcome of that evaluation was so positive.

In performance management settings, social identities will vary by organization, geography and work role. Private, public and not-for-profit sectors in affluent or poorer areas are likely to be different. Schools, dance companies, sport organizations and freelance support services may also vary widely in their commitment to particular training methods or approaches and different regions of the country are likely to be more or less subject to control by external regulations, funding organizations or national governing bodies. In a similar fashion, social identities will vary within a particular organization or work group. Practitioners who work in specific areas such as education, sport performance or performing arts will have discrete identities that differ from others. For instance, a sport physiologist based in a university may have a different identity from a freelance elite coach, although both may be working for the same support team. In a similar fashion, groups will vary in their ideas about how problems should be solved, decisions taken or practice regulated and they may also have identities to do with affiliations with professional bodies, orientations to evidence-based practice or use of research. The type of situation in which such multiple identities may meet in performance situations is highlighted in Chapter 24, where the structure for organizing support teams of different specialists is examined.

It is essential, therefore, that those assuming leadership roles understand the social identities of the various groups and teams they work with. Sound knowledge of the basic beliefs of such groups can be undertaken via questionnaires, open forums and, fundamentally, by listening closely to the group's opinions. On the basis of this information, the leader can then determine the gaps between their characteristics and those of the group. Learning what the leader and group share as common identities and visions for the future can be useful in promoting a strong affiliation between the group and those in leadership roles. Groups often have shared expectations of what they want from a leader and it is important that the leader understands where they can or cannot meet these expectations. In sum, leaders who do not appreciate the values of the group may experience difficulties in influencing them effectively. Of course, some groups have dysfunctional social identities, which may cause harm to the organization or hinder attainment of key objectives. Under these circumstances, one course of action is for the leader to find people whose behaviour and attitude is most supportive for group success and who have significant status in the group and place them in key roles with high levels of communication with others, in the hope that the impetus will change the culture to become more positive (Kerfoot 2007). The work of performance managers is to enable the group to achieve high levels of performance in whatever group configuration they operate. Identifying the social identities of the groups that are part of the organization is therefore an important step in optimizing leadership impact, as the group members, social identity will affect how people perceive themselves, their actions within the team, changes in their motivation or even attempts to leave.

Conclusion

To date at any rate, the application of organizational considerations to performance groups has been somewhat haphazard. Some teams, in possession of an 'obvious' corporate identity, have always employed such ideas; dance companies and *some* football clubs are good examples. Some quite small teams may have thought themselves immune to, or inappropriate for, the use of tools and constructs developed in the far distant land of business. Finally, many performance organizations, sporting national governing bodies being a particular case in point, have been too long dominated by enthusiasts and volunteers to consider the need for such 'professional' concerns. Unfortunately, despite a professional veneer adopted by many, this is still often the case. The main contention of this chapter is that organizational concerns and optimizing group processes are essential considerations for any practitioner involved. I hope this chapter offers useful coverage of these black arts!

References

Baron, R.A., 1989. Personality and organizational conflict: effects on type A behaviour pattern and self monitoring. Organ. Behav. Hum. Decis. Process. 44, 281–296.

Bartlett, A., Ghoshal, S., 1990. Matrix management: not a structure, a frame of mind. Harv. Bus. Rev. 68, 138–145.

Bennis, W., Nanus, B., 1985. Leaders: The strategies for taking charge. Harper & Row, New York.

Berger, B., Pargman, D., Weinberg, R., 2001. Foundations of exercise psychology. Fitness Institute Technology, Morgantown, WV.

Birchall, D.W., 2001. What managers do. In: Crainer, S., Dearlove, D. (Eds.), Financial Times handbook of management, second ed. Prentice Hall, Harlow, Essex, pp. 110–131.

Bowman, C., 1998. Strategy in practice. Prentice Hall, Harlow, Essex.

Brown, L.D., 1979. Managing conflict among groups. In: Kolb, D.A., Rubin, I.M., McIntyre, J.M. (Eds.), Organizational psychology – a book of readings. Prentice Hall, Harlow, Essex.

Buchanan, D., Huczynski, A., 2004. Organizational behaviour – an introductory text, fifth ed. Pearson Education, Harlow, Essex, p. 485.

Butcher, D., 2001. Breaking out of organizational mindsets. In: Crainer, S., Dearlove, D. (Eds.), Financial Times handbook of management, second ed. Prentice Hall, Harlow, Essex, p. 91.

Butcher, D., 2007. The Business Leaders Programme. Cranfield University, Cranfield, Bedfordshire.

Butcher, D., Clarke, M., 1999. Organizational politics: the missing discipline of management? Industrial and Commercial Training 31 (1), 9–12.

Butcher, D., Clarke, M., 2001. Smart management. Palgrave Macmillan, Basingstoke, Hampshire.

Butcher, D., Clarke, M., 2008. Smart management, second ed. Palgrave Macmillan, Basingstoke, Hampshire.

Covey, F., 2004. The seven habits of highly effective people. Simon & Schuster, New York.

Davidson, J., 1990. Competition is healthy if approached correctly – and unhealthy if it isn't. Management Quarterly 31, 42–48.

De Dreu, C.K.W., 1997. Productive conflict: the importance of conflict management and conflict issues. In: De Dreu, C.K.W., Van de Vliert, E. (Eds.), 1997 Using conflict in organizations. Sage, London, pp. 9–23.

Deutsch, M., 1973. The resolution of conflict. Yale University Press, New Haven, CT.

Deutsch, M., 1994. Constructive conflict resolution: principles, training and research. J. Social Issues 50 (1), 13–32.

Drucker, P.F., 2004. The daily Drucker: 366 days on insight and motivation for getting the right things done. Harper Collins, New York.

Duck, J.M., Fielding, K.S., 1999. Leaders and subgroups: one of us or one of them? Group Processes and Intergroup Relations 2, 203–230.

Eaton, J., Johnson, R., 2001. Communicate with emotional intelligence. How To Books, Oxford.

Ellemers, N., De Gilder, N., Haslam, S.A., 2004. Motivating individuals and groups at work: a social identity perspective on leadership and group performance. Acad. Manage. Rev. 29, 459–478.

Feather, N.T., 1990. Reactions to equal reward allocations: effects on situation, gender and values. Br. J. Soc. Psychol. 29, 315–329.

French Jr., J.R.P., Raven, B., 1959. The bases of social power. In: Cartwright, D. (Ed.), Studies in social power. University of Michigan Press, Ann Abor, MI, pp. 150–167.

Friedman, T.L., 2006. The world is flat. Farrar, Straus & Giroux, New York.

George, J.M., 2000. Emotions and leadership: the role of emotional intelligence. Human Relations 53, 1027–1055.

Goleman, D., 1995. Emotional intelligence. Bantam Books, New York.

Goleman, D., 1998a. What makes a leader? Harv. Bus. Rev. 76, 93–102.

Goleman, D., 1998b. Working with emotional intelligence. Bantam Books, New York.

Hall, C.R., 2001. Imagery in sport and exercise. In: Singer, R., Hausenblas, H., Janelle, C. (Eds.), Handbook of sport psychology, second ed. Wiley, New York, pp. 529–549.

Hambrick, D., 2001. Putting the team into top management. In: Pickford, J. (Ed.), Financial Times mastering management, second ed. Prentice Hall, Harlow, Essex, p. 289.

Haslam, S.A., 2001. Psychology in organizations – the social identity approach. Sage, London.

Haslam, S.A., McGarty, C., Brown, P.M., et al., 1998. Inspecting the emperor's clothes: evidence that randomly selected leaders can enhance group performance. Group Dynamics: Theory, Research and Practice 2, 168–184.

Hastings, C., 1993. The new organization: growing the culture of organizational networking. McGraw-Hill, Maidenhead, Berkshire.

Hewstone, M., 1990. The ultimate attribution error? A review of the literature on intergroup causal attribution. Eur. J. Social Psychol. 20, 311–336.

Hogg, M.A., Martin, R., 2003. Social identity analysis of leader member relations: reconciling self categorization and leader-member exchange theories of leadership. In: Haslam, S.A., Van Knippenberg, D., Platow, M.J. et al., Social identity at work: developing theory for organizational practice. Psychology Press, New York, pp. 139–154.

Humphrey, R.H., 2002. The many faces of emotional leadership. Leadership Quarterly 13, 493–504.

Jackson, S., Csikszentmihaliyi, M., 1999. Flow in sports. Human Kinetics, Champaign, IL.

Johnson, G., Scholes, K., Whittington, R., 2005. Exploring corporate strategy, seventh ed. Financial Times/Prentice-Hall, Harlow, Essex.

Kerfoot, K.M., 2007. Leadership: social identity and guiding from within. Nursing Economics 25, 296–299.

Lane, A., Lowther, J., 2005. Relationships between emotional intelligence and psychological skills amongst athletes. J. Sports Sci. 23, 1253–1254.

Lipsett, A., 2006. You'll go far if you can show some emotion. The Times

Higher Education Supplement 24 November. pp. 6–7.

Lyle, J., 1997. Management training and the sport coaching analogy: a content analysis of six management training products. 5th Congress of the European Association for Sports Management, Glasgow. European Association for Sports Management, Vierumäki, Finland.

Lyle, J., 2002. Sports coaching concepts. Routledge, London.

McAuley, E., Blissmer, G., 2002. Self-efficacy and attributional processes in physical activity. In: Horn, J. (Ed.), Advances in sport psychology, second ed. Human Kinetics, Champaign, IL, pp. 185–206.

Mayo, E., 1924. Rivalry and industrial fatigue. Pers. J. 3, 273–281.

Millson, L., 1987. Ballpark figures: the Blue Jays and the business of baseball. McClelland & Stewart, Toronto, Ontario.

Mullins, L.J., 2002. Management and Organisational Behaviour, 7th ed. Prentice Hall, England.

Mullins, L.J., 2005. Management and organizational behaviour, seventh ed. Prentice Hall, Harlow, Essex.

Parker, J.D.A., Creque, R.E., Barnhart, D.L., et al., 2004. Academic achievement in high school: does emotional intelligence matter? Personality Individ. Differ. 37, 1321–1330.

Pedlar, M., Burgoyne, J., Boydell, T., 2004. A manager's guide to leadership. McGraw Hill, Maidenhead, Berkshire.

Pettigrew, A., Fenton, E., 2000. The innovating organization. Sage, London.

Prouty, D.F., 1988. In spite of us: my education in the big and little games of amateur and olympic sport in the US. Vitesse Press, Brattelboro, VT.

Rahim, M.A., 1992. Managing conflict in organizations, second ed. Praeger, Westport, CT.

Reicher, S., Hopkins, N., 1996. Self-category constructions in political rhetoric: an analysis of Thatcher's and Kinnock's speeches concerning the British Miner's Strike (1984–5). Eur. J. Social Psychol. 26, 353–372.

Reicher, S., Haslam, S.A., Platow, M., 2007. The new psychology of leadership. Scientific American Mind 18 (4), 22–29.

Roethlisberger, F.J., Dickinson, W.J., 1939. Management and the worker: an account of a research program conducted by the Western Electric Company Hawthorne Works. Harvard University Press, Cambridge, MA.

Roloff, M.E., 1987. Communication and conflict. In: Berger, C.R., Chaffee, S.H. (Eds.), Handbook of communication science. Sage, Newbury Park, CA, pp. 484–534.

Salovey, P., Mayer, J.D., 1990. Emotional intelligence. Cognition and Personality 9, 185–211.

Senior, B., 2002. Organizational change, second ed. Financial Times/Prentice Hall, Harlow, Essex, p. 87.

Slack, T., 1997. Understanding sport organizations. Human Kinetics, Leeds.

Smith, R., 2001. Positive reinforcement, performance feedback and performance enhancement. In: Williams, J.M. (Ed.), Applied sport psychology: personal growth to peak performance, fourth ed. Mayfield, Mountain View, CA, pp. 29–42.

Spencer Jr., L.M., Spencer, S., 1993. Competence at work: models for superior performance. John Wiley & Sons, New York.

Stewart, R., 1999. The reality of management, third ed. Butterworth-Heinemann, Oxford, p. 190.

Tajfel, H., 1972. Experiments in a vacuum. In: Israel, J., Tajfel, H. (Eds.), The context of social psychology a critical assessment. Academic Press, London, pp. 69–119.

Thomas, K.W., Kilmann, R.H., 1974. Thomas-Kilmann conflict MODE Instrument Xicom Inc, Tuedo, NY.

Thomas, K.W., Schmidt, W.H., 1976. A survey of management interests with respect to conflict. Acad. Manage. J. 19, 315–318.

Tjosvold, D., Chia, L.C., 1989. Conflict between managers and workers: the role of co-operation and competition. J. Soc. Psychol. 129, 235–247.

Turnbull, J.K., Arroba, T., 2005. Reading and carrying: A framework for learning about emotion and emotionally in organisation systems as a core aspect of leadership development. Management Learning 36 (3), 299–316.

Van de Vliert, E., Kabanoff, B., 1990. Toward theory based measures of conflict management. Acad. Manage. J. 22, 199–209.

Weinberg, R.S., Burton, D., Yukelson, D., et al., 2000. Perceived goal setting practices of Olympic athletes: an exploratory investigation. Sport Psychologist 14, 279–295.

Whitaker, D., 1999. The spirit of teams. Crowood Press, Marlborough, Wiltshire.

Zeider, M., Matthews, G., Roberts, R., 2004. Emotional intelligence in the workplace: a critical review. Appl. Psychol. 53, 371–399.

The team perspective: promoting excellence in performance teams

9

Alan C. MacPherson* Patrick W. Howard†

*University of Edinburgh, Edinburgh, UK; †Cromwell, Brisbane, Australia

CHAPTER CONTENTS

Introduction

The success of elite performing teams is lauded and examined across performance domains such as business (Jones 2002) and famous sports teams such as the Chicago Bulls (Jackson 1995) and the All-Blacks rugby team (McConnell 1999). Given this attention, it seems puzzling that group dynamics receives comparatively much less attention in psychology, and sport psychology in particular, than research and understanding of the individual or discrete relationships between two individuals (Hodge 2004). However, the comparative paucity of empirical literature regarding groups may be due to the difficulty in documenting the complex interaction of factors that influence group dynamics, such as those generated from within the group (e.g. conflict), on the part of an individual (e.g. autocratic leadership; Van Vugt 2004), from a quorum within the group (e.g. cliques) or from outside the parameters of the group (media impact or governing body regulations). Despite the difficulty associated with analysing disparate interacting factors, however, it is clear that a wider appreciation of this complex dynamic is critical for all performers who operate as part of a performance team.

In this chapter we examine the way in which fundamental aspects of group dynamics operate in the context of an intact performance team, and the way in which knowledge of these aspects can be used to enhance performance outcome. In many cases, the application of these ideas is exemplified through the considerable experiences of the second author (PH). His experience in rugby union includes top- level professional experience as player, coach and director of performance in both the Northern and Southern Hemispheres and from club to international level with teams such as the Australian national team, ACT Brumbies and Leicester Tigers. These experiences usefully illustrate the way in which ideas can be implemented, and the ideas in this chapter have wide implications for all performance teams. Essentially, the chapter identifies some basic areas in organization, structure and operation to which high-performance teams should attend to achieve the highest level of performance. Contemporary scientific theories from both psychological and business literature are considered in relation to a variety of contrasting real teams to provide an explanation as to how

DOI: 10.1016/B978-0-443-06734-1.00009-2

performance teams can promote and achieve excellence. We start by reflecting on the context of performance environments, then outline a model for understanding the dynamics of groups based on nonlinear principles and consider the key message for successful teams from the theoretical and empirical research. The chapter then moves to more specific detail concerning the development of culture, identity and cohesion, the formulation of strategy, and the way in which organizational structure and leadership both support and deliver strategic goals, with particular reference to the use of power and managing conflicts.

Operating in a performance context

The hard-edged reality of most performance environments is that, in the main, performers and those directly involved in managing (coaching/directing) their performance have relatively short tenure. While the development of the group in 5 years may be of significance at board level and to supporters, in the short term, the coach, director or manager has more immediate priorities in ensuring that the organization is successful and fit to produce consistent, quality performances. Reflecting on this issue in sport settings, Novak (1976, p. 86–87) wrote that:

> It is true for coaches 'winning is the only thing.' No matter how much they enjoy the game, coaches are fired if they do not produce winners. But players go on playing, win or lose; and on the average, all lose as often as they win... Winning is a priceless and lovely thing, but for players it cannot be the only thing, for losing is very much a part of every career.

For those who are charged with improving the performance of the organization, there exists a tension between maximizing current group members' performance and investing in and developing talent that may allow the group to perform, in the future, at a high level. Paradoxically, developing talent and other longer-term investments cannot be a performance director's primary focus – nor can they afford to neglect it. This has profound implications for the dynamic of the group and provides insight into the competing demands that exist in managing group dynamics.

A further tension for managers exists in regard to integrating potential and current group members: as operational demands influence the size of the dynamic, so temporary groups are formed. An example of such a temporary group may be a company for a specific tour, an expedition party or a sport team that is only formed once every 4 years (Olympics, Ryder Cup in golf or British Lions in rugby). Periodically, however, groups of athletes may be asked to train and compete with one another but, whatever the duration of the life-cycle of the group dynamic, if competition for places is fierce and a meritocratic selection policy is in place, there is likely to be little sentiment amongst group members and consequently there is the potential for conflict to be heightened within the group.

An example of such conflict, albeit an extreme one, occurred in Iraq in 2003 when 40 Royal Marine Commandos, combined from various sources as the Manoeuvre Support Group (MSG), was engaged with Iraqi forces near Abu Al Khasib for 19 hours. During this operation both machine gun and antitank sections of the MSG assisted each other to their mutual benefit; from a UK military standpoint the engagement was successful. However, immediately prior to this operation both sections comprising the MSG had fought violently aboard HMS *Ocean* (King 2006). Similarly, with regard to British Special Forces, autobiographical accounts have shown that there is often 'little affection within highly effective primary groups' (King 2006). Whatever the reasons were for the violence prior to entering the theatre of operations, where integration is imposed upon groups with a distinct purpose and identity, conflict may occur (see ideas on role clarity and social identification presented in Chapter 8).

The implications from these examples are that coaching or leading a group to 'perform' is often about organization and providing operational objectives, while accepting that conflict will naturally occur between individuals and subgroups. Management should be aware of the pitfalls that can befall a performance organization when performers are not provided with, or encouraged to develop, goals that coincide with the overall objectives of the parent organization. They may, as in the case of HMS *Ocean*, decide to see who the 'best' troops are on the basis of their own criteria (and again, consider the tenets of social identification).

Within a group, the issue of reward (often financial) and fair treatment is a critical concern for management. When this works well it goes unnoticed but, when the system fails, disharmony, dissatisfaction and conflict are quickly generated, to the detriment of overall group performance. In the extreme, performers will allow team performance to suffer and fail to expose those whom they believe are paid or valued too much by the management. Crucially, in a group setting, when it comes to matters of reward and remuneration, there is a subtle, yet important, distinction between equity and perceived equity. According to Adams (1965), anger is induced by underpayment inequity and guilt is induced by overpayment equity (Spector 2008). Therefore, it is necessary to acknowledge that variable individual factors affect group members' assessment and, therefore, perception of their relationship with their peers; so-called perceived equity (Guerrero et al 2007). For management to intervene effectively, sufficient financial resources may not be the only prerequisite. For example, management can develop explicit roles within the group or performance team that are recognized by group members as positions of responsibility or influence. While these positions may not carry financial reward, they may go some way to controlling the perceived injustices or slights that group members may harbour if perceived equity is dissimilar among peers.

Therefore, to effectively manage the group dynamic of a performance organization, it is necessary to understand and predict the impact of new leadership, to be able to reset group goals in response to altering objectives, to manage changes in performance personnel and to determine and provide satisfactory levels of reward and remuneration. Finally, management requires 'time in' with an organization to gain a vital understanding of the performance culture, the values it holds and the impact of potential solutions on the performance dynamic.

Understanding the performance context is crucial to considering the nature of groups and understanding how interactions will impact on performance levels of the organization. We can now move to examining the way in which scientific research can inform this work, starting with theoretical perspectives on group processes.

Theoretical perspectives

Linear versus non-linear perspectives on the dynamics of performance teams

Insight as to how performance teams operate is dependent on understanding the complex interactions among many different factors and individuals. The traditional conception of group dynamics is most commonly based on a linear model proffered by Tuckman & Jensen (1977), who proposed that groups proceeded through a number of discrete stages referred to as form, storm, norm, perform and adjourn. Simply, groups form through a shared need to tackle a collective goal (form); as the group allocates roles and resources, so conflict is said to occur (storm). Once group structure, roles and normative behaviour are established, a group can focus on maximizing performance. The final stage (adjourn) occurs when the groups objectives have been met and dissolution occurs. This simple model, easy to understand and remember, still features in modern-day training on the subject. However, the term 'group dynamics' alludes to the notion that the social milieu of a group fluctuates more than a linear model has the capacity to depict. Whether these fluctuations are gross or are more accurately termed oscillations is not the point. The way in which change materializes in a group will naturally inform needs analyses and any subsequent interventions that a practitioner may undertake. If the underlying theory does not fit with the reality, then the effectiveness of any intervention will be jeopardized.

For example, a linear view of group dynamics infers that cohesion, and consequently productivity, is optimized when the group arrives at a certain stage ('perform'). However, this conception of group dynamics is arguably of little value to performance teams that have been in existence for some time, albeit with continued turnover of personnel. If the model is considered linear, then a group with well established 'norms' should be approaching the 'perform' stage as this is next in line, but observers of real teams know that this is not necessarily the case. Prolonged failure to perform after significant previous success in a quite well established team may produce internal or external pressures that would equate to 'storming' without this being next in Tuckman's linear chain. Furthermore, the linear model provides little guidance to applied practitioners as to how performance may be improved. So if a team is at a performing stage, there is little the theory can offer other than maintaining the status quo. Equally, if a team is establishing itself and 'norming', no explanation is provided as to how a transition might be achieved toward a performing stage. Unfortunately, it would seem that a linear model may fail to account for quite common real life events in performance teams. Equally, the linear model offers limited utility to applied practitioners and therefore a different approach is required to facilitate an understanding and control of group behaviour.

Another perplexing feature of the dynamics of performance teams is their tendency to change rapidly, making prediction problematic (see the challenges inherent in prediction which are highlighted in Ch. 10). Instead of focusing solely on factors identified as crucial to teams' performance, such as leadership or cohesion, an approach that identifies how these factors interact with each other and influence teams directly is necessary to enhance our understanding of this dynamic process.

McClure (1997) demonstrated that group dynamics contain random (stochastic) variables and recommended that groups be viewed as interacting complex systems. For example, in performance-focused groupings such as sports teams or dance companies, variables that predispose groups to periods of change include fluctuating levels of financial investment, injury/retirement and competing objectives. It seems evident that to work effectively with a performance team it is necessary to understand and consider key factors in relation to each other and their combined effect on performance.

Empirical support for a dynamical systems approach can be found in the area of social psychology, where Vallacher & Nowak (1997) argue that a dynamical rather than linear approach is most appropriate to understanding complex relationships (Kruglanski et al 1997). Support for a dynamical systems approach was shown by modelling how attitude change was arrived at among a group of college graduates, which demonstrated that it took 20 processing steps to change an attitude but only four to revert back to the original pattern (Vallacher & Nowak 1997). If attitude change were purely linear, the number of steps would be the same in both directions. Furthermore, this route to change in one direction as opposed to a different route when the change is reversed is a common feature of complex systems in other environments, most notably nature (the formation then dispersal of cyclones or tidal waves are good examples). This also demonstrates that stochastic (i.e. the current state of the group dynamic can be determined by predictable actions as well as unforeseen random elements) variables are present and operate dynamically in social situations.

Following this same logic, it seems more logical, plausible and in keeping with the evidence that the interactions occurring within performance teams are better explained as complex dynamical systems than linear effects or processes. While the topic considered in the previous paragraph, attitude change, may not seem immediately relevant to team performance, it is worth remembering how many elite managers (see below), coaches and directors cite the need to establish a correct performance culture – 'We score [points] – It's an attitude we have' (Sir Alex Ferguson). As we shall see later, the nature of groups' culture is linked to identity, cohesion and group norms, all of which are dependent on the attitude of group members. As such, changing attitude would seem to share a lot with developing a performance team.

Reversal theory

The previous section suggests strongly that performance groups are best understood as non-linear. One approach that embraces this principle is reversal theory (RT; Kerr 1997), which has been supported with experimental, psychometric, psychophysiological and clinical evidence (Apter 2007). It is important to note that reversal theory recognizes that individuals do not behave in a completely random or haphazard way but rather that they have a series of behaviours that influence the roles that they play in groups. RT links motivation and emotion and provides a series of guidelines for leaders in performance situations to manage and manipulate the emotional repertoire of a group to meet fluctuating performance requirements (Tucker & Rutledge 2007).

The crux of RT is that experience and behaviour are influenced by a set of contrasting alternate states that are related to the environment. Each state is based on a fundamental value or motive (Apter 2007). Specifically, four pairs of such opposite states have been identified and the theory proposes that sudden switches, or reversals, in motivational states can occur in the course of everyday life and under a variety of circumstances (Apter 2007, Kerr 1997). These four pairs of states are detailed below:

- The **serious** state, focused on important goals, and planning ahead, versus the **playful** state, focused on immediate enjoyment and acting spontaneously
- The **conforming** state, focused on obligations and the maintenance of rules and routines, versus the **challenging** style, focused on personal freedom
- The **mastery** state, focused on power, control and dominance, versus the **sympathy** state, focused on kindness, caring and harmony
- The **self**-oriented state, focused on one's own needs, versus the **other**-oriented state, focused on the needs of others.

A crucial skill for an applied practitioner or leader of a group to learn is how to change the motivational (and emotional) focus from, for example, a serious to a playful state – or vice-versa. This might be required to reduce tension 24 hours prior to a performance and a fun/amusing task could be organized by the leader. Conversely, where direction is required to improve productivity, a serious motivational state could be engendered by setting performance targets or revising key performance indicators. Recognizing and having the appropriate tools to manipulate the motivational set of a group is a useful tool in maintaining performance standards.

If we accept that people have a tendency to fluctuate between a state focused on one's own needs (self) and the state focused on the needs of others (other), then this can have major implications for the group dynamic. In a team setting, if an individual is seen to attend to their own need, this may be expected. However, if an individual's needs are already being assisted (e.g. in the number of goal scoring chances provided) and they are not reciprocating in kind, then this will create tension, which may ultimately result in contrary behaviours such as team members not continuing to assist, and lead to a net loss in overall group performance. How members of the team manage such tensions is critical to the success of the team.

If a situation of this type occurs in a performance environment, an applied practitioner may draw attention to the respective strengths of both parties and endeavour to establish a way in which significant individual needs can be met without compromising the needs of others or team goals. By understanding eachothers' needs and providing support and opportunities, both parties can succeed and the performance of the team can be enhanced. In short, the dynamics of performance teams need to be underpinned by an appreciation of essential motivating factors for the individuals involved and the potential tensions that might arise as each strives to meet personal and group goals.

Peak performance organizations theory

In addition to having an effective non-linear theory to understand group dynamics, an additional instructive source of information can be obtained by examining the nature and practices of elite performance teams. Identifying factors that appear common to many successful teams may produce a blueprint of what is required by teams aspiring to long-term success. A systematic study of ten organizations across sport and business has led to the development of peak performance organizations (PPO) theory (Gilson et al 2000), which identifies a number of common principles that might explain how organizations achieve and sustain peak performance. Underpinning PPO theory are three peak performance principles – peak purpose, peak practices and peak flow. A schematic of the theory is provided in Figure 9.1. Peak purpose provides meaning and direction for members of an organization. Peak practices refers to the consistent

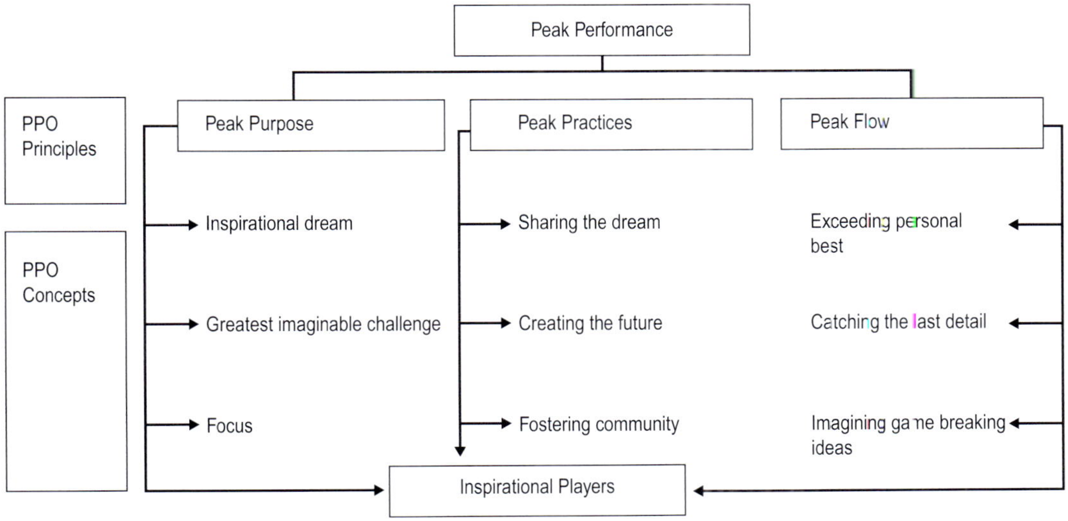

Fig. 9.1 • Schematic of peak performance organizations theory.

best practice of the roles given and accepted by employees or members of a group. Peak flow explains how individuals work together to achieve desired performance outcomes that encompass facets of group dynamics (e.g. leadership, cohesion and social identity). In addition to the three peak principles, the continued role of inspirational performers is considered to be central to the wellbeing of the organization because they provide a model of 'normative' behaviour for aspiring and current performers.

Within the PPO model, each of the peak performance principles is described in more detail. So, for example, peak flow principles include the need to embrace innovative ideas that is crucial for many performance environments. For example, in sport, high media exposure and detailed analysis by rivals often compels directors of performance to constantly develop techniques and tactics that pose novel, significant and unexpected operational dilemmas for rivals/opponents. Innovation was clearly demonstrated through the development of the 'West Coast offence' in American football in the early 1980s by San Francisco 49ers Head Coach, Bill Walsh. This paradigm shift in offence changed the way the game was played and led to the protracted eminence of the 49er franchise over the rest of the NFL. Innovation is also crucial in situations not directly concerned with defeating competitors. For example, dance companies often need to exhibit new interpretations or novel presentations to stimulate both their own performers and public/media interest. Crucially, this demand for innovation must be supported by a group dynamic in which ideas are heard, evaluated and then developed on their merits. It is inevitable that ideas will only be proffered if the perception exists among group members that potential innovations will be received into a constructive environment and the individuals who propose and develop them are subsequently given credit, and their value to the organization is acknowledged.

One aspect of PPO theory that stands outside of the three basic principles is the ongoing link to 'inspirational players'. The reasons for this are interesting: Players or coaches such as Jerry Rice and Joe Montana of the 49ers, Michael Jordan and Phil Jackson of the Chicago Bulls, Kenny Dalglish and Bob Paisley of Liverpool FC are clearly linked to periods of peak success for the organization. As well as the positive historical association for success based on past performance, these individuals also epitomize important traditions and values that, if emulated, help to create a positive performance-orientated group identity and culture. The crucial contribution that such role models can make is considered in the next section.

Group properties

Culture, norms and identity

Understanding, catering for and exploiting the existing culture of a performance team/group is important for any ideas and interventions to be effective. Even if the objective is culture change itself, the route to this lies through utilizing existing elements. The culture of a team is also, in part, bound to the performance context of the team. For example, Leicester Tigers operate in one of the most competitive leagues in world rugby. They are an autonomous commercial enterprise with a very strong fan base of thousands of committed rugby supporters. The organization is not built to finish mid-table and the internal expectation is that, in keeping with their name, the Tigers should be a top-of-the-food-chain predator within the league and Europe. The club is principally focused on achieving success in the domestic league. Beyond domestic competition is the Heineken Cup, a Europe-wide, high-prestige competition. At board level, qualification for the final stages in this is expected by the club. Although Leicester have for many years had many international players from different nations, the senior players give kudos to other players on the basis of what they do for the club, not their country; country comes second.

The culture of a performance team can be beneficial or detrimental to a performance but this is not to say that only one kind of culture equates to success. The point is that recognizing and working within the unique performance culture of a team is an important goal for all practitioners, not just performance psychologists. For example, somewhat peculiarly, Tigers are a working class rugby club. It was no coincidence that, as Director of Rugby, PH drove a battered estate car that might not have been out of place in a stock car race. The message to fellow employees was – don't let your comparative wealth (when contrasted with the supporters, who spend a significant portion of their family income supporting you) conflict with the values of the organization. The performance culture supported a focus on performance levels and accomplishments and opposed team members taking excessive pride in material and financial success. Small behavioural 'norms', while not hugely significant in themselves, reinforce this value.

A social norm is a way of thinking, feeling or behaving that is deemed by the group as appropriate. The most important norms that pertain to any group are those that define the basic values of the group (Bar-Tal 2000, Feldman 1984). Norms do not necessarily refer to clear-cut facts; rather, they refer to certain values that the group agree on and uphold. As previously mentioned, at Leicester Tigers respect is earned from your peers. Players or coaches don't arrive with a big reputation – they develop it when they start to work for that organization. An example of team norms was that no white boots were allowed to be worn in matches or training before March because the individual posturing associated with this did not fit with the all-important team ethic and the shared sense of what it is to be a part of that team. Similarly, the coach let it be known that he didn't get bonuses for winning games or trophies – he negotiated a satisfactory package at the start of his contract and was not going to work harder halfway through a contract for a bonus or less hard because a bonus was not attainable. It is important to recognize that those in positions of influence in the team should exhibit personal values and conform on the whole to the norms that are aligned with the team culture. Equally, the introduction of new team members must be done with these considerations in mind. A team such as Leicester takes time and care to ensure that a person fits well with the club before signing them – individual performance ability alone cannot compensate for the potential damage caused by negative conflict with the team culture. The culture of the team is also inextricably linked with the concept of social identity (see Ch. 8) and also to cohesion, which we will discuss later.

Social identity is defined by Stangor (2004, p. 26) 'as the part of the self-concept that results from our membership in social groups' (Hogg & Abrams 1988, Tajfel & Turner 1986). Generally, the groups that individuals join say something about who they think they are and who they desire to be. Performers will continue to invest part of their identity in a group if their own goals and those of the group are mutually reconcilable. There have been examples of performers in great teams, such as American football's San Francisco 49ers of the 1980s and early 1990s, who did not seek each others' company away from the performance situation. Although the term 'social identity' may suggest that social benefits (camaraderie, friendship, support) are important, in actual fact in this case their self-concept was enhanced because of their association with a successful organization that was task-focused and set up to perform.

Therefore, task-oriented social identity can be derived from membership of a group that acts as a vehicle for personal desires and aspirations (Snyder et al 1986), leading in turn to a desire and motivation to stay with the group until ambitions have been realized or replaced. In a performance environment, self-concept and therefore social identity do not need to be derived from a social group – they can be task-focused and social needs catered for in other facets of an individual's social life. Of course, where a performer is removed from their social setting, such as may happen when recruiting a performer from overseas, then there is an obvious need for and immediate benefit from a supportive social environment.

The point that no one type of culture is the recipe for success is illustrated by comparing Leicester Tigers and the ACT Brumbies (an Australian Rugby Union franchise that now forms part of the Super 14). Unlike Leicester Tigers, the Southern Hemisphere franchise was tasked with recruiting and developing only players who were eligible to represent the national team. This alone is a significant constraint on the recruitment options open to the coach. When the ACT Brumbies started up they were led by a group of influential players who were well educated, very knowledgeable about the sport and from families steeped in the game of Rugby Union. The division of roles in the club emerged from the skills and abilities available at that time; management and directors managed off the field while a self-selected group of players formulated and managed the game plan. By their own admission, the players did not prepare themselves physically as well as they could have, but the techniques and tactics they adopted resulted in successful performances. Their focus was on intelligent planning and use of the performers available, given the recruitment restrictions imposed (as we shall see below in the section on Strategy).

The idiosyncratic nature of effective performance cultures brings significant challenges for practitioners. Firstly, how can entry for a practitioner be successfully negotiated? Secondly, aside from anecdotal material (e.g. accounts by former military Special Forces personnel and successful sports coaches/players following successful outcomes – both notably only available for successes), there is a dearth of balanced empirical evidence on the influence on the overall group dynamic if a team is organized in such a 'bottom-up' fashion.

Recognizing these two contrasting examples of successful teams within the same sport can provide the practitioner with differing propositions and challenges to their expertise, knowledge, manner of working and 'goodness of fit' with such organizations. The implication for applied practitioners is clear: interventions based on standard assumptions about group dynamics are unlikely to deliver. Careful assessment and understanding of a performance culture is central to determining what, where and when interventions should be employed as well as having a clear strategic focus as an overarching guide to all work.

Strategy

As we saw in Chapter 8, a clear strategy represents the core element of group and team performance. Strategy is paramount and should precede and instruct consideration of other components of group dynamics such as structure and leadership. Strategy also influences the dynamical processes such as cohesion and conflict. A tension exists for the management between planning for the duration of a given performance cycle such as a season, tour or period prior to significant performance and longer-term strategic goals with less tangible and immediate impact. These pressures combine to place specific demands on the individual or group responsible for formulating strategy.

With regard to strategy, Sun Tzu wrote that, 'One who knows the enemy and knows himself will not be endangered in a hundred engagements. One who does not know the enemy but knows himself will sometimes be victorious, sometimes meet with defeat. One who knows neither the enemy nor himself will invariably meet with defeat on every occasion'. But what constitutes 'knowledge' in the performance context, and how is it best obtained?

Organizations spend a great deal of time analysing potential capabilities of competitors or rivals. Knowing about others and developing a coherent plan to ameliorate perceived advantage and maintain one's own position does not necessarily reflect an equivalent knowledge of strengths and weaknesses of one's own performance team, as in the above quotation. Team self-analysis has to be purposive and is often uncomfortable, but is necessary if the strategy is to prove effective. The ACT Brumbies team considered both strengths and deficiencies to develop an approach designed to make them competitive and enhance overall performance. ACT routinely played against Polynesian rugby players, who tended to be fast and powerful and used aggressive tackling to win ball. In short, physically the ACT team struggled to dominate the battle; instead they spent a great deal of time learning to collectively 'move the target' and attack at pace on unexpected angles, which placed contact-focused players at a disadvantage. (Between 1997 and 2001 ACT Brumbies played two of the five finals and were Super 12 Champions in 2001.) In other words, strategy should make your disadvantages advantageous!

The importance for a performance team of critically examining its own strengths and weaknesses and the specific challenges it faces seems evident. Unlike typical business strategy formation, which, once completed, may remain static for some time, high-performance teams require more regular 'micro-strategy' sensitive to minor fluctuations in their own performance capability (e.g. a ballet company may have injuries to some key personnel) or the changing challenges (e.g. a sports team may face very different types of opponent in consecutive weeks). However, it is important to note that, while micro-strategy is important to maintain effectiveness in a dynamic environment, if it becomes the predominant goal for the team or group then the immediate success or failures will impact on key group constructs such as cohesion and confidence (efficacy). Micro-strategies combined with, and integrated within, macro-strategies ensure that performances are organized effectively while protecting the team from the vagaries of responding to win/loss or public criticism/acclaim.

In addition to a frank assessment of respective strengths and weaknesses, good strategy apportions effort and resources to the demands of the task facing the organization in the most effective way. Crucially, strategy also needs to be sold to the members of the group. An example of this at Leicester Tigers related to planning how the team could function successfully in concurrent competitions running through the season subject to changing player availability (injury) and additional commitments (international team performances in autumn and spring). Through all of this was the need to protect players from specific detriments (e.g. injury, burnout). To respond to these challenges the Tigers decided to rotate players, a policy that had previously been an anathema. Based on discussion and group goals, however, there were also specific exceptions to this policy of rotation – such as no rotation through the most challenging competition (Heineken Cup). The increased opportunity and experience for more players to perform at the top level extended the pool of talent but also demonstrated who was not able to operate under the pressures that characterized that level. It was important for performers to understand and accept the policy from the outset. Being removed from the starting team was not necessarily indicative of loss of form – it was the rotation policy. Interestingly, the onus was placed on returning international players to regain their place in the starting line-up. Once again, procedures were put in place that resonated with the team's goals, norms and identity.

In terms of the practical strategy of winning the domestic competition from the start of the season, the team aimed for qualification for the top four (the playoffs) – not to finish first. Over the course of 22 games it was determined that 60 points were required, which the team aimed to achieve through 12 wins and 12 bonus points (awarded for scoring four or more tries or being within 4 points of the winner). Thus the bonus points were integral to success and so Tigers developed a bonus point culture, accruing a record amount of 14 points. To promote task cohesion a critical component in developing this strategy was to make the bonus point culture explicit by way of the 'same message, different voices' tactic. For example, rather than have the strategy explained and reinforced repeatedly by the head coach in team meetings, which can tend to be a monologue from an individual, the strategy was communicated by certain trusted 'lieutenants'. This form of communication enabled discussion and understanding more effectively than monologue-style communication. It also enabled the communication to be applied at the most appropriate time in training and to permeate through the performers and organization at other informal times. Letting these lieutenants speak at critical moments also helped to develop their own capacity to make correct decisions and lead or influence other performers at critical, pressured periods of performance. These individuals not only gave the message but modelled it through their own performance.

Once performers accepted the strategy and it was embedded within the team, the strategy was publicly declared to make it common knowledge and to maintain task focus and provide reinforcement from outside the team to keep performers and team 'on message'. This example demonstrates the real detail and focus of strategic planning for a performance team, together with consideration of how it could be implemented. The positive employment of media and public opinion is another notable and very intelligent solution to making strategy real.

The individuals involved in this process of delegation are critical: Sven-Göran Eriksson was lauded in the early days of his tenure as England's soccer head coach as he used 'cultural architects' to introduce and maintain the strategy employed by England (see the work of Willi Railo (1986)). Arguably, it is the personality and aptitude of the lieutenants that govern the successful implementation of the strategy. Within the leadership group of performers that share the coaches' confidence, three players might implement the strategic plan during performance, while other players delivered messages (through verbal, non-verbal and modelling behaviours) on emotional intensity, work rate and the attitude and values integral to the performance team. Coaches need to have the opportunity to develop or recruit performers who can fulfil this type of essential role that goes beyond the basic performance functions. Satisfying such roles is not only a consideration for team games. A performance group in any environment, even a squad of individual extreme sport athletes or dancers, will benefit from an effective and driven environment. Switched-on coaches have long recognized this and recruited training partners and squad members accordingly.

Communicating clear strategy is integral to ensuring that the team maintains high task cohesion. We will revisit this construct again in Chapter 24 but, in short, task cohesion is the extent to which all performers within the team agree with current strategy and understand their own and fellow team members' roles. In addition, they are prepared to work in a mutually cooperative manner in order to pursue performance targets. The need for task cohesion represents familiar territory for performance teams, which are predominantly task-oriented because they are typically evaluated (and funded) on the basis of their performances. In performance environments, until comparatively recently, there has existed doubt as to whether group cohesion improves team performance, or whether performance improves group cohesion. A reason that partly explained this lack of understanding was that the term 'cohesion' had different meanings, which can be differentiated as three subcomponents: interpersonal attraction, group pride and task commitment. Based on these three differentiated types of cohesion, Mullen & Copper (1994), completed a meta-analysis of 49 studies across a variety of settings (military, sport, work, laboratory and nonwork) and found a small but significant relationship between cohesion and performance, with task commitment (analogous to task cohesion) showing the most significant relationship with performance (Carron & Hausenblas 1998). This is an important finding, with important implications. However, it is worth noting that these investigators didn't check that the task features committed to were actually (as opposed to perceived as) common across the group members. So it is critical that practitioners working with groups check such features as role clarity, shared mental models and strategic appreciation and do not merely assume that these are fully understood and agreed by group members.

Organization and group processes

Group structure

Group structure has been defined as the rules that define group norms, roles and status (Stangor 2004). Group structure can be crudely divided into what can be written on paper (formal structure) and implicit structural features (informal structure). The second category is both more important and less accessible. It is often the informal structure and personnel who have been involved for a long period of time that maintain and perpetuate the key norms and values. Top performers, leaders, directors and head coaches may come and go but these key individuals may continue to work for the team/organization provided they do not become too ambitious or suddenly represent a hindrance to the performance of the group, necessitating a clearing out of the 'old guard'.

Developing or maintaining a group structure that maximizes the resources of the group and does not result in the dissatisfaction of its personnel is an exercise in diplomatic relations (see the importance of politics stressed in Ch. 8). A subtle approach to this problem was employed by PH during his time at Tigers (Fig. 9.2). Despite the proposed change being subject to intense scrutiny, his knowledge of the team enabled the change to the group structure to be perceived as complementary to the organization rather than a threat to core values. The approach detailed below is formed using 'silos'; the emphasis is on autonomy for each silo.

At board level, the general manager reports to shareholders. Directly beneath are two operational directors with responsibility for their respective silos and setting performance targets for each self-contained unit. The Director of Rugby attends board meetings and has a direct relationship with the board that is designed to foster direct communication with regard to accountability for team performance.

The Director of Rugby is directly responsible for the performance of the Athletic Performance, Rugby Academy, Rugby Union and Medical support silos. He also has input to the organization and the setting of the performance indicators of the groups represented in the silos, which are under the control of the Director of Operations.

In this structure, the directors appoint personnel and set targets – in essence, assign individuals to specific roles and hold them accountable. Another important consideration is ensuring that individuals are appointed who complement the weaknesses/deficiencies of the individuals in charge. The benefit of a director of performance designing the group structure is that it maintains performance focus as the primary consideration. A clearly identifiable structure and hierarchy is also advantageous for performers and staff, who can be certain from whom they should take instruction. With the group structure in situ, individuals' status is less ambiguous and readily identifiable. This structure offers a good

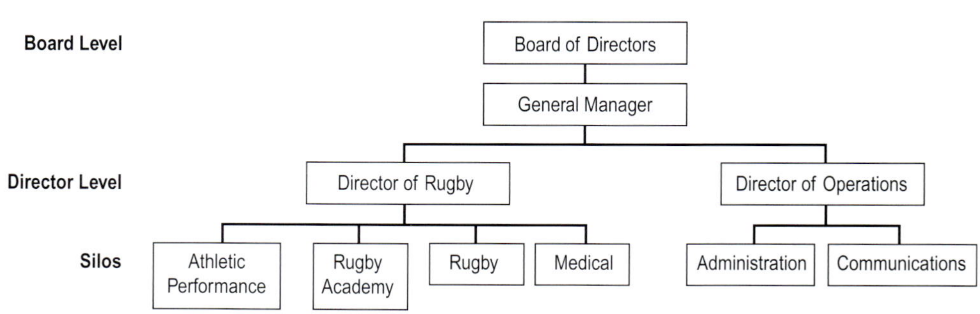

Fig. 9.2 • Leicester Tigers RFC – organizational structure.

example of the matrix management approach identified in Chapter 8.

A vital consideration regarding the imposition of structural change is that alterations affect only targeted areas while leaving intact, and preferably in rude health, the norms and values of the organization with which its members and supporters identify. Would this formal group structure work at another rugby club or in a different sport or domain? It may or may not, but it is not intended as a model to copy but rather as an example that shows how strategy, function and performance-centred considerations were used to dictate the organization of a clear group structure. Therefore, group structures in performance environments display wide variance, but structural changes that might impact on the group dynamic should be sensitive to the values and norms that form part of the identity of the group.

A specific example that highlighted the need for sensitivity was a change in coaching practices that lessened the time each coach had with the first team but was designed to increase the impact of each session (same message – different voices). Unfortunately, among certain coaches personal kudos was governed by the amount of contact time granted by the Director of Rugby. This organizational change had to be managed from a coaching perspective and also a player perspective, as they evaluated the worth of each coach's message according to the amount of time apportioned with the first team. Perceptions are key to this process, and someone somewhere in the structure had to take responsibility for evaluating, allowing for and subtly influencing and evolving perceptions within the team. Fortunately, this responsibility was taken by the Director of Rugby!

Leadership

There are many theories concerning leadership but it is important to keep in mind the observation made by Van Seters & Field (1990), who noted that current modes of leadership style and philosophy, in western culture, are closely related to current economic, political and cultural viewpoints. For example, in the USA in the early 1970s, the civil rights movement gained ground and anti-war protests engendered widespread mistrust of the federal government. As a result, it is interesting to observe the emergence of the anti-leadership era based on widespread dissatisfaction with the hitherto largely unquestioned authority of a government that exercised an unjustifiable (in the opinion of many) mandate to draft young men into the military. This period of political unrest led some to question the supposed qualifications, expertise and mandate that leaders possessed.

In fact, the anti feeling that accrued through this period may have been misplaced on leaders instead of hierarchies. Interestingly, leadership substitution theory (LST; Kerr & Jermier 1978) proposes that, if people in an organization are expert at what they do, then there is no need to create layers of management and bureaucracy to control and manage employees, provided that these individuals are working in synchrony with the overall needs and aims of the organization. This suggestion fits well with the idea of 'flat' structures introduced in Chapter 8.

While LST is an interesting idea, it has not attracted a wealth of empirical investigation. However, LST presupposes that members of a group or organization will be expert and self-regulated. In an applied performance environment it would be ideal to have a group that is motivated and sufficiently trained and experienced to operate without the strictures and threat of sanctions that may be employed by a coach or director of performance if a group underperforms. In other words, a group with traditions that result in self-policing and a constant task focus.

From practical experience, such teams or groups do exist but they have developed organically rather than by design. A good example, already mentioned, was the group of player leaders at ACT Brumbies. Some of these senior players took on and fulfilled tactical roles normally associated with a coach or a director of coaching. The nature of the group dynamic at that time allowed this to occur: the team had a group of bright, well educated rugby players with considerable rugby knowledge, the team was newly formed and there was no dedicated head coach. However, teams where leadership follows an LST approach may be the exception, since the capacity of individuals to self-organize is potentially fraught, as individuals may vie for control and recognition. Also, some members of a group quite reasonably recognize that others around them are better suited to specific roles and may wish to be managed or led. Such 'self-adjusting' target-seeking traditions are common across performance (military exemplars are particularly apparent). Take care, however, since such traditions are easily lost and very hard to regain.

The antithesis of LST is transformational leadership (TL), the essence of which has been neatly summarized by Goethe: 'Dream no small dreams, for they have no power to move the hearts of men.'

TL is based on a charismatic leadership style and assumes that leaders and followers exchange resources: followers receive direction, structure and in some cases expertise from their leader, while the leader gains power and privilege (Baron & Kerr 2003). TL also provides 'ordinary' members of the group with inspiration that seeks to persuade them to buy into the operational goals of the organization. It is the contention of Bass (1998) that transformational leaders encourage innovation and promote a meritocratic performance culture focused on rewarding target behaviours as opposed to punishing incorrect actions. While Bass acknowledged that this style of leadership was hard to achieve, it has been shown to increase creative productivity in groups across a variety of performance settings, e.g. business and military (Bass 1998, Shamir et al 1993).

There is a significant discrepancy between these two theories of leadership, both of which have significant implications for a performance culture. The discrepancy lies between the motivational catalysts for group performance. Simply put: are you part of an organization that relies on inspirational leadership as a motivational catalyst before pursuing peak performance or does the organization of which you are part strive to pursue collectively agreed, performance-orientated goals? Although these are not the only theories of leadership, the differences between them illustrate one of the most important elements that needs to be understood about leadership, which is concerned with the granting, maintenance, influence and dissolution of power.

Power

To lead a successful group, leaders need to learn how to handle and maintain power. One of the primary reasons why groups are organized and structured in particular ways is to allow power to be channelled effectively. Yet striving to maintain an influential group necessitates developing members of the group to become more powerful, whether physically, tactically, technically or mentally. Therefore, crucial to understanding power in a group dynamic is a perception about how power is arrived at and maintained but also how it is given away, to whom and upon what grounds. For example, if a performer is given knowledge and skill this may reduce the power discrepancy between the performer and the director.

In performance groups or teams, power is necessary to deliver change, which is critical to the wellbeing of a healthy group dynamic. Change may be achieved through consultative or autocratic – 'like it or lump it' – approaches. Which of these is appropriate depends significantly on the power position of the leader.

Interestingly, there are numerous examples of individuals appointed to senior roles who do not necessarily become powerful leaders – at least according to the perceptions of group members. This is crucial when you consider that a key aspect of leadership is concerned with influencing others to complete onerous tasks that are enacted to secure the short- and long-term objectives of the organization. As mentioned in Chapter 8, power is a relational concept: people are only powerful because others ascribe and perceive them to have power, and respond and are influenced by them. Therefore, as Veronica Burke points out in Chapter 8, we need to consider the informal means through which leadership and therefore power is wielded.

In an era of flattened management hierarchies and the emergence of new organizational forms, it is clear that leaders require alternative strategies to wield power. As Chapter 8 identified, successful leadership in performance environments requires the recognition of power from peers and followers based upon three facets of personal power; expert power, referent power and connection power. Through expert power a leader's credibility is established and value is placed on competencies in a given performance area; referent power refers to the esteem in which a leader is held by peers and followers and the social attraction that a leader may possess; connection power refers to the social networks that a leader is part of and maintains.

While there are exceptions, it is generally recognized that great performers do not necessarily make great leaders. In performance environments, expert performers have often been appointed at the end of their performance career to lead an organization for which they once performed. The appointment of leading performers to leadership roles is of particular interest as one of the co-authors of this chapter arguably fell into this category! In his second or third season as a professional player PH performed (informal) coaching duties for the team he played for. However, PH had access to elite coaching knowledge gathered by three generations of his family – an interesting example of the utility of connection power.

However, it is important to consider the appointment of ex-performers to leadership roles with caution. They usually want to do it, are confident in their ability and possess immediately credibility and referent power, but their specific expertise power of the performance situation is current for increasingly shorter periods of time. Other, more generic leadership skills presented in this and the previous chapter, such as strategy formation, structural organization and recognizing and utilizing expertise in others must be learned and developed through practice but are not an automatic feature of successful performance in the activity itself. To summarize, expert power may be usefully employed in recognizing expertise in others and organizing their collective response to task demands. The leadership challenge has more facets than this, however, and the full spectrum of skills will be required.

Referent power is the esteem that a leader is held in by peers and followers and, in conjunction with expert power, may get a performance leader an employment opportunity and attract similarly talented significant others to the group. Crucially, however, connection power provides the glue that has the potential to bond the key facets of the group and refers to the social network that a leader is connected with and to. For PH, having trusted advisors to consult with external to the organization was critical. For example, recruiting personnel; keeping abreast (ahead) of technical innovation and having an organizational mentor to assist with the design of the performance dynamic was crucial. Therefore, expert power was not as essential as knowing where to access expertise.

As we saw in Chapter 8, there are a number of different ways of conceptualizing different types of power. In a performance team it is natural to want to assemble a number of experts, so it is likely that many individuals will possess certain types of power, especially expert power. This raises the potential for conflict to occur between a number of individuals who have and wish to exert their expert power to influence the group.

This conflict is neatly illustrated in the case of Leicester, where there were a number of talented assistant coaches vying for recognition and promotion. As previously outlined in the section on group structure, changing the roles of experts can result in conflict if they feel they are competing for resources (e.g. time with the first team and therefore kudos). The rationale for the change was to have a coherent message that was reinforced by several coaches, thereby increasing the likelihood of prolonging the interest and attention of players. Mistakenly, the players and assistant coaches perceived that time with the performance team represented an acknowledgement of the coach's worth and therefore their status, and so time with the team became perceived as the 'currency of power' and was the source of contention and conflict among coaching staff. However, to the Director of Performance, time spent coaching the group/subgroup was not directly related to that coach's expertise. In a situation such as this tensions are inevitable, pitting the perceived wishes/needs of the individuals concerned against the head coach's judgement regarding the most efficient and effective use of time in response to the needs of the group. For the group to remain optimally effective in situations such as this, the structure and leadership must be organized and able to use power (reward, persuade, coerce) to maintain continued success in the face of such conflicts.

Empowerment

The philosophy behind the concept of empowerment is that performers must be encouraged to take responsibility for their performance and development/practice environments. Removing decision making about performance or preparing to perform to a select group of directors, coaches, managers or leading players means that the bulk of performers become merely responsive to their environments and instruction but do not engage proactively by thinking about how they could be better, lay plans to achieve optimum conditions or understand how to modify plans to adapt best to changing conditions. In short, failure to empower performers results in the charge that leaders are not equipping group members for the challenges they will inevitably face during and post career (Kidman 2001). Part of the reluctance to adopt an empowerment approach is that, for many of those responsible for a performance group, their own effectiveness is benchmarked by the success of the group. With this intense pressure to perform, it is understandable why many of those in authoritative positions choose to wield their authority in an attempt to control as many factors as possible that combine to influence their own perceived success or failure.

However, adopting an 'empowerment' approach can have a significant impact on the motivational structure of the group. Advocates of an empowerment approach (Kidman 2001) argue that it can be implemented from the bottom of the organization to the top echelons of the group. To benefit from an empowerment approach, leaders are required to cultivate an environment in which all performers feel they should, and are able to, contribute to the development of the team. For example, if a team member proposes an idea that is adopted by the team and endorsed by those in a leadership position, then they are far more likely to take responsibility for its implementation and performance. Ensuring that ideas are received and considered fairly, as well as making sure that a proportion of them are explicitly seen to be accepted, is, according to Kidman (2001), more likely to engage all members of the performance group.

A performance team adopting the philosophy of empowerment may require a change of group culture currently in existence among performers, leaders and staff. The need to consider change is neatly encapsulated in the reflections of a head coach of a professional rugby team, who acknowledged the need to consider alternative means of working in conjunction with professional performers:

> The role of the coach has changed hugely, and that has been the biggest learning curve for me. Now, I would consider myself as a facilitator of a team and to get players to play to their potential. But it is a facilitating role – it has changed from the finger-wagging, head-banging stuff – you just can't do that – the amount of contact I have with these guys... it has be a totally different approach. From being a sort of authoritarian decision maker on all aspects of how the team play, to moving over to using player empowerment.

Kidman (2001) observed, in sports, that teams who are directive-based and driven by leadership edicts (autocratic) are successful at the start of the season but labour when the pressure increases toward the end of the performance cycle as stakes inevitably increase. An additional factor that may impinge on a team's performance relates to the need to have a consistent emphasis on strategic goals. As discussed previously in this chapter, the principle of same message–different voice is important to increase the effectiveness of communication and so the same message should be delivered coherently by different members of the group and preferably from the operational end. This practice demonstrates trust throughout the group dynamic. If this principle is adopted, it demonstrates the practical application of empowerment and its ability to focus members' attention on the performance task.

In the context of group dynamics in a performance environment, empowerment can have significant motivational benefits for performers, leaders and staff. Identity, commitment, ownership and personal development can be encouraged by the challenge to all members of the team to contribute to the group's ongoing success.

It is important to note that empowerment is not a panacea, nor necessarily appropriate for all performers or teams. In some cases, involving elite performers in decision making and the subsequent evaluation of performance can impact negatively on their performance. While some individuals may demonstrate the capacity to work on a group level and thrive on the execution of responsibility while contributing knowledge and ideas, others may show a marked decline in performance as a consequence. The clear message is: know your individuals before you invite them to participate in debriefs and planning sessions. While empowerment can work where performers are asked to contribute to the continued improvement of technique and acquisition of tactical acumen, experience has shown that this role is not for every performer, despite seniority or their own personal desire to be involved in these aspects of the team dynamic. In simple terms, some performers can only concentrate upon their own role; any further involvement in the operation of the dynamic as a whole can overburden them, leading to a marked decline in performance.

However, performance objectives that focus solely on success may lead the head coach or Performance Director to deem this to be the sole performance indicator. In doing so, Kidman (2001) suggests that the performance team, and in particular those in charge, become accountable for the unaccountable, since many other factors beyond the team can influence outcomes, such as the decisions or performances of others or events such as poor weather conditions. A typical response that may occur as a result of the pressure that an individual can face in this environment is to 'take over' and issue specific directives about how the task should be done (Kidman 2001). The empowered team should react by taking considered action based on the expert judgements of task specialists who are well trained and placed to make the most effective response.

Conflict management

A great deal of attention may be paid to strategy – the continued success of the group may depend on its execution. However, if strategy is not agreed upon and implemented coherently, or if it is undermined by conflict, then performance and success may be significantly undermined. For example, the previously identified situation of several expert staff all seeking contact with performers presents the conditions of a limited resource (time with performers) that provided the potential trigger for conflict. Each member of staff wanted to be as involved as they could, to be able to do their job at the top level, to be valued by the group and to cement their place in the team with a view to continued employment and, potentially, promotion. This need for everyone to have their role, to feel that they too are contributing, is quite understandable but essential to avoid. The informed performance psychologist will be well aware of this possibility and work to ensure that performers are not 'over supported'! In this respect, especially as the time for performance approaches, 'less is more' and 'they truly serve who stand and wait'!

The more successful a performance team becomes, the greater the need for specialist experts to operate in tandem with greater financial resource to employ them such as the support offered to Olympic performers (Fig. 9.3). Therefore, the ongoing development of a team demands commensurate change in the management capabilities of those in key directing roles as the organization becomes more complex, to ensure that the benefits are maximized and minimize the potential drawbacks such as conflict that may occur.

Careful communication, clearly delineated roles and responsibilities and obtaining understanding and acceptance of all individuals is essential. For example, when this situation occurred in a professional rugby team, the communication included clear benefits for those involved. It was emphasized that those involved would benefit in the long term from the opportunity of working with other experts and broadening their own repertoire of innovative practice techniques as well as extending their association with a performance team that aspired to greater achievements than had been achieved already. However, a few of the coaches aspired to be viewed as head coach material, without reflecting upon the state of their own knowledge and, crucially, the needs of the group.

This conflict occurred because of the tension between the needs of the group (as identified by the head coach) and the aspirations of individuals. The currencies that fuelled this conflict were player respect and increased hours of contact. The more contact, the more kudos generated, thus heightening a misplaced self-respect, which in turn propagated the false belief that enhanced reputations and improved career prospects would follow. An insight into this particular conflict can be achieved if it is interpreted in light of realistic conflict theory (RCT; Sherif et al 1961): RCT posits that hostility and aggression will surface when groups (in this case colleagues) are competing for scarce resources or have incompatible and mutually frustrating goals (Baron & Kerr 2003).

The means by which conflicts are either resolved or perpetuated is heavily influenced by the culture of the group dynamic. For example, physical conflict occurring between players in a Rugby Union training environment is not an unusual occurrence and therefore a cultural norm usually exists for managing this. An example norm is that players recognize and adopt two key principles: that conflict must not be allowed to fester and that the individuals must take it upon

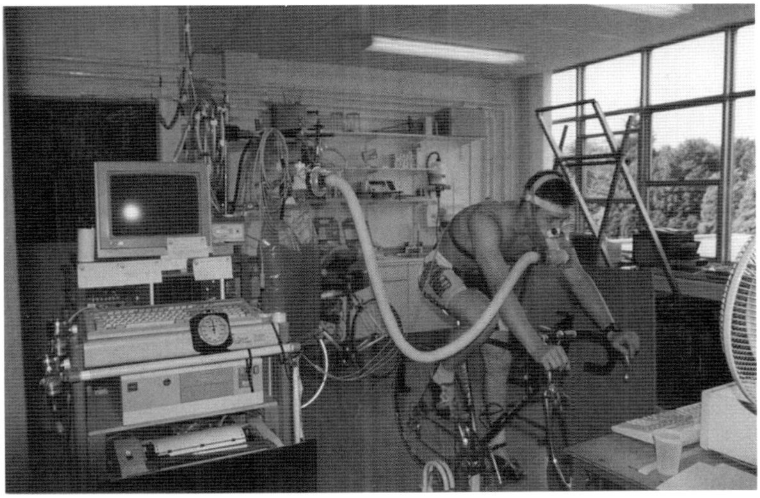

Fig. 9.3 • Performance teams increasingly include a range of scientists. Olympic medallist Nicky Gooch in testing at the British Olympic Medical Centre. Thanks to Alan Luke for the photo.

themselves to sort differences out and not leave the ground until the conflict is resolved. However, if an unanticipated conflict occurs where an existing norm does not exist, as in the case of a French Rugby Union player who struck a coach, then an alternative approach is required. In this case the guilty party, who was deemed to have 'crossed the line', had to take every member of the team out for lunch. The restaurant bill he received when his 'hospitality' was fully exploited served as a peer-enforced deterrent. Thus the coach's authority was reaffirmed by the behaviour of the group.

However, in ordinary circumstances there are practical means by which to foresee and deal with potential conflict. When considering how to handle conflict, the leadership has to decide whether the situation requires immediate or long-term attention (as in the example given of coaching time) or whether it is best left alone. Therefore, three options are readily available: confront it, manage it or ignore it. To use a confrontational style with the person or group it is necessary to make a judgement about the individual/group being dealt with and determine if there are viable alternative solutions, how quickly individuals will return to task focus and the true critical nature of the programme. If there are no apparent solutions to a problem, then it needs to be managed. For example, a performer unavailable because of injury is not directly 'solvable'. In the case of ignoring a problem, it may be that the group experiences a spate of unfavourable media coverage with a particular agenda; in such cases there is usually little point in providing additional comment or response, as this rarely stems the tide and is more likely to provide further ammunition to sustain debate and perpetuate negative attention. Once again, strong steers on conflict management are offered in the previous chapter.

Conclusion

Effectively engaging with and influencing the dynamics of a performance team or group can be thought of as an outcome based initially on accurate knowledge and understanding. This knowledge includes knowledge of others (audiences, stakeholders, competitors), and knowledge of self/team (culture, identity, strengths and weaknesses). Key to successful performance is having knowledge workers – staff and performers who are able to draw on a wealth of knowledge to devise solutions to rapidly changing and fiercely challenging performance environments (Gongla & Rizzuto 2001). A key device to supporting interested and knowledgeable personnel is to have evolving communities where ideas of best practice are shared and developed (Gongla & Rizzuto 2001). These can act as test beds for ideas and concepts or proving grounds for ambitious individuals. IBM –a global organization – recognizes the role of communities as a means of gathering and disseminating knowledge, reporting experiences and retaining and developing intellectual capital (Gongla & Rizzuto 2001). The key component is understanding how to propagate and maintain a healthy group dynamic.

Through this chapter we have combined scientific theory and evidence with applied experience to describe key aspects of developing high-achieving performance teams. In doing so we have supported the view that teams do not operate in linear ways and that alternative models of how to achieve desired performance levels are required, given the complexity of group dynamics. We considered both the theoretical alternative to linear approaches such as reversal theory and the applied evidence of peak performance organizations to provide a more realistic understanding of how excellence could be promoted in performance teams. This emphasized, for example, the role that past performers can have in a performance group by providing continuity between the past and the present. It is interesting to note how some leading performance organizations are beginning to gradually reduce the performance role of exemplary performers and the anticipated levels of productivity each year. This seems to acknowledge that some of the key elements they offer in relation to providing role models and as a source of leadership and decision making are highly valued by the organization. The implicit, informal mentoring provided to young performers is also a hugely beneficial and effective means of educating younger performers that far outweighs the short-term effect of a camp or clinic with an elite performer. These have the correct idea but fail to have a significant or lasting effect because they do not establish a relationship between mentor and performer, nor can they provide the consistency of message that can be delivered by a senior performer through training and during performance.

Many of the important variables we have discussed in this chapter are mediated by the performance culture of the group. For example, the example given earlier of managing conflict in rugby is unlikely to be the same for professional dancers. Good advice and intervention must be based on the specific parameters of what is 'normal', the team's culture, which will dictate how and in which direction change can be effected to enhance performance.

References

Adams, J.S., 1965. Inequity in social exchange. Adv. Exp. Soc. Psychol. 62, 335–343.

Apter, M.J., 2007. Available on line at: http://www.reversaltheory.org/ (accessed 02.09.09).

Baron, R.S., Kerr, N.L., 2003. Group process, group decision, group action. Open University Press, Philadelphia, PA.

Bar-Tal, D., 2000. Shared beliefs in a society: social psychological analysis. Sage, Thousand Oaks, CA.

Bass, B.M., 1998. Transformational leadership: industrial military and educational impact. Lawrence Erlbaum Associates, Mahwah, NJ.

Carron, A.V., Hausenblas, H.A., 1998. Group dynamics in sport. Fitness information technology, Morgantown, WV.

Feldman, D.C., 1984. The development and enforcement of group norms. Acad. Manage. Rev. 9, 47–53.

Gilson, C., Pratt, M., Roberts, K., et al., 2000. Peak performance: business lessons from the world's top sports organizations. Harper Collins, London.

Gongla, P., Rizzuto, C.R., 2001. Evolving communities of practice: IBM global service experience. IBM Sys. J. 40, 842–862.

Guerrero, L.K., Andersen, P.A., Afifi, W.A., 2007. Close encounters: communication in relationships, second ed. McGraw-Hill, Englewood Cliffs, NJ.

Hodge, K., 2004. Sport motivation: training your mind for peak performance. Reed, Auckland.

Hogg, M.A., Abrams, D., 1988. Social identifications: a social psychology of intergroup relations and group processes. Routledge, London.

Jackson, P., 1995. Sacred hoops. Hyperion Books, New York.

Jones, G., 2002. Performance excellence: a personal perspective on the link between sport and business. J. Appl. Sport Psychol. 14, 268–281.

Kerr, J.H., 1997. Motivation and emotion in sport: reversal theory. Taylor & Francis, Hove, East Sussex.

Kerr, S., Jermier, J.M., 1978. Substitutes for leadership: their meaning and measurement. Organ. Behav. Hum. Perform. 22, 375–403.

Kidman, L., 2001. Developing decision makers: an empowerment approach to coaching. Innovative Print Communications, Christchurch, New Zealand.

King, A., 2006. The word of command: communication and cohesion in the military. Armed Forces and Society 32, 493–512.

Kruglanski, A.W., Clement, R.W., Jost, J.T., 1997. The new wave of dynamism: will it engulf the field? Psychological Inquiry 8, 132–135.

McClure, B.A., 1997. Putting a new spin on groups: the science of chaos. Lawrence Erlbaum Associates, Mahwah, NJ.

McConnell, R., 1999. Inside the All-Blacks. Harper Collins, London.

Mullen, B., Copper, C., 1994. The relation between group cohesiveness and performance: an integration. Psychol. Bull. 115, 210–227.

Novak, M., 1976. The joy of sports. Basic Books, New York.

Railo, W., 1986. Willing to win. Amas, Utrecht.

Shamir, B., House, R.J., Arthur, M.B., 1993. The motivational effects of charismatic leadership: a self-concept based theory Organization Science 4, 577–594.

Sherif, M., Harvey, O.J., White, B.J., et al., 1961. Intergroup conflict and cooperation: the robbers cave experiment. University Book Exchange, Norman, OK.

Snyder, C.R., Lassegard, M., Ford, C.E., 1986. Distancing after group success and failure: basking in reflected glory and cutting off reflected failure. J. Pers. Soc. Psychol. 51, 382–388.

Spector, P.E., 2008 Industrial and organizational behavior, fifth ed. Wiley, Hoboken, NJ.

Stangor C., 2004. Social groups in action and interaction. Taylor & Francis, Hove, East Sussex.

Tajfel, H., Turner, J.C., 1986. The social identity theory of intergroup behaviour. In: Worchel, S., Austin, W.G (Eds.), Psychology of intergroup relations. Nelson Hall, Chicago, IL.

Tucker, J., Rutledge, H., 2007. Shaping motivation and emotion in technology teams. CrossTalk Magazine Nov, 10–13.

Tuckman, B.W., Jensen, M.A.C., 1977. Stages of small group development revisited. Group and Organizational Studies 2, 419–427.

Vallacher, R.S., Nowak, A., 1997. The emergence of dynamical social psychology. Psychological Inquiry 8, 73–99.

Van Seters, D.A., Field, R.H.G., 1990. The evolution of leadership theory. J. Organ. Change Manage. 3, 29–45.

Van Vugt, M., 2004. Follow the leader . . . but at what cost? Psychologist 17, 274–277.

Planning for physical performance: the individual perspective

10

Planning, periodization, prediction, and why the future ain't what it used to be!

John Kiely

University of Central Lancashire, Lancashire, UK; UK Athletics, UK

CHAPTER CONTENTS

Introduction

The aim of this chapter is to provide an appreciation of critical factors that influence physical preparation planning within performance environments. Surprisingly, perhaps, a meaningful analysis of this topic requires much more than simply a review of the existing training science literature. It also goes without saying that it is beyond the scope of a single chapter to delve into every crack and corner of such an expansive topic. Nevertheless, we will cover a lot of ground, much of which is previously uncharted within performance science domains, in an attempt to understand the origins and veracity of the methods in common use and, perhaps, how things may be improved.

The objective of the physical preparation plan is to guide the performer towards a state of optimal performance readiness at a specified future date. As such, the preparation plan may essentially be considered an exercise in stress management. As noted by Canadian endocrinologist Hans Selye, the pre-eminent early researcher on the biological effects of stress: 'The goal is certainly not to avoid stress; stress is a part of life. But in order to express yourself fully you must find your optimum stress level and then use your adaptation energy at a rate and in a direction adjusted to the innate structure of your mind and body' (Selye 1956).

In such terms, the planner's quest is to ascertain the *optimum stress level* and impose training stress in both the *magnitude* and *direction* that maximally benefits target performance.

DOI: 10.1016/B978-0-443-06734-1.00010-9

The principle of progressive overload has long been regarded as a fundamental principle of physical preparation planning. From the fable of Milo of Crete's daily squatting of the growing bull calf (lifting the calf every day as it grew heavier gradually made him stronger!), to modern undulating load designs, the critical challenge of preparation planning has been to impose a manageable, progressively challenging stress that elicits optimum positive adaptation. Should imposed training stress be insufficient, optimum adaptation will not occur; alternatively, if stress is excessive then some form of negative adaptation will result. Error within the physical preparation process may be costly. Injury, burnout, disillusionment and failure to realize potential are the likely consequences of an incorrect blending of the various preparation ingredients. Accordingly, preparation plans are a key factor in shaping the destinies and future successes of performers, from the competitive sportsperson to the aspiring ballerina, to the adventurer negotiating a hostile terrain. Reflecting this importance, planners within the realm of physical performance pursuits bear a significant, and at times onerous, responsibility.

Each performance pursuit responds to its own unique set of physical demands, challenges and peculiarities with a tailored set of planning solutions. However, it is also true that there are many aspects of planning custom that are common across the spectrum of physical performance activities: universally shared philosophies, beliefs, traditions and practices. It is these all-pervasive planning commonalities, these collectively shared aspects of planning practice that will be scrutinized and reviewed within this chapter.

We will show evidence that conventional planning approaches owe as much to innate aspects of human psychology and societal planning convention as to physiological training science. Accordingly, this chapter is as relevant to the performance psychologist seeking insight into the biological underpinnings of training planning as it is to the coach, exercise physiologist, conditioning specialist or support team member seeking to understand the psychological forces that have helped shape cultural preparation planning conventions.

The structure of our discussion progresses through four logically consecutive steps:

- A status check on current theory and practice; where we are and how we got here?
- Is there a planning problem? How do we know?
- Why is preparation planning so difficult?
- What can we do?

A status check on current theory and practice: where we are and how we got here?

The published training planning literature emanates predominantly from sport and strength training domains where the universally pervasive planning template is referred to as the periodization of training. As periodization is the only documented, formalized training planning approach, it is worth taking some time to explore both its origins and its basic tenets.

In a series of scholarly works in the 1960s and 1970s, the Soviet training theorist Matveyev described a method of training planning based upon the experiential and scientific knowledge of the time. Matveyev's landmark Russian publication, *Fundamentals of Sports Training*, published in 1977, followed by an English translation in 1981, became the first extensive encapsulation of training planning theory. Matveyev's original work was not widely read in the West. In fact, the cumbersome nature of the English translation makes it quite difficult to discern precisely what is being discussed. What consequently emerged was a collection of various interpretations, based around a couple of core concepts.

What is periodization?

The periodization approach organizes all training in terms of several basic structural units. These are the training session, the microcycle, the mesocycle, the macrocycle, the Olympic (or quadrennial) cycle and the multiyear cycle (Siff 2000). The training plan is consequently represented as the sum of the microcycles aligned in a sequential chain. A specified number of microcycles form a mesocycle, and in turn a specified number of mesocycles form the macrocycle. This structure is described in Box 10.1. Prior to key events there is commonly a planned reduction in training, termed the taper, intended to allow for dissipation of residual fatigue and optimization of performance readiness. So, for example, track and field athletes will attempt to peak for Olympics, team players for important phases of a season, climbers for specific routes, adventurers for expeditions and dancers for an audition or tour.

Box 10.1

Periodization definitions

- **Microcycle**: Shortest sequence of training and recovery days before unit is repeated. Typically between 4 and 10 days.
- **Mesocycle**: A sequence of similarly focused repeated microcycles. Typically 3–8 weeks in duration.
- **Macrocycle**: The overall training period. Typically 6 months to 4 years, dependent on the time-frame of long-term training objectives.

The cornerstones of the traditional periodization model are essentially twofold:

1. Training periods are arranged in a predetermined sequential order so that capacities (e.g. strength or aerobic capacity) developed in preceding periods will enable the development of capacities (e.g. power or anaerobic capacity) in future periods.
2. The preplanned manipulation of training volumes and intensities to realize specific, phasic conditioning goals (e.g. build strength in this phase, develop muscular power in the next).

Classically, this planning template was envisioned as a reduction in training volume accompanied by an associated increase in training intensity as the competitive peak approached. In recent years, however, novel and inventive derivations of the original high-volume/low-intensity to low-volume/high-intensity model have been proposed: more on this later.

Periodization principles have received widespread support in the literature. To illustrate, consider the following sampled snippets from respected planning theorists. Periodization is perceived as 'a logical and phasic method of manipulating training variables to increase the potential for achieving specific performance goals' (Stone 1996), and to provide training planners with a 'methodical, scientific procedure to help athletes achieve high levels of training and performance' (Bompa 1999). Furthermore, 'the development of a precisely controlled training programme is necessary in order to assure that the maximal sports performance is attained at the right moment of the season' (Mujika 1998). Consider the phraseology employed: logical, precisely controlled, productive manipulation, methodical scientific procedure. This is what periodization offers; a rational, scientifically justified planning model that meticulously guides and controls the preparation process. There is an enticing intuitive appeal to such reasoning. The perceived worth of the periodization concept was further promoted by the contemporary success of Eastern Bloc athletes, (periodization frequently being referred to as a Soviet training secret). As a consequence, and in the absence of any significant competing theories, periodization entered the lore of physical performance cultures as the pre-eminent training planning model for physical performance.

It must be noted here that Matveyev was certainly not solely responsible for formulating the periodized training approach. Within the general sports training literature there have been a number of influential, predominantly ex-Soviet, theorists who have published widely, and frequently argued widely, on the topic. Furthermore, most performance pursuits have influential practitioners who have shaped philosophies within that domain. So for example, endurance running culture has been heavily influenced by planning methodologies employed by legendary coaches such as Jack Daniels and Arthur Lydiard. However, regardless of the individual twists and quirks advocated by individual practitioners, the underpinning planning rationale is remarkable consistent. Why? Essentially because they share a common planning ancestor.

The historical context

So, what is this common heritage? Consider the similarities between periodization philosophy and the industrial and political planning approaches of the early-to-mid 20th century; for example, the stylized mechanistic planning approach typified by the works of industrial theorists such as Henry Gannt and Frederick Winslow Taylor. In particular, Taylor's influential work *The Principles of Scientific Management* applied strict scientific principle to the management of the production industry. Taylor combined the scientific knowledge of the day, his pioneering 'time and motion' studies and what is best termed contemporary management's prejudice towards workers ('all we want of them is to obey the orders we give them') to construct the first great planning paradigm of the modern era.

Taylor believed that there was a 'one best way' to organize, manage and plan: that optimal practices were deterministic in nature. In other words, once optimal practices were uncovered, they remained stable and did not change. Hence, once the 'best' plan is formulated, all that's required is for it to be repeatedly implemented. Taylor therefore believed in the strict segregation of plan and process. Step one, formulate the plan; step two, execute the plan. Henry Ford readily embraced the principles of this classical perspective, to the extent that this approach was frequently referred to as Fordism. Scientific management precepts were famously endorsed by Lenin and Stalin and are considered by historians to have been a formative influence on the Soviet Five-Year Plans of the 1920s and 1930s.

A concern with this approach is that it is based on a number of simplifying assumptions:

- Control of a limited number of factors controls the behaviour of the system
- Progress is determined through measurement and quantification
- Factors that are measurable are of greater importance than those that are not readily measurable.

Now, the problem with this set of assumptions is that 'what can be measured' and 'what's important' become confused (see the Introduction to this book). Peripheral factors that are easily measured can assume ill-deservedly elevated hierarchical positions. Conversely, critical factors that are not readily quantifiable tend to occupy a planning blind spot and may be largely ignored. This presents a significant theoretical weakness. For example, consider the gross inefficiencies of the Soviet Five-Year Plans and China's Great Leap Forwards – all the hyperbole of strong leadership, a firm direction, a motivated population, simple, straightforward objectives. True, some objectives were achieved, but not at an acceptable cost considering the human collateral damage. Is this an example of good planning with laudable firm resolve or a grossly oversimplified interpretation of reality bordering on criminal negligence?

The purpose of this diversion is to highlight the fact that the early training planners were heavily influenced by this historical planning template. So in essence, when the Soviet training theorists sought to construct training planning templates, they combined the cultural planning blueprint (as per Taylor and the philosophy of the Five-Year Plans) with training records and contemporary scientific knowledge. For example, the historically influential Matveyev collated training data from the 1950s and 1960s, in swimming, running and weightlifting, and applied these records to the pervasive mechanistic planning blueprint. Thus the original periodized concept was a reincarnation of the industrial planning template, with the same strengths, weaknesses and assumptions.

In industrial and political planning domains, the inefficiencies of such regimented approaches gradually became apparent. Today, the Ford Motor Company no longer manufactures cars in the strictly segregated production-line fashion of Henry Ford's day. Similarly, modern governmental agencies realize the dangers that assumptions and generalizations present to project planning. In areas where many factors interact to influence outcome, planning approaches that ignore both minor and unmeasurable system components are excessively vulnerable to error. Consequently modern governments, policy makers and industries, no longer employ rigid 'reduce and resolve' planning solutions. Unfortunately, physical training principles may not have been examined with equal rigour and, in consequence, may not have evolved to quite the same extent.

Scientific support for periodization planning

The next step in our investigation is to briefly review the empirical evidence supporting the periodization approach. Again, the published peer-reviewed literature emanates exclusively from sporting and strength-training domains.

Stone and colleagues (1999a) reviewed 15 studies of mesocycle length (7–24 weeks). 13 of these studies suggested that periodized models produced statistically superior results in performance measures when compared with models that consisted solely of linear increases in training loads. However, in the majority of these studies (11), there were no controls in place to equalize measures of total work performed. Consequently, intergroup differences in derived training benefits may have resulted from the differing training volumes performed. The authors concluded that the review strongly suggested that a periodized approach, even over a short term, produced superior results, especially in previously trained subjects, compared with constant-repetition programmes (Stone et al 1999b).

In a similar review, Graham (2002) cites 10 studies demonstrating that periodized strength-training models provided statistically significant improvements in one or more of a variety of performance standards when compared with linear non-periodized models (Graham 2002). A more recent meta-analysis comparing the effectiveness of periodized and non-periodized strength training programmes concluded that periodized training structures were more effective for both males and females, for individuals of varying training backgrounds and for a range of age groups (Rhea & Alderman 2004).

In one of the few studies that did not support the efficacy of periodized training regimes, Baker et al (1994) found no differences between an undulating periodized group and a non-periodized control group when volume and relative intensity were equated over a short-term training period (Baker et al 1994). Similarly, DeBeliso and colleagues (2005) concluded that a fixed repetition strength training protocol was as effective in promoting strength gains as a periodized programme in elderly, untrained subjects.

In a rare training study of extended duration (9 months), Kraemer and colleagues (2003) compared the effectiveness of two equitable volume training schemes, demonstrating that the strength and motor performance of female collegiate tennis players was preferentially enhanced in the periodized, as compared to the non-periodized, training group. The authors concluded that the superiority of the periodized training protocol was a consequence of (1) the greater variation of training variables and (2) the periodic exposure to higher training loads afforded by the periodized nature of the programme (Kraemer et al 2003).

In recent years published articles have suggested novel and creative derivations of the original periodized scheme (e.g. non-linear (Brown 2001, Rhea et al 2002), conjugate sequence (Plisk & Stone 2003), block (Issurin 2008), and fractal (Brown & Greenwood 2005)). Furthermore, Plisk and Stone (2003) have inventively equated preparation planning to concepts of game theory and advocated the need for planned unpredictability within the training programme (Plisk & Stone 2003).

In summary, the vast bulk of the published literature concludes that periodized is more effective than non-periodized training. There have been studies that have failed to demonstrate a significant benefit of periodized over non-periodized structures. However, these investigations typically have two design characteristics in common: first, subject groups of low initial fitness and second, a short time-frame of investigation.

Scientific validity

Based on the reviewed evidence it seems reasonable to conclude that periodized planning models are effective. However, there is an interesting point to note here. Studies such as these are commonly presented as evidence of the efficacy of periodization principles. However, this may be a somewhat over-elaborate conclusion. What is strongly supported is that training variation is a beneficial factor in programme design, but the question of how this variation is best achieved remains largely unexplored.

This is worth noting, as the term 'science of periodization' is one that frequently crops up in the sports science and coaching literature. Unfortunately, the use of such language portrays an illusion of scientific propriety. It generates a sense that more is known about training planning than is actually the case; in short, that periodization principles have been empirically validated. On the basis of the evidence so far, the only valid conclusion to be drawn is that variation is an essential component of good training design.

A further point to note is the group-based nature of both the training records upon which periodization is justified and the empirical investigations offered as proof. These group-based conclusions discount the possibility that an individual's response to any given training input and/or method of organization may vary widely from the average group response. As we will see later, this assumption is called into question by contemporary evidence. Other obvious but often by necessity unavoidable limitations of such studies are the use of subelite populations as subject cohorts, the habitually short duration of training studies and the lack of sensitive fitness assessment measures.

A final point before moving on: the term 'periodization' has become so ubiquitous in sporting parlance that many now commonly neglect its original meaning and use the term interchangeably with 'training plan'. Thus the term has the potential to conjure up different interpretations for different practitioners. This chapter will consider the term in its originally intended context as representing training schemes that are segregated into sequential, distinct, pre-planned training blocks.

Summary

So before we proceed, a quick summary of the key points so far:

- Preparation planning throughout the physical performance domains has been heavily influenced by the historical culturally pervasive planning paradigm
- The planning process is essentially an exercise in stress management

- The nature of the conducted periodization studies means that current training philosophies for individuals are heavily based on averaged, group-based empirical data
- Regular variation of training parameters over the course of the training programme is broadly supported as a prerequisite of good planning
- Differing planning structures have been proposed as means to providing appropriate training variation. However, there is little empirical evidence to aid discrimination between the worth of the various schemes
- The principle of gradual progressive overload appears an eminently sensible guideline. However, the issue of whether or not progress can be adequately modulated solely through manipulation of training 'numbers' (sets, reps, intensities, etc.) will be addressed later in this chapter.

Is there a planning problem? If so, how do we know?

That preparation planning models are in need of refinement may be a contentious assertion. A standard defence against such an accusation is to point to celebrated performers who have reached the heights of their profession using conventional, periodized preparation plans. Such reasoning is a very understandable human reaction to visible facts. However, despite its instinctive appeal, such rationale does unquestionably present a damaging logical inconsistency. Employing isolated examples to support any stance, as is frequently the norm in performance environments, is a one-sided and ultimately irrational argument. A valid assessment of the worth of any training scheme necessitates that both the scheme's successes and 'failures' be factored into analysis. This peculiar aspect of human cognition is pervasive throughout domains and has been extensively documented elsewhere (e.g. Taleb 2005). Accordingly, great care must be taken to avoid the temptation to employ isolated individual examples to confirm the worth of any planning scheme while neglecting to consider all those who adhered to a similar planning framework yet 'failed'.

That a performer achieved previous success does not provide evidence that this was the most efficient preparation scheme. How can we know whether or not following a different plan would have led to still greater achievement? To less injury or illness? To a longer, healthier, more productive career? Our inability to run counterfactual, alternative reality strategies that originate from the same starting point means that we cannot answer such questions.

Accordingly, in the absence of any direct 'proof' of preparation planning problems, further exploration of the topic requires consideration of two distinct lines of indirect evidence. To shed light on the question of whether or not training planning conceptions would benefit from refinement, let's consider the problem from two perspectives. First, we will briefly review evidence of planning problems in other domains of human endeavour and second, we will consider circumstantial evidence emerging from within physical performance environments.

Evidence of a general planning problem?

The pervasiveness of human planning inadequacies has been extensively documented. High-profile examples include the construction of Denver International Airport (16 months late, costs 300% greater than forecast), the development of the Eurofighter jet (5 years late, $25 billion above predicted cost), the Scottish Parliament building (3 years late, with projected cost of £35million escalating to £414 million) and, most famously, the Sydney Opera House (a scaled-down version completed 10 years late, with estimated costs of $7 million eventually amounting to $102 million). What is startling about such examples is that these projects were not entered into lightly and were not planned by inexperienced amateurs short on resources, yet all still floundered spectacularly. Military planners have often been the butt of ridicule, yet planning in this domain has typically been conducted by intelligent, highly trained, highly experienced groups of individuals. However, factual evidence indicates that, despite high levels of resource, planning in such environments habitually goes awry. Exempting combat examples, consider that the US General Accounting Office estimated that only 1% of major military high-tech purchases were delivered on budget and on-time (Buehler et al 2002).

As far back as the 1950s, psychologist Paul Meehl investigated discrepancies between expert clinical prediction and prediction based solely on simple mathematical formulas. His research revealed that such basic methods of prediction almost always outperformed those of clinicians. Meehl's conclusion, that statistical prediction consistently outperforms clinical judgment, has stood up extremely well for over half a century. Surprisingly, Meehl also discovered a sharp discrepancy between clinicians' rating of their personal performance and their actual record of success (Meehl 1954).

Subsequent evidence of planning and predictive inadequacies has been gathered across a spectrum of domains, from large-scale governmental projects to personal tasks such as completing Christmas shopping. For example, when asked to predict how long it would take to finish their honours thesis 'if everything went as poorly as it possibly could', psychology students significantly underestimated completion time (Buehler et al 1994). Buehler and colleagues (2002, p. 252), commenting on this and other work, wrote: 'Even when asked to make a highly conservative forecast, a prediction that they felt virtually certain that they would fulfil, students' confidence in their time estimates far exceeded their accomplishments'. In similar fashion, Newby-Clark and colleagues (2000) found that asking subjects for predictions based on realistic 'best guess' scenarios and for their hoped-for 'best case' scenarios, produced indistinguishable results. This neatly illustrates that when people think of their 'most probable' outcome they typically envision everything going exactly to plan! Ironically however, the empirical evidence suggests that what actually happens is typically worse than the predicted 'worst case' scenario. In fact, there is a mismatch between our illusion of capability in planning tasks and the reality of our documented performance. This is commonly termed the planning fallacy (Newby-Kahneman & Tversky 1979) and is pervasive across domains and cultures.

In the most extensive examination of human predictive ability to date, Philip Tetlock of the University of California at Berkeley collated the precisely specified predictions of a large cohort of experts. This 20-year study involved 284 professionals, all of whom made their livelihood through the prediction and analysis of political and economic trends. All experts were given regular lists of questions and asked to forecast future outcomes. All had access to extensive information, had extensive experience, had high levels of relevant education and were considered leaders in their respective fields. Yet, when the results of the many thousands of predictions were collated, it became blatantly obvious that their ability to predict was universally poor. No single expert came remotely close to being consistently right. In fact, only in certain cases were expert predictions better than what researchers termed 'dart-throwing chimps' – in other words, randomly generated guesses (Tetlock 2005).

Finally, in closing this quick review it is worth noting that researchers have previously concluded that it is impossible to find any domain in which humans can outperform even crude predictive algorithms, far less sophisticated ones (Grove & Meehl 1996).

Evidence of a specific performance planning problem?

A line of circumstantial evidence that is suggestive of potential planning inadequacies within performance environments relates to the widespread proliferation of the various 'stress mismanagement' syndromes that plague performance domains.

Overuse injury has been defined as an imbalance caused by overintensive training and inadequate recovery leading to a breakdown in tissue reparative mechanisms (Cosca & Navazio 2007). Overuse has been identified as a major mechanism for injury in a wide diversity of physical pursuits, e.g. multisport athletes (Villavicencio et al 2007), cross-country skiing (Smith et al 1996), elite Olympic weightlifting (Calhoon & Fry 1999), professional soccer (Waldén et al 2007), various dance disciplines (Bronner et al 2003, Brown and Micheli 2004, Garrick & Lewis 2001, Quirk 1994, Shan 2005) and professional ballet (Nilsson et al 2001). Some examples are shown in Box 10.2.

Further evidence of potential programming deficiencies comes from the variously labelled manifestations of chronic imbalance between psychophysiological stress and recovery, such as staleness,

Box 10.2

Sample findings illustrating the extent of overuse within physical performance contexts

- Overuse accounted for 37% of all injuries to Swedish professional football teams (Waldén et al 2007)
- Half of over 500 elite junior figure skaters surveyed reported repeat occurrence of overuse syndrome (Dubravcic-Simunjak et al 2003)
- 64% of professional dancers need to stop performing for extended periods due to overuse syndrome (Shan 2005)
- In a retrospective study of a Swedish professional ballet company, most injuries were considered overuse in nature, and 95% of dancers suffered injuries over the 5-year study period (Nilsson et al 2001)

burnout and overtraining syndrome. Previously, burnout has been described as a 'psychological syndrome' (Maslach & Jackson 1984) but it may be more appropriately considered a clinically complex stress-imbalance condition of indeterminate cause with a range of physical, psychological and social symptoms. Overtraining syndrome has been defined as long-lasting performance incompetence due to an imbalance of training load, competition, non-training stressors and recovery (Smith 2003). In ballet, manifestations of burnout and overtraining phenomena have been described (Koutedakis et al 1999, Koutedakis & Jamurtas 2004), and staleness, burnout and overtraining syndrome have all been identified as widespread problems among athletes and sportspeople (e.g. Junge et al 2002).

The proliferation of stress mismanagement syndromes throughout the physical performance domains is certainly, in and of itself, suggestive of cultural planning inefficiencies. The counterpoint to this argument is that, in high-performance settings, when both body and mind are consistently being stretched to their absolute limits, some form of physical or psychophysiological damage is inevitable. There is surely an element of truth in this perspective: an inevitable byproduct of negotiating fine margins of error is that, occasionally, thresholds will be exceeded.

However, stress mismanagement need not be an inevitable byproduct of high-performance preparation. This is effectively illustrated by a number of studies that have successfully reduced the incidence of 'stress syndromes' through the introduction of simple, easy-to-implement management strategies (Box 10.3).

Box 10.3

Impact of programme management interventions in reducing incidence of overuse injuries

- Case management and an early intervention programme reduced the annual number of compensation cases from 81% to 17%, and decreased the number of days lost by 60%, over a 3 year time span in a professional corps de ballet (Bronner et al 2003)
- A significant decrease (21%) in sports injury incidence following an intervention based solely on education and increased supervision (Junge et al 2002)
- Monitoring of ratings of perceived exertion has previously been associated with avoidance of under-recovery, e.g. in rowing (Maestu et al 2005) and sprinting (Suzuki et al 2006)

Why is preparation planning so difficult?

Two strands of evidence have been presented thus far, serving to question our current planning capabilities and paradigms: specifically, the clear demonstrations of the planning fallacy that have emerged from studies within social, behavioural and cognitive psychology, and also the provocative circumstantial evidence of a proliferation of stress mismanagement syndromes emerging from within performance environments.

In order to evolve strategies to redress the observed planning deficiencies, we will first need to unravel the psychological and biological considerations that interact to predispose to planning error.

Innate psychological considerations

An extensive literature has provided illustrations demonstrating that, as a species, we universally struggle with planning and prediction tasks (Fig. 10.1). Paradoxically, in both the seminal work of Meehl and the extensive study of Tetlock, experts with the lowest rates of forecasting accuracy were simultaneously the very ones with the greatest confidence in their predictive abilities. It would appear that this misplaced overconfidence made experts increasingly vulnerable to decision-making error. In contrast, their less dogmatic peers, who resisted the temptation to employ the cognitive shortcut of predicting the future exclusively on the basis of past observations and who refined their perspectives against the emerging evidence, consistently outperformed their more confident peers.

The key factors driving such behaviours are innate, instinctive ego-protective mechanisms, which habitually rationalize our successes as resulting from our superior intuition but failure as being consequent to events outside our control (for more on this, see Tetlock 2005).

A direct implication of this is that we commonly fail to update our beliefs even when confronted with contradictory evidence. An immediate implication of such reflexive tendencies is that we frequently fail to learn from past mistakes, because we fail to self-critique dispassionately and in an unbiased manner. As previously noted, 'when faced with the choice between changing one's mind and proving that there is no need to do so, almost everyone

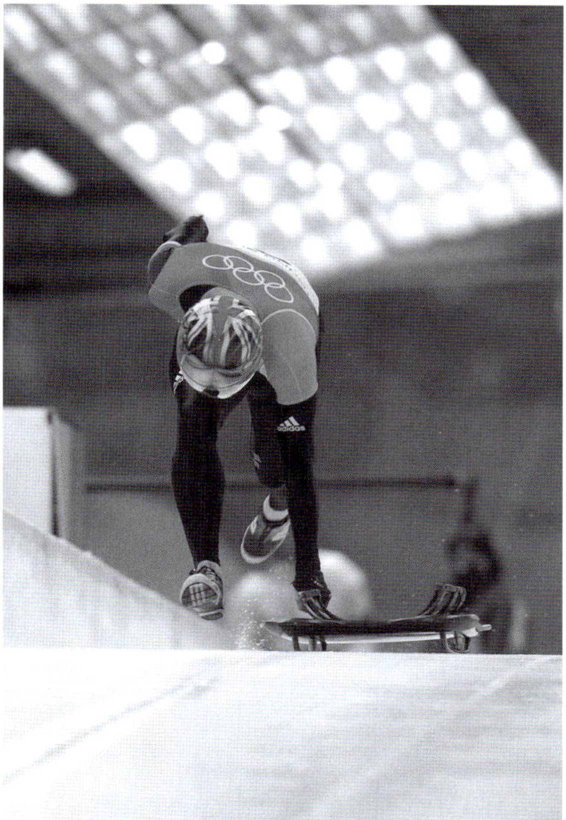

Fig. 10.1 • Kristan Bromley at the top of a skeleton bobsleigh run – always a 'hard to predict' challenge. With thanks to Kristan Bronley.

gets busy on the proof' (Gilovich & Griffin 2002). However, research has also revealed that such irrational tendencies can be overridden and consequent decision-making ability enhanced. For example, chess masters actively seek to falsify potential next-move decisions. In contrast, experienced novices primarily seek evidence that confirms the perceived worth of their next move (Cowley & Byrne 2004). In other words, masters sought to objectively pick holes in their own theories, whereas novices sought evidence that positively supported their initial opinions.

Within the literature, our planning and prediction limitations are commonly attributed to a number of innate psychological traits. Tetlock (2005) has described four key contributing factors:

- A strong preference for simplicity
- An aversion to ambiguity and dissonance
- A deep-rooted need to believe we live in an orderly world
- A lack of appreciation of the laws of chance.

These cognitive characteristics are most commonly explained as a consequence of our evolutionary past. Simple, rule- based decision making is highly functional in environments where survival is dependent on quick, instinctive, fight-or-flight-based choices. Accordingly, there is a discrepancy between the nature of the problems that now confront us and those that evolution equipped us to solve. Our performance suffers when faced with convoluted, multifactorial problems, as we are fundamentally deterministic thinkers with a demonstrated aversion to probabilistic reasoning (Tetlock 2005). The significance of this problem is illustrated by a report by the US Institute of Medicine estimating that between 44 000 and 94 000 patients die each year in US hospitals as a result of medical error (Institute of Medicine of the National Academies 1999), and major causes of error in medical decision making have been identified as physicians' lack of competency in probabilistic reasoning and a faulty conceptual knowledge (Patel 2000). Accordingly it would seem that, as previously noted, 'our brains are made for fitness, not for truth' (Pinker 1997). We actively seek out simple, straightforward answers. Such a habitual preference for simplistic, rule-based decision-making is a predisposition that is especially exposed when we attempt to plan in unpredictable, complex environments.

Biological complexity – a further complication

An essential requirement for any efficient planner is a conceptual model that is optimally reflective of the true nature of the system under consideration. Put more plainly, in order to plan effectively there must be an incisive understanding of how the system works. If the conceptual model, or paradigm, for understanding the system is flawed, then all subsequent decision making will be compromised. In relation to performance planning, the most obvious system to consider is the performer's biological system.

The predominant historical model for conceptualizing biological function has been the mechanistic paradigm. This mechanistic conception of 'human being as machine' is widespread and deeply ingrained in our conceptual system (Karaliute 2007). This classical perspective depicts the biological system as analogous to a well maintained, well oiled machine. Accordingly, the covert conceptual lens through which we have historically rationalized human functioning envisions our biology as a highly intricate, advanced but ultimately mechanical system.

If the biological system is indeed characterized by machine-like functioning, then enhancing performance is a relatively straightforward process. Mechanical systems are predictable, with stable functioning in which a known intervention results in a predictable output. When dealing with mechanistic systems we can use linear, deterministic logic to derive appropriate plans. In such circumstances, periodized training schemes would be eminently sensible. Frustratingly, however, reality intervenes to spoil the party.

One of the great tectonic shifts in science over the course of the 20th century was the realization of the explanatory inadequacies of the mechanistic world-view when applied to real-world systems. This shift was not sudden, nor can it be accredited to the work of any single person or scientific discipline. In a slow, meandering journey that started in physics and mathematics in the late 19th century and progressed through various scientific disciplines, mechanistic concepts have gradually been supplanted by a more reflective paradigm that has only recently been embraced by biologists and the medical professions.

The term 'complex adaptive system' was coined to describe systems that are composed of multiple component subsystems that interact in non-linear, non-periodic and non-proportional ways. These systems are adaptive, as they undergo temporary or permanent modification in response to imposed stress. The global behaviour of such systems is impossible to track in terms of its elements and so, unlike the simple 'billiard-ball' systems of classical mechanics, complex adaptive systems cannot be decomposed to a series of proportionate cause and effect reactions. Chaotic properties are a fundamental component of complex systems. Many have encountered chaos theory primarily through the butterfly metaphor. However, chaotic systems are not necessarily chaotic, and the butterfly metaphor is not very good at explaining how such systems work. Much of the time, chaotic systems remain relatively stable. In fact, it is a hallmark of such systems that imposed shocks reverberate through the component subsystems and are dissipated throughout the network. Accordingly, such systems are typically robust to perturbation.

However, this is not the case if the system is sufficiently delicately poised. In this condition, a single minute occurrence may be all that is necessary to push the system past its tipping point. Alternatively, the ripples of a number of seemingly innocuous occurrences may interact, being exponentially amplified as they propagate through the system, eventually resulting in large-scale disruption. There is a bifurcation (a dramatic and sudden change) in behaviour. Minor episodes can rapidly mushroom into major events. As we have no means of adequately assessing current states of the component subsystems, of knowing which are the most important subsystems or of unravelling the dynamic relationships between the subsystems, a defining feature of complex adaptive systems is that future behaviour is impossible to predict.

Consider weather systems: despite the meticulous study of meteorology, despite all the technical advances and efforts of scientists and space agencies, we will never have complete predictive capability. Why? Because we cannot measure to a fine enough scale, because infinitesimally small measurement errors can rapidly upset any prediction and because the various component elements of weather systems interact in complex and unpredictable ways.

The current global credit crunch offers an excellent example of how the behaviour of a seemingly stable, 'tamed', complex adaptive system can rapidly and unpredictably diverge from the expected path. Complete control of such systems is ultimately illusory. We can influence, we may nudge in a given direction but we cannot completely regulate and hence need to be aware of the pitfalls and avoid complacency.

One of the hidden implications of the mechanistic perspective of biology is that appropriate plans, and appropriate solutions can be advance-planned through a process of deduction and prediction. However, in the light of complexity theory it is evident that this would require an extensive knowledge of the innumerable causal connections that exist between the components of the system, a knowledge that clearly does not exist (van Regenmortel 2007).

Evidence of biological complexity?

A defining characteristic of periodized training plans is the implicit assumption of stable, cyclic, underpinning biological processes. For example, consider the rationale supporting the logic of fixed duration planning blocks. The most prevalent scheme, as documented in the published literature, organizes training programmes into phases of 4 weeks' duration. Plisk & Stone (2003) cite the rationales of three noted periodization theorists in advocating 4-week cycles:

- To correspond with natural monthly biocycles (Matveyev 1972)
- To correspond with the half-time of training effect involution (Viru 1995)
- In order to super-impose delayed training effects (Zatsiorsky 1995).

Such rationale was eminently logical given the level of insight provided by the mechanistic model of biological functioning. However, if we consider this rationale through the lens of the complexity paradigm, a very different picture emerges. It is without question that distinct but mutually interactive biological rhythms underpin all aspects of the human life cycle, health and response to applied training stress.

Consider: complex bodily rhythms are ubiquitous in all living organisms (Glass 2001). Organisms have evolved timing mechanisms, commonly referred to as biological clocks, that assimilate cues from multiple sources and modulate oscillations accordingly (Rensing et al 2001). These rhythms interact with eachother through myriad feedback and feedforward linkages while also being subjected to the influence of environmentally generated cues and perturbations. It is the seemingly orderly behaviour emerging from this multiplicity of interactive, fluctuating constraints that characterizes the functioning of complex biological systems (for further review, see Foster & Kreitzman 2005).

The interactive effects of various forms of stress have been shown to affect biological functioning. For example, emotional stress has been observed to downregulate the immune system (Aubert 2008, Rogers et al 2001, Venkatraman et al 2000). Loneliness has been established as a predictor of morbidity and mortality (Cacioppo et al 2002). Sleep disruption has been shown to have substantial negative effects on a range of capacities such as motor and cognitive performance, mood, metabolism, hormonal health, and immune function (Ferrara & De Gennaro 2001, Himashree et al 2002). Academic stress has been noted to have a negative effect on the mood scores of swimmers (Carl et al 2001). Mood has been shown to affect the training performance of cross-country skiers (Mahood et al 2001) and personal, economical, psychological and physical factors have been proposed to increase the stress levels of ballet dancers, resulting in elevated injury risk (Kelman 2000).

As a further illustration, consider the variety of factors that have been demonstrated to affect the release characteristics of the androgenic hormone testosterone. Observed patterns of testosterone release have been variously noted to modulate in males in response to the time of day (Bird & Tarpenning 2004), week, month and female partner's cycle (Hogg 2002), in response to cycles of light and dark (Luboshitzky 2000, Takagi 1986), in accordance to ratings of work satisfaction (Axelsson et al 2003), in response to motivational and assertiveness levels (Schultheiss et al 1999, Schultheiss & Rohde 2002), and in response to training stress (Filaire et al 2003).

In summary, the body of evidence demonstrating the mutual inter-connectivity and inter-activity between psychophysiology, cognition, emotion, brain function, and genetic predisposition continues to grow, emphasizing both the extent of biological complexity and the limitations of mechanistic conceptual frameworks (for review, see Lovallo 2005).

Biological complexity and physical fitness

Physical fitness is influenced by a variety of environmental and genetic factors. Consider the evidence emerging from the HEIRITAGE Family Studies, a linked series of investigations focused on uncovering the genetic underpinnings of individual responses to exercise and disease risk factors.

Studies have demonstrated a considerable heterogeneity in the responsiveness of individuals to regular physical exercise (Bouchard et al 2000). For example, training induced changes to VO_2max were established to vary widely among subjects in response to identical training parameters. High, medium and low responders existed among all age groups, in both sexes, among blacks and whites and at all levels of initial fitness. When $\dot{V}O_2max$ was adjusted for age, sex, body mass and composition; genetic factors explained about 40% of interindividual variation. The average increase in $\dot{V}O_2max$ was 19% but it was the range of training responses that was truly surprising. 5% of subjects had no change in $\dot{V}O_2max$ consequent to training and 5% had an increase of over 50% (Skinner et al 2001). Of course, it must be noted that subjects were previously untrained. Nevertheless, such extremes of outcome in response to identical training parameters serve to illustrate the uncertainty associated with any attempts to forecast the effects of prescribed training interventions.

Elsewhere, an investigation employing a cohort of professional rugby players established that prescribed resistance training sessions produced a range of individually-specific hormonal responses in subjects (Beavan et al 2008a). Individuals with broadly similar training backgrounds responded differently to the same training stress. Individual players were high responders to a certain session but not to another, while team-mates displayed the opposing pattern. In an aligned study, the hormonal responses of players to four differing resistance training sessions were determined. Then, in a 3-week crossover design, players alternated between the sessions that elicited their maximum and their minimum testosterone responses. All players demonstrated significant gains in strength after 3 weeks of training using the protocol that elicited their maximum testosterone response. In contrast, when subjects performed the protocol that occasioned their minimum response, either no change or a significant decline in tested strength measures resulted (Beavan et al 2008b).

When we consider these converging streams of evidence, it seems logical to conclude that adaptation, and consequent retention, rates of differing aspects of fitness are highly individual-specific. Taken as a whole, the presented evidence suggests that any training loading interacts with intrinsic and environmental factors to occasion a unique adaptive response.

The key mutually interactive factors dictating this response are:

- Training loading parameters
- Genetic inheritance
- Transient states of biological functioning
- Habituation to previous stress exposures (i.e. training history)
- Transient psychological states
- Transient social and environmental factors.

Accordingly it can be concluded that:

- Identical training parameters will always elicit a unique adaptive response for each individual
- An individual will respond uniquely each time identical training sessions are repeated
- Generalized conclusions from group-based observations may be seriously misleading in guiding individual training
- It is highly improbable that there are universal 'best' loading schemes for any given pursuits or objectives.

How should we cope? what can we do?

Design and management of dynamic adaptive preparation planning systems

To err is very definitely an unavoidable aspect of the human condition. However, it is also within the compass of human ingenuity to create solutions, find alternative ways of working and devise strategies serving to offset human planning and decision-making errors. An understanding of the factors at the root of our habitual planning inadequacies permits the formulation of such pre-emptive strategies. Training theorists whose work contributed to the formulation and popularization of periodization concepts were certainly intelligent, experienced and insightful. Their conclusions were eminently sensible when contextualized against the pervasive conceptual frameworks and knowledge base of the past. However, our exploration and synthesis of relevant emerging evidence thus far highlights a number of conflicts between current scientific knowledge and traditional practice.

Specifically; three critical assumptions of the traditional periodization planning model are challenged:

- It is possible to predict the effects of any given training intervention and/or training organizational structure
- It is feasible to optimally advance plan preparation programmes
- Prescribing training in empirical terms is an adequate means of controlling imposed stress.

In the discussion thus far we have shown the mismatch between our innate predisposition for rule-directed, pre-formed planning solutions and the complex reality of the planning problem. Evidence from other planning pursuits, as well as circumstantial evidence from within performance domains, has been offered to illustrate the potential consequences of this mismatch. Accordingly, the challenge of appropriate planning has shifted from a process of mathematically manipulating and segregating future training into preformed schemes to the design of dynamically adaptive training systems.

Consequent refinements to convention can be categorized under the following four headings:

- Paradigm
- Process
- Planning structure
- Prescription.

Paradigm

The planning paradigm is the conceptual model, the implicit set of assumptions and core beliefs that defines our framework for understanding the planning task. A clearly defined conceptual knowledge is an essential aspect of appropriate planning decision making.

Within this chapter, strands of evidence questioning habitual planning perspectives have been examined. The key conceptual sources of error may be broadly summarized into two sections; human cognitive limitations and the underlying task complexity.

Human cognitive limitations

Awareness of our human fallibility in forecasting and predictive realms should foster a healthy planning and decision making paranoia. Recall the evidence. Despite having an extensively documented poor track record in planning and predictive tasks, simultaneously we have a demonstrated tendency to be over-confident in these pursuits.

This over-confidence, our habitual over-commitment to favoured strategies, our ingenuity in rationalizing inconvenient facts in ways that deflect self-critique, are all factors that limit learning from, and predispose towards, repeated error.

These peculiarities lead to an evident paradox. The values we typically admire in 'experts' – assertiveness, undoubting self-belief and an unswerving confidence – are the very characteristics that appear to predispose to decision making error. Yet, ironically, the evidence suggests that our predictive confidence when functioning in complex environments is unjustified and ultimately delusional. There is an evident dissonance in that the values we find laudable in decision makers are not necessarily those that facilitate good management and planning. This presents a conundrum to those responsible for directing physical preparation programmes; an apparent contradiction between cognitive approach and self-presentation style. On one hand there is the cautious, questioning, consultative, consistently checking and re-checking, cognitive style required to enable good planning decision making; on the other, the confident, assertive and self-assured facade necessary to engender performer trust, generate expectation and strengthen commitment to the chosen path.

Understanding our innate reasoning tendencies is an important first step in conquering them. While we cannot re-write our evolutionary programming, we can be aware of our habitual cognitive blind-spots and devise remedial strategies.

Underlying task complexity

Within this chapter we have uncovered evidence of a mismatch between, on the one hand, our innate desire for parsimony, simplicity and explanatory closure, and on the other, the inherent complexity of the preparation process. When faced with complex reality, the human mind rationalizes the threatening unpredictability of the environment by searching for observable patterns. When patterns are observed, 'rules' are extrapolated. Review of periodization rationale clearly illustrates the covert shaping influence that this mechanistic philosophical legacy has exerted on training planning philosophies. Simplistic questions, eliciting simplistic answers: What is the ideal duration of a training phase? How long is the optimal taper? How frequent, how hard, how many, what percentage of maximum? Broad, generalized, averaged answers offered as solutions to individual-specific and context-specific problems. Much of physical performance science has been absorbed in this quest for 'golden' rules, focused on uncovering idealized solutions, uncovering the 'answer'. If we truly were mechanical systems, this approach would be valid. However, yet again reality fails to cooperate.

The complex, highly sensitive, nature of the biological system will ensure that the progress of physical fitness will not be an orderly, uniformly incremental, predictable process. The adaptive responses to any given training 'input' will not result in a readily predictable fitness 'output'. An approach that proved successful for one individual will not necessarily work for another, and what worked for an individual in the past may not work for them in the future. Furthermore, and critically, you cannot determine the most appropriate strategy in advance. Consider this: would you buy next year's shoes for your 9-year-old child based on the average shoe size for 10-year-olds? Of course not! You would be relying on a very broad predictive algorithm based on averaged observations with large sample deviations. What you would do is wait until the child is 10, measure their feet, and buy a pair of shoes that you know will fit. You would also monitor the fit carefully as your child grew, to anticipate and avoid the problems inherent in unforeseen and sudden changes in growth. Responses to training are infinitely more variable, less predictable and more subject to change over short-time scales than a growing child's foot-size. So why would we assume that we can prescribe future optimal organizational schemes, training modes or loading variables?

The traditional planning model presents sweeping generalizations in relation to the 'best' structure, phase duration, sequential order, offering planners idealized training solutions. Although periodization theorists have variously championed and debated the relative worth of differing organizational schemes, the evidence suggests that such arguments are, to a large extent, irrelevant. Rather than searching for notional universal 'best' answers that are then cobbled together to formulate plans, a more perceptive approach is the design of processes that facilitate the emergence of context-specific training solutions.

The key take-home message is that automated planning approaches ignore the extreme specificity arising from individual biological systems interacting with ever-changing, dynamic contexts.

Process

Earlier in the chapter it was suggested that traditional training planning approaches were directly descended from the historically pervasive mechanistic planning paradigm. There are a number of hangovers from this formative philosophy still readily apparent in modern training planning conceptions. Recall that Taylor's conception of planning was essentially 'plan' then 'execute'. This approach promoted rigid adherence to the plan, and devalued the importance of review and revision. Consequently, sticking to the plan was considered an ideal to be aspired to, and deviating from the plan was ultimately a sign of weakness.

Although classical articles on periodization have frequently made reference to the need for flexibility, it tends to be treated more as a necessary evil than a virtue to be embraced: a sometimes unavoidable, frustrating deviation from the chosen path. However, a main thrust of this chapter is that the correct path cannot be chosen ahead of time. Accordingly, what now takes on added significance is the design of a sensitive and responsive preparation process: sensitive to emerging threats and opportunities; responsive so as to enable swift modification of training in order to alleviate risk and capitalize on unforeseen progression.

The following are offered as hallmarks of a sensitive and responsive training process.

Information gathering

Information that is relevant to organizing and planning preparation can be collected through both formal and informal means and should include the collation of both objective and subjective data (Fig. 10.2). The worth of performer-generated subjective information has surprisingly been largely ignored within the traditional periodization literature. This should be considered a major oversight, essentially neglecting the primary source of pertinent feedback, i.e. the performer him/herself. The value of subjective feedback as a training modulating factor has been clearly demonstrated elsewhere in the literature. For example, a clinical diagnosis of an athlete's state of

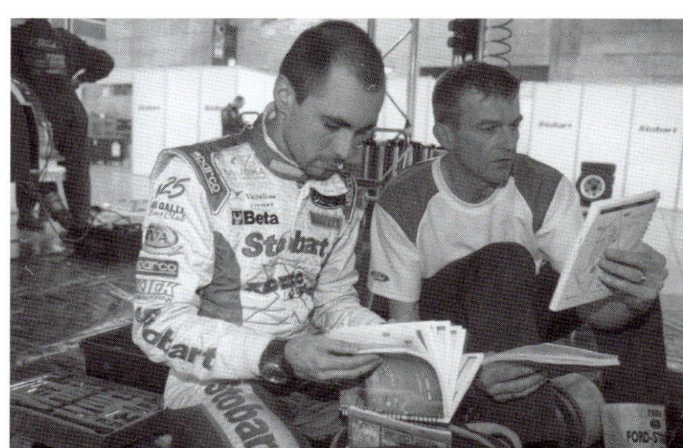

Fig. 10.2 • Support specialists in action. Rally driver Giovanni Bernacchini making last-minute checks with his engineer. © Stobart Motorport. With thanks to the Royal Automobile Motor Sports Association.

stress and recovery is possible through consideration of relevant subjective parameters (Steinacker & Lehmann 2002). Various tools for eliciting such information have been offered in the literature, e.g. the Profile of Mood States (Armstrong & VanHeest 2002), Recovery-Stress Questionnaire for Athletes (Kellmann & Kallus 2001), Mental States of Readiness and Satisfaction (Hogg 2002) and the Psycho-behavioural Overtraining Scale (Collins 1995). In order to optimize the efficacy of such protocols, the performer should be fully aware of the purpose and rationale underpinning subjective data collection. Furthermore, accuracy of subjective ratings is likely to be greatly enhanced by clear definition of rating systems, and consistent application.

Trend analysis

The belief that effective preplanning is possible, that adherence to preplanned schemes is desirable and that plans may be adequately described in sparing empirical terms creates a system that is particularly insensitive to what may be termed 'weak signals'. Weak signals may be considered low-level background information that may herald future major changes in function. These bifurcations in behaviour may take the form of unexpected favourable shifts in condition that may present unforeseen training opportunities or may provide early indication of elevated risk. For example, muscular strain injuries may be preceded by persistent localized fatigue, which in turn may only be detected through a process of regular information gathering and routine in-training 'readiness' assessments.

Failure to respond accordingly to pertinent low-level information is likely to increase the prospect of unfavourable outcomes such as illness, injury and under- or overloading. Hence system sensitivity to weak signals facilitates the pre-emption and avoidance of potentially unfavourable events and enables the adaptive readiness necessary to respond and capitalize on unforeseen opportunities. An unforeseen training opportunity may take the form of an unprojected improvement in training performance, which in turn may facilitate the positive readjustment of training goals.

Within the sports science literature, much time and energy has been devoted to finding reliable markers of physiological function, variables that may serve as indicators of the performer's readiness to train. The uncovering of such markers would greatly enhance the preparation process.

Although many objective markers have been investigated, none have proved to be universally applicable. When we look at the problem from the perspective of biological complexity it makes sense that such a 'one size fits all' measure would prove elusive. In addition, given the range of both inter- and intraperformer variation, coupled with the diversity of demands of the various performance pursuits, the search for a single definitive marker may ultimately be unrealistic.

However, what does suggest itself as a perceptive and practical way forward is the collation of both objective and subjective information and the periodic trend analysis of such data. The linking of a number of low-level 'weak signals may pre-empt future biological events more effectively than any single marker. Linked indicators are likely to vary on both a discipline and on an individual basis, and yet again, frustratingly, we are unlikely to be able to predict which trends are most critical until we have longitudinally collated and analysed the data. Hence what is required is an attention to recording detail, regular review of training and performance trends, and an ongoing search for clues. Ultimately, the effectiveness of the training process is likely to be largely dictated by this capacity to readily anticipate positive or negative trends and adapt accordingly (see Table 10.1). A final point of note: when operating in complex environments it is very difficult to learn unless, first, we observe with an open mind as devoid as possible of preconception and, second, we have some definitive means of checking projections against outcomes. In performance training contexts, the collation of a broad range of subjective and objective data and the consequent trend analysis of this information is the best tool available to provide such sorely needed reality checks.

To summarize:

- Data collection and trend analysis should be an integral part of the training process
- It takes time to build a coherent picture. For data collection to be optimally useful it needs to be conducted over prolonged periods so that trends can be identified and tracked
- Introduce data collation from the start of the training process; it is too late when injury, illness or overtraining have already occurred
- Use training data to learn lessons. Check projections against outcomes
- Establishing trends may prove helpful in determining appropriate endpoints for return to exercise programmes following injury or illness.

Communication, consultation and challenge

Optimized communications are an essential component of any effective management process. Accordingly, due consideration must be given to enhancing networking between the performer, the training director and performer-centred support team. Everyday communication checks should promote clarity throughout the team:

- Is the performer clear on why they're doing what they're doing?
- Does the performer understand exactly how a certain mode of training should feel?
- Is the performer confident of the efficacy of conducted training and on how training modes will positively impact on future event specific performance?
- Is the support team clear on their responsibilities and the expectations placed upon them?
- Is the language used to communicate critical concepts shared, clear, and precise? Are you sure? Check and recheck!

In complex environments there are always innumerable potential perspectives on the best way forward and innumerable ways to justify a preferred course of action. Therefore it is important that, in exploring the worth of a proposed way forward, the training director seeks dissonant, rather than concurring, perspectives. As a protocol, this may take the form of asking support team members to play devil's advocate in critiquing proposed training plans; perhaps reversing roles and arguing opposing positions may prove a useful strategy. External consultants can also offer a new perspective and honest appraisal without the reticence frequently demonstrated by team members. Whatever strategies are employed, it should be borne in mind that the greatest learning opportunities are unlikely to emerge through the vision of a single mind or, indeed, through cosy agreement among group members who share strongly held but similar convictions. Instead, appropriate solutions are more likely to evolve through informed, un-entrenched debate and consideration of differing perspectives. In environments where human learning is severely curtailed by our tendency to seize on the first available perceived pattern and from then on to see only confirming evidence, dissonance is the friend of learning.

These approaches support the use of case conferencing and other methods highlighted in Chapter 24. Directors, managers, coaches and senior staff all need to play a part in developing a performance culture that optimizes benefit from this kind of communication.

Built-in review and revision

Traditional project planning and management tools can frequently deal with minor uncertainties in relatively stable environments. In more dynamic environments, conditions may rapidly evolve beyond the assumptions made in preplanning, requiring major deviations from the path initially selected. Consequently, rigid planning strategies designed solely on the basis of 'hoped-for' or most likely outcomes, which do not incorporate mechanisms enabling swift modification, are unlikely to yield optimal results. Given the unpredictability and chaotic behaviour of biological systems, contingency-planning processes should be considered an important component of preparation planning.

Performers and team members should be aware that regular review and training redirection is a necessary and planned aspect of effective plan management.

Planning structure

The implications of biological complexity suggest there is little if any logical rationale supporting the existence of universal 'best' phase duration. However, this does not necessarily imply that programmes should not be planned in segmented blocks. The keypoint is that phase duration should be decided on the basis of logistical constraints and not on any perceived biological imperative. Accordingly, if it suits the specific logistical situation, or a particular performer's preferred approach, or just happens to make the most sense for a specific period, then planning in blocks may be a judicious solution. However, most convenient does not necessarily equal optimal: the longer the time-lag between review and redirection, the greater the uncertainty. Therefore it would appear sensible to review and debrief training progress on a routine and regular basis and to refine training direction accordingly on as frequent a basis as logistically feasible.

Training monotony has been proposed as an important concept in the management of training plans (Bosch & Klomp 2005, Foster 1998, Kreider et al 1998). Monotony has been defined as the variability of practice over the course of a season (Anderson et al 2003) and is suggested as a training error that increases the risk of overtraining syndromes (Kellmann 2002). High training monotony has been linked to poor performance and an increased frequency of banal infections, whereas a reduction in monotony was related to attainment of personal best performances (Foster & Lehmann 1997, Suzuki et al 2003). Accordingly, an index of training monotony, calculated using performer ratings of perceived exertion, has been employed as a useful training-monitoring tool in rowing (Suzuki et al 2003) and sprinting (Suzuki et al 2006).

Long-term physical training schemes that do not provide sufficient diversity of both loading and movement characteristics are likely to expose performers to heightened risks of stress disorders. For example, in ballet, evidence suggests that supplementary (non-ballet) training led to improvements in fitness parameters and reduced injury occurrence without interfering with key artistic and aesthetic requirements (Koutedakis & Jamurtas 2004). Koutedakis & Jamurtas suggest that, even at the height of their professional careers, dancers' aerobic power, muscular strength, muscular balance, and bone and joint integrity are the 'Achilles heel' of the dance-only selection and training system.

Consequently, it would appear sensible to minimize training monotony. However, it is important to recognize that occasionally concentrated phases of replicated training stress may serve to induce rapid development of a particular fitness component. Conversely, it should also be noted that, if training is too widely diverse for extended periods, then gains in fitness parameters are likely to be blunted. Hence there is an evident trade-off that must be negotiated and a delicate balance that must be struck between training monotony, training variation and diminishing training returns resulting from habituation to an unvarying training stressor. The most perceptive solution to this trade-off problem is once again to adopt a sensitive and responsive management approach. The effective training process will monitor, record, gather relevant information, analyse the trends, and can thus facilitate informed training decisions (see Table 10.1).

Prescription

A hypothetically 'ideal' training load is one that occasions the greatest performance adaptation at the lowest possible cost in terms of energy, residual fatigue and risk of injury. If training load is too low, minimal or suboptimal adaptive response results; conversely, if load is too great then some form of damage will occur. Traditionally, training is prescribed solely using empirical descriptors. How many sets, how many times, at what numerical expression of intensity? Given the extent of biological sensitivity explored earlier, prescribing training in such terms must be considered a crude attempt at providing the precision required in gauging optimal loads. In essence, this approach can be seen as attempting to control the adaptation of a very sensitive system using a technology that is grossly insensitive.

But perhaps the advance planning of 'ideal' training parameters is not always necessary? For many sessions a crude prescription is adequate. Recall that it is the nature of the chaotic biological system to buffer shocks, to self-organize to accommodate stress; our biology is remarkably able to absorb and adapt. So unless the capability of a performer is grossly over-estimated then an inappropriate imposition of stress, for a single session, will be accommodated. However, during periods of elevated stress, the capacity of the system to cope is pushed to its limit. The investment of both physiological and psychological resource is substantial and draining. Though the potential gains are high, so too are the potential risks. In such circumstances optimally accurate prescription and management of training takes on an added significance.

Similarly, slight but chronic training errors may insidiously creep ever closer to critical threshold levels. Maybe hormonal health is compromised; perhaps immune function is gradually suppressed; muscular biases, imbalances and irritations grow. The pressure of a confluence of negative changes in several factors may gradually mount and, unless this pressure is vented, illness or injury will inevitably result.

A counterclaim to this charge may be that such means of prescription are the only available option and that performers are not expected to stick rigidly to the plan as presented on paper. However, the plan does set the tone. It does serve to constrain the field of possibilities.

A final implication of the traditional numerical means of prescribing training is its surreptitious insinuation that conforming to empirical preplanned variables is important. Such a perspective promotes the fallacy that non-adherence to empirically prescribed, preplanned loading is a form of failure, essentially a sign of weakness. It would appear likely that such a belief structure is at the root of prevalent issues such as overtraining, burnout and staleness.

What can we do? Simple tools for dynamic adaptive planning

The implications of the evidence presented, and the key thrusts of this chapter, are essentially threefold:

- Each planning task presents a distinct challenge, and hence optimally efficient planning solutions are inevitably unique and cannot be empirically pre-planned
- The unpredictability inherent in the physical preparation process demands that expectations are consistently monitored against the progress data. Hence, information gathering and insightful assessment tools should be considered a fundamental component of appropriate planning
- Traditional periodization concepts founded in deterministic logic can no longer be considered scientifically valid. Instead, training planning is more appropriately perceived as the design of systems that facilitate the evolution of optimal training structures based upon emerging information and challenges (Box 10.4).

> **Box 10.4**
>
> **Characteristics of an effective dynamic adaptive planning system**
>
> - Appropriate conceptual model
> - Optimized systems functioning
>   - Shared objectives and ethos
>   - Communications and networking
>   - Organizational learning
>   - Data collation and trend analysis
> - Logistical planning constraints
>   - Optimized contact time with training director and access to support team
>   - Experience and relevant education of performer
>   - Frequent consultation, review, debrief and redirection
>   - Minimized planning horizon
> - Practical delivery
>   - Contingency planning and preparatory strategies
>   - Provision of Focused Diversity (Monotony V's Variation trade-off)
>   - Subjective/objective monitoring combinations
>   - Cross-referenced training prescription
> - Optimized system sensitivity and responsiveness to emerging threats and opportunities

As exemplars of ways to meet these challenges, consider Table 10.1, which presents a sample menu of various monitoring tools, many of which have been previously advocated in the literature. These tools are being offered solely as examples of easily applied subjective/objective assessments. To reiterate a previous point, use of any of these tools in isolation is likely to be less effective than the use of monitoring combinations. As with all the key messages in this chapter, indeed in this book, appropriate solutions can only be unravelled after exploration.

The prescription of training variables is an aspect of traditional practice that may also benefit from additional precision. Consider the following: in a previous survey, investigators examined the relationship between the training prescribed by 123 coaches and the self-reported training of their best runners (Hewson & Hopkins 1995). The results illustrated that the association between the coach's prescription and the actual training performed by the runners was generally poor. This was attributed to insufficiently clear communication between coach and athlete. Athletes did adhere to the coach's prescriptions with regard to training volumes but the intensities described by the coaches and performed by the athletes were substantially different. Similar findings have been documented in swimmers (Stewart & Hopkins 2000).

A practical means of optimizing clarity in the communication of training intensities is through triangulation of training variables. In other words, for any desired training adaptation, appropriate training descriptors are cross-referenced. For example, this is how much work should be done, this is how the work should feel and this is the necessary quality of execution. (Compare this with the idea of performance criteria described in Ch. 23.)

The triangulation of variables enables a more accurate prescription of training parameters, thus helping to eradicate some of the pitfalls inherent when describing training loadings in solely empirical, unidimensional terms (Table 10.2).

Summary

The objective of this chapter was to provide an appreciation of both psychological and biological considerations that affect our ability to formulate and manage preparation plans. It is clear from the arguments and

Table 10.1 Some suggested monitoring methods

When	What	Who says
Pre-pretraining	• *Subjective indicator of 'general' well-being*, e.g. RESTQ, POMS, recovery-cue; abbreviated versions of same • *Objective measure* Morning HR/HR variability	Collins 2000 Kellmann 2002
Pretraining	• *Subjective rating (Score 1–10) of key indicators*, e.g. Mood Sleep quality Readiness to train Residual muscle soreness/fatigue Site specific soreness rating Perceived readiness rating • *Objective measure (readiness check)* Psychomotor speed/reaction time Measure system readiness, e.g. countermovement jump (height); drop jump (contact time/height)	Collins 2000 Nurmekivi et al 2001 Rietjens et al 2005 Nederhof et al 2006, 2007
In-training	• *Prescriptive accuracy* Rate desired intensity (how it should feel) Technical execution (required quality) Empirical range (load and repetition limits) • *Recording detail* Empirical descriptors RPE (per effort, set, or session)	
Post-training	• *Post-session objective measure* Repeat pre-session readiness check • *Session RPE*. Retrospectively calculate associated measures, e.g. Monotony (weekly average load/standard deviation) Strain (mean weekly load × monotony) Training load (RPE × training time) CPS (category ratio pain scale) TQR (total quality recovery) • *Weekly training 'stress' assessment* Daily and/or individual session RPE = week total	 Suzuki et al 2003, 2006

HR, heart rate; POMS, profile of mood state; RESTQ, recovery-stress questionnaire for athletes; RPE, rating of perceived exertion

evidence presented that many aspects of our customary planning approaches lack both an empirical evidence base and an underpinning conceptual logic.

The illusory security of assumed 'rules' and the associated simplistic vision of the preparation task should be rejected, and the reality of biological complexity and the implications of human cognitive limitations acknowledged. Critically, a dynamic adaptive planning approach demands that the elemental uncertainty and ambiguity inherent in training planning is recognized and appropriate counteractive strategies devised.

Unfortunately, as with so many of the things that are good for us, this approach is also more difficult and more challenging than traditional preformed planning recipes. The management skills required are also not necessarily those historically promoted. Formal, pedagogical planning skills are of limited value within such a dynamic environment. Instead, of more pivotal importance is the organizational ability to create support team networks, to develop communications systems, to implement information gathering processes and to optimize organizational learning. The planning

Table 10.2 Triangulation of training prescription parameters

Construct	Training parameter	How to quantify
Volume	Recommended range of sets and reps	Numerical prescription
Subjective feel	How efforts should feel during execution	Performer rating (e.g. 1–10)
Quality of effort	Expected technical quality *or* speed *or* power output/ distance/ height, etc.	Coach rating (e.g. 1–10) Timing system Measurement

process now becomes centred on facilitating the seamless emergence of training strategy in response to unfolding events, within the boundaries imposed by logistical factors, the stated programme objectives and the time frame imposed by the performance schedule.

And finally...

Mike Tyson once said, 'everyone has a plan, until they get punched in the face', and that's quite an insightful comment. If we plan on the basis of optimistic, 'hoped for' outcomes, neglecting contingencies, our plans become fragile, vulnerable to unexpected events and consequently easily disrupted and derailed. Conversely, a planning paradigm founded on the principles of consistent assessment and rapid adjustment enables the evasion of potential stumbling blocks, facilitating robust and sustainable preparation processes. Effective preparation plans identify and circumnavigate potential pitfalls, are sensitive to emerging threats and respond with considered and timely action.

References

Anderson, L., Triplett-McBride, T., Foster, C., et al., 2003. Impact of training patterns on incidence of illness and injury during a women's collegiate basketball season. J. Strength Cond. Res. 17, 734–738.

Armstrong, L.E., VanHeest, J.L., 2002. The unknown mechanism of the overtraining syndrome: clues from depression and psychoneuroimmunology. Sports Med. 32, 185–209.

Aubert, A., 2008. Psychosocial stress, emotions and cytokine-related disorders. Recent Patents on Inflammation and Allergy Drug Discovery 2, 139–148.

Axelsson, J., Akerstedt, T., Kecklund, G., et al., 2003. Hormonal changes in satisfied and dissatisfied shift workers across a shift cycle. J. Appl. Physiol. 95, 2099–2105.

Baker, D., Wilson, G., Carlyon, R., 1994. Periodization: the effect on strength of manipulating volume and intensity. J. Strength Cond. Res. 8, 235–242.

Beavan, C.M., Gill, N.D., Cook, C.J., 2008a. Salivary testosterone and cortisol responses in professional rugby players after four resistance exercise protocols. J. Strength Cond. Res. 22, 426–431.

Beavan, C.M., Cook, C.J., Gill, N.D., 2008b. Significant strength gains observed in rugby players after specific resistance exercise protocols based on individual salivary testosterone responses. J. Strength Cond. Res. 22, 419–425.

Bird, S.P., Tarpenning, K.M., 2004. Influence of circadian time structure on acute hormonal responses to a single bout of heavy-resistance exercise in weight-trained men. Chronobiol. Int. 21, 131–146.

Bompa, T.O., 1999. Periodization training: theory and methodology, fourth ed. Human Kinetics, Champaign, IL.

Bosch, F., Klomp, R., 2005. Running: biomechanics and exercise physiology in practice. Churchill Livingstone, Edinburgh.

Bouchard, C., Rankinen, T., Chagnon, Y.C., et al., 2000. Genomic scan for maximal oxygen uptake and its response to training in the HERITAGE Family Study. J. Appl. Physiol. 88, 551–559.

Bronner, S., Ojofeitimi, S., Rose, D., 2003. Injuries in a modern dance company: effect of comprehensive management on injury incidence and time loss. Am. J. Sports Med. 31, 365–373.

Brown, L.E., 2001. Nonlinear versus linear periodization models. National Strength and Conditioning Association 23 (1), 42–44.

Brown, L.E., Greenwood, M., 2005. Periodization essentials and innovations in resistance training protocols. J. Strength Cond. Res. 27 (4), 80–85.

Brown, T.D., Micheli, L.J., 2004. Foot and ankle injuries in dance. Am. J. Orthop. 33, 303–309.

Buehler, R., Griffin, D., Ross, M., 1994. Exploring the' planning fallacy': Why people underestimate their task completion times. J. Pers. Soc. Psychol. 67, 366–381.

Buehler, R., Griffin, D., Ross, M., 2002. Inside the planning fallacy: the causes and consequences of optimistic time predictions. In: Gilovich, T., Griffin, D., Kahneman, D. (Eds.), Heuristics and biases: the psychology of intuitive judgement. Cambridge University Press, New York, pp. 250–270.

Cacioppo, J.T., Hawkley, L.C., Berntson, G.G., et al., 2002. Do lonely days invade the nights? Potential social modulation of sleep efficiency. Psychol. Sci. 13, 384–387.

Calhoon, G., Fry, A.C., 1999. Injury rates and profiles of elite competitive weightlifters. J. Athletic Training 34, 232–238.

Carl, D.L., Tyree, B., Strasser, S., 2001. Effect of environment and training on mood states of competitive swimmers. Med. Sci. Sports Exerc. 33 (Suppl. 5), abstract 1252.

Collins, D., 1995. Early detection of overtraining problems in athletes. Coaching Focus 28, 17–20.

Collins, D., 2000. The 'Zulu' principle: avoiding staleness and overtraining with your athletes. FHS 9, 3–7.

Cosca, D.D., Navazio, F., 2007. Common problems in endurance athletes. Am. Fam. Physician 76, 237–244.

Cowley, M., Byrne, R., 2004. Hypothesis testing in chess masters' problem solving. In: Fifth International Conference on Thinking, Leuven, Belgium, 22–24 July 2004.

DeBeliso, M., Harris, C., Spitzer-Gibson, T., Adams, K.J., 2005. A comparison of periodised and fixed repetition training protocol on strength in older adults. J. Sci. Med. Sport 8, 190–199.

Dubravcic-Simunjak, S., Pecina, M., et al., 2003. The incidence of injuries in elite junior figure skaters. Am. J. Sports Med. 31, 511–517.

Ferrara, M., De Gennaro, L., 2001. How much sleep do we need? Sleep Med. Rev. 5, 155–179.

Filaire, E., Lac, G., Pequignot, J., 2003. Biological, hormonal, and psychological parameters in professional soccer players throughout a competitive season. Percept. Mot. Skills 97, 1061–1072.

Foster, C., 1998. Monitoring training in athletes with reference to overtraining syndrome. Med. Sci. Sports Exerc. 30, 1164–1168.

Foster, R.G., Kreitzman, L., 2005. Rhythms of life: the biological clocks that control the daily lives of every living thing. Yale University Press, New Haven, CT.

Foster, C., Lehmann, M., 1997. Overtraining syndrome. In: Guten, G.N. (Ed.), Running injuries. WB Saunders, Philadelphia, pp. 173–188.

Garrick, J.G., Lewis, S.L., 2001. Career hazards for the dancer. Occup. Med. 16, 609–618.

Gilovich, T., Griffin, D., 2002. Introduction – heuristics and biases: then and now. In: Gilovich, T., Griffin, D., Kahneman, D. (Eds.), Heuristics and biases: the psychology of intuitive judgement. Cambridge University Press, New York, pp. 1–18.

Glass, L., 2001. Review article: synchronization and rhythmic processes in physiology. Nature 410, 277–284.

Graham, J., 2002. Periodization: research and an example application. J. Strength Cond. Res. 24, 62–70.

Grove, W.M., Meehl, P.E., 1996. Comparative efficiency of informal (subjective, impressionistic) and formal (mechanical, algorithmic) prediction procedures: the clinical-statistical controversy. Psychology, Public Policy and Law 2, 1–31.

Hewson, D.J., Hopkins, W.G., 1995. Prescribed and self-reported seasonal training of distance runners. J. Sports Sci. 13, 463–470.

Himashree, G., Banerjee, P.K., Selvamurthy, W., 2002. Sleep and performance – recent trends. Indian J. Physiol. Pharmacol. 46, 6–24.

Hogg, J.M., 2002. Debriefing: a means to increasing recovery and subsequent performance. In: Hirschenhauser, K., Frigerio, D., Grammer, K., Magnusson, M.S. (Eds.), 2002 Monthly patterns of testosterone and behaviour in prospective fathers. Hormonal Behaviour, vol. 42, pp. 172–181.

Institute of Medicine of the National Academies, 1999. To err is human: building a safer health system. National Academy of Sciences, Baltimore, MD.

Issurin, V., 2008. Block periodization versus traditional training theory: a review. J. Sports Med. Phys. Fitness 48, 65–75.

Karaliute, E., 2007. Mechanistic conception of the human being: the machine metaphor. J. Young Scientists 1, 12.

Kellmann, M. (Ed.), 2002. Enhancing recovery: preventing underperformance in athletes. Human Kinetics, Champaign, IL, pp. 181–198.

Kellmann, M., Kallus, K.W., 2001. Recovery-Stress Questionnaire for Athletes: user manual. Human Kinetics, Champaign, IL.

Kelman, B.B., 2000. Occupational hazards in female ballet dancers. Advocate for a forgotten population. Am. Assoc. Occu. Health Nurses J. 48, 430–434.

Junge, A., Rosch, D., Peterson, L., et al., 2002. Prevention of soccer injuries: a prospective intervention study in youth amateur players. Am. J. Sports Med. 30, 652–659.

Koutedakis, Y., Jamurtas, A., 2004. The dancer as a performing athlete: physiological considerations. Sports Med. 34, 651–661.

Koutedakis, Y., Myszkewycz, L., Soulas, D., et al., 1999. The effects of rest and subsequent training on selected physiological parameters in professional female classical dancers. Int. J. Sports Med. 20, 379–383.

Kraemer, W.J., Hakkinen, K., Triplett-McBride, N.T., 2003. Physiological changes with periodized resistance training in women tennis players. Med. Sci. Sports Exerc. 35, 157–168.

Kreider, R.B., Fry, A.C., O'Toole, M.L., 1998. Overtraining in sport: terms, definitions and prevalence. In: Kreider, R.B., Fry, A.C., O'Toole, M.L. (Eds.), Overtraining in sport. Human Kinetics, Champaign, IL.

Lovallo, W.R., 2005. Stress and health: biological and psychological interactions, second ed. Sage Publications, Thousand Oaks, CA.

Luboshitzky, R., 2000. Endocrine activity during sleep. J. Pediatr. Endocrinol. Metab. 13, 13–20.

Maestu, J., Jurimae, J., Jurimse, T., 2005. Monitoring of performance and training in rowing. Sports Med. 35, 597–619.

Mahood, N.V., Kenefick, R.W., Kertzer, R., Quinn, T.J., 2001. Physiological determinants of cross-country ski racing performance. Med. Sci. Sports Exerc. 33, 1379–1384.

Maslach, C., Jackson, S.E., 1984. Burnout in organizational settings. Applied Psychological Annual 5, 133–153.

Matveyev, L., 1972. Periodisierung des sportlichen Trainings. Fizkultura i Sport, Moscow

Matveyev, L., 1977. Fundamentals of sports training. Fizkultura i Sport, Moscow

Meehl, P.E., 1954. Clinical versus statistical prediction, University of Minnesota Press, Minneapolis, MN.

Mujika, I., 1998. The influence of training characteristics and tapering on the adaptation in highly trained. Int. J. Sports Med. 19, 439–446.

Nederhof, E., Lemmink, K.A., Visscher, C., et al., 2006. Psychomotor speed: possibly a new marker for overtraining syndrome. Sports Med. 36, 817–828.

Nederhof, E., Lemmink, K., Zwerver, J., Mulder, T., 2007. The effect of high load training on psychomotor speed. Int. J. Sports Med. 28, 595–601.

Newby-Clark, I.R., Ross, M., Buehler, R., Koehler, D.J., 2000. People focus on optimistic scenarios and disregard pessimistic scenarios while predicting task. J. Exp. Psychol. Appl. 6, 171–182.

Newby-Kahneman, D., Tversky, A., 1979. Intuitive prediction: biases and corrective procedures. TIMS Studies in Management Science 12, 313–327.

Nilsson, C., Leanderson, J., Wykman, A., Strender, L.E., 2001. The injury panorama in a Swedish professional ballet company. Knee Surg. Sports Traumatol. Arthrosc. 9, 242–246.

Nurmekivi, A., Karu, T., Pihl, E., et al., 2001. Blood lactate recovery and perceived readiness to start a new run in middle-distance runners during interval training. Percept. Mot. Skills 93, 397–404.

Patel, V.L., 2000. Conceptual and procedural errors in medical decision making. In: Slips, mistakes and faulty reasoning: the nature of human errors in medicine, Proceedings of the AMIA Symposium.

Pinker, S., 1997. How the mind works. WW Norton, New York.

Plisk, S.S., Stone, M.H., 2003. Periodization strategies. J. Strength Cond. Res. 25, 19–37.

Quirk, R., 1994. Common foot and ankle injuries in dance. Orthop. Clin. North Am. 25, 123–133.

Rensing, L., Meyer-Grahle, U., Ruoff, P., 2001. Biological timing and the clock metaphor: oscillatory and hourglass mechanisms. Chronobiol. Int. 18, 329–369.

Rhea, M.R., Alderman, B.L., 2004. A meta-analysis of periodized versus nonperiodized strength and power training programs. Res. Q. Exerc. Sport 75, 413–422.

Rhea, M.R., Ball, S.D., Phillips, W.T., Burkett, L., 2002. A comparison of linear and daily undulating periodized programs with equated volume and intensity. J. Strength Cond. Res. 16, 250–255.

Rietjens, G.J., Kuipers, H., Adam, J.J., et al., 2005. Physiological, biochemical and psychological markers of strenuous training-induced fatigue. Int. J. Sports Med. 26, 16–26.

Rogers, N.L., Szuba, M.P., Staab, J.P., et al., 2001. Neuroimmunologic aspects of sleep and sleep loss. Semin. Clin. Neuropsychiatry 6, 295–307.

Schultheiss, O.C., Rohde, W., 2002. Implicit power motivation predicts men's testosterone changes and implicit learning in a contest situation. Hormonal Behaviour 41, 195–202.

Schultheiss, O.C., Campbell, K.L., McClelland, D.C., 1999. Implicit power motivation moderates men's testosterone responses to imagined and real dominance success. Hormonal Behaviour 36, 234–241.

Selye, H., 1956. The stress of life. McGraw-Hill, New York.

Shan, G., 2005. Comparison of repetitive movements between ballet dancers and martial artists: risk assessment of muscle overuse injuries and prevention strategies. Res. Sports Med. 13, 63–76.

Siff, M.C., 2000. Supertraining, fifth ed. Supertraining Institute, Denver, CO.

Skinner, J.S., Jaskólski, A., Jaskólska, A., et al., 2001. Age, sex, race, initial fitness, and response to training: the HERITAGE Family Study. J. Appl. Physiol. 90, 1770–1776.

Smith, D.J., 2003. A framework for understanding the training process leading to elite performance. Sports Med. 33, 1103–1126.

Smith, M., Matheson, G.O., Meeuwisse, W.H., 1996. Injuries in cross-country skiing: a critical appraisal of the literature. Sports Med. 21, 239–250.

Steinacker, J.M., Lehmann, M., 2002. Clinical findings and mechanisms of stress and recovery in athletes. In: Kellmann, M. (Ed.), Enhancing recovery: preventing underperformance in athletes. Human Kinetics, Champaign, IL, pp. 103–118.

Stewart, A.M., Hopkins, W.G., 2000. Seasonal training and performance of competitive swimmers. J. Sports Sci. 18, 873–884.

Stone, M.H., 1996. Periodization, Presented at the NSCA National Conference, June, Atlanta, GA.

Stone, M.H., O'Bryant, H.S., Schilling, B.K., et al., 1999a. Periodization. Part 1: Effects of manipulating volume and intensity. J. Strength Cond. Res. 21, 56–62.

Stone, M.H., O'Bryant, H.S., Schilling, B.K., et al., 1999b. Periodization. Part 2: Effects of manipulating volume and intensity. J. Strength Cond. Res. 21, 54–60.

Suzuki, S., Sato, T., Takahasi, Y., 2003. Diagnosis of training program for a Japanese rower by using the index of monotony. Can. J. Appl. Physiol. 28, 105–106.

Suzuki, S., Sato, T., Maeda, A., Takahasi, Y., 2006. Program design based on a mathematical model using rating of perceived exertion for an elite Japanese sprinter: a case study. J. Strength Cond. Res. 20, 36–42.

Takagi, T., 1986. [Longitudinal study on circadian rhythms of plasma hormone levels during Japanese Antarctic Research Expedition.]. Hokkaido Igaku Zasshi 61, 121–133 [In Japanese].

Taleb, N.N., 2005. The black swan. Random House, New York.

Taylor, F.W., 1911. The principles of scientific management. Harper Bros, New York.

Tetlock, P., 2005. Expert political judgment: how good is It? How can we know? Princeton University Press, Princeton, NJ.

Van Regenmortel, M.H.V., 2007. The rational design of biological complexity: a deceptive metaphor. Proteomics 7, 965–975.

Venkatraman, J.T., Leddy, J., Pendergast, D., 2000. Dietary fats and immune status in athletes: clinical implications. Med. Sci. Sports Exerc. 32, S389–S395.

Villavicencio, A.T., Hernández, T.D., Burneikiene, S., Thramann, J., 2007. Neck pain in multisport athletes. J. Neurosurg. Spine 7, 408–413.

Viru, A., 1995. Adaptation in sports training. CRC Press, Boca Raton, FL.

Waldén, M., Hägglund, M., Ekstrand, J., 2007. Football injuries during European Championships 2004–2005. Knee Surg. Sports Traumatol. Arthrosc. 15, 1155–1162.

Zatsiorsky, V.M., 1995. Science and practice of strength training. Human Kinetics, Champaign, IL.

Practical dimensions of providing for excellence: views from the performer's panel

11

Dave Collins

Grey Matters/UCLan

CHAPTER CONTENTS

Introduction

As I said in Chapter 7, consideration of these performance environment issues has been comparatively sparse in the literature. In contrast, the content of the preceding three chapters has highlighted the important issues and illustrated how these can be used to enhance performance management and the support systems of teams, companies and groups aspiring to 'be all that they can be'.

The apparent diversity of performance environments may make it hard to see what common managerial problems may accrue. This made the common thread to the PP comments all the more interesting. Their observations and exemplars seemed to come from three 'categories' of organization. The first, and smallest, related to practice and training groups; sometimes fairly loose, convenience or semiformal assemblies of performers and supporters just working together towards (presumably and hopefully) common aims. The second were professional teams or companies: named organizations with performance as the most central and easily identifiable aim. The third is a particularly British situation (although similar structures are increasingly apparent worldwide): the national governing body (NGB) or blanket organization with several responsibilities, one of which is performance. For simplicity, unless the point relates to a specific case, I will use 'group' as meaning any one of these three.

You should keep your own situation in mind as you consider the advice in this chapter. It may be a more complex environment, involving a combination of characteristics from two or even all of these types. Whatever the case, however, one must always examine things from the 'other side' of the system; in short, what the performer has to do to secure support and how effectively those services are allocated and deployed.

Key practical issues

The most important managerial issues to emerge from the section, almost irrespective of which of our three categories is considered, are the need for common and overriding aims for the group, plus a clear and coherent strategy designed to make this happen. Almost inevitably, these issues relate to

DOI: 10.1016/B978-0-443-06734-1.00011-0

leadership of and belief in the plans implemented, as the culture within the group is refined and sharpened towards a performance focus.

B****y politics

The role of leadership and power in cultural change is important, whatever the size of the group. Most will be familiar with the form, storm, norm, perform and adjourn sequence described in Chapter 9. However, a key quote from Chapter 8 says a lot about the interpersonal challenges that typify the 'high ego involvement' world of performance.

> Above all what this ignores is the self-interest and partisan mentality that is not only inherent in organizations, but if seen as destructive, becomes just that. Unwavering adherence to the principles of rationality, then, is eventually self defeating.
>
> Butcher & Clarke 2001, p. 11–12

One key aspect of group dynamics that is illustrated in this is the apparently central role of politics. In business, there is an increasing recognition that 'management is politics... all about reconciling different stakeholder interests' (Butcher & Clarke 2008, p. 1). Clearly, when making essential and rational change to any group, there is a need to take people with you while taking notice of the existing culture. One important implication is the avoidance of 'one size fits all' solutions. For example, at the time of writing, cycling, sailing and rowing represent every UK sport administrator's favourite organizational setup and management style. However, without critical appreciation of a given performance group's specific, internal cultural challenges, this attempt to clone one successful approach to another situation can lead to the erroneous but prescribed uptake of all the successful sport's characteristics. This cloning will, to some extent, almost inevitably run completely counter to the extant culture and what most people believe. In short, direct copying is almost always doomed. Careful and considered adoption of key principles, on the other hand, should almost be de rigueur.

Evolve or die

Another point to emerge very strongly from the PP was the need to constantly strive to improve; excessive comfort was seen as the precursor to a fall from grace. Exploring the need for change, KB pointed out the need for constant 'renewal' to stay ahead; especially pertinent in team sports where increasingly effective scouting means that your methods are rapidly analysed, understood and countered by your opposition. One relevant point here is the timing of change, and I am indebted to Wayne Goldsmith, Australian Performance Consultant extraordinaire, for the model of the regeneration cycle presented in Figure 11.1.

The idea is based on the (almost) inevitable cycle of peak performance, slump and regrowth. The point is when one should think about regeneration and working towards the next cycle. Ideally, someone is planning the next cycle (or at least thinking about it) even while the current incumbents are at their peak. At the very least, however, plans must be in place as the current group goes 'off the boil' so that the swing down, through 6 o'clock and back up towards the next peak, is as quick and smooth as possible. Loiter around after 2 o'clock, as many very successful teams have displayed a tendency to do, and delay the inevitable changes that take you forwards, and your slump is elongated and harder to climb out of.

Other implications include the consequences for when new team members are appointed and the challenges they will face. Just after 1 o'clock is when the new cohort is most commonly started; obviously better if they have been 'blooded' while the team is performing well, but at least the new influx will help to speed the swing back to good levels, so long as time is allowed. If the team has got

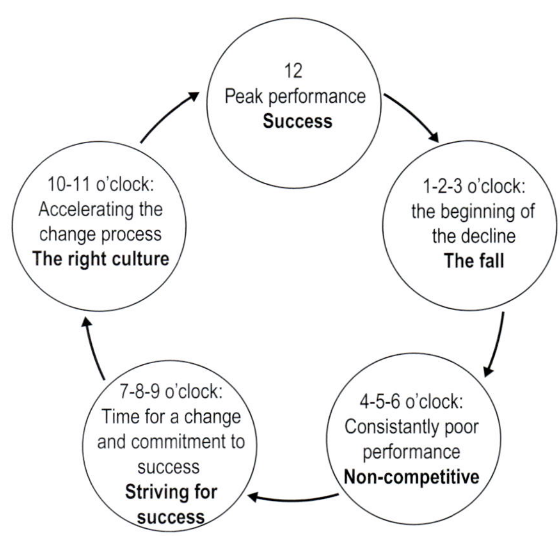

Fig. 11.1 • The 'Clock Model' of the performance cycle. With kind permission of Wayne Goldsmith, www.sportscoachingbrain.com

comfortable and complacent already, however, the introduction of new blood around the 3–5 o'clock mark sets them a horrendous challenge. You can 'kill off', or at least stunt the development of promising young performers by appointing them to an 'in the doldrums' team: much better to introduce good ones while the team is still firing on most, if not all, cylinders. This model can apply to performance teams in almost any domain. I'll leave you to insert your own examples here, but you won't have to think very hard to come up with some!

Another important point is whether this cycle is truly inevitable or if skilful management can avoid or minimize it even further. Both SB and KB believed in the possibility of more consistent and long lasting 'peaks' achieved by an almost constant process of tweaking and refinement (see planning ideas in Ch. 10). As an individual athlete for example, SB would complete an annual review of everything he had tried over the previous year, looking to introduce new ideas and almost reinvent some components to keep things fresh. In teams, long tenure managers always seem to be 'shaking the tree' somewhat, ensuring that team members must continue to evolve. Sir Alex Ferguson at Manchester United provides a perfect example of this; consider his public statements on particular 'star' players, or the decision to purchase players into positions of already established strength. The bottom line is the need to maintain a level of uncertainty; not too much but sufficient to prevent complacency.

Organizational evolution is hard, however, and requires careful management to ensure that the members stay on board and 'aligned' with the new aims. As Chapter 8 explains, the leaders' emotional intelligence (EI) can be a big factor here, especially in smaller team/group environments and/or where the leader/teacher/coach lacks an already established and credible reputation in that particular domain, necessitating greater leadership through others who do have one. As a result of good EI, old-school autocratic leadership will give way to greater 'differentiation', making more allowances for individual needs within the overall plan in order to benefit most from each individual's potential contribution.

The politics and mechanisms of change

Political considerations are important in changing a group at all levels from the micro level, between factions or friendship groups, right up to competing departments within what Veronica describes as a corporate setup. In NGBs, for example, there are often tensions between the performance department and other sections of the organization (e.g. the first team and academy challenges highlighted in Ch. 9). When these exist, the organization is practically hamstrung, as the departments need to interact effectively for each to achieve their prescribed role. For example, performance functions must rely on grassroots/development providing appropriately trained potential elites (see above) while, vice versa, grassroots will benefit from clear and successful role models at the 'top' of the sport. Performance and development must depend on effective coaches/teachers/ instructors who must be educated and competent to operate at both these extremes and all the levels in between. In short, the departments are at least as interdependent as the sales, research & development and finance units of a major corporation. In the absence of clear and concise leadership, integrated within commonly understood and accepted goals, the various units will fail to contribute to meeting the overall goal. This may be either because they were too successful in pursuing their own goal to the detriment of others or because they failed to adequately meet their own target. KB and SM stressed the need for performance objectives and methods being understood by and coherent with the management team, especially in situations where the management board may lack genuine appreciation of the performance challenge. This point is emphasized later in the section on vertical coherence.

The next consideration is to identify who does what within the setup. In a small group with a single 'clear' leader, this comes down to his/her personal skills and the extent to which the leader stays in touch with and responds to the 'rumblings' (both positive and negative) coming from within. Keeping your ear to the ground is a very useful aphorism, and this constant progress check also fits in well with the advice from Chapter 10. It is just too easy to lose your way and misinterpret the signs to fit what you want to see. Several PP members stressed that well defined roles plus responsibility generate individual ownership, ensuring that the leader stays involved in what is now his/her own task.

Things get macro very quickly in groups, however, and there is usually a need for subgroups and/or members with leadership roles to fulfil some of the political functions. As a result, most notably in larger, multi-aim groups such as professional dance companies, sports teams and NGBs, message sending will need to be agreed and coordinated 'in private' to ensure consistency. Ensuring that change is encouraged, exemplified and facilitated from a number of different directions within and outwith the organization will also help to keep things on track. Although this is a 'pan-group' function, it also needs each individual 'change agent' to keep an eye on what messages are being sent and hopefully to ensure that things are working in the same direction. Accordingly, the lead coach, Artistic Director or Performance Director will take time to ensure that each individual performer is receiving a consistent and clear message on expectations and actions for improvement (see Chs 5 and 24 for examples).

Political acumen is equally important for any specialist support professional working in a performance environment, or at least 'knowing someone who can' to get advice and guidance from on such issues. It is also important for the specialist (coach, scientist, performance manager) to ensure that they are completely up to date, and preferably in tune, with the aims and strategy of the group. Ideally, they will be contributing to its evolution, and fostering and implementing feedback mechanisms to ensure the group remains coherent and on track. One useful habit identified by both KB and RR is to 'audit' your own/your subunit's goals and actions against the group's mission statement. Things should fit coherently (see vertical coherence, below) but if they don't, and the actions are seen as really necessary, you might want to revisit and tweak your mission!

Interestingly, small units within bigger organizations can act as 'agents of change' on their own: research into the dynamics of culture change shows how a single unit, acting as a 'beacon of excellence' or 'pocket of good practice' (Clarke & Meldrum, 1999) can attract the attention of others. In a formal sense, this provides leaders with a role model for other groups, one of the three key aspects of culture change. So if you have a part that is doing this well, then flaunt it! At the informal level, an effective and clearly socially tight unit acts as a 'beacon' for others in the organization, be they leaders or not. Once again, fellow workers can use this as a role model, but in this case as a way to 'win over' other colleagues or even management. So, acting as a personification of organizational values, tight and effective groups can offer lower-level management with the chance to exemplify what could be – to win over top management to new ways of working. Wherever you are in the performance setup, your motivation to improve can be a genuine catalyst for change. Switched on leadership at the top can fully exploit this important 'alternative route to greatness'. So, given that top-down change can often stall, sensible and sensitive leaders will build pockets of excellence and utilize them in the political battle for development and the bigger win.

Role clarity, common goals and coherence

As a second practical concern, consider the points John makes in Chapter 10 on the difficulties of genuine prediction and hence accurate manipulation of the future. We have already addressed some of these challenges in the previous section, showing how hard it is for genuine talent identification in a specific activity. Obviously, as performers get older and closer to peak maturity (when they should be at their best) this prediction/manipulation of the future becomes easier. However, someone somewhere is going to be upset if the goals each individual is working towards are not commonly understood and operationalized by the support group; without this agreement up front, the performer is going to be pulled in different directions by the different support elements. With regard to the performance group itself, each individual's development plan can be effectively facilitated if the aims are understood and acknowledged as relevant for group performance; in short, the team acts as a motivator for each individual. In similar fashion, selection within a group will also depend on a similar set of aspirations, and the means of 'getting there' being common knowledge within the members trying to get chosen. Those in leadership roles must ensure the widest possible publicity and greatest possible clarity for selection criteria if these are to make an effective contribution to team performance.

Successful achievement of this common knowledge and understanding is absolutely essential to interactions across the performance group. Assumptions are all too common and all too fatal to eventual achievement. Therefore, ensuring an openness and commonality to support providers' plans is central to the leader's role and will require the deployment of several concepts from Chapter 8, particularly the conflict management and EI skills. 'Case conferencing', when well prepared for, executed and followed through, is the key tool here; we consider it in more detail in the last part of this chapter. In similar fashion, effective leaders will ensure the dissemination of selection criteria by every means at their disposal. So long as the message is consistent, it is almost impossible to communicate this through too many channels. Once again, we cover this in slightly more detail later.

Things to think about

Almost all of the organizational issues, and the associated, often politically-motivated, disputes, can usefully be addressed by a 'back to basics' approach. SB was particularly strong on this point, reporting a rapid side-step whenever politics was mentioned throughout his career. His point is a good one: define 'performance' up front (what it looks like, how it is measured, etc.) then address all the issues against a performance focus. So, if 'performance' is measured against world and Olympic medals, lower-level team events or competitions must take second place. Although this sounds simplistic – and, having been in the hot seat myself, I know that there are a variety of pressures (political and financial to name but two) that are brought to bear – SB's point remains valid. Many directors, performance managers, coaches and instructors spend a great deal of their time acting as an 'umbrella' to enable their performers to stay focused on the correct picture. Of course, these challenges and distractions are often avoided by performers, coaches and administrators working to a common and agreed plan; this is also known as 'vertical coherence'.

Vertical coherence

Ideas on coherence and consistency should have rung loudly throughout this section in the book and the previous statements in this chapter. Examples of a lack of coherence, or conflict between potentially competing aims, are quite common in performance environments. Consider, for example, the short-term performance versus long-term development conundrum faced by almost all coaches/managers in teams or companies. Those charged with creating high performance are often on a limited lifespan in that, while the establishment of longer-term talent development strategies is both central to the role and essential for the organization, very, very few are afforded the luxury of development activity that does not show immediate return or the opportunity to be present when the seeds sown bear fruit. Vertical coherence, ensuring a smooth and effective pathway for talent, is an important long-term aim, but one that may get buried under the short-term need for success.

The convenient answer is to cover these two agendas with two distinct support teams, often under separate management and leadership. Such a situation is common in premiership football, for example: academy setups for young player development often have no point of contact with the elite end of the business, even to the extent of being on separate sites. We think that some separation is inevitable, but there are considerable benefits to harmonizing the efforts of the two units.

It is worth considering situations where the two units are integrated, to see some of the benefits that may accrue. Interestingly (especially in light of the luxurious status inferred in the previous paragraph), genuine integration, and hence productivity of the development unit, seems to be a characteristic of organizations with more mature, well established leadership. In football, for example, Arsène Wenger at Arsenal and Sir Alex Ferguson at Manchester United seem completely in touch with their respective 'youth' programmes, with a (consequent?) steady stream of young players into the first team from their own academy who have been groomed and selected into the appropriate performance style and culture. Nor is this the sole preserve of very big, rich organizations. Consider Dario Gradi at Crewe, until his retirement the manager of the single most productive development academy in British football.

Examples of this 'coherence between' and 'flow upwards' situation are not that common but, when they occur, they represent an integration of aims, philosophy and conduct that is almost inevitably successful. As such, this integration should be a feature of effective pathway systems of any size and explicit consideration of ways to achieve this is given in the final part of this chapter (see also Ch. 5). At the Central School of Ballet in London, SM ensures integration by inviting artistic directors from professional dance companies to sit as artistic advisors. This keeps the school on the same track as the people who employ their students, a situation that is often not the case in many apparently better integrated sports settings.

Horizontal coherence

As highlighted earlier in this chapter, integration between specialists working at a certain level (e.g. elite or development) within an organization is as important as integration between the levels. Role clarity is key to ensuring this important factor, together with consistent leadership messages from a variety of sources (through case conferences, for example, or wherever else the integration takes place). Some considerations on clarifying responsibilities between specialists are examined in Chapter 24. I'll consider the leadership messages aspect here.

The point is that different domains (e.g. dance versus team sports versus individual sports versus extreme sports) have completely different mores and expectations on leadership and degree of perceived control. Such issues are particularly apparent when people of a highly individual nature must collaborate and act together as a group. My own experiences in track and field athletics exemplify this well. Forming a group identity in people whose whole sport is traditionally built around rabid individuality was often like herding cats. Such problems have also beset expeditions from time immemorial; from Robert Falcon Scott through Chris Bonnington, extending to the most recent alpine-ascent-style teams, interindividual conflict is common and can be lethal. The need for clarification and consistent implementation, especially in cases of culture change, is well presented as a feature of role compliance against commitment.

Considerations of group identity are well demonstrated by these examples, and they are of much greater importance than many practitioners think. Considering the leader behaviours, carefully observing the group and talking through past incidents with members are other important tools for getting sorted. Especially in the short term, it comes down to seeing who the group thinks are (or even should be) the leaders, then trying to involve them in sending messages and leading change as much as possible. So, concentrating attention on these leaders and trying to get and keep them on board with the new direction is a key management function.

Of course, the leaders will not always, or exclusively, be the people nominated as in charge. Getting inside the group dynamic will reveal some 'informal' leaders (cf. the idea of cultural architects explored in Chs 8 and 24) who play a central role in shaping attitude and setting behaviour within the group. These people are not always easy to spot but you might start with senior performers, those with 'central' roles (e.g. playmakers in basketball or setters in volleyball), those with high status and power or those with more successful personal profiles (senior performers, for example). Forming a separate relationship, which doesn't undercut the nominated or formal leader, is another important strand of influence to lead change. Related to these ideas, all members of the PP commented on the importance of 'role models' in promoting coherence down and across the development pathway. Modelling research (e.g. McCullagh & Weiss 2001) tells us that role models are most successful when close enough to be perceived as 'like me'. So SB commented very positively on the strong role model offered to him by Mick Hill, another excellent international javelin thrower two years his senior. Mick's taking SB 'under his wing' on a first international training camp had a strong influence on him. SM had a similar experience on joining the Rambert Dance Company; in fact, such mentoring is an accepted feature of many companies.

Good leaders will structure this strong but usually informal influence, by scheduling practice 'downwards', for example, so younger performers are provided with strong role models as they prepare. This idea is enshrined in traditional martial arts, particularly karate, where students line up and practise in grade order. As a result, those in the back-line, lower-grade ranks are provided with a constant role model of what it should look like. Such simple approaches are often far more effective than the blanket use of expensive and sometimes ego-laden retired performers as formal mentors, although these too can make an excellent contribution if selected correctly and used sensitively (see Ch. 6).

Finally, you might also look for an often separate category of group members, which I have called 'weathercocks'. Often quite distinct from the leadership system, these members offer a particularly sensitive 'group-empathic' or 'group-representative' response to change or current status. In simple terms, keeping an eye on how they are doing will give you a quick insight into the group's moods and confidence in what is currently occurring.

Recognize that each subgroup within your performance team/company/organization may have its own leaders, architects and weathercocks, so keeping your ear to the ground is going to take a lot of listening in multiple stereo surround sound. Be careful, however, that, in listening to all these different tracks, you don't get confused by the cacophony! Indeed, there will be occasions when you need to persist with a direction even though there is strong and vociferous opposition. In such a case, think carefully and concisely through your options and use trusted lieutenants or peers as sounding boards to 'audit' your thinking – in short, get an external check on whether the decision or line taken is a good one. As John demonstrates in Chapter 10, we are notoriously good at fooling ourselves that everything in the garden is rosy and that we are, of course, in the right!

So what should you do?

This chapter and the preceding chapters in this section on Provision demonstrate the complexity of issues that must be considered in the development and leadership of an effective performance system. The need for regular and frequent evaluation and refinement should also be clear from the perspectives offered in Chapter 10. So, with these challenges in mind, I will try to offer a set of simple guidelines and actions, each designed to address a subset of the important factors and considerations.

Ensure the best environment by open, critical and accepted debate

There is general recognition that, notwithstanding the political issues highlighted earlier, the best performance environments are characterized by 'gloves off but nothing personal' debates! As such, a key question is: How does your organization handle and ensure benefit from the 'Zone of Uncomfortable Debate' (ZOUD)?

Note that this characteristic is essential in any group focused on peak performance, whether a few specialists employed on one performer, a professional performance grouping or a multilevel/ multiactivity performance and development organization (see earlier comments on NGBs). Once again, the importance of EI and conflict management skills is obvious, but equal importance must be placed on how the debates are contextualized (timing, location, participants, etc.) and effort should be made to develop a culture where this is expected and accepted (model it and reinforce it). In this regard, SB made an interesting point; if 'performance' is defined up front, and the debate is clearly focused on performance, what is there to be uncomfortable about? This willingness, even eagerness, to overtly consider anything that may help performance is, in my personal opinion, a mark of elites. You might like to refocus attention on this superordinate goal when someone gets 'precious' about well founded and reasonably expressed criticism.

In group settings, especially where all may not be so open-minded, use of performers' panels (not like this one!) drawn from within the group is a good way to test the waters on new ideas and ensure a group input to new direction. A group of representative performers, drawn from different levels in the group, offers a forum for ideas to be sounded out and 'perceived rumblings' of discontent to be clarified. Some care is needed, however, especially in performance domains that are highly individual by nature. In such activities, you are more likely to get an individual slant than a 'representing the group' response. Of course, people will almost always consider their own interests first but gently returning the focus to the aims and benefits of the group will be an important bit of micro leadership when working with the panel. Ensure also that membership of the panel is widely publicized and use of this communication pathway consistently encouraged. Human nature means that most will only concern themselves with

Scientific support offers a lot of data, but this needs to be part of the planning picture rather than the whole story. Thanks to Alan Luke for the photo.

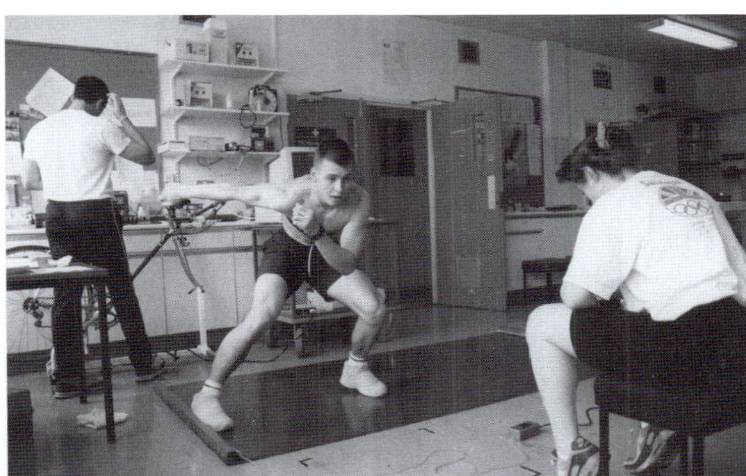

the route when they have a personal gripe, at least until the panel gets recognized and accepted in its 'people's parliament' role. Furthermore, as SM stressed, team members need to accept and enact their own responsibility to express their moans in the correct direction. In short, if you whinge under your breath, ain't nothing gonna change!

Of course, some groups will be small enough, or the issue big enough, that a full team meeting is called for. Start of the season planning meets, addressing a current crisis or setting a new direction are common examples of such meetings. But don't take the meeting as sufficient to determine the group's involvement and buy in. Setting up the meeting through tactical conversations with architects and evaluating responses post-meet with weathercocks are essential parts of ensuring maximum return from this time-consuming but essential activity. Note also the old but well established ideas on polarization. The meeting may well accentuate views in line with pre-existing subtle preferences or tendencies. If this is likely to happen, consider alternatives to sell the idea and get buy-in. One such technique, 'lobbying', has even become a profession, at least in British political circles. The big issue here is the need to be completely aware of the hidden agendas around the table prior to going into the meeting.

Finally, and reflecting the earlier comments about natural groups or families, recognize that this whole strand of communication and debate is often best delegated downwards. More open communication, more honest opinion and more complete buy-in and acceptance are benefits that might accrue. Establishing performance 'units' on this common business approach, the quality circle method, will optimize the benefits of existing structures while pushing through the necessary change to further enhance the system. Be careful to keep the number of such units to a minimum, however. Each one should ideally involve three or more of the existing subgroups; more than one to promote greater integration and natural 'challenge' to existing practice, and more than two to prevent 'us and them'-style standoffs. The main point here is that ZOUD is essential, but unlikely in a group where everyone has established a set hierarchy and way of getting along. Discombobulation (a useful term and a great word for Scrabble!), system perturbation, avoiding the comfort zone or just 'shaking things up'; however you term it, this is an essential part of striving for and maintaining peak performance (as per earlier comments in this chapter).

One final word about the conduct of meetings, especially in team or other performance group environments, which are increasingly recognized as important and used for enhancing performance effectiveness. Unfortunately however, importance and commonality are often not accompanied by the necessary skills. Getting the most from such meetings is a definite skill, which needs to be learned and developed, most effectively with some external coaching or other input. Performance psychology practitioners should be useful resources for such facilitation, so long as they have done the necessary development work themselves.

Concentrate on case conferencing – before, during and after

Getting everyone concerned with a performer or performance group together is often a long-winded operation. Accordingly, many group leaders shy away from this, except as a crisis response measure by which time the fan is firmly clogged! I would see this as a big mistake: not only are such 'problem only' meetings reactive and unlikely to work, they also don't enable you to fully exploit the case conference for wider benefits, such as ensuring the coherence of all the specialists concerned.

Accordingly, case conferences are a good idea; not too often but certainly on an annual basis as a minimum, depending on your performance cycle. Dance companies should, at the very least, conduct a case conference at the start, mid-cycle and towards the end of a dancer's contract. Not just good and caring practice; it may also help to prevent litigation for constructive dismissal. The conference is not a standalone item, however, and its impact will be enhanced by attention to the right priming, meeting conduct and follow-up procedures. To prevent the case conference turning into a talking shop or points scoring exercise, all concerned should be asked to provide upfront a report that focuses on actions and issues in their own discipline, together with what they see as the key issues for the performer, across the disciplines. This cross-disciplinary element is really important, as it prevents negative aspects of the 'silo' culture that is often evident in performance organizations – 'Well, *we* are doing our job, it must be...!' is evidence of such a problem. Managers can prompt this by identifying (backed by objective data) what they think the current hot issues are.

So, for example, case conferences on an individual can be focused by reference to more general challenges; win/loss data, injury records, lack of progress on development programmes or poor reviews. Based on feedback from the different individuals, an agenda can be distributed that addresses the key factors, with unidisciplinary concerns often 'noted at the meeting' but addressed through one-on-ones off-line.

The meeting itself needs to be, or at least to be evolving towards, an 'equal expertise' model. In short, everyone must (and be seen to) bring something performance-relevant to the meet and all must listen with equal regard. This is a big challenge to establish in systems where one specialist is seen (or even practically is) dominant. For example, coaches, choreographers, performance or artistic directors or managers can dominate these meets with generally negative repercussions. It is worth considering the need for criticality and openness as a characteristic of individuals in these lead roles; this idea is covered in more detail in Chapter 15. In the meantime, however, the political and EI skills of the leader will be usefully deployed in increasing, albeit gradually, the balance of such meetings to ensure an open but friendly disagreement wherever necessary.

Finally, the time-linked action points that should result from such a meeting (much better than minutes – for example, 'Dave to establish costed options for our winter training camps and distribute by 1 August') must be seen to be followed through. Methods for keeping this process on track are explored in Chapter 24. In the current context, however, the various feedback channels espoused in this chapter (both formal and informal, overt and semi-covert) should be used to follow up and check on actual and perceived progress with each of the factors identified.

All this is quite labour-intensive, and best achieved by someone who is in constant contact with the training environment. This is the case for smaller or more specialized performance groups, and also represents one of the major advantages for successful units such as rowing or cycling, which was hinted at earlier. Unless the overall leader/director is to suffer 'death by driving' however, larger or more complex groups will require careful but clear delegation. The bottom line is that meetings must be run by someone proximate to but distinct from the support team, with auditing from a separate source either through line management or by an evolved process of peer review (e.g. where the manager for the north shares outputs with the manager from the south, and so on). In fact, peer review offers another good way to disseminate the messages and keep everyone coherent. So long as it is purposeful and on task, it is almost impossible to have too much interaction, so long as there is time for your day job too!

Maximize coherence between different sections of your group

Coherence must be both vertical and horizontal, as shown above. To help you achieve this, I'll consider exemplars of both in a little more detail. The necessity within and outwith the group is for a well articulated and common plan, which all can agree to. Mission statements are a common modern method to satisfy this need. Unfortunately, however, they are frequently just part of the paper chase that accompanies modern structures; something that has to be written (though Lord knows why) but then sits unaddressed on a website or in a filing cabinet until the next strategic upheaval.

If well done, by contrast, the mission statement is an expression of the philosophy and values of the organization (gosh... lapsing into 'management-speak' too, but I genuinely mean this!), which is accompanied by clear operationalizing actions that are goal-focused and keep it both real and practically relevant. Consider some of the examples provided by Pat in Chapter 9. Part of his philosophy was clearly to enhance the 'squad' approach. This mission statement (even if it wasn't formally written down) was disseminated across the organization and made real by a number of actions such as one-on-ones with lower-level performers (ensuring both their own personal motivation and a constant upwards pressure on established players) and a clearly stated and consistently followed rotation policy. Taking this example, you might ask yourself the following questions:

- Can I provide members with a clear statement of the group's philosophy?
  - Does the philosophy consistently guide actions on important issues such as selection, contract renewal and perceived equitable reward of members?
  - Are policies as open as they can be, given the necessary practical, ethical and legal constraints?

 - If so, this enables all to follow a simple but effective 'Do – Test – Move on' check to ensure their actions are on the right track
- Are the philosophy, ways of working and standards expected consistent vertically within the organization?
  - For example, are there clear and public pathways for developing performers to get to the top?
  - Are these provided through an appropriate combination of objective and 'evidenced subjective' measures (see the APPT in Chapter 24)
- Do we have systems that enable group members to articulate and address concerns, of both a personal and group nature?
  - For example, does each performer have a clear 'line manager' who has responsibility for enhancing this individual's performance?
  - Is this 'Performance Manager' the person who can quickly action resources to support the performer?
- Do support teams regularly review and revise each performer's development plans?
  - For example, are there regular case conferences, at least on a small scale?
  - Do systems of reward, review and rehire relate to these?

Not rocket science, I know, but this simple checklist represents where I would start when consulting with a group. You should be able to see how these are addressed by your group and give examples of these in action if your group is firing on all cylinders. In fact, checking these basics, effectively and often, should be seen as a core function in the management of performance environments.

Conclusion

Managing performance environments is a complex and multifaceted job. We have only scratched the surface with this section, but nevertheless have offered some useful direction and immediate checks that can be achieved relatively easily. For support professionals, especially psychologists, this area is obviously a rich vein for performance enhancement. You should not leave this alone but rather, deploying the political acumen and EI inherent in your training (one hopes), gently squeeze the nettle of structures and systems that have a significant and direct impact on the ultimate performance of the group and the individuals you work with. Increasingly open interaction between leader/managers and appropriately qualified and experienced psychologists will bring benefits to your group.

As a final word, and a summary to the ideas in this section, I am grateful to KB for pointing out the PERFORM acronym from Blanchard et al (2006). A summary of the approach is presented in Table 11.1. You might care to use it as a checklist, to check the coherence and contributory structures in your own team.

Happy managing!

Table 11.1 The PERFORM acronym as a checklist for the advice in this chapter

P	Purpose	Team members can articulate, and are committed to, a common purpose
E	Empowerment	Team members feel able to express opinions and take independent action
R	Relationships	Team members engage in, and act on, Zone of Uncomfortable Debate conversations
F	Flexibility	Team members are open and adaptable to new ideas
O	Output	The team are performing, as measured against the upfront definition of performance
R	Recognition/reward	Team members feel that their contributions are recognized and rewarded appropriately
M	Morale	Team members feel good about membership – we feel we are getting somewhere and we are enthusiastic about the journey

Source: based on Blanchard et al 2006

References

Blanchard, K., Carew, D., Parisi-Carew, E., 2006. One minute manager builds high performance teams, Harper-Collins, London.

Butcher, D., Clarke, M., 2001. Smart management, Palgrave, Basingstoke, Hampshire.

Butcher, D., Clarke, M., 2008. Politics and worthy management agendas. Management Online Review, August. Available on line at: www.morexpertise.com

Clarke, M., Meldrum, M., 1999. Creating change from below: early lessons for agents of change. Leadership and Organization Development Journal 20, 70–82.

McCullagh, P., Weiss, M.R., 2001. Modelling: considerations for motor skill performance and psychological responses. In: Singer, R.N., Hausenblaus, H.A., Janelle, C.M. (Eds.), Handbook of sport psychology, second ed. John Wiley, New York, pp. 205–238.

Section 3

Practice

Introduction: practice regimens for excellence

12

Dave Collins

Grey Matters/UCLan

The contents of this next section are crucial for the design and implementation of an effective performance support system. Given this importance, it is very surprising that, to date at any rate, skill acquisition and control aspects have been a neglected part of the performance psychologists' armoury.

In Chapter 13, Chris Button, Clare MacMahon and Rich Masters look at the control of movement. Understanding the mechanisms of control and why they break down under pressure is fundamental, as this is the primary way in which pressure acts to limit performance. Chris, Clare and Rich also explore some ways in which these breakdowns can be countered. This theme is continued in Chapter 14 by Joan Vickers, who looks at the ways in which practice environments can be tweaked to optimize them. Her suggestions are eminently practical and backed by a thorough consideration of relevant research... just what this book is about.

In the next chapter, Andy Abraham (with some input from me) considers the second most crucial feature of the performance practice environment, the coach. The messages here draw from many of the same principles used by Joan, so it is unsurprising that, nomenclature apart, readers should get a double dose of how learning environments and coaching practice may be enhanced. The repetition is merited, however. Despite the strong base for the guidelines offered in these chapters, the methods espoused are hardly common; in fact, many coaches of quite advanced status would not recognize some of the terminology. As such, these guidelines represent a 'goldmine' for all concerned in performance coaching.

Chapter 16 looks at arguably the most important tool in the performer's armoury: mental practice. Paul Holmes and Clare Camels offer a new integrated approach to this key mental skill, taking it forwards through application of the neurologically 'close cousin' construct of observation. Once again, the practical implications of their ideas are considerable.

Duncan Mascarenhas and Nick Smith cover the cognitive aspects of practice in Chapter 17. There are a lot of ideas here with wide implications. For example, decision making is not only important for games players but also impacts on the total performance process through a wide variety of processes including performer planning, coaching, selection and refereeing. As such, this chapter has implications for all the physical domains, albeit more on the support than the doing front for some of them.

Finally, the PP chapter considers the implications and applications of these ideas when designing and managing your performance environment.

DOI: 10.1016/B978-0-443-06734-1.00012-2

'Keeping it together': motor control under pressure

13

Chris Button* Clare MacMahon[†] Rich Masters[‡]

*School of Physical Education, University of Otago, Dunedin, New Zealand; [†]School of Sport and Exercise Science, and Institute of Sport, Exercise and Active Living (ISEAL), Victoria University, Melbourne, Australia; [‡]Institute of Human Performance, The University of Hong Kong, Hong Kong, China

CHAPTER CONTENTS

Introduction

Performers must learn to coordinate their actions in pressured situations to achieve success. In comparing themselves to equally talented but less successful performers, elites often cite their ability to perform under pressure as the key distinguishing factor. At all levels of performance, maintaining effective skill execution when placed under pressure is undoubtedly a desirable attribute. Pressure manifests itself in many different forms and across different timescales. For example, common sports tasks such as passing a ball or participating in a race present pressure in the form of rapidly changing spatial and temporal demands to be satisfied within the performance environment. Performing in the presence of spectators can also introduce varying levels of pressure in terms of meeting social expectations. Furthermore, success can yield a multitude of rewards in the form of recognition, prize money, travel, etc. It has been acknowledged in a number of chapters in this book that perceived pressure can lead to decreased performance. Therefore, an important question for this book and this chapter concerns how performers learn to deal with these different sources of pressure when preparing for an event, whether a competition or a performance before an audience. The way in which coaches design and structure practice has a strong influence upon a performer's ability to move effectively and to cope with these inevitable pressures. So what can coaches do during practice to develop mentally resilient performers whose technique will not wilt under pressure?

This chapter reviews key research findings from the sport psychology and motor learning literature in order to address some of the questions posed above. We begin by providing a brief overview of some of the key principles of skill acquisition and the theoretical influences responsible for their emergence. We then discuss motor control and learning in relation to the influence of anxiety on coordination and performance stability. In the second half of the chapter we describe how the cognitive processes used during practice can influence learning effectiveness. Finally, we concentrate on a number of learning strategies that coaches may consider when planning practice activities.

DOI: 10.1016/B978-0-443-06734-1.00013-4

How the control of movement changes as we learn skills

The process of skill acquisition is distinct from the process of skill execution (i.e. motor control) in that skill acquisition is a gradual process that occurs over many performance attempts, resulting in behaviour that is less vulnerable to transitory factors such as fatigue, audience effects and anxiety. However, as we shall explain later in this chapter, this does not imply that temporary factors, such as performance anxiety, do not influence the learning process at all. Motor skill acquisition has traditionally been described as the 'changes in internal processes that determine an individual's capability for producing a motor task' (Schmidt & Wrisberg 2004, p. 12). Broadly speaking, for learners, skill acquisition involves gaining an understanding of the performance goal, engaging appropriate sets of muscle groups at the right times to move the body, and modifying action on the basis of feedback.

Researchers have grappled with understanding how humans learn to perform motor skills for over 100 years, and different theories have evolved. While it is beyond the scope of this chapter to explain each theory (for historical overviews see Davids et al 2007 or Summers 2004), it is useful to be aware of the two dominant theoretical approaches that currently coexist, i.e. the cognitive and ecological approaches. The cognitive approach regards the brain as the central organ underpinning movement organization. Cognitive psychologists suggest that the brain plays a crucial role in perceiving information from the world and using such representations to construct and release sophisticated motor programmes to bring about movement (e.g. Willingham 1998). From a quite different perspective, ecological psychologists prefer to consider human movement as the result of dynamic, self-organization processes in which coordination results from the confluence of task, individual and environmental constraints (Chow et al 2006). This approach has led to the belief that humans have evolved 'intelligent' sensory systems that can be used to directly couple environmental information on to action possibilities with only limited input required from conscious brain processing (Gibson 1979). While each approach has its own strengths and weaknesses (Summers 2004), there is no debate about the importance of using a theoretical model to explain motor behaviour and the relative contributions of the cognitive and ecological approaches to the study of motor learning should become apparent as we proceed through the chapter.

It is important to consider how the control of movement changes as we learn a motor skill, as a number of unseen, inter-related processes are happening inside the learner. One can begin to understand more about these processes by considering how they are manifested at the behavioural level in different stages of learning (Fitts & Posner 1967). Initially, learners' movements are often slow, discontinuous, inefficient and riddled with errors (just watch a novice trying to juggle!). It is also very obvious that novice performers need to concentrate very hard to achieve a performance goal. This is perhaps not surprising, as initial learning of action sequences predominantly relies upon the creation of new neural pathways within areas of the brain's motor cortex that are largely under conscious control (Kennedy 1990). Trial and error processes dominate the learner's initial attempts to perform a skill, leading to the gradual repetition of a functional movement pattern, which in turn causes certain neural connections to become strengthened or reinforced in favour of others (Sporns & Edelman 1993). Luckily for the learner, considerable performance gains can occur quickly once a fledgling coordination pattern is discovered.

Bernstein (1967) recognized that early learners typically restrict the movement of many joints of the body to exert control over their limbs (although recent research has questioned the generality of this observation to a number of tasks, e.g. Chen et al 2005, Chow et al 2006). In practical terms, this often means that early learners move in an awkward and uneconomic manner while striving to satisfy a task goal. Interestingly, some similarities have been observed in the coordination characteristics of early learners and more skilled performers in high-pressure situations, which we shall return to later in the chapter. One might ask what advantage early learners gain from 'freezing' joint coordination in this way. It has been argued that such a control strategy relieves the processing burden upon learners of simultaneously regulating all their available biomechanical degrees of freedom at once (Vereijken et al 1992).

As a skill is learnt, the responsibility for moment-to-moment movement control is thought to pass deeper into subconscious regions of the brain stem, the spinal cord, and local muscular feedback loops (Badgaiyan 2000, Manoonpong et al 2007). As depicted in Figure 13.1 the gradual delegation of motor control to lower levels frees up the conscious brain for other activities that may be important for performers, such

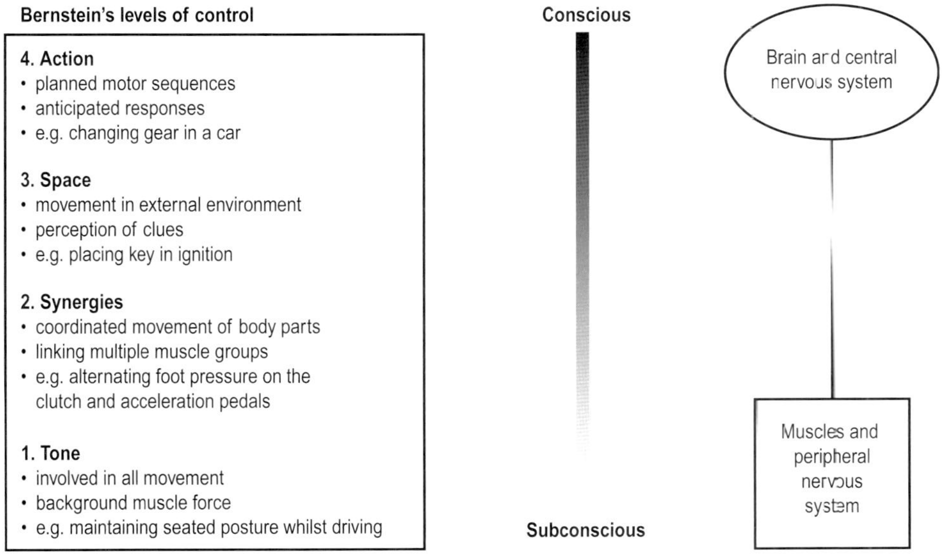

Fig. 13.1 • Simplified diagram depicting different levels of human movement control. Adapted from Bernstein 1967.

as anticipation and planning (Abernethy et al 2007). Accordingly, the next challenge for learners is to identify important sources of environmental information that allow their coordination to be modified and improved even further.

With practice, 'intermediate learners' typically become more selective over which joints need to be actively controlled, thereby permitting a smoother, more efficient action (e.g. Chen et al 2005). Achieving good coordination involves establishing a close relationship or fit between the way that our limbs move and the specific environmental circumstances in which we perform. Intermediate learners have started to identify the key sources of information that are used to guide their actions (e.g. visual feedback from an approaching ball or a canoeist's location on a rapid). By becoming more attuned to these perceptual cues and ignoring irrelevant information, learners become able to adapt their movement patterns to each unique situation in which they find themselves.

An insight into how attentional processes change as a function of learning is provided through research measuring differences in visual scanning behaviours in performers at different skill levels (e.g. Land & McLeod 2000). For example, experienced performers typically show less erratic scan-paths with longer fixations on critical cues than their less experienced counterparts (for an example in ice-hockey, see Martell & Vickers 2004). It seems that performers learn to identify anticipatory information from the behaviour of opponents, team-mates, their own movement and other relevant cues that can be used to attune the most appropriate responses at the right times.

Advanced or skilled performers have typically participated in large amounts of practice and consequently are able to freely adapt their movement patterns to a wide range of situations. The control of a skilled performer's movement has become seemingly automatic, manifested by the ability to share attentional resources and perform multiple tasks simultaneously. Movement patterns are more fluid and draw upon surrounding energy flows in the environment to enhance their effectiveness (e.g. consider a skilled tennis player using the speed of a fast serve to play an effective return). Skilled performers achieve outcome goals to a high standard very consistently and, of particular relevance to this chapter, they have an ability to focus and ignore distractions. Under pressure, while climbing a high-grade route, for example, experienced climbers seem to have more time and control; in short, to be less 'hassled' than their less experienced peers. However, while the movement patterns of an expert may at times seem very similar, recent research is revealing that even expert performers display variability from one performance to the next (e.g. Chow et al 2006). As Bernstein (1967) acknowledged, variability of movement patterns is a necessary byproduct of skilled performance. The key for most athletes is being able to use movement variability to their advantage in a functional manner (Davids et al 2007).

Skill development models, such as the one proposed by Fitts & Posner (1967), reveal that learners generally progress through different behavioural stages, which allows us to make inferences about the processes that underlie skill acquisition. A series of levels of control has been suggested in which learners initially consciously process motor control for new or novel motor skills (Bernstein 1967). With practice, the responsibility for control of movement is relegated to subconscious levels of the central nervous system, which frees up attentional resources for other tasks. Indeed as learning progresses, humans become better at identifying and using relevant sources of environmental information, thus benefiting from improved performance. While the findings of development models such as these are of interest, it is still not clear how anxiety can bring about changes to performance during skill execution, which is where we turn our attention in the next section.

Anxiety and skill execution

A considerable amount of research effort has been invested in understanding the relationship between anxiety and skilled performance (for an overview see Beilock & Gray 2007). For example, Chung et al (2005) wanted to verify whether increased anxiety actually leads to a decline in performance among early learners. A group of trainee army rifle-shooters had their performance assessed and completed questionnaires probing their affective feelings of worry and anxiety. The commonly employed CSAI-2 inventory (Martens et al 1990) was used to identify cognitive and somatic anxiety among the trainees. It was shown that affective measures such as state worry accounted for a significant amount of the variance in shooting performance levels. While the statistical analysis was only correlational and therefore can not be used to indicate causality, the study seems to indicate that worrying too much about skill execution can interfere with performance among early learners.

As this field of research has progressed, a number of increasingly sophisticated performance models have acknowledged the multidimensional and non-linear nature of the anxiety–performance relationship (Eysenck & Calvo 1992, Hardy 1996). For example, relatively small increases in perceived anxiety may initially result in gradual improvements in performance, but at certain transitional phases small changes in anxiety can lead to 'catastrophic' performance drops. Furthermore, anxiety-performance profiles can differ considerably depending on the individual's trait and state predispositions towards anxiety-inducing conditions. Such modelling is helping to improve our understanding of common phenomena such as 'choking' during sports performance. However, as Higuchi et al (2002) point out, surprisingly little attention has been directed to the question of how anxiety affects the movement features of skill execution. Such information could throw more light upon how athletes can learn to cope with pressured situations.

One of the few studies that has considered how anxiety impacts upon movement execution was conducted by van Gemmett & van Galen (1997), who examined coordination during writing and aiming tasks performed under moderate levels of stress. They proposed a model of stress in which physical and cognitive stressors were suggested to increase the level of 'neuromotor noise' present in the information-processing system. A series of studies were performed in which cognitive stress was introduced by having participants perform a secondary, arithmetic task, and physical stress involved exposure to a loud auditory stimulus (up to 95 dB). Interestingly, both positive and negative effects of the different types of stress were found. High levels of either cognitive or physical stress resulted in unnecessary increases in the pressure exerted by the participants on the writing implement. This reduction in movement economy was attributed to the introduction of neuromotor noise creating below-optimal values of the perceptual threshold at which participants can distinguish signal from noise. In terms of timing, the physical stress actually improved reaction time but the cognitive stress resulted in delayed responses. For easier writing tasks, stress resulted in quicker overall movement times; however, for difficult aiming tasks longer movement times were found in the high-stress conditions. While the levels of actual stress experienced by the subjects were not verified in the study, these preliminary findings showed that there are differential outcomes of increased anxiety depending on both the task undertaken, and the nature of the stressor.

Recently, Higuchi et al (2002) verified some of the movement responses to anxiety shown by van Gemmett & van Galen (1997). These authors manipulated perceived stress during a computer-simulated baseball batting task by 'punishing' poor performance with mild electrical shock treatment. When participants were worried about receiving a shock they exhibited delayed movement initiation, smaller movement amplitudes and a trend towards lower trajectory variability across trials. Interestingly, these findings were similar to those found in the task when high accuracy demands were imposed. The authors argue that psychological stress induces the production of more constrained movement patterns even when task difficulty changes. A number of explanations for the effect were suggested, including increased reflex activities (such as coupled body and eye movements, e.g. the vestibulo-ocular reflex), impaired working memory and a shift in attentional bias towards threatening information.

Court et al (2005) used a stressor common to sports performers by introducing an evaluative audience to induce moderate anxiety levels in subjects performing a two-handed coordination task. Previous research has shown that two stable coordination patterns typically exist for such tasks (where the hands move symmetrically or in a synchronous fashion) and that spontaneous transitions from symmetrical to synchronous movements can occur as movement frequency is increased. While the overall structure and quality of the movement pattern was not significantly altered by the elevated anxiety levels, it was shown that the 'natural' transition to synchronous coordination was delayed (i.e. occurred at a higher movement frequency). The authors interpreted this finding as evidence that additional attentional resources are recruited during anxious situations, which, in this case, led to enhanced stability of movement. In tennis, a similar effect might be observed for a player who prefers a certain type of shot (e.g. two-handed backhand) and typically relies most heavily upon this coordination pattern during crucial points. In other words, participants can actually benefit from experiencing moderate levels of anxiety through enhanced task-related focus of attention. This suggestion also fits well with 'processing efficiency theory' (Eysenck & Calvo 1992), where it is acknowledged that worry can motivate performers to produce extra on-task effort with either positive or negative consequences.

Summarizing so far, it is known that moderate to high levels of anxiety may be accompanied by movements that are less smooth, less efficient in terms of time and energy, and less variable (see also Beuter & Duda 1985). However, in the research described thus far, the ecological validity in relation to sports performance was typically low, hence one might question the generality of the findings. Collins et al (2001) addressed this concern by examining 'real world behaviour' in anxiety-inducing conditions. In one study, soldiers were asked to complete a stepping task along a narrow bar at ground level and at a height of 20 m. The results showed that the same task performed at height typically produced elevated levels of anxiety and it took longer to cross the bar. Furthermore, when anxious, the soldiers exhibited reduced variability, as indexed by increased joint coupling, although they did not later report any awareness of changing their action. One can think of several similar situations in everyday life such as walking over icy ground or when carrying a heavy object down a flight of steps, in which our stepping rate and length decreases in response to the increased risk of falling.

In a second study, Collins et al (2001) compared the coordination of elite weightlifters performing snatch lifts in training and competition conditions. Once more, the cognitive and somatic anxiety induced by competition was also associated with alterations in the lifters' techniques. Interestingly in this case, the more experienced elite performers reported being aware of the modifications, suggesting that they were consciously mediated to help enhance performance. Each study reported considerable individual differences in the degree of kinematic responses. This finding highlights how individual characteristics, such as previous experience, task expertise and self-confidence, can mediate the anxiety response.

Pijpers et al (2003) extended one of the studies of Collins and colleagues (2001) by asking experienced climbers to negotiate a traverse in low anxiety-inducing (near to the ground) and high anxiety-inducing (far from the ground) conditions. It was expected that the high-anxiety climb would lead to performance and movement execution decrements similar to some of the typical coordination characteristics associated with early learners (see above). In the high-anxiety climb, subjects reported feeling more anxious and had higher heart rates (22 beats per minute higher than low-anxiety climb) and increased muscular fatigue (indicative of higher muscle tension). Interestingly, Pijpers et al (2003) also assessed movement time and relative fluency by calculating the amount of variation (or entropy) of each climber's centre of gravity.

As expected, movement time was longer, and hence climbing performance was poorer, in the high-anxiety climbs. Also, movement entropy was increased, indicating less trajectory smoothness (partly attributable to more explorative hand and foot movements) over a reduced solution space. Therefore, the data confirmed that when experienced performers are anxious they exhibit some of the behavioural features one might expect of early learners. An interesting addition to previous work is that increased movement anxiety in certain real-world tasks can lead to the performer using more exploratory, variable behaviour. It is likely that the appearance of this behavioural feature is strongly related to its functionality within the task. For example, the climbing wall (Pijpers et al 2003) provides enhanced opportunity to explore alternative movement solutions in comparison to the stepping task (Collins et al 2001) and therefore more degeneracy within the available task constraints.

In summary, anxiety appears to influence coordination in a number of different ways and its influence is also mediated by several key factors. Skill execution of highly anxious performers may become less fluent and less efficient and, in some cases, coordination may regress back to some of the characteristics first associated with learning the skill. Performers typically apply more on-task effort when anxious, as a consequence of redirecting attentional focus toward the accomplishment of the goal. As we shall discover in the next section, an important implication for practitioners is that performers can benefit from an increase in perceived anxiety (e.g. moving from training to competitive environments) by clarifying where their attention should be allocated.

While anxiety can act as a powerful constraint on coordination, the degree of its influence depends on the previous experiences of the performer, their ability to cope and maintain focus and, importantly, the nature of the task itself. For example, where the task permits it, performers can learn to modify their actions when anxious in a positive, functional manner by exploring alternative coordination solutions, as shown previously in rock-climbing. In highly constrained tasks, such as weightlifting or the 100 m sprint, which have relatively less tolerance for movement variability, performers may exhibit a reduction in moment-to-moment adaptation. In the following section we explain why such characteristics can occasionally have devastating effects for high-performance athletes.

'Keeping it together': attentional focus

It is clear so far that, as performers learn movement skills, they also must develop the ability to deal with pressure and anxiety. When a skill that is normally performed at a high level breaks down under pressure, we say that the performer has 'choked'. One of the first places to begin, before discussing methods or strategies for dealing with choking, is with an understanding of what it is about pressure and anxiety that seems to result in the loss of automated movement control. The previous section pointed to attentional focus as a potential mechanism for the impact of anxiety and pressure on performance. Furthermore, a breakdown of the temporal patterns (or rhythm) underlying movement may explain some of the behavioural characteristics described above (MacPherson et al 2009). In the second half of this chapter, we will review these concepts and discuss some of the implications for skill training.

Deautomatization of movement: reinvestment theory

Masters (1992) elucidated a hypothesis, based on work by Baumeister (1984) and many others (e.g. Boder 1935, Deikman 1969, Fitts & Posner 1967), in order to explain skill failures under pressure conditions. Masters argued that performers, be they surgeons, athletes or musicians, can suffer from disrupted performance under pressure, as a consequence of directing their attention mainly to how to execute the individual components of the skill. A surgeon who reflects upon the survival chances of a patient, or a tennis player who reflects on the prospect of losing a first round match, may attempt to ensure the quality of his or her movements by consciously monitoring and controlling the movements on-line, as it were. Reinvestment theory (Masters 1992, Masters et al 1993, Masters & Maxwell 2008, Maxwell et al 2006) or the conscious processing hypothesis, as it has been called (Hardy et al 1996), suggests that, under psychological pressure to perform well, performers can over-reflect specifically on the biomechanical aspects of their movements, which causes 'deautomaticity' or disruption of the normally automatic, on-line control of those movements (Fig. 13.1). Deikman (1969,

p. 31) described 'deautomatization' as the 'undoing of automatization, presumably by reinvesting actions and percepts with attention'.

Masters et al (1993) proposed that reinvestment is a relatively stable characteristic of personality. They developed a 20-item Reinvestment Scale to test this idea, and showed that high scores on the scale are associated with disrupted motor performance under conditions of anxiety. Squash and tennis players, for example, who were rated by their coach as likely to 'choke under pressure' possessed higher reinvestment scores than those rated unlikely to choke ($r = 0.64$, $p < 0.01$). Other research has also shown this association (e.g. Jackson et al 2006, Maxwell et al 2006). Further support for the concept of reinvestment is available in a variety of recent research findings. For example, Gray (2004) showed that, during slumps in performance, skilled baseball hitters were better at performing a secondary task that required them to make a judgment about the whereabouts of the bat when a tone sounded than they were during hot streaks in their performance. An implication of this finding is that anxiety brought about by the slump in performance caused certain batters to direct their attention towards the mechanics of their movements, which improved their awareness of the whereabouts of the bat when the tone sounded. It seems that how learners allocate their attention during skill acquisition has a profound effect on their ability to avoid skill failures under pressure.

Shifting attentional focus

William James (1890, p 403) famously described attention as 'the taking possession by the mind, in clear and vivid form, of one out of what seem several simultaneously possible objects or trains of thought... [implying] withdrawal from some things in order to deal effectively with others'. This description applies very much to sport, where attention is generally considered to be a process of becoming aware of a stimulus array and processing only selected information from that array (Abernethy et al 2007). For example, a point guard may become aware that an open (unguarded) team mate is a good option for a pass while ignoring the photographer at the back of the court, or a rugby player may focus only on catching a ball even as the opposition forwards approach en masse.

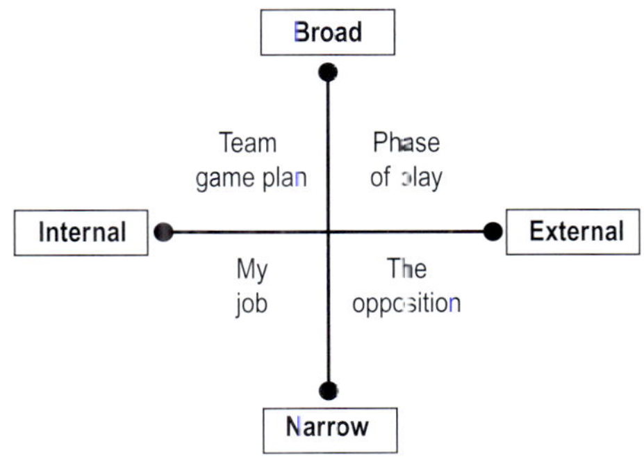

Fig. 13.2 • Dimensions of attentional focus. Adapted from Nideffer 1976.

The classic work of Nideffer (1976) defines four different types of attentional focus, based on dimensions of width (broad, narrow) and direction (internal, external) (Fig. 13.2). A *broad external* focus of attention is used to assess the environment, such as when an ice hockey 'point man' on a power play assesses the positions of offensive and defensive players. A *broad internal* focus of attention is used to analyse and plan, like when a quarterback thinks about the defensive formations in relation to choosing the next play. A *narrow external* focus is typical in the case of a penalty shot on goal in soccer – for both the shooter and the goalie. In this case, both players are focusing on a limited number of cues. And finally, a *narrow internal* focus of attention is used to rehearse upcoming performances or focus on the self, such as imagining an upcoming jump ball in basketball, or thinking about your level of fatigue in a game.

Clearly, different types of attentional focus are suited to different tasks. Indeed, a key mental skill of top athletes is attentional control: the ability to switch focus to suit needs. Recent approaches, however, have been concerned with the way in which attention and attentional needs change as we learn a skill. Wulf and colleagues (e.g. Wulf et al 1998, Wulf et al 1999), for example, have argued that paying attention to the effects of a movement or skill generally improves learning. Wulf et al (1998) tested participants learning to balance on a ski simulator. In an internal focus of attention, the learners were instructed to concentrate on their movements by focusing on the force exerted by their feet. In an external focus of attention, the learners concentrated on the effects of their movements, or the apparatus, by focusing on the wheels of the apparatus. The external focus of attention on the wheels of the platform, or the effects of the movement, showed superior learning. The focus of attention effects have also been replicated for a number of field-like conditions such as learning the golf pitch shot (Wulf et al 1999) and a basketball free-throw shot (Zachry et al 2005).

In search of an explanation for these findings, Wulf et al (2001) proposed the constrained action hypothesis. This hypothesis reframes 'reinvestment theory' by proposing that an internal focus of attention on movements (rather than their effects) interferes with automated processes such as balance, which typically do not require control. This interference effect was expected for both novel and well-learned skills, and was supported by the results of tests of dynamic and static balance by Wulf et al (2003). Clearly, the constrained action hypothesis would also predict many of the effects of anxiety on movement execution discussed above.

The attentional focus effect is moderated by skill level

A natural conclusion emerging from the work of Wulf and colleagues might be to promote an external focus of attention by all performers as they practise and execute skills. However, in reality this statement seems a little over-simplified. Work by Beilock et al (2002) has shown that the impact of attentional focus is moderated by skill level. This was shown in two ways using a task in which participants were asked to dribble a soccer ball through a course as quickly as possible. First, experienced soccer players performed better when they were asked to simultaneously perform a word monitoring task (extraneous focus) than when they were asked to indicate which foot had last touched the ball in response to a tone (skill focus). On the other hand, the opposite pattern was found for novice soccer dribblers, who performed better in the skill-focus than in the extraneous focus condition. Second, testing both the dominant and non-dominant foot showed that, although experienced soccer players performed better overall, performance using the non-dominant foot was disrupted by the extraneous focus and facilitated by the skill focus, showing a pattern similar to that found in novices. In other work, Perkins-Ceccato et al (2003) showed that performance of a pitch shot in golf was better for skilled golfers who employed an external focus of attention, but for unskilled golfers performance was better if an internal focus was employed.

Ford et al (2005) attempted to manipulate the relevance of the skill focus that is used. Expert and novice soccer players dribbled a soccer ball through cones in one control condition and three experimental conditions. In a relevant internal skill focus, participants paid attention to their foot by indicating which side (inside, outside) had touched the ball in response to a tone. In an irrelevant internal skill focus, participants paid attention to their arm by indicating which arm was closest to a pylon in response to a tone. Finally, in an extraneous focus condition, participants dribbled while listening for target words on an audio tape. Experts were disrupted in both the relevant (foot) and irrelevant (arm) skill focus conditions but not in the extraneous (word monitoring) condition. On the other hand, novices were disrupted by the extraneous focus and the irrelevant skill focus (arm) conditions but not by the relevant skill focus condition.

Clearly, the direction in which attention is focused has an impact on learning and performance and may explain why some experienced performers can choke under pressure. Once a skill has been developed to a high level of proficiency, performance is best left to run off automatically without attention to the component parts of the skill, but in the furnace that is high-performance sport it is not easy to avoid paying attention to the skill. Even Freud (1922, p. 23) referred to this: 'many acts are most successfully carried out when they are not the object of particularly concentrated attention... mistakes may occur just on (those) occasions when one is most eager to be accurate'.

It seems likely that those who do not fully trust their capability to perform optimally in stressful situations are particularly susceptible to reinvestment (Moore & Stevenson 1991). Indeed, as previously discussed, the concept of reinvestment implies that some performers are predisposed to think about the control of movement when highly anxious, which can lead to deautomaticity and possibly to 'choking'. Fortunately for such performers, there are cognitive strategies that both prevent inappropriate thoughts and promote effective movement, as we shall discover in the next section.

Practical strategies to prevent deautomatization of movement

In the previous section of this chapter it was acknowledged that skill failures under pressure often occur as a consequence of an inappropriate attentional focus or destructive thoughts that lead to deautomatization of movement. However, this is not to imply that any thinking or self-reflection during skill execution is necessarily harmful. For example, it is known that a significant advantage that distinguishes expert from less able performers is their ability to act upon the large base of 'explicit' knowledge they have collected over many years of practice (e.g. Bennett 2000). Indeed, this extensive knowledge base is arguably very important as it underpins advanced skills (such as anticipation, planning, strategizing and decision-making), so clearly attention can at times be allocated internally to benefit performance. The key message seems to be that performers should try to avoid harmful thoughts that interfere with motor control; however, cognitive reflection at certain times is beneficial (indeed vital) for skilled performance.

So how can performers avoid unwanted thoughts when they get anxious? Wegner and colleagues (Wegner & Erskine 2003, Wegner & Schneider 2003) have demonstrated that simply trying not to think consciously about a particular topic (such as one's movements) causes an 'ironic' rebound effect where one unwittingly produces an action that is the exact opposite of the one intended (e.g. trying not to overshoot the hole in a golf putting task). During the ironic rebound effect, explicit processing is used to monitor the suppression but implicit processes continue to act upon information associated with the topic. In fact, Wegner and his colleagues argue that there are only a limited number of methods by which to avoid unwanted thoughts: (1) process information that is more emotionally attention-grabbing than the thoughts to be avoided or (2) process distracting tasks such as riddles or arithmetic. However, both of these techniques make substantial demands of working memory (Boyer & Lienard 2006) and are likely to disrupt performance as much as directing attention internally (reinvestment). In this section we discuss three training alternatives that appear promising, focusing primarily on techniques relating to implicit motor learning (see Jackson & Beilock 2008 for discussion of further techniques and MacPherson et al 2009 for a consideration of relevant causative processes).

Pre-performance routines

One option for performers is to employ pre-performance routines (see Chs 22 and 23) in a highly ritualized manner. Skilled performers in sports such as tennis, golf and basketball demonstrate highly consistent and individual-specific behavioural routines prior to significant moments, such as serving at match point, in their respective sports. Boyer & Lienard (2006) argue that stereotypical, rigid, repetitive rituals have evolved in humans as part of a 'hazard precaution system' that, when activated by stress, promotes per-formance of 'correct' actions from the repertoire of rituals available. Using the terminology of Boyer & Lienard, focusing on ritualized behaviours might temporarily swamp working memory, causing a moderately efficient form of thought-suppression. If ritualized behaviours are incorporated into a pre-performance routine, effective motor behaviour, without cognitive interference, can occur (Jackson & Masters 2006). Furthermore, it is possible that pre-performance routines can act as a form of rhythmical guide that primes the movement system into producing well practised sequences of action (MacPherson et al 2009). This idea is intuitively appealing, as the phenomenon of choking is commonly associated with a breakdown of the temporal sequencing (or rhythmicity) of an action.

Focusing more specifically on training the performer's focus of attention, Singer et al (1993) proposed a five-step routine to perform self-paced skills such as the basketball free throw or golf shots. Consistent with the research outlined in this book, the strategy includes an instruction to focus, with effort, on an external cue. Interestingly, in this study Singer et al (1993) demonstrated that learners could be taught to adopt the attentional strategies frequently reported by experts, and outperformed a group who were instructed to focus on their body movements.

Cognitive strategies to prevent reinvestment

A second alternative is to reduce the predisposition to interfere with the control of action. For example, Marnassis & Doganis (2004) used a season-long intervention to train a group of young tennis players in cognitive strategies that discouraged them from reinvesting, including positive thinking, concentration, imagery and arousal regulation. The intervention group showed improved performance and better self-confidence at the end of the season in comparison to a group with similar skill levels who received no mental training. Another strategy designed to reduce the tendency to think too much is to try to gradually familiarize (or 'acclimatize') the performer to potential triggers of this process (Lewis & Linder 1997). For example, if a dancer typically becomes overanxious in the final moments before their entrance on stage, an instructor could include and potentially modify this period of time in the dancer's normal practice routine. A practice activity such as this will encourage the dancer to develop effective coping strategies at the time when pre-performance anxieties are peaking.

Although little research currently exists to support the strategy, many performers report that using temporally structured cue-words can facilitate the timing of their actions. For example, a golfer may say to themselves '1–2–3' to correspond with the set-up (1), the end of the backswing (2), and ball-contact (3) (another pertinent example would be Gallwey's (1986) simple 'bounce-hit' cue in tennis). Arguably, attending to the sequence and timing of the cue-words prevents reinvestment by the performer, which may explain the potential training benefits to be gained with self-paced skills. Further research concerning practical strategies to enhance rhythm and timing in movement production is required (MacPherson et al 2009).

Implicit motor learning

A third and perhaps innovative alternative is to learn the skill to be performed under pressure without explicit verbal awareness of the knowledge structures that underlie and support the skill. Considerable evidence now counsels against practice strategies that focus on the accumulation of explicit knowledge during motor skill learning (e.g. Bayley et al 2005, Hardy et al 1996, Hodges & Lee 1999, Masters 1992, Maxwell et al 2000, Maxwell et al 2003, Mullen et al 2007, Poolton et al 2004, Wulf & Weigelt 1997). A large body of research demonstrates that 'we' can acquire implicit knowledge of abstract underlying rules of a task without 'consciously' being aware of what we have learned (e.g. Stadler & Frensch 1998). The research shows that these unconscious processes are faster and supported by more structurally sophisticated mechanisms than consciously controlled processes and tend to exhibit resilience 'in the face of disorders and dysfunctions that compromise explicit knowledge' (Reber 1993, p. 88).

Masters (1992) showed that practising a golf putting task in conjunction with a secondary task, in this case random letter generation (Baddeley 1966), resulted in improved putting skill but little or no describable knowledge of how each putt was executed (implicit motor learning). The secondary task was employed specifically to distract working memory so that the learners would be less aware consciously of how they were carrying out the putting task. The findings also showed that putting performance remained robust under psychological stress when compared to the performance of those who had learned explicitly. Masters argued that the implicit motor learners were less able to 'reinvest' under pressure because they had less conscious knowledge to reinvest. Interestingly, recent studies suggest that implicit motor learning may even result in stable performance under physiological stress (Masters et al 2008, Poolton et al 2007).

Masters and colleagues (2008) argue that implicit motor learning should take place in an environment that discourages conscious hypothesis-testing behaviour, on the grounds that explicit knowledge accumulates as a consequence of the testing of hypotheses. That is, each time a performer tries something different, they will retain in memory a recollection of what to do or what not to do. As all golfers know, to try consciously to 'not move the head when teeing off' is not wise, especially on the first hole, which is usually positioned for the viewing pleasure of the members in the clubhouse.

While it may not be possible (or practical) to constrain the skill-learning environment to provide an uninterrupted implicit motor-learning experience, techniques have been developed that help to dissuade the learner from testing hypotheses. Maxwell et al (2001), for example, showed that, in an environment that reduces the likelihood of performance errors, learners are unlikely to test hypotheses or become acutely conscious of the way in which they are carrying out the skill because the lack of errors implies that performance is satisfactory (motivation to change a movement that is already effective is likely to be considerably less than to change a movement accompanied by many errors). A number of studies have now confirmed that a relatively error-free performance environment can lead to learning that is implicit and unaccompanied by verbal knowledge (Masters & Maxwell 2004, Poolton et al 2005). One interesting finding to come out of these studies is that, as long as performance is error free in the initial stages of practice, the performance advantages of implicit learning are not lost if verbal knowledge is later acquired. Poolton et al (2005) specifically confirmed the presence of this phenomenon in a brief initial period of errorless learning in golf putting (as few as 150 trials carried out from distances ranging between 25 cm and 75 cm), and concluded that an initial period of errorless learning may be enough to lock the learner into a mode of motor control that is disassociated from explicit control of movement. This speculation has its merits, given that, as we mentioned earlier, it is early in the discovery of coordination patterns that most of the neural pathways for movement are laid down (Sporns & Edelman 1993).

The concept of error-free learning should not be taken to imply that the learner be required to produce repetitive drills to avoid errors completely (e.g. play forehands from the same place on the court on each attempt) as this strategy would discourage exploration and discovery, which are also important elements of learning. Instead, drills should be carefully designed to encourage subtle (non-conscious) and progressive adaptations, which have the potential to cause implicit motor learning. There are simple, yet surprisingly elegant ways in which the practice environment can be adapted to cause this kind of implicit motor learning. A good example can be seen in the differences in racket grip and movement pattern that exist in tennis players who learn the game on grass courts compared to those who learn on clay courts. The relatively subtle difference in height of the bounce on the two different playing surfaces encourages the use of predominantly different types of grip. On grass, an Eastern forehand grip dominates because it allows the player to more easily play shots to a low bouncing ball (with greater use of underspin a consequence). On clay, a full or semi-Western grip dominates because it allows the player to more easily bring the racket over the higher bouncing ball, imparting topspin. Anyone who has played on both surfaces will recognize the difficulties associated with adapting to the differences in height of bounce – for the first few games (or sets) a player who has just switched surfaces will be highly conscious of the differences in the environment and will probably perform in an explicit manner, testing numerous hypotheses. If, however, the height of the bounce is gradually changed over several weeks (or months), without the conscious awareness of the player, it is likely that the player will implicitly adapt their movements to the conditions without an explicit component. Eventually, the player will notice that the bounce height has changed but, given that the benefits of implicit motor learning occur in the early stages of learning, such explicit awareness would by then be of no importance.

One other method to encourage a mode of learning that is implicit is analogy learning (Law et al 2003, Masters 2000, Poolton et al 2006). For example, a swimming teacher may use the image of a shark's fin to conceptualize a high elbow recovery for the learner. The use of analogy for instructional purposes is common in coaching, and allows the coach to instruct the performer implicitly without resorting to verbal instructions. Most coaches probably employ analogies not because they wish to use implicit motor learning but rather because they find that the analogy is a rapid, economical method in which to describe the biomechanical principles or coordination patterns that they wish the learner to accomplish. Wulf et al (1999) also employed an analogy in their studies of internal and external focus of attention ('let the club perform a pendulum-like motion') so it is possible that the analogy underlies the benefits associated with an external focus of attention.

Most of the research into implicit characteristics of analogy learning has examined the right-angled triangle analogy proposed by Masters (2000). The research has shown that this particular analogy can be used in both tennis and table tennis to teach beginners a topspin forehand shot implicitly. The learner is instructed to first draw a right-angled triangle with the bat or racket. Once this is accomplished the learner is instructed that when striking the ball he or she is to sweep the racquet/bat up the hypotenuse (longest side) of the right-angled triangle. The result in all of the research has been that learners quickly achieve movement patterns that are fundamentally satisfactory, without becoming aware of much of the complex knowledge that underlies a successful topspin movement. The movements tend to be resilient to pressure (Law et al 2003) and stable under conditions that call for complex decision making while performing (Poolton et al 2006).

A number of practical strategies to enable athletes to cope with anxiety have been suggested in this section. Of course, practitioners may think of, or indeed already employ, a number of similar strategies within their practice sessions. The important common theme underlying much of this chapter has been to promote a learning environment in which robust and effective movement patterns are learned. To deal with pressured performance environments, athletes must learn to gain attentional control to prevent distractive thought processes, which can lead to choking and other related phenomena.

Summary and conclusion

This chapter has considered why athletes can experience drops in performance in anxiety-inducing or pressured situations. We started by discussing the various behavioural stages that learners progress through during skill acquisition. It was noted that, with practice, the responsibility for movement control is gradually passed into subconscious regions of the brain. In other words, skilled movement becomes increasingly automated, enabling athletes to engage in other important activities such as anticipation and decision making (see Chs 14 and 17). However, when the athlete experiences high levels of anxiety these feelings may be accompanied by a regression (reinvestment) to conscious control of action in which attention is redirected to movement production. This phenomenon can result in skill execution that is less smooth, less efficient in terms of time and energy, and more or less variable (depending on the nature of the task) than required. Disrupted performance under pressure is thought to occur as a consequence of additional on-task effort and/or via over-reflection on how to execute the individual components of the skill.

In the second half of the chapter we discussed how the athlete needs to gain attentional control in order to 'keep it together' when performing under pressure. Gaining attentional control can be defined as shifting attentional focus appropriately so that skill execution is not affected by distractive thought processes. A considerable body of sport-related research has emerged that suggests that adopting an external focus of attention during practice generally seems to help prevent athletes from reinvesting under pressure. However, the performer's skill level may well mediate external focus benefits, with less-skilled performers needing to focus upon skill production at certain times.

A number of practical strategies have also been suggested that practitioners and athletes could employ to avoid choking under pressure. For example, a Movement Specific Reinvestment Scale (Masters & Maxwell 2008) could be used to gauge the propensity of the athlete for deautomatization of movement. Such a tool might be useful to managers trying to decide who should take the kicks during penalty shootouts at the World Cup. For those athletes who show a high likelihood of reinvestment, coaches might consider developing targeted practice activities to account for this individual characteristic. One common-sense option would be to rehearse or acclimatize in the presence of typical stressors (e.g. evaluative audience, prospect of rewards, rapidly changing spatio-temporal demands). By making practice 'feel' like performance, the athlete is able to develop appropriate attentional control to transfer into realistic situations. It has also been suggested that an initial period of error-free practice may be beneficial for early learners. For example, this might involve practice environments in which no performance feedback or only bandwidth feedback is provided (see Ch. 14). Other implicit learning techniques have been discussed such as analogy learning, introducing subtle (subconscious) variations in the performance environment, and practising while performing a secondary task. Each has been tested in research studies and is intended to prevent the learner from developing reliance upon explicit rule-based knowledge accumulated during practice. The challenge facing practitioners now is to develop such strategies further into effective practice activities within their own sports or physical activities.

References

Abernethy, B., Maxwell, J., Masters, R.S.W., et al., 2007. Attentional processes in skill learning and expert performance. In: Tenenbaum, G., Eklund, R.C. (Eds.), Handbook of sport psychology, third ed. John Wiley, London, pp. 245–263.

Baddeley, A.D., 1966. The capacity for generating information by randomisation. Q. J. Exp. Psychol. 18, 119–129.

Badgaiyan, R.D., 2000. Executive control, willed actions, and nonconscious processing. Hum. Brain Mapp. 9, 38–41.

Baumeister, R.F., 1984. Choking under pressure: self-consciousness and paradoxical effects of incentives on skilful performance. J. Pers. Soc. Psychol. 46, 610–620.

Bayley, P.J., Frascino, J.C., Squire, L.R., 2005. Robust habit learning in the absence of awareness and independent of the medial temporal lobe. Nature 436, 550–553.

Beilock, S.L., Gray, R., 2007. Why do athletes choke under pressure. In: Tenenbaum, G., Eklund, R.C. (Eds.), Handbook of sport psychology, third ed. John Wiley, London, pp. 425–444.

Beilock, S.L., Carr, T.H., MacMahon, C., et al., 2002. When paying attention becomes counterproductive: impact of divided versus skill-focused attention on novice and experienced performance of sensorimotor skills. J. Exp. Psychol. Appl. 6, 6–16.

Bennett, S.J., 2000. Implicit learning: should it be used in practice? International Journal of Sport Psychology 31, 542–546.

Bernstein, N.A., 1967. The control and regulation of movements. Pergamon Press, London.

Beuter, A., Duda, J.L., 1985. Analysis of the arousal/motor performance relationship in children using movement kinematics. Journal of Sport Psychology 7, 229–243.

Boder, D.P., 1935. The influence of concomitant activity and fatigue upon certain forms of reciprocal hand movement and its fundamental components. Comparative Psychology Monographs 11, 4.

Boyer, P., Lienard, P., 2006. Why ritualized behavior? Precaution systems and action-parsing in developmental, pathological and cultural rituals. Behav. Brain Sci. 29, 595–693.

Chen, H.H., Liu, Y.T., Mayer-Kress, G., et al., 2005. Learning the pedalo locomotion task. J. Mot. Behav. 37, 247–256.

Chow, J.Y., Davids, K., Button, C., et al., 2006. Organisation of motor system degrees of freedom during the soccer chip: an analysis of skilled performance. International Journal of Sport Psychology 2–3, 207–229.

Chung, G.K.W.K., O'Neil, H.F., Delacruz, G.C., et al., 2005. The role of anxiety on novices' rifle marksmanship performance. Educational Assessment 10, 257–275.

Collins, D.V., Jones, B., Fairweather, M., et al., 2001. Examining anxiety changes in movement patterns. International Journal of Sport Psychology 32, 223–242.

Court, M.L.J., Bennett, S.J., Williams, A.M., et al., 2005. Effects of attentional strategies and anxiety constraints on perceptual-motor organisation of rhythmical arm movements. Neurosci. Lett. 384 (1–2), 17–22.

Davids, K., Button, C., Bennett, S.J., 2007. The dynamics of skill acquisition: a constraints-led approach. Human Kinetics, Champaign, IL.

Deikman, A.J., 1969. Deautomatization and the mystic experience. In: Tart, C.T. (Ed.), Altered states of consciousness. Wiley, New York.

Eysenck, M.W., Calvo, M.G., 1992. Anxiety and performance: the processing efficiency theory. Cognition and Emotion 6, 409–434.

Fitts, P.M., Posner, M.I., 1967. Human performance. Brooks/Cole, Belmont, CA.

Ford, P., Hodges, N.J., Williams, A.M., 2005. Online attentional-focus manipulation in a soccer-dribbling task: implications for the proceduralization of motor skills. J. Mot. Behav. 37, 386–394.

Freud, S., 1922. Introductory lectures on psychoanalysis. George Allen & Unwin, London.

Gallwey, T.W., 1986. The inner game of tennis. Pan Books, London.

Gibson, J.J., 1979. The ecological approach to visual perception. Lawrence Erlbaum Associates, Hillsdale, NJ.

Gray, R., 2004. Attending to the execution of a complex sensorimotor skill: expertise differences, choking, and slumps. J. Exp. Psychol. Appl. 10, 42–54.

Hardy, L., 1996. Testing the predictions of the cusp catastrophe model of anxiety and performance. Sport Psychologist 10, 140–156.

Hardy, L., Mullen, R., Jones, G., 1996. Knowledge and conscious control of motor actions under stress. Br. J. Psychol. 87, 621–636.

Higuchi, T., Imanaka, K., Hatayama, T., 2002. Freezing degrees of freedom under stress: kinematic evidence of constrained movement strategies. Hum. Mov. Sci. 21, 831–846.

Hodges, N.J., Lee, T.D., 1999. The role of augmented information prior to learning a bimanual visual-motor coordination task: do instructions of the movement pattern facilitate learning relative to discovery learning? Br. J. Psychol. 90, 389–403.

Jackson, R.C., Beilock, S.L., 2008. Performance pressure and paralysis by analysis: research and implications. In: Farrow, D., Baker, J., MacMahon, C. (Eds.), Developing sport expertise: researchers and coaches put theory into practice. Routledge, London, pp. 104–118.

Jackson, R.C., Masters, R.S.W., 2006. Ritualized behavior in sport. Behav. Brain Sci. 29, 27–28.

Jackson, R.C., Ashford, K.J., Norsworthy, G., 2006. Attentional focus, dispositional reinvestment and skilled motor performance under pressure. Journal of Sport and Exercise Psychology 28, 49–68.

James, W., 1890. Principles of psychology. Holt, Rinehart & Winston, New York.

Kennedy, P.R., 1990. Corticospinal, rubrospinal, and rubro-olivary projections: a unifying hypothesis. Trends Neurosci. 13, 474–479.

Land, M.F., McLeod, P., 2000. From eye movements to actions: how batsmen hit the ball. Nat. Neurosci. 3, 1340–1345.

Law, J., Masters, R.S.W., Bray, S., et al., 2003. Motor performance as a function of audience affability and metaknowledge. Journal of Sport and Exercise Psychology 25, 484–500.

Lewis, B.P., Linder, D.E., 1997. Thinking about choking? Attentional processes and paradoxical performance. Pers. Soc. Psychol. Bull. 23, 937–944.

MacPherson, A., Collins, D., Obhi, S., 2009. The importance of temporal structure and rhythm for the optimum performance of motor skills: a new focus for practitioners of sport psychology. Journal of Applied Sport Psychology 21 (Suppl. 1), S48–S61.

Manoonpong, P., Geng, T., Kulvicius, T., et al., 2007. Adaptive, fast walking in a biped robot under neuronal control and learning. PLoS Comput. Biol. 3 (7), 1–16.

Marnassis, G., Doganis, G., 2004. The effects of a mental training program on juniors pre-competitive anxiety, self-confidence, and tennis performance. Journal of Applied Sport Psychology 16, 118–137.

Martell, S.G., Vickers, J.N., 2004. Gaze characteristics of elite and near-elite athletes in ice hockey defensive tactics. Hum. Mov. Sci. 22, 689–712.

Martens, R., Burton, D., Vealey, R., et al., 1990. Development and validation of competitive state anxiety inventory-2. In: Martens, R., Vealey, R., Burton, D. (Eds.), Competitive anxiety in sport. Human Kinetics, Champaign, IL, pp. 117–190.

Masters, R.S.W., 1992. Knowledge, knerves and know-how: the role of explicit versus implicit knowledge in the breakdown of a complex motor skill under pressure. Br. J. Psychol. 83, 343–358.

Masters, R.S.W., 2000. Theoretical aspects of implicit learning in sport. International Journal of Sport Psychology 31, 530–541.

Masters, R.S.W., Maxwell, J.P., 2004. Implicit motor learning, reinvestment and movement disruption: what you don't know won't hurt you? In: Williams, A.M., Hodges, N.J. (Eds.), Skill acquisition in sport: research, theory and practice. Routledge, London, pp. 207–228.

Masters, R.S.W., Maxwell, J., 2008. The theory of reinvestment. International Review of Sport and Exercise Psychology 1, 160–183.

Masters, R.S.W., Polman, R.C.J., Hammond, N.V., 1993. 'Reinvestment': a dimension of personality implicated in skill breakdown under pressure. Journal of Personality and Individual Differences 14, 655–666.

Masters, R.S.W., Poolton, J.M., Maxwell, J.P., 2008. Stable implicit motor processes despite aerobic locomotor fatigue. Conscious. Cogn. 17, 335–338.

Maxwell, J.P., Masters, R.S.W., Eves, F.F., 2000. From novice to know-how: a longitudinal study of implicit motor learning. J. Sports Sci. 18, 111–120.

Maxwell, J.P., Masters, R.S.W., Kerr, E., et al., 2001. The implicit benefit of learning without errors. Q. J. Exp. Psychol. 54A, 1049–1068.

Maxwell, J.P., Masters, R.S.W., Eves, F.F., 2003. The role of working memory in motor learning and performance. Conscious. Cogn. 12, 376–402.

Maxwell, J.P., Masters, R.S.W., Poolton, J.M., 2006. Performance breakdown in sport: the roles of reinvestment and verbal knowledge. Res. Q. Exerc. Sport 77, 271–276.

Moore, W.E., Stevenson, J.R., 1991. Understanding trust in the performance of complex automatic sport skills. Sport Psychologist 5, 281–289.

Mullen, R., Hardy, L., Oldham, A., 2007. Implicit and explicit control of motor actions: revisiting some early evidence. Br. J. Psychol. 98, 141–156.

Nideffer, R.M., 1976. Test of attentional and interpersonal style. J. Pers. Soc. Psychol. 34, 394–404.

Perkins-Ceccato, N., Passmore, S.R., Lee, T.D., 2003. Effects of focus of attention depend on golfers' skill. J. Sports Sci. 21, 593–600.

Pijpers, J.R., Oudejans, R.R.D., Holsheimer, F., et al., 2003. Anxiety-performance relationships in climbing: a process-oriented approach. Psychology of Sport and Exercise 4, 283–304.

Poolton, J., Maxwell, J., Masters, R.S.W., 2004. Rules for reinvestment. Percept. Mot. Skills 99, 771–774.

Poolton, J.M., Masters, R.S.W., Maxwell, J.P., 2005. The relationship between initial errorless learning conditions and subsequent performance. Hum. Mov. Sci. 24, 362–378.

Poolton, J.M., Masters, R.S.W., Maxwell, J.P., 2006. The influence of analogy learning on decision-making in table tennis: evidence from behavioural data. Psychology of Sport and Exercise 7, 677–688.

Poolton, J.M., Masters, R.S.W., Maxwell, J.P., 2007. Passing thoughts on the evolutionary stability of implicit motor behaviour: Performance retention under physiological fatigue. Conscious. Cogn. 16, 456–468.

Reber, A.S., 1993. Implicit learning and tacit knowledge: an essay on the cognitive unconscious. Oxford University Press, New York.

Schmidt, R.A., Wrisberg, C.A., 2004. Motor learning and performance, third ed. Human Kinetics, Champaign, IL.

Singer, R.N., Lidor, R., Cauraugh, J.H., 1993. To be aware or not aware? What to think about while learning and performing a motor skill. Sport Psychologist 7, 19–30.

Sporns, O., Edelman, G.M., 1993. Solving Bernstein's problem: a proposal for the development of coordinated movement by selection. Child Dev. 64, 960–981.

Stadler, M.A., Frensch, P.A., 1998. Handbook of implicit learning. Sage Publications, London.

Summers, J.J., 2004. A historical perspective on skill acquisition. In: Williams, A.M., Hodges, N.J. (Eds.), Skill acquisition in sport: research, theory and practice. Routledge. Oxfordshire, Abingdon, pp. 1–26.

Van Gemmett, A.W.A., van Galen, G.P., 1997. Stress, neuromotor noise, and human performance: a theoretical perspective. J. Exp. Psychol. Hum. Percept. Perform. 23, 1299–1313.

Vereijken, B., van Emmerik, R.E.A., Whiting, H.T.A., Newell, K.M., 1992. Free(z)ing degrees of freedom in skill acquisition. J. Mot. Behav. 24, 133–142.

Wegner, D.M., Erskine, J.A.K., 2003. Voluntary involuntariness: thought suppression and the regulation of the experience of will. Conscious. Cogn. 12, 684–694.

Wegner, D.M., Schneider, D.J., 2003. The white bear story. Psychological Inquiry 14, 326–329.

Willingham, D.B., 1998. A neuropsychological theory of motor skill learning. Psychol. Rev. 105, 558–584.

Wulf, G., Weigelt, C., 1997. Instructions about physical principles in learning a complex motor skill: to tell or not to tell. Res. Q. Exerc. Sport 68, 362–367.

Wulf, G., Höß, M., Prinz, W., 1998. Instructions for motor learning: differential effects of internal versus external focus attention. J. Mot. Behav. 30, 169–179.

Wulf, G., Lauterbach, B., Toole, T., 1999. The learning advantages of an external focus of attention in golf. Res. Q. Exerc. Sport 70, 120–126.

Wulf, G., McNevin, N.H., Shea, C.H., 2001. The automaticity of complex skill learning as a function of attentional focus. Q. J. Exp. Psychol. A 54, 1143–1154.

Wulf, G., Weigelt, C., Poulter, D., et al., 2003. Attentional focus on supra-postural tasks affects balance learning. Q. J. Exp. Psychol. 56, 1191–1211.

Zachry, T., Wulf, G., Mercer, J., Bezodis, N., 2005. Increased movement accuracy and reduced EMG activity as the result of adopting an external focus of attention. Brain Res. Bull. 67, 304–309.

Skill acquisition: designing optimal learning environments

14

Joan N. Vickers

University of Calgary, Calgary, Alberta, Canada

CHAPTER CONTENTS

Cognitive principles of motor learning

People engage in motor learning when they go through a number of phases, stages, steps or transitions on their way to becoming proficient in a motor skill. Motor learning requires physical practice and is affected by age, maturation, the amount of time devoted to practice, plus a host of other factors. In contrast, a person is engaged in motor performance when most of the learning of the skill has been done and the challenge is now one of motor control, or the ability to produce a movement that successfully achieves a particular goal. The outcome of the skill is important, as is determining the reasons why one is successful or unsuccessful. There is no single point where motor learning ends and motor performance begins. This is because a person may be an elite performer in one aspect of an activity and still be a novice learning a particular skill in another. For example, it is not unusual for a golfer to be good at putting and poor with the driver, or vice versa.

Cognitive psychology offers a formal way to study how the brain functions during motor learning and performance. Sternberg (2003, p. 527) defines cognitive psychology as 'the study of how people perceive, learn, remember, and think about information'. Solso (1995, p. 2) explains that 'cognitive psychology is the scientific study of the thinking mind and is concerned with how we attend to and gain information about the world, how that information is stored in memory by the brain and how that knowledge is used to solve problems, to think and to formulate language'. Summers (2004, p. 7) explains that when a cognitive approach is used, 'the processing of information occurs through discrete stages that can be isolated and studied through appropriate chronometric methods. Using flow-diagram techniques borrowed from computer programming, the flow of information is typically traced through three primary stages involving perceptual processes, decision making and response selection, and response programming and execution.' Button et al (in Ch. 13) explain that 'the brain plays a crucial role

DOI: 10.1016/B978-0-443-06734-1.00014-6

in perceiving information from the world and using such representations to construct and release sophisticated motor programmes to bring about movement'.

In all these definitions of cognition the critical word is 'information'. To this day we do not have a concrete way of measuring the information used in cognitive processing in the same way that we can measure the oxygen levels in the blood, the strength of a muscle or the pressure under our feet. It is for this reason that cognitive psychologists and researchers in motor learning study the effects of different conditions on the flow of information and how this affects motor performance. For example, if a novice performer is asked to press a key as fast as possible when a light appears, then at first it will take about 180–200 ms, which is the average for visual reaction time. With practice, however, an expert can perform the same task in closer to 120 ms. Is the gain in time due to a faster finger movement? Generally no; instead, the gain is due to a more efficient processing of information in the brain prior to the command to perform the key press. Reaction time, or the time it takes to process the information before a movement occurs, improves the most, while time required to move remains relatively constant. The above is also true for more complex tasks.

Cognitive psychology is comprised of many areas. Below are listed some of the ones that play an important role in motor learning.

- **Perception**. Explains how we process sensory information in very short periods of time, usually less than 100 ms
- **Attention**. Explains how we select information for more extensive processing in thresholds that minimally range from 120 to 200 ms, depending on the sensory modality – vision, hearing, touch, smell or taste
- **Anticipation**. Explains how we direct attention to a stimulus prior to its presentation, thus better preparing the body and mind to act
- **Pattern recognition**. Explains how we are able to discern meaning from configurations of stationary or moving objects (such as players in a team game), as well as when navigating a cluttered environment
- **Memory**. Describes how information is stored in the brain, how we access it and represent it as knowledge, and how we use it to guide our actions
- **Problem solving**. Explains how we use perception, attention and other cognitive abilities to arrive at solutions in both old and new situations
- **Decision making**. Explains how we choose from the many alternatives that are available.

An understanding of these constructs and how they differ from one another will help to determine the design and execution of optimum learning environments. Obviously, the various constructs will hold more or less importance for different activities.

The scientific foundations of decision training

Decision training incorporates into the regular practice environment high levels of cognitive effort and decision making within simulated and real performance contexts. Decision training brings the science of how we think, or cognition, to the fore of preparation. It is designed to improve the performer's perception, attention, anticipation, concentration, memory and problem-solving skills through practices where cognitive training is incorporated with physical and technical training. The overall goal is the development of a performer who is able to make effective decisions under all the pressures of competition or other high level challenge.

The first foundation of decision training comes from recent advances in cognitive psychology and research in gaze control in sport. Thanks to the development of light mobile eye trackers, what athletes see when they perform is now known and this information serves as a basis for understanding the focus of attention and decision making when performing (Vickers 2007, Williams et al 1999). Understanding how gaze and attention function in real world environments opens a new level of understanding of what underlies decision making in human performance. The link between gaze, attention and decision making in motor skills is now possible because of emerging research from cognitive and neural science which shows a strong relationship between shifts of gaze and shifts of attention, thus opening a window that objectively explains how focus and concentration (or lack thereof) contribute to motor performance.

The second foundation comes from motor learning and the emergence of a paradoxical finding in research on practice design, feedback and instruction. Extensive research in all three areas indicates that our traditional forms of teaching and coaching (which are collectively called behavioural training in this chapter) are very successful in the short term, but athletes trained exclusively under these conditions are unable to perform at a high level in the long term, especially when under pressure (for reviews see Christina & Bjork 1991, Farr 1987, Lee et al 1994, Schmidt & Lee 2005, Vickers 1994, Wulf et al 2001). This topic is addressed in more detail in Ch.15.

The third foundation of decision training comes from its extensive use in the field. Decision training has been used for more than 15 years by coaches at all levels in a wide variety of sports and with all age and ability groups. During this time, the literature underlying decision training has been put to the test in terms of its applicability to real world environments. In some cases it has been found wanting in terms of transferring from the laboratory to the practice and competition setting, and so successful adaptations of this valuable research have been made in the decision training model that allow the concepts to work in the field (Chambers & Vickers 2006, Raab et al 2005, Vickers et al 1999, 2004 Vickers 2000, 2003, 2007).

Foundation 1: cognitive and gaze research

We know that performers must be able to anticipate what is most important in the environment and attend to critical cues. They must be able to retrieve from memory the information that is needed at the right time and concentrate at appropriate moments. They must be able to recognize complex patterns in the display, whether on a pitch, court or river rapid, solve problems and make the right decision under all kinds of time constraints. It is the ability to implement these cognitive skills at the right moment that often separates the elite performer from the near-elite or lower-skilled performer. Gaze research in sport provides an objective body of knowledge about how athletes fixate or track objects and/or locations in their sports environment and how this information underlies the decisions they make. Gaze control research therefore provides a valuable source of information that can be used to aid skill acquisition and performance.

There are two main methods used to study the gaze of athletes, called the visual search and vision-in-action paradigms. When the visual search paradigm is used, the gazes of novice and elite athletes are compared as they view video stimuli derived from a specific sports task. Considerable progress has been made in defining how novices and experts differ, using this approach. Williams & Ward (2003) summarize some of the differences as follows: expert athletes have superior recall and recognition of sport-specific patterns of play; they are faster in detecting and recognizing objects, such as a ball within the visual field; they have an enhanced ability to effectively pick-up advance (pre-event) visual cues, particularly from an opponent's postural orientation; experts have greater attunement to relative motion information when presented in the form of point-light displays. Finally, experts have more accurate expectations of likely events based on the refined use for situational probabilities.

The visual search paradigm has provided valuable insights into how novice and expert athletes differ but it is limited in that the physical skills associated with the process are rarely performed in these test conditions. Limited insight is therefore gained into the gaze, attention and decision-making characteristics of athletes as to whether they succeed and fail. Although the visual search paradigm is very good at detecting skill differences (novices versus experts), it is not able to determine how differences in gaze control and cognition affect performance outcomes (success and failure).

The visual search paradigm also requires participants to look straight ahead at displays presented on monitors or screens placed directly in front of them. In the real world of performance, athletes carry their head and gaze in ways dictated by the inherent constraints of the task. For example, when a golfer performs a putt, he or she looks down at the green and the gaze shifts from the ball to the hole (or other areas of the green) and back. At least two visuomotor workspaces are used, one in the vicinity of the ball and the club and the other in the vicinity of the hole. In soccer, ice hockey, basketball and other team sports, players not only look straight ahead, they also look left, right, up, down and all around. In all forms of goaltending, the gaze is oriented upward and located at a distance on the object being shot or kicked or thrown, and then, as the object approaches, the gaze moves downward as the object is stopped, caught, hit or otherwise controlled. In some sports, such as basketball shooting and dart throwing, the athlete's limbs actually occlude the visuomotor workspace as the skill is performed. In climbing, the visuomotor space is constantly changing as alternative plans are considered and rejected, or implemented. Finally, for dancers, gaze behaviour may be used for completely different purposes; in short, the dancer may actually not be looking at anything.

The visual-search paradigm, by design, often negates or ignores the task and organismic constraints inherent in sport tasks. Although the visual-search paradigm tells us much about sport expertise and provides intriguing insight into the perceptual and cognitive characteristics of elite performers compared with novices, it does not identify the specific characteristics of gaze control under all task constraints, nor does it identify the gaze and attentional characteristics that are found when an athlete is successful or not.

The vision-in-action paradigm (Vickers 1996) differs from the visual search paradigm in four main ways:

- The athlete's gaze is recorded as he or she physically performs well-known sports tasks in environments very similar to those found in the real world – there is always a coupling of perception/attention and action
- The athlete performs a well-known sports task for which there are established international standards (e.g. race times, shots made, goals saved), thus permitting a comparison of athletes according to performance levels
- The athlete's gaze and motor behaviour is determined within an experimental environment that is similar to that found in the sport
- The athlete performs the task until an equal number of successful and unsuccessful trials are accomplished.

The vision-in-action paradigm therefore recognizes the factors found in the constraints-led model – the task, the environment, the organism and perception-action coupling within realistic perceptual motor workspaces (Newell & McDonald 1994, Vickers 2007, Williams et al 2004).

Figure 14.1 shows a frame of vision-in-action data as collected in short-track speed skating (Vickers 2006). The skater is shown wearing a light eye tracking system that measures eye-line-of-gaze with respect to the field of view. On the left are shown the skater's movements, which were recorded by two external video cameras at each end of the oval. The scene on the right was recorded by cameras on the eye tracker and shows the location of the skater's gaze (circle) with an accuracy of 1° of visual angle. By coupling both images precisely in time the performer's gaze is coupled with his skating actions at a rate of 30 frames per second or 33.33 ms per frame of data. From this coupled gaze and motor data can be derived the characteristics related to lap speed. To see other examples of vision-in-action data in selected sports tasks, go to www.quieteyesolutions.com.

Gaze, attention and performance

Studies using vision-in-action methods have increased during the past few years for three reasons. Until recently, it was thought that it is very easy to separate, or dissociate, the locus of our gaze from the locus of attention (Posner 1980); therefore, eye movement data were not considered a strong indicator of an athlete's attention. Recently, there has been a major shift in the literature and new evidence that shows that a shift in the gaze is invariably preceded by a shift in attention (Corbetta 1998, Deubel & Schneider 1996, Henderson 2003, Kowler et al

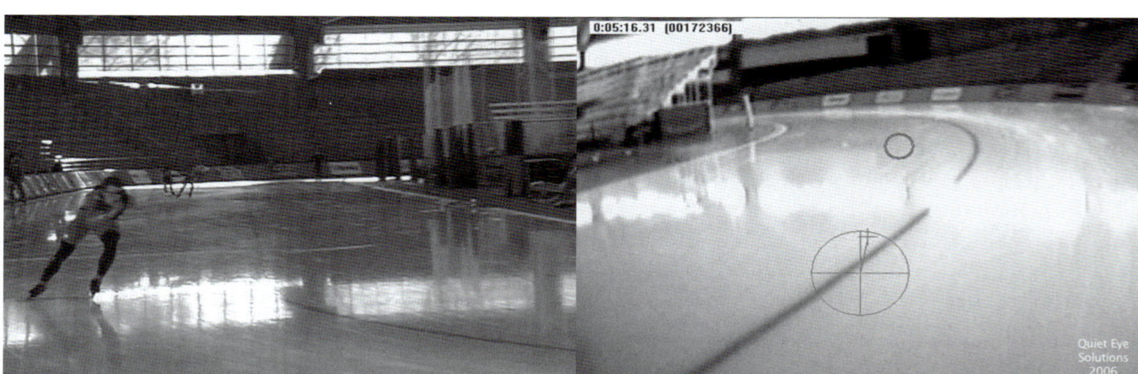

Fig. 14.1 • A frame of vision-in-action data as collected in speed skating. With kind permission of Quiet Eye Solutions, Inc.

1995, Shepard et al 1986). When an athlete shifts the gaze to a specific part of a perceptual–motor workspace then we can assume that a shift in attention has also occurred. Second, advances in eye tracking technology have improved so that the gaze of the athlete can be recorded in most live sport settings. Research methods have also evolved that make the coding and analysis of gaze and motor data both easier and more meaningful. Third, a number of gaze training studies show that training athletes how to control their gaze and attention leads to significant increases in performance (Adolphe et al 1997, Harle & Vickers 2001, Oudejans et al 2005, Vickers 2007). It is clear that elite athletes not only control their gaze in the more efficient ways described earlier in the visual search studies but also define a spotlight for their visual attention (Treisman 1986) that is both measurable and trainable. This spotlight is called *the quiet eye* (Vickers 1996).

The spotlight of attention: the quiet eye

Typically, when a gaze study is carried out, all the gaze behaviours (fixations, pursuit tracking, saccades, blinks) to all the objects and locations in the visuomotor workspace are analysed in an effort to determine which most affects performance. One gaze, called the quiet eye, has emerged as central to success in a wide range of sport tasks. The quiet eye has been shown to underlie higher levels of skill and/or performance in golf (Vickers 1992, 2004, 2007), basketball (Oudejans et al 2002, 2005, Vickers 1996), volleyball (Adolphe et al 1997, McPherson & Vickers 2004, Vickers & Adolphe 1997); darts (Vickers et al 2000), rifle shooting (Janelle et al 2000, Vickers & Williams 2007), billiards (Williams et al 2002), table tennis (Rodrigues et al 2002), ice hockey tactics (Martell & Vickers 2004) and ice hockey goaltending (Panchuk & Vickers 2006). A recent meta-analysis by Mann et al (2007) also shows the quiet eye being one of three predictors of perceptual–motor expertise out of 42 studies meeting the inclusion criteria from a total of 180 papers originally retrieved.

The quiet eye is a fixation or tracking gaze that is directed to a specific location in the sports visuomotor workspace within 3° of visual angle (or less) for a minimum of 100 ms. The quiet eye has an onset that occurs prior to a critical final movement in the task and an offset that occurs when gaze deviates off the location by more than 3° degrees (or less) for 100 ms. The quiet eye may therefore extend beyond the task (as in golf) or be terminated prior to it (e.g. basketball free throw). Many of the studies listed above show that the quiet eye of elite athletes is both earlier and longer than that of non-elite athletes; it is also longer during successful versus non-successful performance. The quiet eye is also trainable and has been shown to contribute to unusually large increases in performance in a number of sports (Adolphe et al 1997, Harle & Vickers 2001, Oudejans et al 2005, Vickers 2007). As is evident, there has been a tremendous growth in the number of vision-in-action studies completed that offer new insights about elite athlete gaze, attention and decision-making skills. This information provides a valuable resource that can be used to enhance athlete decision making. In the next section, the second foundation of decision training is presented, which is a dramatic change in the central message of motor learning research over the past 20 years.

Foundation 2: the paradox of modern motor learning research

Extensive motor learning research in the areas of practice design, feedback and instruction show that our traditional forms of teaching and coaching (which I collectively call behavioural training) are very successful in the short term, but athletes trained exclusively under these conditions are unable to perform at a high level in the long term, especially when under pressure. Figure 14.2 presents an overview of this research and the paradox in performance that has emerged from research on instruction, practice and feedback (Doane et al 1996, Goode & Magill 1986, Hall et al 1994, Shea & Morgan 1979, Sherwood 1988, Sidaway & Hand 1993, Swinnen et al 1990, Weeks & Kordus 1998). Shown on the vertical *y*-axis is the amount of improvement achieved in a skill or tactic, while on the horizontal *x*-axis is the amount of progress made over both the short and long term. The dotted line shows the progress of performers who have been trained using traditional behavioural methods, while the solid line shows the progress of those trained using the newer methods advocated by motor learning and gaze research, which I call decision training. Notice that, during behavioural training, positive

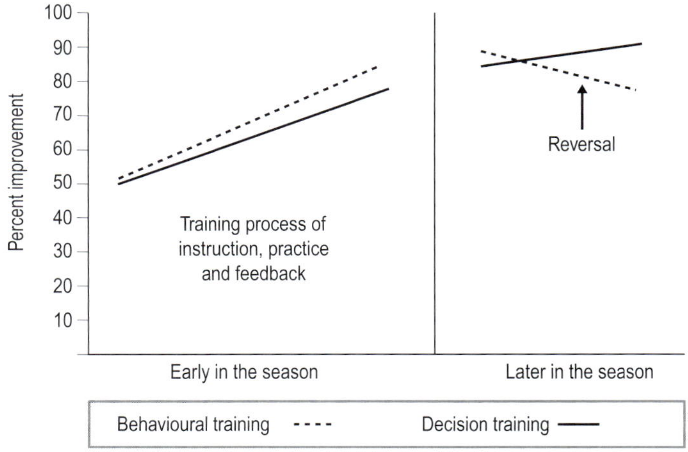

Fig. 14.2 • Overview of motor learning research and the reversal in results when decision training and behavioural training are used.

gains occur immediately; this type of training is therefore appealing to many coaches and athletes. Coaches assume they are training their athletes correctly and athletes feel they are mastering the many skills and tactics in their sport; but notice what happens in the long term. When behavioural methods are used, performance declines in the long term, especially when difficult and stressful conditions are encountered. In contrast, the solid line shows the progress of those who have experienced decision training. When decision training methods are used, performance may be depressed initially but in the long term athletes continue to improve and ultimately perform at a higher level (cf. the toolbox approach described in Ch. 15).

Table 14.1 presents the main characteristics of decision training and behavioural training. During behavioural training, the main emphasis is on the acquisition of technical and physiological skill and there is little regard for the development of cognitive skills during practices. Behavioural coaching promotes high levels of physical effort but ignores the development of the athlete's perceptual and cognitive processes within regular practices. Instruction follows a path of part-to-whole learning using simple to complex drills. Basic skills are taught before more advanced ones, using high levels of repetitive blocked practice. The intent is to build the sport gradually so that more complex skills and tactics are introduced only after the basic skills have been achieved. Practice drills are normally blocked, with the same drills often performed over and over. Technical and physical perfection is the goal.

Table 14.1 Characteristics of behavioural training and decision training

Behavioural training (physical, technical, non-cognitive)	Decision training (physical, technical, cognitive)
Instruction	
Part-to-whole training	Tactical whole training
Simple to complex drills	Competition-like drills
Easy-first instruction	Hard-first instruction
Technical emphasis	Technique within tactics
Internal focus of instruction	External focus of instruction
Low use of video models	High use of video models
Practice	
Blocked practice	Variable practice
Low variability	Random practice
Feedback	
Abundant coach feedback	Bandwidth feedback
Low use of questioning	High use of questioning
Low use of video feedback	High use of video feedback
Low athlete detection and correction of errors	High athlete detection and correction of errors
Overall	
Low levels of athlete cognitive effort	High levels of athlete cognitive effort

Coaches who use a behavioural approach immediately provide abundant feedback whenever possible. Athletes are rarely questioned about their performance or expected to detect or correct their own errors or provide solutions. Instead, this is viewed as the primary function of the coach or teacher. There is limited use of video models, where the athletes view other athletes in order to gain insight into how to perform better, or video feedback, where the athletes view themselves in order to detect and correct their own errors.

Behavioural training promotes an internal focus of attention, since coaches continually draw the athletes' attention into their own bodies. Often there is an active attempt to switch the athlete's mind off in favour of the attainment of rapid automaticity. But this approach may be hit and miss, where performance is exceptionally good one day and terrible the next. Both the athlete and coach are usually at a loss to know why. Athletes trained in this way do not develop the higher-order cognitive skills needed to understand what underlies their own higher (or lower) levels of performance. Ericsson (2003) states that experts in any field rarely let their actions become fully automatic but constantly find ways to improve, involving high levels of cognitive effort and decision making. This is one reason why they are unable to retain the skill or tactics over long periods of time. Contrary to popular belief, there is no such thing as muscle memory. Instead, all memories about movements are stored in the brain. In order for the long-term retention and transfer of skills to occur, the athlete has to lay down new neural networks that underlie gains in motor performance.

Characteristics of decision training

When a decision-training approach is used, the same emphasis is placed on technical and physiological excellence but the cognitive skills underlying higher levels of performance are trained at the same time. Instead of using simple to complex drills, tactical whole training is used, where skills are trained within tactically oriented drills that simulate parts of the game or the whole game. A technique-within-tactics approach is used, where the same technical perfection is sought, but within tactical contexts. Hard-first instruction is used, where higher-level tactical concepts are taught in advance of specific skills training. Instead of emphasizing an internal focus of instruction that continually draws the athletes' attention into their bodies and their emotional processes, an external focus is trained where athletes are taught to direct their attention outward to the critical objects, locations and tactical events in their sport. The quiet eye, presented earlier, provides an objective indicator of where externally the visual focus should be directed, thereby providing coaches with a valuable coaching aid. Communication between the coach and athlete changes from one where the coach tells the athletes what to do to one where the athletes are asked questions that help them think about and analyse their own performance and provide corrective solutions. This is achieved by deliberately withdrawing and reducing feedback using a bandwidth approach. In order to maintain communication and increase cognitive effort, the athletes are asked questions that probe their understanding and knowledge of the specific skills, tactics and activities they are engaged in.

When a decision-training approach is used, learning is inferred when there is evidence of two things: there is evidence that the correct decision has been made, and the decision contributes to higher levels of physical performance. As a result, a decision trainer conducts practices where athletes learn to make decisions under the many conditions encountered in the sport or activity. Practices with a decision-training focus help athletes anticipate events, attend to critical cues, retrieve the best response from memory, focus on the appropriate events at the right time, and make effective decisions in both low- and high-pressure settings. Decision training therefore incorporates higher levels of cognitive effort into the practice environment while preserving or increasing the amount of physiological, technical and tactical training that occurs. Cognitive effort is defined as the mental work that 'leads to high levels of decision making… anticipation, planning, regulation and interpretation of motor performance' (Lee et al 1994, p. 328–329). Permanent gains are only achieved when cognitive and physical training occurs in concert.

The three-step decision training model

In order to facilitate the training of decision-making skills in sport, the model presented in Figure 14.3 shows three steps that coaches can use to improve decision making in sport. The decision-training model can be applied to any sport, age or ability group, thus

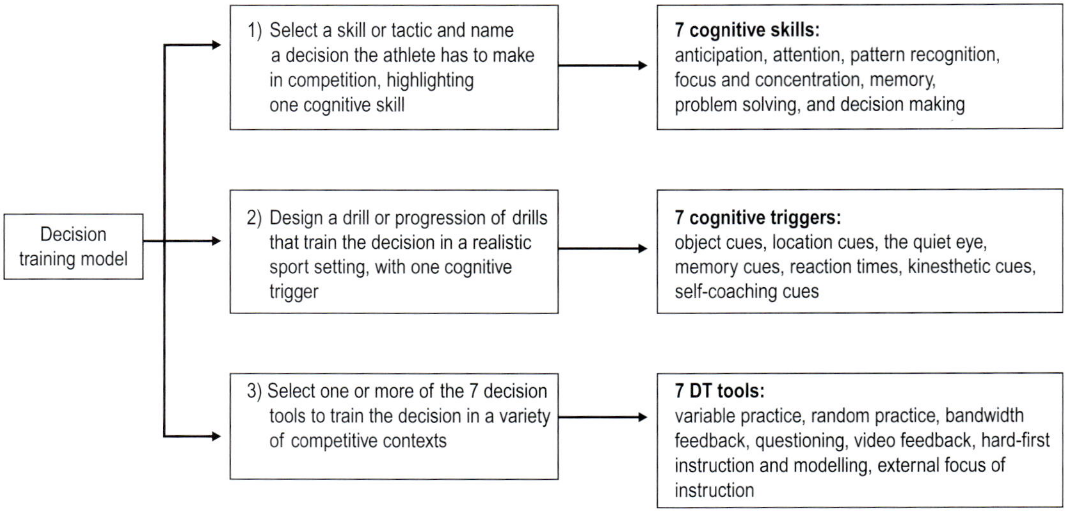

Fig. 14.3 • The decision training model, showing the three steps, seven cognitive skills, seven cognitive triggers and seven decision training tools.

offering a universal approach to coaching science that has been lacking thus far.

In step 1, it is necessary to identify a decision that the athlete has to make in competition. These decisions should come from objective sources whenever possible, e.g. the gaze and quiet eye research presented earlier that not only reveals what athletes see but also how they make decisions when performing at a high level (Martell & Vickers 2004, Oudejans et al 2002, 2005, Panchuk & Vickers 2006, Vickers 1996, 2007, Williams et al 2002). Other sources of decisions that can be used come from the extensive knowledge base found in each sport, as well as anecdotal reports provided by elite performers. In framing a decision that is to be trained, it is critical that only one cognitive skill be identified that the athlete can concentrate on while performing one specific skill or tactic in the sport. This is because attention is limited and it is important not to overload the athlete. That is, it is important to isolate one of the seven cognitive skills of anticipation, attention, focus and concentration, memory, pattern recognition, problem solving, and decision making and to do this in a specific task drill.

In step 2, a drill or progression of drills or activities is designed to train the decision within a simulated sport setting. As a part of designing the drill, it is important to identify a 'cognitive trigger'. An effective cognitive trigger tells the athlete (and coach) if the correct decision has been made as the skill or tactic is performed.

In step 3, one or more of the seven decision tools are used to train the decision in a variety of simulated competitive contexts. The seven tools come from motor learning and gaze research and include: variable practice, random practice, bandwidth feedback, questioning, video feedback, hard-first instruction and modelling, and an external focus of instruction.

Foundation 3: evidence showing the effectiveness of decision training

Decision training has been used extensively in the field and has been shown to be effective in improving athlete performance (Chambers & Vickers 2006, Raab et al 2005, Vickers et al 1999, 2004, Vickers 2000, 2003, 2007). In this section, we look at two studies, the first, by Raab et al (2005), shows its effectiveness with athletes and the second with coaches (Vickers et al 2004).

Raab et al (2005) compared the effectiveness of decision training and behavioural training on elite junior level table tennis players. At the outset they described decision training as having

> integrated the existing motor learning literature and emphasized the training of cognitive aspects involved in decisions rather than only movement execution. In short, this approach proposes that skills should be acquired as a gestalt whole that does not separate declarative from

> procedural, or technical from tactical, because performance requires efficient integration of all sources of information/knowledge.... However, the effectiveness of combining both behavioral and decision strategies into a single training regime has not been assessed. It is possible that behavioral training exerts its influence primarily on 'how' to perform an action, whereas decision training benefits 'what' movement should be performed.
>
> Raab et al 2005, p. 328

The purpose of the study was to determine which training method (behavioural training or decision training) would produce the best shot selection in table tennis both in training and also later in game play. A total of 20 table tennis players (mean age 11.4 years) were recruited from the German Olympic Training Centre and assigned quasirandomly to two groups (behavioural and decision training) so that their performance levels were equivalent. Both groups received the same number of hours of training over 9 weeks. The behavioural group received technical training at regular intervals, emphasizing targeting accuracy in the forehand and backhand strokes. The decision group received the same training for the first 4 weeks but in the remaining 5 weeks they were also provided with video feedback and video modelling oriented toward improving their transitions from the backhand to forehand (or vice versa). Table tennis is a sport where technically hitting the ball takes about 400 ms but about 550 ms is needed to select a shot and make a hit (Rodrigues et al 2002). The training was therefore designed to improve not only the ability to hit the ball but also to tactically select the best shot as quickly as possible.

Videotapes were taken of all the athletes during competitive matches and rated by two national-level table tennis coaches before, midway and twice after the training period. The groups were assessed both on how well they technically performed the strokes and their ability to make the best tactical decisions in terms of shot selection. The final results showed that the behaviour group were not able to make tactical decisions but were better in terms of technique, while the decision-trained group were better at tactical decision-making skills and performed at a lower level technically. This study therefore shows that athletes are affected by the training they receive in terms of how well they perform tactically and technically. Since both technique and tactics are important in sports performance, a successful training system is one that leads to the optimum development of both.

While the study by Raab et al (2005) provides research support for using decision training in tactical sport settings, it is also important to study the extent to which coaches will use decision-training methods in the long term. Vickers et al (2004) studied 13 coaches involved in an elite coaching certification programme. The critical question they asked was whether the coaches would continue to use decision-training methods after their programme was finished.

All the coaches were level 3 coaches enrolled in the four-level system used in Canada. All were full-time coaches (four females and nine males) enrolled in a level 4 coaching certification programme. The sports they coached included badminton, cross-country skiing, short- and long-track speed skating, squash, men's and women's ice hockey, track and field, and wrestling. Their athletes ranged in age from 11 to 30 years old, the athletes' skill levels ranged from developmental to seasoned international and Olympic competitors

The coaches were videotaped during three regularly scheduled practices (P1, P2, P3) spaced across the season. Practice 1 (P1) occurred in the first month of their programme and was videotaped before the coaches received any formal education in decision training. In month 2, the coaches took a 1-week course where the three-step decision model was presented. The first 2 days were spent covering the underlying theory and research in a workshop setting, followed by 3 days of micro coaching where each coach assumed three roles: coach, athlete and peer evaluator. By experiencing these three roles, the coaches were able to learn how to implement decision training as a coach, experience decision training as an athlete and develop skills in observing peer coaches and providing constructive feedback. Practice 2 (P2) occurred 1 month after the course, during the coaches' regularly scheduled practice with the athletes. Practice 3 (P3) then occurred in months 5 or 6, after all course requirements were completed and no evaluation pressures were present. It was expected that the coaches would improve from P1 to P2 as a result of taking the decision-training course. The critical comparison was therefore from P1 to P3, where no evaluation pressures or observers were present and the coaches were free to conduct their practices as they deemed appropriate.

Two coders familiar with decision training coded the videotapes using the decision-training instrument (Vickers 2000). This instrument was developed over many years of working with the coaches and included the three-step decision-training process and the seven decision training (DT) tools. A five-point Likert scale was used in which a score of 5 was deemed excellent, 4 good, 3 above average, 2 below average, and 1 unacceptable.

No significant differences were found in any of the practice-management skills. All percentages obtained were within the ranges expected (Vickers 1990, 2000), allaying fears that increasing cognitive effort during practices would take away from the time devoted to physical training (Douge & Hastie 1993).

Significant improvements were found from P1 to P3 in using variable and random practice, as well as bandwidth feedback and questioning. The coaches reduced the frequency of corrective feedback while at the same time increasing the number of questions asked. Of all the tools, the coaches consistently commented that questioning was the most valuable. One of the coaches put it best when he stated

> If an athlete comes up to me and asks a simple question, I know he or she is looking for a simple answer and the athlete does not understand how decision making operates in our sport. I know now that this also translates into a bad or inconsistent performance in competition. On the other hand, if an athlete asks for verification of their own discovery, then I know that athlete is engaged in developing the decision-making skills needed. Decision training encourages the process of self-discovery and starts the athletes on coming up with well-thought-out questions and solutions and not just looking for answers.

From P1 to P2 there was an increase in the use of hard-first instruction and modelling, but there were no increases from P2 to P3. During hard-first instruction, the athlete is taught higher-level concepts in their sport at the beginning of the season. This is appropriate, as by definition hard-first instruction should be provided early in the season and not later, in order to maximize the amount of time the athletes have to cognitively incorporate new tactical concepts into their motor performance. The use of modelling also increased from P1 to P2 but not from P2 to P3. This again was expected, since modelling should occur more often in the early part of a season as a method of developing analytical and cognitive skills that are sport-specific and most effective after long-term use. Overall, the increased use of decision-training methods was observed to help the athletes develop the anticipation, attention, memory and problem-solving skills needed to perform under all competitive conditions. In the opinion of the observers, the coaching environment improved significantly in that high-level decision-making abilities were developed. Another benefit of decision training about which coaches and athletes often commented was that it improved communication between them, leading to better decisions being made later in competition. The coaches were followed for 3 years after the study in terms of their employment and success as coaches. Of the 13 who took part, four coached athletes at the 2002 Salt Lake Olympics and two of their athletes won medals, even though they were relatively junior coaches at the time of learning about decision training. In addition, eight went on to coach successfully at the national or provincial level, three at the university or college level and two at the professional or club level.

We now look at three examples of the Three-Step Decision Training Model. The first two examples come from long-track speed skating and the last from freestyle skiing jump training. These drills were selected as many of the decisions trained can also be applied to other sports. The freestyle skiing drill was developed by Murray Cluff, coach of Jennifer Heil, Gold Medal winner at the Turin Olympics and Julie Stegall, Team Canada Coach, while the speed skating decision-training drills were developed with Debra Fisher, director of developmental skating at the Olympic Oval, Calgary, along with Marcel LaCroix, Olympic Speed Skating Head Coach, Team Canada.

Speed skating decision-training drill 1: the start

Speed-skating races are won in milliseconds; therefore any time that can be saved is critical. A successful start in speed skating (and in many other races) is dependent on who has the best reaction time and movement time. Most coaches concentrate on the movement time of the start, but an equally good place for an athlete to reduce time is the reaction-time phase. This is the 150–200 ms that occurs from the time the gun sounds until the skater's first observable movement. This drill presents the type of decision making required to minimize reaction time.

Step 1: Define a decision that athletes have to make in competition. The decision should name at least one key perceptual or cognitive skill the athlete needs to master while performing a specific skill or tactic. The seven perceptual/cognitive skills are anticipation, attention, focus and concentration, memory, pattern recognition, problem solving and decision making.

Buckolz & Vigars (1987) determined whether a sensory set (sound) or a motor set provided faster reaction times. An athlete who starts using a motor set is focusing internally on the muscles and limbs responsible for an explosive start. Motor sets tend to be slower because they encourage the performer to focus internally on the details of response execution, which slows reaction time, while an auditory set tends to be fastest of all. The decision to be trained, therefore, is attention to the auditory cue, even as the gaze is focused externally on the entrance to the turn. This gives the racer total visual control over the entry to the turn, even as they devote their attention to the starter's gun.

Step 2: Design a drill or progression of drills to train the decision in a competition-like situation. As a part of designing the drill, it is necessary to identify a cognitive trigger that lets both the athlete and coach know if the athlete has made the right decision Some cognitive triggers include object cues, location cues, memory cues, reaction times, and self-coaching cues (see Vickers 2007 for a fuller explanation).

The drill is similar to the start in other races, complete with a starter who calls the correct commands. Three commands are normally given: go to the start, ready and go. The goal is to have the athletes experiment with different attentional sets, which serve as different cognitive triggers.

- Auditory cue: attend to the 'go' signal (voice, gun, other sound)
- Visual cue: attend to the movements of the skater beside you
- Motor set: think about pushing off the back skate.

The coach begins the starting drill by asking the skaters to completely clear their minds of all thoughts and focus on each cue only as the starting commands occur. The skaters go through a number of starts with the coach presenting various cues on the command of 'go.'

Step 3: Select one or more of the seven decision tools to train the decision in a variety of simulated competitive contexts. The seven decision-training tools are variable practice, random practice, bandwidth feedback, questioning, video feedback, hard-first instruction and modelling, and an external focus of instruction.

The DT tools used in this drill are external focus of instruction, bandwidth feedback and questioning. Each start is videotaped so that both reaction time and movement time can be determined. Reaction time occurs from the sound of the gun (or the smoke) to the racer's first observable movement. Movement time is from the first observable movement until the completion of one full stride. Following the three sets, the skaters are shown their starts and asked questions about what they thought was the cue that allowed them to have a faster start. They also determined their own reaction time and movement time from their videotapes. Over a series of starts, the athletes were trained to attend to the auditory cue, even as they held their gaze on the entry block to the turn.

Speed training decision-training drill 2: entering the turn

Speed skaters have to enter each turn and begin the crossover steps that allow them to build speed as they skate the apex and exit the turn. In Vickers (2006) the gaze of elite speed skaters was described as they entered and exited the turn. This drill is derived from the results of that study and may be used in both long- and short-track speed skating. Short-track speed skating differs from long-track in that the racers can move out of their lanes and obstruct one another within certain limits.

Step 1: Define a decision that athletes have to make in competition. The decision should name at least one key perceptual or cognitive skill the athlete needs to master while performing a specific skill or tactic. The seven cognitive skills are anticipation, attention, focus and concentration, memory, pattern recognition, problem solving and decision making.

The decision to be trained is 'concentration and visual focus on the correct entry point of the turn'. It is critical that the athletes learn to focus on the correct point of entry well before they reach the turn so anticipation and attention to a specific cue is important.

Step 2: Design a drill or progression of drills to train the decision in a competition-like situation. As a part of designing the drill, it is also necessary to identify a cognitive trigger that lets both the athlete and coach know if the athlete has made the right decision. Some cognitive triggers include object cues, location cues, memory cues, reaction times and self-coaching cues.

The skaters do two sets of three starts from different positions on the starting line looking toward the entry of the turn. The cognitive trigger is different blocks placed at different locations on the entry, each with a number. The blocks act as cues for the athletes' external focus and attention, but they also serve as a cue for when the first crossover steps begins.

Step 3: Select one or more of the seven decision tools to train the decision in a variety of simulated competitive contexts. The seven DT tools are variable practice, random practice, bandwidth feedback, questioning, video feedback, hard-first instruction and modelling, and external focus of instruction.

The DT tools used in this example are variable practice, bandwidth feedback, questioning and video feedback. The skaters perform a number of entries, focusing on a different block and entry point each time. After each entry, the coach probes the athletes' understanding of the best entrance cue and optimal focus and concentration points after the start. The athletes are also required to do an assignment where they analyse their best and worst entrances on videotape.

Speed training decision-training drill 3: freestyle skiing jumps

We now look at a third example of the decision-training model applied in a task where the athlete has to be able to retrieve the best movement under temporal, environmental and competitive pressure. Gaze research in locomotion (Patla & Vickers 1997) shows that information must be acquired 200–300 ms in advance of stepping over the obstacle in order to successfully walk over and around obstacles. If this amount of time is needed when simply walking, then even more time is needed to detect critical cues on the course when skiing downhill at high speed. This example from jump training in freestyle skiing was designed to help the athletes learn to make decisions about the best jump to perform under extreme variable time pressure. It was also designed to develop the ability to retrieve skills from memory under different environmental and temporal constraints.

Step 1: Define a decision that athletes have to make in competition. The decision should name at least one key perceptual or cognitive skill the athlete needs to master while performing a specific skill or tactic. The seven cognitive skills are anticipation, attention, focus and concentration, memory, pattern recognition, problem solving and decision making.

In freestyle skiing, competitors are required to complete two jumps at strategic locations on the course. In order to be successful, the athlete has to complete the entire run with both precision and speed. Each run is usually choreographed in much the same way as occurs in gymnastics, dance, figure skating, kayak racing, diving and other judgement sports – by a coach who has high expectations that the jumps will be executed as planned. Coaches often expect their athlete to stay as close to the preset choreography as possible, but this creates tremendous stress for many athletes because of the variable conditions that are present on any day of competition. The course may be rutted from previous skiers; there may be low light, poor snow and a host of other distractions. The athlete may also experience difficulties due to equipment, anxiety or other causes. This decision-training drill is designed to help athletes attend to the conditions in the course well in advance, under different reaction-time pressures, selecting the best jump from a number of preset alternatives stored in memory.

Step 2: Design a drill or progression of drills to train the decision in a competition-like situation. As a part of designing the drill, it is also necessary to identify a cognitive trigger that lets both the athlete and coach know if the athlete has made the right decision. Some cognitive triggers include object cues, location cues, memory cues, reaction times and self-coaching cues.

Figure 14.4 shows a freestyle skiing drill located on a slope similar to that used in competition. This decision-training drill has been used effectively with children as young as 11 up to Olympic gold medalists. The drill helps athletes make decisions under challenging performance conditions that are created by the coach in practice. The figure shows the location of the athletes and coach and the jump site on the hill. The coach first asks the athlete to name a double jump to be performed. The coach then asks the athlete to select a second single jump that is to be held in memory. As the athlete begins the in-run, if the coach calls 'single,' then the athlete has to throw the double jump out from memory, prime the single, and perform it under temporal pressure. The call to change to a single jump under reaction-time pressure is the cognitive trigger. If the coach says nothing, then the original jump (the double) is performed. This drill teaches athletes how to mentally switch quickly

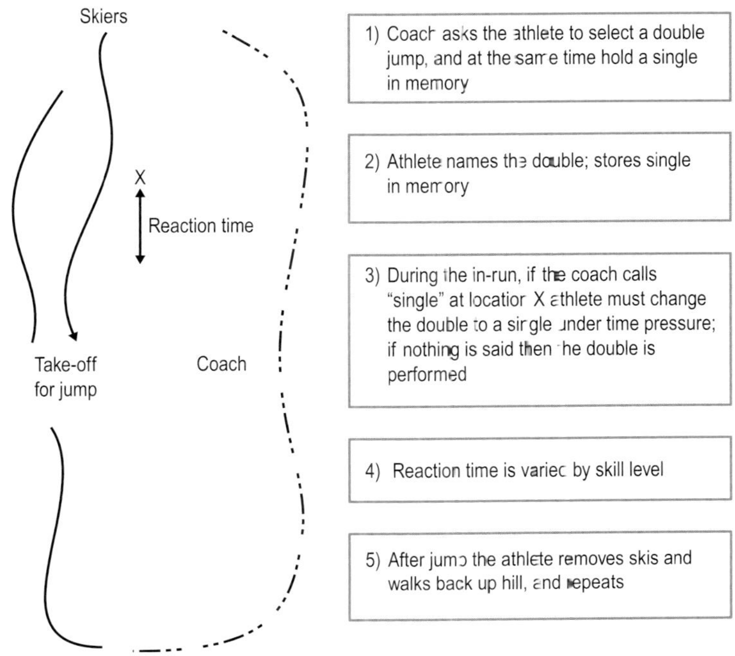

Fig. 14.4 • Decision-training drill in the freestyle jump.

to a different move, as well as how to inhibit moves and carry through with the original plan no matter what the conditions. It also teaches the athlete how to work with their coach in making this kind of decision over many practices.

This drill uses auditory reaction time to manipulate the amount of reaction time provided. The reaction-time period is the amount of time from when the coach calls 'single' until the jump is first initiated. If the skier is a beginner, then the reaction-time period will be longer and therefore the cue to change should occur early in the in-run. More experienced athletes enjoy a shortened reaction-time period and find this drill both challenging and stimulating. The skier therefore learns to anticipate the conditions in the run, prime the best jump alternatives in memory, and select and execute the best alternative under variable time pressure, and they learn to do all of this with the aid of their coach. In this example, an auditory/verbal cue is given, as the goal is to manipulate the athlete's reaction time during the in-run. A visual cue can also be used (such as high and low stubby gates) that directs the athlete's gaze to a specific entry to the jump, or to a certain line on the course (among a number that are painted on the course). But in these later examples, the decisions being trained are different; they relate to reading the in-run and making the best choice among alternatives. They also relate to the location of the quiet eye and its optimal onset and offset, which have not been identified yet (to my knowledge).

Step 3: Select one or more of the seven decision tools to train the decision in a variety of simulated competitive contexts. The seven DT tools are variable practice, random practice, bandwidth feedback, questioning, video feedback, hard-first instruction and modelling, and external focus of instruction.

The types of jump that are trained can be increased or reduced in complexity by using variable and random practice. Variable practice is present when the same jump is stored in memory but different degrees of complexity are trained (single to double, double to single, double to triple, and so on). Variable practice is also used when the coach varies the reaction-time period from early to later on. A later cue is more challenging. Random practice occurs when the athlete stores completely different jumps in memory and thus has to learn to quickly shift or transition from one motor programme to another.

The drill in Figure 14.4 also includes time for bandwidth feedback and questioning. After each jump, the skiers remove their skis and climb up the hill to the location by the coach. This gives them time to think about their performance and also how they will answer the questions their coach will ask. The coach asks questions about the choice of jump, the athlete's ability to handle the time pressure and uncertainty. It is during this time that the coach and athlete work on their communication skills in terms of the types of jump to be performed. Together they develop strategies on how to physically and mentally handle challenging conditions. Through decision training, the athlete develops the ability to communicate with the coach and make the decisions required to perform at a high level. Having the athletes climb back up to the location of their next jump also adds a physiological training component that is lost if a lift is used. This drill design also increases the number of jumps that an athlete takes in each practice session relative to the training that occurs when the ski lift is used.

It is through this decision-training process that athletes begin the process of being responsible for their own decisions relative to the choreography of the run. Flexibility rather than rigidity is the goal; exploitation and optimization are the focus rather than artificially imposed restrictions or limitations. To perform well in freestyle skiing under the stress of competition, the athlete has to learn to assess the terrain and retrieve the best jump from memory – and do this under incredible time pressure. Regardless of whether the conditions are poor or excellent, the athlete learns to retrieve the optimal jump and execute it at a high level. Overall, the goal is to exploit the conditions to full advantage on a daily basis. The coach and athlete work together during practices to develop the best decisions together. Over time, this type of decision-training drill improves athlete–coach communication and instils confidence all around.

Conclusion

Decision training is a new method of teaching and coaching that has a number of strong research foundations. Decision training incorporates into the regular practice environment high levels of cognition and decision making within simulated and real sport contexts. Decision-training drills improve the athlete's attention, anticipation, concentration, memory and problem-solving skills in drills where cognitive training is incorporated with physical and technical training. The end result is the development of athletes who are able to make effective decisions under all the pressures of competition (Fig. 14.5).

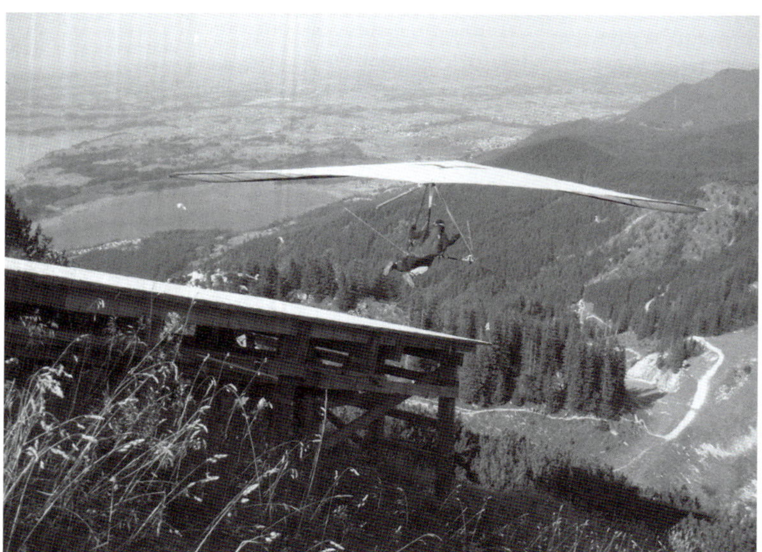

Fig. 14.5 • In extreme sports, effective skill acquisition is the key to safe participation. With thanks to Martin Colclough for the photo.

References

Adolphe, R.M., Vickers, J.N., LaPlante, G., 1997. The effects of training visual attention on gaze behaviour and accuracy: a pilot study. International Journal of Sports Vision 4, 28–33.

Buckolz, E., Vigars, B., 1987. Sprint start reaction time: on the advisability of sensory vs motor sets. Can. J. Sport Sci. 12, 51–53.

Chambers, K.L., Vickers, J.N., 2006. The effect of bandwidth feedback and questioning on competitive swim performance. Sport Psychologist 20, 184–197.

Christina, R.W., Bjork, R., 1991. Optimizing long-term retention and transfer. In: Druckman, D., Bjork, R.A. (Eds.), In the mind's eye: enhancing human performance. National Academy Press, Washington, DC, pp. 23–56.

Corbetta, M., 1998. Frontoparietal cortical networks for directing attention and the eye to visual locations: identical, independent, or overlapping neural systems? Proc. Natl. Acad. Sci. U. S. A. 95, 831–838.

Deubel, H., Schneider, W.X., 1996. Saccade target selection and object recognition: evidence of a common attentional mechanism. Vis. Res. 36, 1827–1837.

Doane, S.M., Alderton, D., Sohn, Y., et al., 1996. Acquisition and transfer of skilled performance: are visual discrimination skills stimulus specific? J. Exp. Psychol. Hum. Percept. Perform. 22, 1218–1248.

Douge, B., Hastie, P., 1993. Coach effectiveness. Sport Science Review 2 (2), 14–29.

Ericsson, K.A., 2003. Development of elite performance and deliberate practice: an update from the perspective of the expert performance approach. In: Starkes, J., Ericsson, K.A. (Eds.), Expert performance in sports: advances in research on sport expertise. Human Kinetics, Champaign, IL, pp. 370–402.

Farr, M.J., 1987. The long-term retention of knowledge and skills. Springer-Verlag, New York.

Goode, S., Magill, R., 1986. Contextual interference effects in learning three badminton serves. Res. Q. Exerc. Sport 53, 308–314.

Hall, K., Domingues, D., Cavazos, R., 1994. The effects of contextual interference on college level baseball players. Percept. Mot. Skills 78, 838.

Harle, S.K., Vickers, J.N., 2001. Training quiet eye improves accuracy in the basketball free throw. Sport Psychologist 15, 289–305.

Henderson, J.M., 2003. Human gaze control during real-world scene perception. Trends Cogn. Sci. 7, 498–504.

Janelle, C.M., Hillman, C.H., Apparies, R.J., et al., 2000. Expertise differences in cortical activation and gaze behavior during rifle shooting. Journal of Sport and Exercise Psychology 22, 167–182.

Kowler, E., Anderson, E., Dosher, B., et al., 1995. The role of attention in the programming of saccades. Vis. Res. 35, 1897–1916.

Lee, T.D., Swinnen, S., Serrien, D., 1994. Cognitive effort and motor learning. Quest 46, 328–344.

McPherson, S.L., Vickers, J.N., 2004. Cognitive control in motor expertise. International Journal of Sport and Exercise Psychology 2, 274–300.

Mann, D.T.Y., Williams, A.M., Ward, P., et al., 2007. Perceptual–cognitive expertise in sport: a meta-analysis. Journal of Sport and Exercise Psychology 29, 457–478.

Martell, S., Vickers, J.N., 2004. Gaze characteristics of elite and near-elite ice hockey players. Hum. Mov. Sci. 22, 689–712.

Newell, K.M., McDonald, P.V., 1994. Learning to coordinate redundant biomechanical degrees of freedom. In: Swinnen, S., Heuer, H., Massion, J. et al., (Eds.), Interlimb coordination: neural, dynamical, and cognitive constraints. Academic Press, New York, pp. 515–536.

Oudejans, R.R.D., van de Langenberg, R.W., Hutter, R.I., 2002. Aiming at a far target under different viewing conditions: Visual control in basketball jump shooting. Hum. Mov. Sci. 21, 457–480.

Oudejans, R.R.D., Koedijker, J.M., Bleijendaal, I., et al., 2005. The education of attention in aiming at a far target: training visual control in basketball jump shooting. International Journal of Sport & Exercise Psychology 3, 197–221.

Panchuk, D., Vickers, J.N., 2006. Gaze behaviours of goaltenders under spatial temporal constraints. Hum. Mov. Sci. 25, 733–752.

Patla, A., Vickers, J.N., 1997. When and where do we look as we approach and step over an obstacle in the travel path? Neuroreport 8, 3661–3665.

Posner, M.I., 1980. Orienting of attention. Q. J. Exp. Psychol. 32, 3–25.

Raab, M., Masters, R.S.W., Maxwell, J.P., 2005. Improving the 'how' and 'what' decisions of elite table tennis players. Hum. Mov. Sci. 24, 326–344.

Rodrigues, S.T., Vickers, J.N., Williams, A.M., 2002. Head, eye and arm co-ordination in table tennis: an exploratory study. J. Sports Sci. 20, 171–186.

Schmidt, R.A., Lee, T.D., 2005. Motor control and learning: a behavioral emphasis, fourth ed. Human Kinetics, Champaign, IL.

Shea, J., Morgan, R., 1979. Contextual interference effects on the acquisition, retention, and transfer of a motor skill. J. Exp. Psychol. [Hum. Learn.] 5, 179–187.

Shepard, M., Findlay, J.M., Hockey, R.J., 1986. The relationship between eye movements and spatial attention. Q. J. Exp. Psychol. 38 (3A), 475–491.

Sherwood, D.E., 1988. Effect of bandwidth knowledge of results on movement consistency. Percept. Mot. Skills 66, 535–542.

Sidaway, B., Hand, J., 1993. Relative frequency of modeling effects on the acquisition and retention of a motor skill. Res. Q. Exerc. Sport 64, 122–126.

Solso, R., 1995. Cognitive psychology, fourth ed. Allyn & Bacon, Boston, MA.

Sternberg, R., 2003. Cognitive psychology, third ed. Thompson & Wadsworth Barnes, Belmont, CA.

Summers, J.J., 2004. A historical perspective on skill acquisition. In: Williams, A.M., Hodges, N.J. (Eds.), Skill acquisition in sport: research, theory and practice. Routledge, London, pp. 1–26.

Swinnen, S., Schmidt, R.A., Nicholson, D.E., et al., 1990. Information feedback for skill acquisition: instantaneous knowledge of results degrades performance. J. Exp. Psychol. Learn. Mem. Cogn. 16, 706–716.

Treisman, A., 1986. Properties, parts and objects. In: Boff, K.R., Kaufman, L., Thomas, J.P. (Eds.), Handbook of Perception and Human Performance. John Wiley, New York, pp. 1–70.

Vickers, J., 1990. Instructional design for teaching physical activity: a knowledge structures approach. Human Kinetics, Champaign, IL.

Vickers, J.N., 1992. Gaze control in putting. Perception 21, 117–132.

Vickers, J.N., 1994. Psychological research in sports pedagogy: exploring the reversal effect. Sport Sciences Review Journal 3, 28–40.

Vickers, J.N., 1996. Visual control when aiming at a far target. J. Exp. Psychol. Hum. Percept. Perform. 22, 342–354.

Vickers, J.N., 2000. Decision training: a new approach in coaching. Coaches Association of British Columbia, Richmond, BC.

Vickers, J.N., 2003. Decision training: an innovative approach to coaching. Canadian Journal for Women Coaches 3 (3). Available online at: http://www.coach.ca/WOMEN/e/journal/feb2003/pg1.htm#Roots (accessed 14.02.09).

Vickers, J.N., 2004. The quiet eye: it's the difference between a good putter and a poor one, here's proof. GolfDigest 96–101. January Online Available http://findarticles.com/p/articles/mi_m0HFI/is_2004_Jan/ai_112104116?tag=content;col1 (accessed 14.02.09).

Vickers, J.N., 2006. Gaze of Olympic speed skaters while skating at full speed on a regulation oval. Perception-action coupling in a dynamic performance environment. Cogn. Process. 7 (Suppl. 1), S102–S105.

Vickers, J.N., 2007. Perception, cognition, decision training: the quiet eye in action. Human Kinetics, Champaign, IL.

Vickers, J.N., Adolphe, R.M., 1997. Gaze behavior during a ball tracking and aiming skill. International Journal of Sports Vision 4, 18–27.

Vickers, J.N., Williams, A.M., 2007. Performing under pressure: the interactive effects of physiological arousal, cognitive anxiety, and gaze control in elite biathlon shooters. J. Mot. Behav. 39, 381–394.

Vickers, J.N., Livingston, L., Umeris, S., et al., 1999. Decision training: the effects of complex instruction, variable practice and reduced delayed feedback on the acquisition and transfer of a complex motor skill. J. Sports Sci. 17, 357–367.

Vickers, J.N., Rodrigues, S.T., Edworthy, G., 2000. Quiet eye and accuracy in the dart throw. International Journal of Sports Vision 6, 30–36.

Vickers, J.N., Reeves, M.A., Chambers, K.L., et al., 2004. Decision training: cognitive strategies for enhancing performance. In: Williams, A.M., Hodges, N.J. (Eds.), Skill acquisition in sport: research, theory and practice. Routledge, London, pp. 103–120.

Weeks, D.L., Kordus, R.N., 1998. Relative frequency of knowledge of performance and motor skill learning. Res. Q. Exerc. Sport 69, 224–230.

Williams, A.M., Ward, P., 2003. Perceptual expertise: development in sport. In: Starkes, J.L., Ericsson, K.A. (Eds.), Expert performance in sport. Human Kinetics, Champaign, IL, pp. 219–251.

Williams, A.M., Davids, K., Williams, J.G., 1999. Visual perception and action in sports. E & FN Spon, London.

Williams, A.M., Singer, R.A., Frehlich, S., 2002. Quiet eye duration, expertise, and task complexity in a near and far aiming task. J. Mot. Behav. 34, 197–207.

Williams, A.M., Janelle, C.K., Davids, K., 2004. Constraints on the search for visual information in sport. International Journal of Sports Psychology 2, 301–318.

Wulf, G., Shea, C., Park, J.H., 2001. Attention and motor performance: preferences for and advantages of an external focus. Research Quarterly for Exercise and Health 72, 335–344.

Effective skill development: how should athletes' skills be developed?

15

Andrew Abraham* Dave Collins†

*Leeds Metropolitan University, Leeds, UK; †Grey Matters/UCLan

CHAPTER CONTENTS

Introduction

From the moment we are born we engage in skill development, moving from a set of involuntary reflexive and spontaneous movements to the development of grasping, posture control and locomotion to more complex linked movements such as running, jumping, throwing, kicking, hitting, etc. (Haywood & Getchell 2005). Much of this initial development occurs through trial and error, influenced by implicit copying behaviours, explicit guidance from significant others (parents, siblings, etc.) and environmental factors, all of which are underpinned by physiological developments in the neuromuscular system. There are some very obvious influences on a child's early development through the provision of environmental stimuli such as mobiles, shape sorters, trolleys, etc. that parents can use to encourage children to develop skills.

Although this is correctly categorized as skill acquisition, we would be hard pushed to call this a planned skilled development programme! Furthermore, other than toddlers/children hitting broadly defined development goals it would be very difficult to identify if a child had gone through an 'effective' skill development programme, even if we wanted to, until several years after completion. By contrast, case history evidence from elite sports players (e.g. Côté et al 2003) would suggest that, at some point in an athlete's development, effective skill development becomes linked with, or even dependent on, a planned and deliberate skill development programme. Indeed, recent research examining the long-term development of talent (Abbott & Collins 2004, Bailey & Morley 2006, Balyi 2002) would suggest that planned skill development programmes are important from as early as 6 or 7 years if children are to gain the early motor, cognitive and emotional skills crucial for a successful lifetime association with physical activity. Unfortunately, as we will show later in this chapter, there appear to be real problems across the coaching spectrum of novice to expert in coaches' capacity to optimally plan for and implement effective skill development programmes.

Consequently, our aim in this chapter is to provide well evidenced and practical advice that can facilitate the development of effective skill development programmes. In delivering this aim, and in accordance with the principles presented, we provide reasons for (and sometimes against) the guidelines espoused, leaving you, the reader, to reach your own conclusions while also knowing why you have done so.

DOI: 10.1016/B978-0-443-06734-1.00015-8

The first section sets out to explain why a coach is essential in an effective skill development environment. We go on to identify how effective/expert coaches are known to operate and deliver effective skill development environments through setting and solving problems. In effect, we create an argument that skill development is an ongoing and goal-defined decision-making (DM) process. We conclude the first section with a modus operandi for coach DM. This shows that a thorough understanding and systematic consideration of the athlete, the sport, and pedagogy (the learning environment), in combination with an effective integration of these three domains, can facilitate the design and implementation of effective skill development environments.

The second section focuses on helping coaches and practitioners gain an understanding of the most neglected of these three domains, namely pedagogy, and thence the factors that should be considered when setting up a learning environment. We begin by identifying the inherent dangers of learning solely through experience – a common source of pedagogical knowledge for many effective/expert coaches. We argue that, because of this method of developing pedagogical knowledge, expert coaches often lack the essential 'deep understanding' of pedagogy. Consequently, even though expert coaches are generally 'effective' in developing the skills of their athletes, the lack of deep understanding of pedagogy ultimately limits their ability to be innovative within this domain. In order to provide some solution to these issues we offer an exemplar 'toolbox' of ten coaching tools, which provides a framework to assist coaches in deliberate DM.

To avoid unnecessary repetition, we will use the term 'coach' throughout. Dance teachers, canoeing instructors and martial artist sifus and senseis should consider this to be a blanket term!

Three components and two types of knowledge for more than one answer

During the 20th century, the Russian psychologist Lev Vygotsky wrote about a concept termed the zone of proximal development (ZPD; Vygotsky 1978). Central to this concept was the idea that a test of a learner's ability will give the tester an account of current unaided completed learning. However, should a teacher offer advice, leading questions or potential solutions through feedback and instruction, the learner's performance can quickly improve the suggestion is that the new performance is indicative of the learning that can be achieved in the future, subject to the appropriate opportunities. We will show later how such rapid performance increments (improvements within a single session for example) are often mistaken for evidence of learning as opposed to learning potential; in other words, very little, if any, learning may have actually occurred. This often leads to frustration for both coach and athlete when retrieval of a skill is expected but is not forthcoming!

Implicit within the concept of ZPD, therefore, is the notion of 'added value' that an educator can bring to the development of skills (cognitive, motor or emotional) in a learner that they would not (or at least be less likely to) have achieved in their absence. Indeed, the need for input from a quality coach in order to promote improved performance has been confirmed by various authors (Abraham & Collins 1998a, Côté et al 2003). The crucial issue here is what does effective practice look like? Is it just the outcome (i.e. improved performance) or must we consider aspects of the coaching process itself?

The coaching schematic – modelling effective practice

Effectiveness is always difficult to define in such a subjective area as coaching simply because the outcome, athlete development for example, can be so variable. Indeed, it is possible for a 'poor' coach to work with a good athlete and vice versa and yet a simple assumption about coach effectiveness is often made on the basis of athlete performance. This point was made by Gilbert & Trudel (2004a), who identified that too much emphasis is placed on win/loss record when selecting coaches as models for investigation. Basing a judgement of coaching quality on performer outcome is a risky business but is a trap that almost everyone falls into at one time or other. Another tacit but equally risky assumption is that expert/good coaching is a unitary concept; in other words, what works at one developmental stage or with one performer will be equally effective elsewhere (Côté et al 2007). In exposing such misapprehensions, we like the analogy of the maths teacher – will the same one take a primary school child all the way through to PhD? This is somewhat unlikely, so don't expect Sir Alex Ferguson to be an expert coach for your child's under-7s football team; equally, youth soccer coaches should avoid trying to be Sir Alex Ferguson.

In an effort to bring some resolution to this problem, a number of coaching models have been developed. Lyle (2002) and Cushion et al (2006) categorized these models as being either 'for' or 'of' the coaching process. The 'for' models were generated through critical thought and review of literature but not necessarily tested against coaching practice, while 'of' models were grounded in practice but not always tested against previous theoretical ideas. In addressing this dichotomy, we took a 'middle way' (Abraham et al 2006); an approach that developed a model 'for' coaching and then tested the model through grounded then led interviews with expert coaches selected upon the basis of the recommendations of Gilbert and Trudel (2004a, b).

Our model drew on three major ideas that seemed to underpin effective coaching. The first was that effective coaching requires the application of knowledge from several linked domains to develop optimum learning environments (Berliner 1991) in order to develop and then achieve set goals. As such, effective coaches must draw from and balance often contradictory ideas derived from different theoretical and experiential perspectives. For example, experience and research suggest that many (but not all!) children like competition but, equally, experience and research can tell us that focusing on competition can create barriers for many children and/or develop inappropriate long-term motivational associations (Chen & Hancock 2006). Consequently, the decision to introduce or remove competition is not as black and white as it is often painted.

The second was that effective problem solving and DM require the development of high-level thinking that enables several sometimes competing ideas to be considered, often leading to several potential solutions (Abraham & Collins 1998a, Abraham et al 2006, Biggs & Collis 1982) that the coach will have to 'orchestrate' (Jones & Wallace 2006) into meaningful actions. Furthermore, the highest level thinking relates to selecting the best option from these several solutions and being able to commit to, take responsibility for and justify that decision, while also acknowledging that the solution is likely to evolve over time (Perry 1988).

Finally, in order to support such higher-order thinking, the coach will need to develop at least a conceptual competence or, preferably, a declarative expertise in the range of required knowledge bases in order to more accurately identify, define and solve athlete development barriers through a DM process (e.g. Rutt-Leas & Chi 1993).

Consequently, the schematic was built on the premise that the design of effective coaching environments is based on an ongoing series of 'pros and cons', trade-off decisions taken at a micro, meso and macro (e.g. activity that minute, versus work in that session, versus programme for that month) level. The final schematic is displayed in Figure 15.1.

The design of the schematic was informed by categorizing required knowledge in two ways. The first categorization (columns 1 and 2) focuses on required knowledge from a declarative or knowledge source point of view (column 1) and application or procedural (see below)/conceptual point of view (column 2). Within both of these columns is the second knowledge categorization method, splitting knowledge into that which helps the coach to:

- understand the athlete (scientific disciplines – -ologies and their applications);
- understand the sport (sport specific, technique and tactics); and
- understand the learning environment (pedagogy, drills, communication).

Finally, the set of arrows displays the need to seek and consider links within and between domains of knowledge – i.e. the process and practice of coach decision making.

Potential limitations of the schematic ... and other research on coaching

Throughout this chapter we will challenge performance psychologists, coaches and performers to critically examine the way they coach or are coached, and to be equally critical about reading research-based chapters/papers such as this one. However, if this is our goal we must be up to this task ourselves and practise what we preach when introducing ideas such as the schematic. Therefore, while Abraham et al (2006) provide strong evidence for the validity of the schematic it is important to acknowledge the limitations of this work. Indeed, there has been criticism of using models in coaching in general (Cushion et al 2006) and the schematic in particular (Cushion 2007). The main thrust of the argument is that two dimensional models of coaching cannot accurately reflect the complexity of a coaching process underpinned by the three key ideas identified earlier

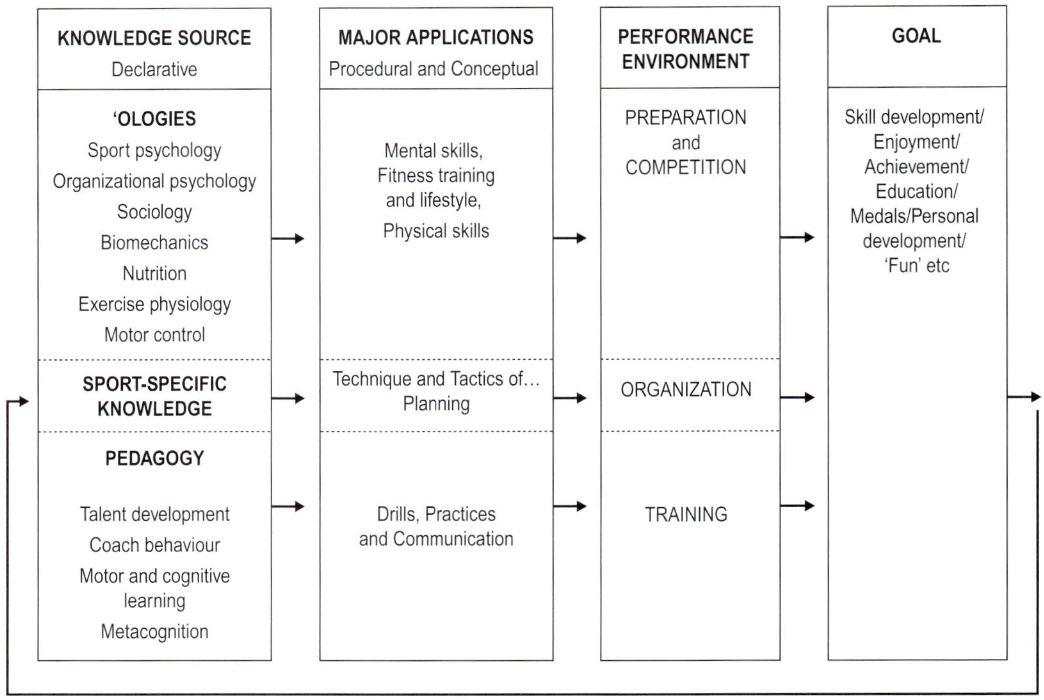

Fig. 15.1 • The coaching schematic, illustrating the comprehensive and required emphasis to establish and promote effective coaching practice in performance environments. Arrows indicate level of cross linkage within thinking and DM processes. Adapted from Abraham et al 2006.

(i.e. drawing knowledge from linked domains, effective problem solving and decision making, conceptual competence and/or declarative expertise, etc.) and including a coach, an athlete, other coaches, other athletes and the environment within which all these key people operate. Furthermore, there are significant others such as parents and teachers who can further impact on the coaching process (see Ch. 4). Such complexity led some researchers to conclude that coaching is not as planned and systematic (e.g. Cushion et al 2006, Saury & Durand 1998) as others would suggest (e.g. Lyle 2002). In fact, coaching may well be similar to occupations such as social work, which have to contend with the 'swampy lowlands' of practice – where the randomness of human behaviour can lay waste to the best laid plans (Thompson 2000).

While there is some truth in these interpretations, we would argue (and do so in the next and subsequent sections) that (good) coaching is, and indeed must be, systematic. We just had/have to get better at identifying and developing the systems that can and do cope with the 'swampy lowlands'. For example, how does an expert coach of youth athletes keep a session on track when one or two seem intent on disruption? How does an expert coach of elite athletes keep a group of headstrong performers focused when jealousy can quickly lead to confrontation? Expertise research in coaching would suggest that good coaches will spot these sorts of problems earlier, understand the problems better and draw on knowledge to solve them (Abraham & Collins 1998a, Schempp et al 2006). However, such descriptions don't actually describe the DM systems within each of these stages at both an explicit and implicit level (Nash & Collins 2006), making it difficult to pass this vital metacognitive activity on to less expert or even novice coaches.

Given that the schematic presented was validated by a group of expert coaches (Abraham et al 2006) and further pilot testing (Abraham & Collins 2006, Collins et al 2003) has supported the explanatory power of the schematic, we would suggest that the approach of explicitly considering

- the athlete;
- the sport; and
- the learning environment

in a structured manner holds much for understanding and developing the coaching/skill development DM process even at the swampy levels (see also the arguments built around Fig. 15.4). In summary therefore, the outcome of a process based around the schematic leads to a holistic approach to coaching and skill development that goes much further than drills and a pitch, track, court, pool or studio in or on which to execute them.

The goal-driven nature of coaching

To conclude the discussion relating to the original schematic, the work of Abraham et al (2006) and Smith & Cushion (2006) has shown that good coaches are constantly setting and solving goal-based problems, in line with the final column of Figure 15.1. However, while there is a great deal of applied work examining goals from a 'SMART' perspective (e.g. Weinberg & Gould 2003 – see also applied content in Section 4 of this book), goals should perhaps be more realistically viewed as our attempt to formalize a problem that then needs to be tackled. Reclassifying goals in this way identifies how professionals cope with the evolving nature and swampiness of their practice (Bowes & Jones 2006). In consequence, goals can occur on a moment-to-moment basis within a training session that are probably just as indicative of a coaching process as a long-term 5 year SMART goal, if not more. This does not mean that we feel long-term plans are unnecessary or that SMART goal setting is not important. It is, however, recognition that effective coaching is not just the unchanging implementation of a carefully crafted and well considered set of plans (it's March, so the plan says you should be...). Rather, the whole process has to be flexible by the minute, session or month, with both goals and the means of achieving them subject to considered refinement throughout the process (it's March so the plan says you should be..., but you're doing very well, so...). This need is echoed by the increasing recognition that physical preparation schedules must be flexible and varied according to individualized measures of progress (see Ch. 10).

Reflecting this imperative for a constant 'test and adjust' approach, problem-based learning has been identified as one way that education can begin to prepare professionals such as coaches and doctors for working in an environment where new problems and goals commonly occur (Jones & Turner 2006, O'Neill et al 2002). Consequently, a coaching process can be viewed as an ongoing series of goal-related problem solving and DM that can occur on a macro, meso and micro level. Furthermore, these goal-pursuit process refinements can occur in both a systematic (e.g. Lyle 2002) and non-systematic (e.g. Saury & Durand 1998) manner. We will exemplify how this process works in the Modus operandi for DM section later in this chapter. The main point is that 'goal-directed' should not mean 'stick rigidly to the plan'; the best performances accrue from keeping the goals firmly in mind but varying the route so as to fully exploit the challenges and opportunities that emerge along the way.

Optimizing coach decision making – providing a theoretical platform

Thus far we have outlined our arguments about how and why effective coaching, and therefore skill development, should be viewed as an ongoing goal-led, problem-solving and DM process. We have also identified a schematic designed to reflect this process. The next key issue is to consider how coaches can implement this work in their own practice. In order to answer this question it is worthwhile exploring some of the underpinning theory of DM further before concluding with a method for structuring this process in coaching.

Procedural and declarative knowledge – the underpinning theory

In order to understand DM it is worth understanding 'knowledge' and how it is acquired and ultimately used within problem solving. Anderson (1982) developed a theory that identified how knowledge could be split into two broad domains: declarative knowledge and procedural knowledge. Declarative knowledge can be defined as the 'why' knowledge or the knowledge of understanding, while procedural knowledge is 'doing' knowledge or knowing how to do something (see Abraham & Collins 1998b for a more in-depth discussion of this topic within the coaching environment). This separation is important since it explains how it is possible to have one without the other, i.e. the coach who does something (procedural) without knowing why (declarative), or the researcher who knows why (declarative) something works but cannot apply that knowledge practically. Similarities can be drawn here with the theory–practice link (or lack thereof) that should underpin all work in performance – indeed, all parts of this book.

In explaining his theory, Anderson (1982) further defined procedural knowledge into two categories: broad proceduralized knowledge and specific proceduralized knowledge. Specific proceduralized knowledge is knowledge specific to very few or just one situation(s). In contrast, broad proceduralized knowledge enables us to approach similar problems in a standard way (even if this standard way is not always particularly useful, i.e. trial and error). For example, in teaching English you could provide a general rule that to make a noun plural requires the addition of 's'. However, there are specific occasions when this general rule does not apply, i.e. the plural of 'sheep' is 'sheep' while the plural of 'coach' is 'coaches'. Similarly, in coaching you could provide the general rule that athletes should be taken out of their comfort zone; however, there may be a specific occasion when this could be negative for performance and so a specific alternative approach may be required (Fig. 15.2).

Returning to Figure 15.1, therefore, it becomes more obvious why broad procedural rules are useful in structuring and understanding complex environments. For example, mental skills techniques and drills (see column 2) are obviously important broad procedural ideas in coaching. However, if the underpinning theory/declarative knowledge is absent, use by coaches is ultimately limited to doing without truly understanding. This situation arises because it is the declarative knowledge, or understanding of a situation that allows broad procedural rules to be used to search out the most appropriate action in each individual instance (i.e. specific procedural knowledge). The alternative is to rely on the same general approach in a catchall manner for a whole range of similar but not exactly the same problems (Abraham & Collins 1998b, Pennington et al 1995) and accept that things may be missed, i.e. 'I see-ed lots of sheeps in the field, daddy' is cute from a 4-year-old but indicative of poor English grammar education in a 36-year-old! Or put another way, a smart coach knows why SMART doesn't work for everyone.

Perhaps crucially, declarative knowledge strongly contributes to our ability to transfer learning from one environment to another (Pennington et al 1995). In fact, taken to its extreme, declarative knowledge ultimately underpins our ability to be consistently innovative (as opposed to getting lucky once or twice), since this is the ultimate form of transfer, i.e. coming up with an idea that is completely new to us that hasn't been provided by someone else. Thus, as a current and pertinent example, consider the theoretical content (declarative knowledge) we are presenting, hopefully with useful exemplar applications (i.e. procedural knowledge) but certainly lacking a completely comprehensive set of implications for your own specific environment, even if such a thing were possible. In essence, innovation is the goal of this chapter by providing the reader with declarative knowledge that provides the basis for new ideas and practice.

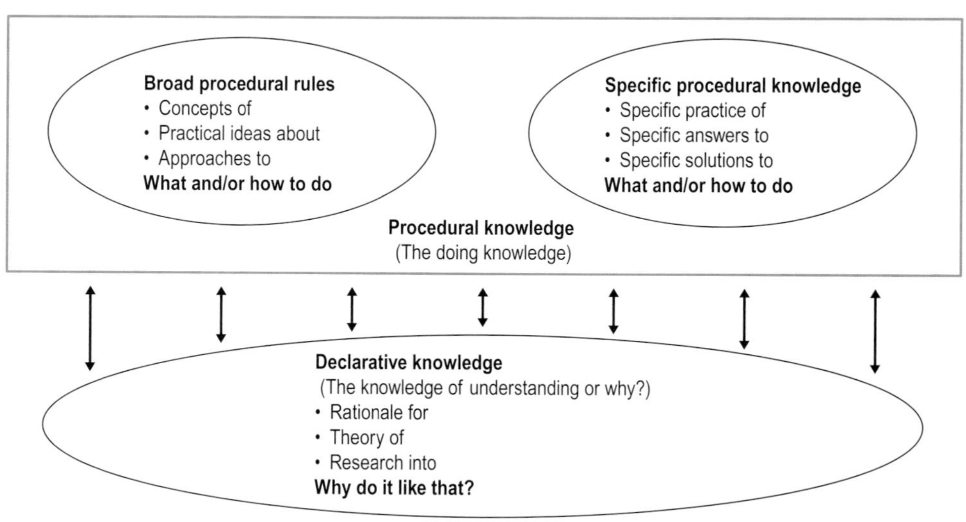

Fig. 15.2 • Summary of Anderson's (1982) theory of procedural and declarative knowledge and the relationships between them.

A useful analogy actually comes from gastronomy. The innovative chef is the one with a full declarative knowledge of why different foods, spices and herbs taste like they do and why different cooking approaches change the final flavour and texture, etc. of the food. This enables the chef to create new dishes and sell recipe books to exploit this creativity. By contrast, the willing, enthusiastic but lower-level cook who goes out and buys the book can follow a procedural recipe to recreate a dish like the innovative chef so long as everything goes smoothly. However, if even a small part of the procedural recipe starts to go wrong in practice, the enthusiastic cook is soon at a loss as to what to do, since they lack the declarative knowledge needed to solve the problem. To complete the analogy in coaching, therefore, beware the book of drills unless you understand where they come from and why they work – or know someone who does!

Finally, it may appear that we are claiming that theory and empirical knowledge (i.e. research) is declarative knowledge – but this would be inaccurate. In fact our personal declarative knowledge is best developed through our own explicit cognitive elaborations of experience (Pennington et al 1995), albeit reading is one of those experiences. What we are saying is that theory and research represent an existing, comparatively valid and reliable source of declarative knowledge that, if experienced through use, challenged, reflected and elaborated upon, can result in a highly effective knowledge base for practitioners to use in future decisions. This theory–practice link is perhaps most eloquently and succinctly summarized by Lewin (1952), who stated that 'There is nothing more practical than a good theory' (cited in Vansteenkiste & Sheldon 2006, p. 63). Indeed, this approach would suggest that the concept of a 'theory–practice gap' doesn't actually exist, at least for coaches who reflect, since they will have reasons (theory) for doing what they do. The gap is probably better explained as lying between the academic theory of research and the personal theory of the practitioner. Consequently, really critical reflective practice should involve being aware of and reflecting on personal theory against the 'standards' that academic theory brings (Strean et al 1997).

To conclude the discussion on knowledge, we must consider the role of tacit knowledge in action. Thus far we have referred to good coaching as an explicit and thought-through process that is learned in an explicit manner: i.e. reflective practice is an explicit and conscious activity that encourages the development of new declarative knowledge, and so on. In contrast, implicit learning 'is the acquisition of (tacit) knowledge that takes place largely independently of conscious attempts to learn and largely in the absence of explicit knowledge about what was acquired' (Reber 1993, p. 5) (see Ch. 13). There is little doubt that much of human behaviour is directed by tacit knowledge acquired through implicit learning that occurs by simply operating and immersing ourselves in social settings. Indeed, this learning underpins many of our assumptions and deep-seated beliefs that we are, consequently, not particularly aware of (Strean et al 1997). It is also why, almost unconsciously and automatically, social norms are developed; in other words, footballers act like footballers, dancers act like dancers, etc. and 'boxes that should be thought out of' are cast in stone. Given such a theoretical standpoint, there is an argument that explicit education has only a limited impact on behaviour until it actively links and engages with these beliefs and assumptions gained, in part, through implicit learning (cf. our earlier comments about academic theory needing to link with personal theory). One of the keys to this is for coaches to understand and critique the way they think about their athletes, their sport and learning, indeed even themselves! In fact, this is why coach educators should understand their coaches, subject matter and the learning process equally well. Accordingly, as pointed out by Strean et al (1997), it is not until we become aware of these assumptions (tacit knowledge) that we become truly critically reflective and consequently more able to think through our explicit decisions. In short, while tacit knowledge is unavoidable in any setting, not least coaching, it is those coaches who gain an explicit awareness of, and critically reflect on, this tacit knowledge who are best able to make the most use of it – declarative knowledge is still key.

Linking academic theory to personal theory to practice

It is from this theoretical position that we believe a more complete understanding can be developed of learning and practice within coaching. Coaching has often been viewed as being defined through 'doing' (Abraham & Collins 1998b), which can, in turn, be conceptualized through competencies. Consider, for example, the British application of National Vocational Qualification (NVQ) systems developed in bricklaying and hairdressing to the assessment and certification of coaches. Such an assessment process would evaluate knowledge of, say, health and safety, by confirming that the coach completed a series of pre-session checks on the environment (e.g. checking the surface for slippery or damaged sections, inspecting equipment, etc.). Consequently, and expanding on this comparatively simple but easily justified approach, the focus has been on what coaches behaviourally do – we only need to look at the vast number of books that are based around drills. While such outcome-based coaching competences, i.e. the ability to produce a session plan, manage a group or demonstrate a skill, are obviously important, it has meant that other, probably more key characteristics, such as reflective practice, problem solving, DM and innovation, have been missed in the education and evaluation of coaches (see Thompson 2000 for a more in-depth review of the competency vs professionalism debate). In essence, the focus has been on what, and to a lesser extent, how, coaches do (procedural) as opposed to why (declarative) they do it.

This dichotomy between what (how) and why is exemplified by an unexplored key point made by rugby coach Ian McGeechan (within Jones et al 2004), which linked the practice and personal theory of coaches against academic theory. During the reported interview, McGeechan identifies his frustration in teaching coaches tactics that are already out of date. In essence, his frustration appears to be born out of telling what he *did*, i.e. out of date procedural knowledge. So the answer is to teach more up-to-date tactics? Maybe; however, Anderson's theory would suggest that it would be more beneficial to identify what broad procedural rules Ian adheres to in critically thinking about tactics and why those procedural rules work so effectively – in short, revealing the underpinning declarative theories that structure his problem solving and DM. We would argue that this would be far more beneficial to coaches in enabling them to develop their own tactics in the future.

In simple terms, therefore, any educational sessions with a 'master' (or mistress) coach must explore the whys (not least because this may reveal that the master coach doesn't know why, because his/her behaviour is based on tacit knowledge) as well as the wherefores. You can listen to, watch and apply the methods of a successful coach, assuming of course that what s/he is doing is genuinely causing the high-quality achievements of their performers (cf. our earlier comments). Unless you know why this, and why not that, method was used, however, you lack the knowledge to adapt the advice to your own circumstance. Consequently, a whole series of problems will accrue from uncritical and uninformed acceptance of advice from someone who has, by definition, been successful in a different set of conditions with a different type of performer. Declarative knowledge structures, and their application and elaboration, are a coach's best protection against such problems and the way in which they can grow their own creativity so that they can design their own new answers to their own pertinent questions.

A modus operandi for decision making in coaching

To facilitate the theory to practice process, there is a need to 'operationalize' all these ideas into an approach that can be used practically. This process usually benefits from thinking through, and often simplifying, the advice to generate a set of procedures/guidelines for practice. Coaches and performers typically like such 'clear cut and practical advice' and question more complex approaches as 'academic' or 'impractical'. Be careful, though: simplification is seductive: often what practitioners crave but, unless you understand the nuances and qualifications underpinning the bland statements, you can fall into the same trap of blindly following a recipe. This won't inevitably be wrong, but it will inevitably provide you with suboptimum answers and also limit your own development by inhibiting your ability to generate new wrinkles to more effectively meet your own challenges. So beware unthinking acceptance of simple, straightforward models – 'That way lies danger' (Master Yoda, *Star Wars Part IV*).

So, remembering this caveat but in pursuit of clear advice, let's start by developing a simple version of the coaching schematic in Figure 15.1. Figure 15.3 presents the essence of the original in simple form; note that:

- this whole process is goal-directed; a combination of one goal for the total process (session, programme, etc.) and desired outcome goals that accrue from the various options from each domain and combinations thereof;
- the coach's behaviours are based on decisions that draw on a blend of three domains of knowledge;

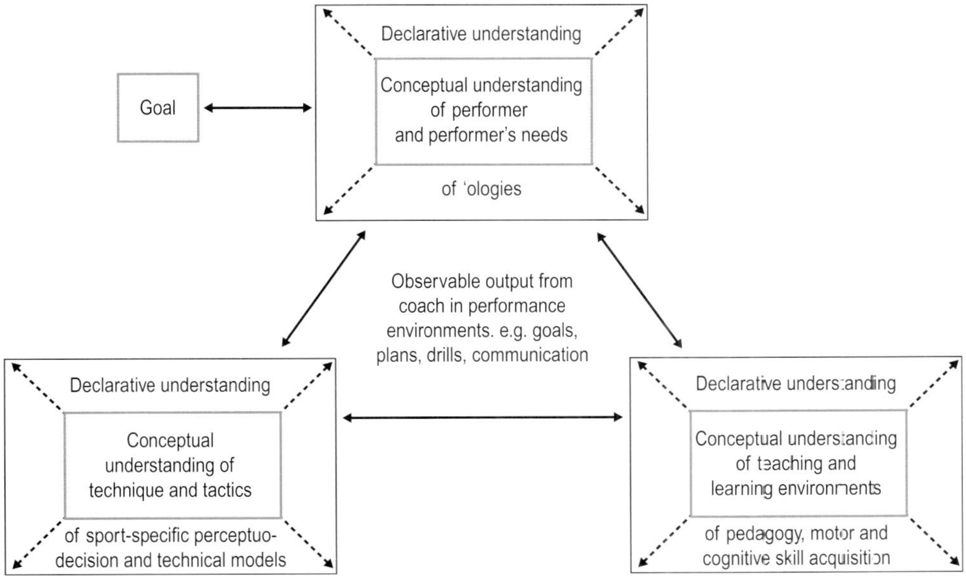

Fig. 15.3 • The redrawn coaching schematic, showing a conceptual view of goal-based coach problem solving and decision making (for the sake of brevity the term 'conceptual' has been used in place of 'broad procedural').

- the three are distinct, and may offer different or differing answers;
- the science of coaching lies in knowing and understanding the implications of each domain, and their interactions; and
- the art lies in developing, refining and deploying the optimum 'blend' from these domains.

In fact, redrawing the schematic in this manner is in keeping with the tone of this chapter in that Figure 15.3 reflects what research says about effective problem defining and solving. Anderson (1987) has described how, as humans, we can rely on a range of weak problem-solving methods such as trial and error or heuristic approaches such as working backwards from the solution in the absence of more effective and efficient methods. They are termed weak because these methods lack a coherent strategy to DM and can lead to people working hard but not necessarily smartly. In contrast to these approaches, research in disparate DM environments such as coaching (Abraham et al 2006) computer programming (Davies 1994, Zeitz & Spoehr 1989) and medicine (Johnson et al 1981) displays how experts who are strategic in their thinking take a similar, breadth-first and hierarchical approach that deliberately draws on knowledge from several interrelated domains in order to understand and solve a problem. As eloquently described by one of the coaches in the Abraham et al (2006) study:

> Are you familiar with the move towards synoptic papers at A level [an optional national examination taken in England and Wales by 18-year-olds]? Synoptic papers basically draw knowledge from all areas to answer a central question. That is what the good coach does. They have to be good at the synoptic work. They have to be able to draw things from different sports. They have to be able to bring different sciences, etc. to answer the central question or problem. That's what good coaches can do. You can't pigeon-hole things for a coach and if I was looking for an elite coach that's what I would be seeing, somebody who could bring a whole lot of different knowledge to solve problems.
>
> Team sport coach, Abraham et al 2006, p. 558

Consequently, the redrawn schematic in Figure 15.3 represents a breadth-first approach to coach problem solving and DM. There is, however, one further bonus of drawing the schematic in this fashion. The centre of the triangle shows the observable output from the DM process. These outputs are essentially solutions to problems, or specific procedural knowledge. As such, these outputs become a knowledge source in themselves that can be called on again in the future to answer similar problems, a process termed tactical learning by Anderson (1990). These 'personal favourite' solutions are different to the recipe approach we described earlier, as they are arrived at through critical reflection and are justifiable against theory. Even here though, regular revision is important if the coach isn't to fall into the comfort trap of unthinkingly providing the same set of sessions off pat.

So how is this approach deployed in practice? Clear guidelines are both possible and extremely useful, but please remember the cautionary approach highlighted at the start of this section. Practically, the coaching process can be viewed as a series of decisions, initiated by and then finally checked against a goal, which generate the best-fit option plan for that particular setting. This process is repeated ad infinitum, as aspects of the situation change, across any timespan, micro, meso or macro. Figure 15.4 displays how this DM process is one that occurs constantly and is both cyclical and linear in nature. This DM cycle is repeated many times within a session, in developing then continuously refining a programme of work on a weekly/season/quadrennial basis or in planning/refining a development plan across the performer's total lifespan.

A quick word about the genesis and scope of this model. We have already shown how research in several professions is increasingly focusing on the cognitive and metacognitive strategies of experts as a means of informing the development of novices and intermediates. For this cyclic approach, research suggests (Abraham et al 2006) that thinking through options in this way is a characteristic of expert thinking in planning a coaching session or programme. When expert coaches think through plans in slow time (as opposed to using tacit knowledge, as described earlier) they demonstrate this three-domain approach rather than merely thinking through things in a chronological flow. Accordingly, and reflecting the 'expert thinking' approach, we would suggest that novices or intermediates benefit from exposing their thinking and reasoning based on this structure, and talk through the DM process as a structured part of their development. Applying this approach in a 'whole–part–whole' fashion is particularly valuable for ensuring the ongoing development of already proficient practitioners. When 'forced' to critically consider and choose between options, experienced coaches are encouraged to expand their repertoires and explore the applicability of new ideas. In fact, we would suggest that this style of 'critical reflection' should be a consistent part of the repertoire for any aspiring expert coach. Without it, they won't stay expert for long!

A specific focus on pedagogy

Thus far we have focused on a holistic or 'whole' approach to examining coaching. However, as indicated in the overview at the start of this chapter we would also like to focus on the pedagogical 'part' of this holistic picture. Our reasoning for this is that pedagogy and its application represents an area that is both ripe and overdue for further attention within coach education and practice. In short, our research suggests that, as the weakest area, attention here may provide the greatest gains, at least in immediate return.

Perhaps a good place to start, therefore, would be defining what pedagogy actually is. At its simplest, pedagogy is the science and art of teaching (Reber 1985). Given such a broad definition it could be argued that the schematic presented in Figure 15.1 is a 'pedagogical' model as it has been designed to reflect a teaching and learning process. Indeed, such a broad approach is used by Armour (2004), who calls for pedagogical environments to consider coaches, learners, knowledge and the learning environment. For the purpose of this chapter, however, we would like to delimit pedagogy to focusing on the science of learning and the subsequent impact this knowledge can have on coaching.

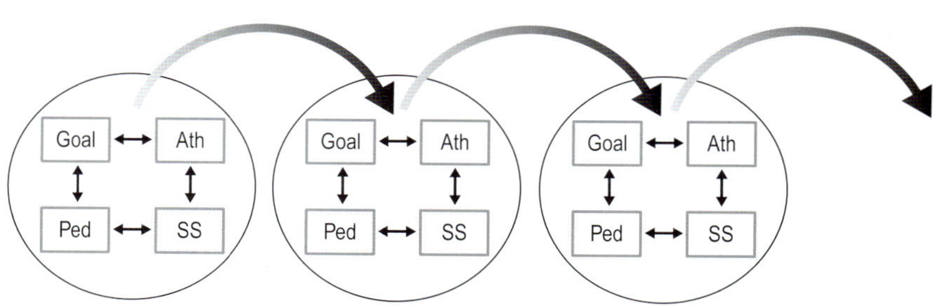

Fig. 15.4 • A holistic view of an ongoing series of goal-based decision making based on the three knowledge domains (Ath, athlete; SS, sport specific; Ped, pedagogy).

Some authors (e.g. Potrac et al 2000) have questioned the role and impact of sport sciences in coaching, perhaps because of its reductionist nature and narrow view of athlete development. There is little doubt, however, that many coaches have made use of research in the parallel domains of physiology, psychology and biomechanics, e.g. strength and conditioning, fitness, periodization, technique analysis, mental skills and nutrition (Abraham et al 2006). In so doing, coaches have attempted to make judgements and decisions (Martindale & Collins 2007) that are more objective and less prone to the vagaries of trial and error or other 'weak' problem-solving approaches (Anderson 1987). However, there are real and empirically justified concerns that similar advances haven't been made in breaching the theory–practice gap in skill acquisition and learning (Abraham & Collins 1998b, Collins et al 2003, Morgan 2006, Potrac et al 2000, Potrac & Cassidy 2006, Vickers et al 2004, Williams 2006). Given the somewhat self-evident relevance of learning to the coaching process, this represents a serious concern since knowledge derived from empirical studies (e.g. Chambers & Vickers 2006) and conceptual work (Vygotsky 1978) in the area of learning offers the opportunity to plan, deliver and review learning opportunities against a valid and reliable knowledge base. In short, the declarative knowledge base can drive both innovation and personal development.

The problem of only reflecting on experience

So, if knowledge derived from learning research isn't being used, what is? We know from various studies (e.g. Gilbert & Trudel 2001, 2005, Nelson & Cushion 2006) that experience is the major source of coach learning and that this learning often occurs through a process of reflection. However, work in sport psychologist development by Martindale & Collins (2007) highlights the dangers of learning solely through experience, since the reflective practice underpinning experiential learning is only informed by a set of conditions distinctive to that individual's own experience. In other words, there is no opportunity for reflection back on theoretical and empirical standards (Strean et al 1997) to challenge and understand the experience, a method that is the basis of development in other professions such as medicine (O'Neill et al 2002). Or, put even more simply, how can you know what you have never experienced or been shown? Consequently, problem setting, solving and DM with respect to learning environments for many coaches are likely to be based on experientially gained knowledge at best or, at worst, on an unthinking, implicit and/or direct copy of how the coach was coached as an athlete.

The lack of awareness of this issue is fairly far-reaching. For example, Abraham et al (2006) noted that, on examination of the work by Côté et al (1995a), there was an apparent lack of awareness of communication behaviours used by the expert gymnastic coaches interviewed in their study. Such a lack of awareness has also been supported in behavioural observation studies showing that coaches have poor recall of behaviours that they have used during a coaching session (Smith & Smoll 1996). However, what is not clear from these studies is whether this is poor recall or just a lack of awareness; in other words, it is very difficult to recall an event if you are not even aware that one has occurred. In the case of very experienced but infrequently self-reflective coaches, the fact that DM is mostly tacit serves to almost completely eliminate opportunities for self-development, or even a structured contribution to others through mentoring. It's hard to suggest what you don't know you do! More recent work, however, has begun to reveal the issues involved in whether or how coaches consider the development of learning environments.

Evidencing the problem

Potrac & Cassidy (2006) discuss the unfortunately common coach who can't understand why athletes are not picking up the skills being taught; one who often refers to the athletes as being uncoachable. This implies that the coach does not consider or is not even aware of his/her role in the athlete's development. While Potrac and Cassidy offer only anecdotal evidence of the problems caused by coaches who lack pedagogical knowledge, other work offers some level of empirical evidence. For example, when investigating the DM of expert coaches in planning and running a coaching session, Collins et al (2003) found that, out of a sample of 13 coaches, only one explicitly referred to considering the educational environment when describing how they planned a recorded coaching session. Interestingly and more positively, however, when talking through their sessions, all of the same coaches did refer to at least one of the following learning-focused constructs: retention and transfer, player understanding and/or the need to introduce difficulties to the learner. This would suggest that the pedagogical element in session planning is being considered in a tacit or semitacit manner – in other words, the need for these forms of learning environment is so automated that the coaches do not actively consider them in planning a session. While it is important to note that the pedagogical practice of these coaches was being directed by learning ideas that would equate well with learning literature, the lack of explicit thinking about the area would make it difficult to reflect on this element of their practice, or discuss it with other coaches.

A further study by Abraham & Collins (2006) investigated the problem-solving skills of a group of athletics coaches. In this study, groups of event-specific coaches were given the following scenario, with the scenario contextualized to the specific event:

> You have a situation where a talented 14-year-old athlete has an ongoing technical problem causing poor:
>
> - stride rate in the 800M *or*
> - take off and sequencing in the triple jump *or*
> - start out of the blocks and first 20 m in a 100 m sprint/sprint hurdles *or*
> - consistency in throwing distance in the javelin.
>
> What would you do to resolve the problem?

Initial approaches to solving the problem were focused on what the athlete was doing wrong and why, with justifications made through reference to sport-specific and -ology models. In contrast, however, there was very little reference to examining the role to be played subsequently by the coach in developing and administering an appropriate learning environment – findings that support the anecdotal evidence from Potrac & Cassidy (2006). When each of the focus groups was specifically prompted to discuss what they would do in a typical session designed to resolve the problem, there was once again a lack of declarative reasoning to drill design and communication methods. The interventions discussed would often rely on constraining the environment in a way that would logically lead to and behaviourally reinforce the correct technique but not, significantly, on what active interactional strategies could be used with the learner. While there is evidence that supports the use of a constraints-based approach (e.g. Davids et al 2008) in designing practices, the depth of understanding revealed by these coaches was more based on treating the athlete as a passive participant who was part of an 'if–then' relationship that would lead to the required behaviour. These approaches had more to do with the consistent and solution-focused drills discussed by Schmidt & Wriseberg (2004) than a process where the athlete would be an active self-determined participant in their own discovery learning.

Of course, at a certain level these methods are effective. For example, they can often lead to short-term and rapid changes in behaviour (see our earlier comments regarding the difference between learning potential and learning), but they can also prolong ongoing technical problems, as little genuine learning (a relatively permanent and observable change in behaviour) actually occurs (Schmidt & Bjork 1992). This didn't seem to be a consideration for the coaches in the Abraham study described above, however. In fact, some coaches wanted to go straight to drill design before any real consideration of the factors underpinning the scenario; in essence, trying to solve the problem before they had understood it. Again, this would be reflective of our own experiences in coach education, where novice and even some quite experienced coaches often want to dive straight in, designing drills before spending any significant time working on the aims and goals of a session, a series of sessions or even a longer-term plan from an individual, sport-specific or pedagogical point of view.

A further series of studies completed by Morgan (2006) with football academy coaches identified a number of pertinent findings. For example, Morgan found that the content of feedback provided to players was delivered on a 2:1 ratio of general non-informational to specific informational feedback. While similar findings have been found in behavioural observation literature, the more important finding from Morgan's work was that, irrespective of the skill acquisition value (or lack thereof) of their feedback, coaches were not even aware of their differing use of the different types. Furthermore, while significant probing did reveal that the coaches had a semi-awareness of the effect the differing approaches to feedback could have (mirroring Abraham et al's 2006 ideas that much of a coach's behaviour operates at a semitacit level), there was certainly no explicit planning relating to the use of feedback or the impact that this would have on an athlete's development. Interestingly, most of the coaches had a greater awareness of their use of questioning; however, only a minority had a specific understanding of how and why this tool could enhance athlete learning. The remaining coaches viewed questioning as a method to test players as opposed to encouraging problem solving, cognitive development and transfer. Irrespective of their understanding of how and why questioning works, none of the coaches referred to any strategic approach to planning for, delivering and critiquing learning environments.

More encouragingly, Smith & Cushion (2006), in a similar fashion to Morgan (2006), investigated the behaviours and cognitions of academy football coaches in the UK. In this instance, however, the setting was in-game as opposed to training behaviours. This study showed that these coaches had indeed considered the effect their behaviour would have on the learning of their athletes, providing excellent insight into the way good coaches are very rarely cognitively silent even if their behaviour is! Smith & Cushion (2006) deductively ascribed the behaviours and cognitions of these coaches to taking a constructivist approach to athlete learning, such that athletes must be allowed to develop their own knowledge and skills through a structured and live learning process. However, in common with the Collins et al (2003) study, there are no reported findings relating to the DM used by the coaches to shape the learning environment and whether their approach would change dependent on the context of the games. Irrespective of this, any lack of a priori DM would reduce the likelihood of self-analysis after the event. In fact a contradiction is revealed in the reported cognitions and behaviour. The coaches reported a wish to get players to 'work things out for themselves and to learn through the experience'. Yet a level of importance was attached to using pre-instruction in order to pre-empt mistakes happening, essentially limiting the athletes' ability to learn from their mistakes. Interestingly, coach participants from Martindale et al's (2007) study examining effective talent development environments revealed an opposite inclination: to try and avoid using pre-emptive instructions in order to more effectively achieve this 'think for yourself' goal.

While such contradictions are always going to be observable in coaching, as in other non-exact sciences (Abraham & Collins 1998b), we should not necessarily be trying to work out who is right and who is wrong. Rather, the focus should be on examining the DM processes and underpinning rationale that leads to such behaviour. In general terms, where there is an obvious and explicit DM process that draws on a knowledge base influenced by relevant theory, evidence and experience, then the solution and resulting behaviour are likely to be of higher quality than if the solution was informed by only one or two of these sources (Strean et al 1997). Furthermore, an explicit DM process is more likely to be associated with the use of a more critically informed approach. For example, even though a constructivist approach was ascribed to the coaches' approach in the Smith & Cushion (2006) study, at no point did the authors suggest that such a philosophical/theoretical underpinning was identified by the coaches – so was there a thorough DM process and rationale leading to the behaviour of the coaches or was it guess work or experientially gained, belief-led DM?

Is this problem really a problem?

An obvious question at this point may be: does it matter what approach is being taken so long as goals are being reached? The evidence supplied so far suggests that the coaches from the Smith & Cushion (2006) study were certainly using a worthwhile and conscientious approach to athlete development, which appeared to tie in with pedagogical ideas of constructivism or empowerment/athlete-centred learning (Kidman et al 2005). In the light of this clear progress and commitment to empowerment, it may seem a little churlish to criticize/critique the practice of these coaches. In response, however, we would return to the argument that, in the absence of an explicit DM process and an accessible theoretical and empirical knowledge base, reflective practice must rely heavily, if not exclusively, on experientially based interpretations, thus limiting the explanatory power of that reflective process. Furthermore, as mentioned earlier, the absence of such declarative knowledge also limits the coach's ability to develop their own innovative new teaching and learning approaches.

Finally, and as previously mentioned, we are promoting the metacognitive (i.e. thinking about why you think/behave the way you do) approach and associated/consequent cognition and behaviour, which is increasingly acknowledged as a characteristic of superior performance. Coaches involved in both the Smith & Cushion (2006) and the Collins et al (2003) studies all identified general approaches that sit well with theoretical ideas of learning, albeit there was an apparent lack of depth to their explanations. However, these were all high-quality coaches, most of whom were graduates, which led Smith and Cushion (2006, p. 364) to eloquently ask 'whether their behaviour and their ability to *intellectualize* the coaching process in this way would be common to all coaches working at this level within sport?'

As revealed at the beginning of this section, we are by no means the first to recognize the problem of transferring pedagogical theory into coal-face practice. However, we would hope that, by examining this problem within a holistic structure, we can gain a better understanding of the challenges facing practitioners and researchers involved in coach education and coaching practice. In summary, while there is still a lack of peer-reviewed studies examining the development of learning environments in situ (almost certainly exacerbated by the difficulties in achieving methodological consistency and/or transferable messages from both quantitative and qualitative studies), the weight of evidence available suggests a generic problem in pedagogical reasoning, problem solving, planning and delivery for coaches across the spectra of activity, qualification level and athlete age/abilities.

Addressing the pedagogy problem

Given such a problem, our intention is to transfer research from the skill acquisition domain into a usable form for coaches. To do this we often utilize a 'toolbox' of applied learning tools, the goal being that, when a coach plans a session (micro), a month of sessions (meso) or a longer term plan (macro), they have an explicit DM process that can integrate the pedagogical element with the sport-specific and athlete elements of Figures 15.3 and 15.4. In short, the toolbox offers a 'rough guide' on what to do and why in the pedagogy area.

Structuring the toolbox

Bowes & Jones (2006) identified that coaches spend a great deal of their time working at the edge of chaos. The coaching environment is affected by so many factors that developing a systematic, 'production line'-like approach is simply impossible. In our experience, coaches typically take one of two approaches to dealing with this problem: to control the chaos through a very rigid and autocratic approach or, as advocated by Jones & Wallace (2006), to work with the chaos to facilitate an optimized pathway. Ultimately, the second of these two approaches must surely be the goal of coach education. The first does offer a quieter life, but only the second approach will develop athletes who are equally able to deal with the chaos encountered in performance environments. In order to work with potentially chaotic environments, coaches must be able to make decisions that are based on a fine balance of pros and cons. As previously indicated, we know from expert coaches (Abraham et al 2006) that their courses of action are always based on a compromise or 'best fit possible'. So, when making coaching decisions, all coaches should be aware of the pros and cons, and be prepared to justify what they are doing against an awareness of other alternatives.

But how is this complex and intricate metacognitive skill achieved? We have already discussed how a number of broad procedural rules or concepts can be used to structure educational environments to guide planning and reflective practices. It is into this structure that more in-depth declarative knowledge gained from experience and other sources (written text, workshops, etc.) can be integrated, thus establishing an understanding that links theory and research to a coach's own beliefs and ultimately the chaotic 'swampy lowlands' of practice. So, for example, Figure 15.3 is designed to give a theoretically valid, broad procedural overview to the coaching process that is designed to guide the initial planning and reflective (both in and on action; Gilbert & Trudel 2005) processes of coach DM. The toolbox (Fig. 15.5) offered has been designed to take this overview to a deeper level of knowledge, by structuring a tool within the pedagogical domain that is based around three further broad rules.

- Make the content as personally relevant for the performer as possible – for example, how does it tie in with their development plan?
- Promote understanding whenever you can, especially when working towards long-term development – for example, does the performer know why they are doing what they are doing? Do you need to check?
- For rapid short-term results make the session (mentally) easy for your performer, for long-term development make it harder.

Each of these rules is then associated with further in-depth procedural and declarative knowledge in the form of the coaching tools.

Several key ideas were used to identify the tools that should be included within the toolbox. The first

Whilst using these tools try to remember the **three golden rules** of developing a learning environment:

1. Make the content as **personally relevant** for your player as possible – for example, does it tie in with their development plan?
2. Promote player **understanding** whenever you can, especially when working towards long-term development. For example, does the player know why they are doing what they are doing? Do you need to check?
3. For **rapid short-term** results make the session (mentally) easy for your player, for long-term development make it harder. Consider the continuum overleaf.

1 Knowing Your Player-K • Aids development of an effective coaching relationship • Helps coach understand desires and wants of the player • Used in an ongoing fashion helps coach understand lifestyle and circumstances of player • Individualization of information - therefore greater effect • Enables information to meet the expressed needs of learners	**2 Assessment-A** **Formal assessment best when:** • Objective - quantifiable • Specific to goals • Individualized Informal assessment is a constant process, so good for: • Keeping coaching directed towards player's needs	**3 Goal Setting-G** **Recognized as being a major tool to improve motivation** Goals should be • Short and intermediate term goals which provide a logical progression toward a realistic long-term goal. **Any goal set should be:** • Objective and/or quantifiable • Individualized – Is your player able to achieve the goals set? Are there sub goals that also need setting? Does the player agree with the goal? • Situation specific: Time of year, practice or match, matched to developmental requirements • Consistently reviewed so that progress is reinforced	**4 Physical Guidance-PG** **Good for** • Getting the idea of a movement • Developing the 'correct feel' • Prevents information overload **Against** • Provides a crutch for the player • Inhibits the player's problem solving • Little use if the player is totally passive when being guided; ask them to resist the movement a little **BE CAREFUL** • Be aware of child protection issues
5 Verbal Instruction-I • This is the preferred approach for many learners as they are used to being told what to do • When instructing a technique emphasize: 1.Sequencing of the technique 2.Timing of the technique • When instructing on game play/tactics emphasize: 1.Structure/whole game sense 2.Where current tactic fits in **But** • Be careful not to always provide a constant 'answer' to problems • Consider using **Tool - QA** **If used incorrectly** • Overload of **I** can confuse your player • Keep to a maximum of 3 or 4 key points	**6 Demonstration-** **Expert Demo DE** Performed by coach, and good for • Short tern effect and rapid skill acquisition – gives an overall idea of what is required • Focusing attention, and motivation **Negative Demo DN** Demo of wrong technique, good for: • Increasing awareness of weakness • Improving understanding of what was done well and what needs to be changed • Consider using with QA instead of Feedback to promote problem solving	**6 Coping Demonstration CD** Players watch each other, with a structured purpose and attention directed to specific elements of a technique or section of play • Useful when coaching groups • Helps promote and check the understanding of the observer • Can increase confidence in non-threatening environment • Encourages self and peer coaching (buddy coaching) • Consider use in conjunction with QA, i.e. direct the player to a certain aspect of the demonstration and ask them for a description of what they saw	**7 Question and Answer-QA** Obtaining a considered and accurate answer from your player can: • Test and improve understanding • Provide an alternative to tools I and KR/KP • Emphasize and improve the DM process • Increase player self-confidence • Promote problem solving • Focus attention • Generate, secure and use player's own 'language' But avoid excessive and inappropriate use. • Can the player provide an answer? • Do you have time to ask?

Fig. 15.5 • The coaching toolbox. Identifying three golden rules of pedagogical rules to guide pedagogical decision making and ten coaching tools to support the decision-making process and subsequent practice. Note: the version of the toolbox reproduced here was designed for use in tennis. Coaches and coach educators should feel free to modify it for their own performance environment.

(Continued)

8 Command Words-C	9 Feedback-KP/KR	10 Practice-P
Word/phrase association with a movement or series of movements. **Good for** • Reducing complex instructions • Being used in association with **Tool-PP** • Can be used by coach and or player • Increasing understanding and so learning **Against** When used as feedback - not specific enough - reduces learning	**Informational (Can be verbal, visual or 'feel' based)** • About what he or she is doing **correctly** (try to avoid only saying good, excellent etc. Why was it good or excellent?) • Provides reinforcement to continue making successful attempts • About what he or she is doing **incorrectly** • Becomes the basis for trying to make some adjustments on the next practice attempt through the use of **Instruction** • Enhances acquisition of the skill • Time saver = increased efficiency • Can address whole or part of the skill **Motivational** • Lets the learner know that they are improving/progressing towards set goals Tool **G**, even when improvement is not detectable by the learner watching their own performance = Continue to Practice • Provides Competence information - helps to increase self-esteem BUT Consider **how much** feedback is given and **when** it is given • **More** feedback encourages quick improvements as the coach solves performance blocks • **Less** feedback may slow acquisition but can encourage player problem solving (especially if prompted by the coach). Good for retention and transfer • **Immediate** feedback allows for quick change • **Delayed** feedback can promote considered thinking by the player Consider using Tool 5 **QA** as an alternative (i.e. instead of telling the player how well they did ask them how well they thought they did and even what they think they need to do next time) **Problem** Too much feedback results in overload (the learner feels too busy) and may cause dependence on the coach, thus discouraging problem solving • Keep to a maximum of 3 or 4 key points	**WPW - Whole Part Whole** • Try to make sure the player knows where the part fits in with the 'big picture' to maintain meaningfulness • Practise whole skill early in process. • Break down the skill only into meaningful units **Random/Distributed./Variable PRDV** (More Challenging for Player) **Random:** several skills practised randomly in one drill **Distributed:** skill practised in short bursts – i.e. 10 mins on drill 1 then 10 mins on drill 2 then return to drill 1; encourages players to retrieve from previous attempts. Intervening time can be increased to make retrieval process harder **Variable:** one skill practised in a variety of ways All three can be mixed to create one drill – often forming constrained games **Good/Appropriate for** • Long-term development as it encourages the player to think for themselves and/or develop skills that are adaptable and transferable • Talented or experienced players • Training for match play/transfer **Blocked/Massed/Structured PBMS** (Mentally Easier For Player) **Blocked:** several skills practised in blocks (1-1-1, 2-2-2, 3-3-3) **Massed:** skill practised for long period of time **Structured:** skill practised in a very controlled way **Good/Appropriate for** • Rapid improvements as the player can get in a 'groove' but note that if they fall out of the groove or have even small amounts of time where the skill isn't practised the rapid improvement can disappear quickly • Beginners & younger players • Early gains provides motivation **BUT** • Can quickly become boring **Overlearning PO** Continued practice after a skill has been learnt • Grooves technique • Possibly Stress resistant techniques N.B. Overlearning = up to 100% of learning time

Fig. 15.5—Cont'd

(Continued)

SHORT TERM	CONTINUUM	LONG TERM
Expert demonstration	versus	Coping demonstration
More	versus	Less feedback
Instruction	versus	Question and answer
Consistent	versus	Varied practice
Massed	versus	Distributed practice

Fig. 15.5—Cont'd

returns to Figure 15.3, which identifies how the skill development process should consider the sport-specific requirements and individualization of the coaching process. Reflecting this link, tools 1–3 in Figure 13.5 relate to how a coach can develop a positive and individualized coach–athlete relationship through knowing and understanding the player and planning programmes that are relevant to their needs through appropriate assessment and goal setting.

Tools 4–10 relate much more to the actual skill development environment that a coach will establish. From an experiential and empirical point of view, we know that coaches communicate verbally and non-verbally with athletes and that they design drills and practices (Côté et al 1995b) that draw on these two modalities. Consequently, it is these two approaches, *communication* and *physical practice*, that form the basis of a coach's approach to skill acquisition in training settings. In keeping with the message throughout this chapter, though, we needed to declaratively unpack these two ideas. What is communication? What is physical practice? How do they relate to athletes acquiring skill and learning?

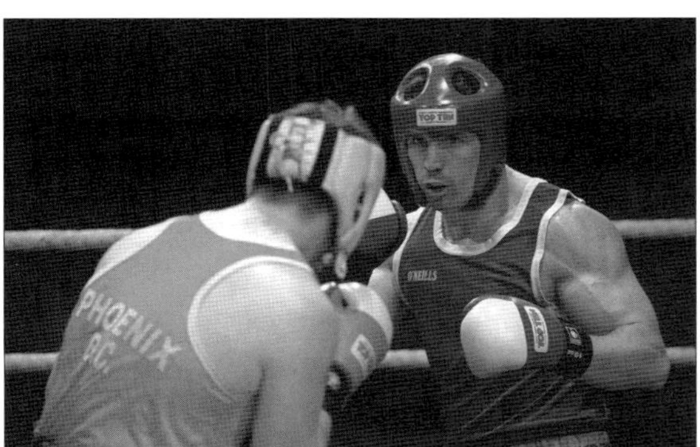

Pressure is never much greater than in combat sports. John Kiely maintains composure at the National Championships. Photo © Sportsfile. Reprinted with kind permission.

A review of coach behaviour research (e.g. Claxton 1988, Smith & Smoll 1996) reveals that coaches use a large range of verbal and non-verbal communication methods. We chose to condense these verbal and non-verbal behaviours into tools 4–9 in Figure 15.5. The additional declarative information included with the tool is sourced from research examining how communication strategies facilitate the acquisition, learning, retention and transfer of cognitive and motor skills. There is obviously only a limited amount of declarative information, but this is deliberate. There is a host of additional information that can be found to further inform a coach's DM process; some is listed as 'further reading' at the end of this chapter and in essence serves as the bibliography used to develop the content of the toolbox

The final tool, *practice*, is probably the most important tool to get right for any coach. It also means that if an athlete consistently practises a 'wrong' technique, that is what will be learned – practice makes permanent. Only perfect practice makes perfect. As coach educators we have watched both novice and experienced coaches preside over coaching sessions where incorrect technique and/or DM has gone unnoticed and unremedied. Again, therefore, we have provided various options for the coach to choose from, depending on what they want their players to achieve from a particular session or set of sessions. It is worth noting here that we have used language associated with the skill acquisition work of authors such as Magill (2007) and Schmidt & Wriseberg (2004). However, there are other approaches to understanding the practice environment such as the games for understanding approach (e.g. Oslin & Mitchell 2006) or dynamical systems approach (e.g. Davids et al 2008) that coaches should investigate in order to identify areas of agreement and difference between the approaches. It is our contention that the information included within this chapter focuses on areas that are broadly agreed upon across the approaches.

Working with the toolbox

Even though we went through a 'condensing process' prior to its development, the toolbox deliberately provides a number of methods of interacting with the athlete in a skill development environment. This is because we know that coaching is a complex process (Bowes & Jones 2006) where there is rarely one right answer (Abraham et al 2006). Consequently, the toolbox needs to help coaches cope with such a dynamic environment, encouraging them to at least consider broader alternatives rather than falling back on the same traditional answer of 'it's worked for me in the past'. However, the sheer number of tools available makes this process potentially daunting to coaches who are new to both coaching and/or the approach espoused by the toolbox. Therefore, and in keeping with the ideas presented earlier in this chapter, we help coaches make sense of this complexity through the provision of three broad procedural rules to guide the selection and use of the tools. We'll go through each of these rules in order to display how they can be applied and how they link to the tools.

'Rule' 1: Make the content as personally relevant as possible. While this is to a large extent self-explanatory, it is worthwhile considering some of the issues delivered in this book. Section 1, for example, emphasizes the individual nature of development and performance. In short, it is extremely unlikely that the learning and development needs of two athletes are going to be exactly the same. Obviously, true individualization of coaching is extremely difficult unless there is a low coach : athlete ratio. However, the more individualization of coaching is set as a goal, the more successful the skill development process will be (Martindale et al 2007, Smith et al 2001). In order to achieve personally relevant content, the coach must know and understand the individuals. There are obvious means of achieving this goal, e.g. simply talking to the athlete about their goals, lifestyle, likes and dislikes (i.e. Tool 1: Knowing your athlete). Furthermore, there are more complex methods within the broad realm of performance analysis (e.g. Hughes & Franks 2004). However, the usefulness of performance analysis is ultimately limited by the knowledge of the coach undertaking this analysis. It is fortunate, therefore, that there is a whole host of texts, both research- and practice-based, that can accurately enhance assessment process (i.e. talent development models; Abbott & Collins 2004, Martindale et al 2007) and performance specifics (e.g. psychology (Orlick & Partington 1988), physiology (Bompa 1999), technique (Knudson & Morrison 2002) and sport-specific (Bangsbo & Peitersen 2004); see Tool 2). Finally, formulating the ideas gained from this assessment process into SMART goals (Tool 3) will promote motivation, optimize progress and help to develop the open and honest relationship that typifies most good coach–athlete teams.

'Rule' 2: Promote performer understanding whenever you can. We have previously identified that declarative knowledge is the knowledge of understanding, and that understanding is crucial for coaches. However, research in sport performance reveals that the same is true for athletes. The most effective athletes have a thorough understanding of their own performance and its effect by and on team mates or opponents (McPherson 1994, Williams & Davids 1995). While there will obviously be times when the coach needs to take control, be authoritarian and tell the player what to do, coaches should mostly, and especially in coaching for long-term development, aim to 'educate' the athlete as much as possible, emphasizing his/her understanding of what is involved and why this is the better option. Such an approach can be achieved through open question and answer (Tool 7) sessions, or enhanced by encouraging buddy coaching using athletes to demonstrate the required skill and asking the watching athletes to learn from and provide feedback on the skill observed (Tool 6: Coping demonstration).

'Rule' 3: For rapid, short-term results make the session (mentally) 'easy' for the player; for longer-term development focused on retention/transfer make it 'harder'. This golden rule is probably the one that requires most explanation in order for the linked tools to make sense. In order to achieve this goal we will draw heavily on a piece of work by Schmidt & Bjork (1992) that was written to summarize key findings in skill acquisition research and stimulate the reader to critically think about how they design learning environments.

Based on a synthesis of varied research findings, Schmidt & Bjork (1992) identified that skill acquisition can (apparently) be speeded up by providing a learning environment that allows repeated attempts at a skill with high levels of feedback. However, retention and transfer tests indicate that these performance increments don't last. In contrast, learning environments that

- decreased repetition;
- increased unpredictability; and
- reduced feedback

slowed the acquisition rate of skills but produced better performance in retention tests (cf. decision training ideas in Ch. 14). The underpinning rationale is that learning occurs through active involvement in a challenging environment where learners are required to think through and solve problems for themselves and/or recall similar solutions to previous problems. In contrast, the rapid performance increments seen in environments characterized by high levels of skill repetition and feedback are more due to the coach setting easy 'questions' and/or providing the answers. There are, however, five important points of clarification required that reflect the 'no right answer' basis of the toolbox.

First, even though easy practice with lots of coach-led problem solving may not encourage learning, the rapid changes in skilled behaviour may provide a useful confidence boost or display the athlete's potential (Vygotsky 1978) to a novice or athlete anxious for a quick fix when there isn't time for the athlete to discover the answer for themselves. By contrast, if things are too easy in the early stages of development, the learner is likely to receive a nasty (and demotivating) shock when the fan clogs up and the genuine difficulties involved become obvious. A 'problems early' approach can often eliminate the low-motivation 'play at it' individuals while facilitating the genuinely interested and committed performer who is there for the long haul.

Second, the term 'challenging environment' needs careful consideration, since what is challenging for one athlete may be easy or even anxiety-producing for another. This becomes a much easier decision once the coach has spent time getting to know their athlete, as suggested in Rule 1.

Third, and following on from the previous point, coaches should consider the variety and intricacy of skills required in their sport, the type and number of decisions required, and the randomness of conditions (task, environmental and personal (Davids et al 2008)) under which all these skills and decisions are produced and made. This should lead the coach to question and consider how much variety and randomness is required in the practices they employ. Furthermore, since learning does not happen immediately, this consideration should take account of the learning environments required over a long period of time and sessions, not just one or two sessions. Perhaps just as importantly, the coach should stick to this plan and avoid, as far as possible (bearing in mind our earlier comments that plans should not be set in stone), firefighting problems that may arise from competition settings, especially if they are working with children or developing athletes. If a programme has been planned properly, the problems that occur in competition settings should already be catered for and will be taken care of in the completion of a programme of learning.

Fourth, developing a random and variable skill environment often means that game-like situations are developed. However, the coach will need to be careful that all participants in these practices actually get to practise the skills required – especially in team sports. For example, Fenoglio (2007) identifies how asking young football players to engage in games any larger than 5 v 5 will lead to many players not actually getting enough touches of the ball to effect learning. In fact, Fenoglio (2007) recommends that, for children under 12, small-side games of; 3 v 3, 4 v 4 or 5 v 5 are probably optimal in terms of creating an environment where a balance of technical and tactical skills is developed. It may also be worth asking if one or two sessions a week are enough for skill development to occur or whether homework is required.

Fifth, research in talent development (Abbott & Collins 2004, Martindale et al 2007) clearly identifies that expert coaches are concerned with developing their athletes' ability to become effective, self-aware and self-reinforcing learners. Consequently, the long-term approach to skill acquisition refers as much to developing learning and mental skills in the athletes as it does to getting the athlete to practise the full range of skills needed to cope with variable and random performance environments, be they a game of tag or an Olympic final.

To summarize, therefore, the third golden rule should lead to coaches asking questions of themselves along the lines of:

- what and how many problems am I providing in this learning environment?
- are the problems specific to the needs of my athletes?
- who is solving the problems, me or the athletes? and
- have I taught my athletes how to solve problems?

If there are few problems in the practice environment (i.e. a structured practice) and lots of problem solving being done by the coach through feedback and instruction, a 'short-term benefits' environment is likely to be in place. If, by contrast, there are multiple problems in the practice environment (i.e. random and variable practice) with minimal help from the coach, then a long-term learning environment will result.

Finally, while we have identified 'short-term' and 'long-term' approaches to skill development, there is, as identified in Figure 13.5, a continuum between short- and long-term approaches. The application of this continuum can, in essence, become the 'art' of coaching, which mixes and matches communication strategies with approaches to practice design in order to set a learning environment that is appropriate for the athlete and the achievement of their individual goals. For example, a random practice supported with lots of problem-solving feedback from the coach, or using a previously successful practice with only minimal input from the coach, thus encouraging the athletes to recall prior successful performances (distributed practice), are both examples of how a coach can mix and match 'short-term' tools with 'long-term' tools in order to decrease and/or increase the challenge or 'mental workload' on the athlete. In an ideal world, such decisions should/would be made in accordance with the goals of that athlete, the state of the athlete and the time frame within which a change in skill is required. Typically however, we would hope that coaches, especially those working with athletes who are not operating at an elite level, would be guided by a need to encourage learning as opposed to meeting short-term performance goals. Our experience would suggest that this may require a substantial change in coaches' attitude and behaviour.

Common vocabulary

The final consideration within the design of the toolbox is that, even though most behavioural studies illustrate that coaches are already using most of the tools described, research (e.g. Côté et al 1995a) has also highlighted that coaches may not actually be aware of these tools beyond the idea of 'communication' (Morgan 2006). The toolbox is, therefore, also useful in distinguishing between different methods of communication and practice design and the effects that these methods can have. While educating coaches in the functional jargon included in the toolbox may seem to be intuitively good practice, there is another powerful knock-on effect. If all coaches begin to plan the 'pedagogical' aspect of their sessions using the same vocabulary, they can also reflect/think critically using the same vocabulary. This becomes all the more powerful if the reflection is based on the reality of their practice. Our experience has been that getting coaches to analyse their own behaviour through video, using the golden rules and the individual tools of the toolbox, can prove to be a truly enlightening and developmental experience. In addition to this form of self analysis, the toolbox can also prove effective in coaches checking ideas and practice with colleagues. At present this is difficult for coaches to do in the pedagogical area since there is currently no comprehensive and accurate common vocabulary used by coaches in this domain (Lyle 2002). As a result, discussions between coaches referring to coaching performance tend to centre on 'drills' and the content of drills, i.e. techniques or tactics developed. In addition, these will almost certainly be judged heavily on the successfulness of athlete performance in the drill, leading to a short-term approach. Encouraging a philosophy of peer critiquing against the framework of the toolbox can aid the development of a truly functional community of practice among coaches (Culver & Trudel 2006).

Conclusion

Our aim at the beginning of this chapter was to offer some procedural advice in tandem with declarative explanations in order to help practitioners understand and better develop learning environments so as to subsequently achieve more effective skill development. We provided three linked models of the coaching process in Figures 15.1, 15.3 and 15.4 to display how having and applying a knowledge of the athlete, the sport and the learning environment can lead to a holistic approach to problem setting and solving. Our argument is that taking such an approach can lead to a more comprehensive approach to skill development – this would certainly be backed up by the coaches in the Abraham et al (2006) study.

We also provided evidence from a number of sources that identified how there was an apparent problem with the problem solving and DM of coaches within the 'understand the learning environment' domain. So, while very good coaches appeared to be working to useful conceptual ideas, their lack of declarative knowledge in this area was probably limiting their capacity to be innovative in developing their own bespoke effective learning environments. The logical conclusion from this finding was that this problem is even worse with not-so-good coaches. All this evidence pointed to the need for some level of intervention that introduced declarative knowledge in the area of skill acquisition that didn't simply resort to suggesting that coaches should read a range of journal articles or text books. Consequently, we provided a toolbox of behaviours that coaches are known to use but linked these with introductory declarative ideas of skill acquisition and associated 'golden rules' to guide the use and implementation of these tools. The suggestion is that once coaches have become comfortable with this level of theory they may then wish to engage more with journal articles and text books identified in the 'further reading' associated with the toolbox.

Consequently, our ultimate aim is to encourage coaches and athletes to improve their own declarative understanding of skill development such that they develop their own procedural guidelines and perhaps even critique those supplied by us as authors. In fact, our aim is very much in keeping with the proverb: 'Give a man a fish and feed him for a day, teach a man to fish and feed him for a lifetime'. We hope you don't starve as a result of reading this chapter!

Further reading for toolbox

Bjork, R.A., 1993. Memory and metamemory considerations in the training of human beings. In: Metcalfe, J., Shimamura, A.P. (Eds.), Metacognition: knowing about knowing. MIT Press, Cambridge, MA.

Chambers, K.L., Vickers, J.N., 2006. Effects of bandwidth feedback and questioning on the performance of competitive swimmers. Sport Psychologist 20, 184–197.

Christina, R.W., Bjork, R.A., 1991. Optimizing long term retention and transfer. In: Druckman, D., Bjork, R. A. (Eds.), In the mind's eye: enhancing human performance. National Academy Press, Washington, DC, pp. 23–56.

Davids, K., Button, C., Bennett, S., 2008. Dynamics of skill acquisition – a constraints led approach. Human Kinetics, Champaign, IL.

Griffin, L.L., Butler, J.I. (Eds.), 2005. Teaching games for understanding. Human Kinetics, Champaign, IL.

Hodges, N.J., Franks, I.M., 2002. Modelling coaching practice: the role of instruction and demonstration. J. Sports Sci. 20, 793–811.

McCullagh, P., Weiss, M.R., 2001. Modelling: considerations for motor skill performance and psychological responses. In: Singer, R.N., Hausenblas, H.A., Janelle, C.M. (Eds.), Handbook of sport psychology. John Wiley, New York, pp. 205–238.

Magill, R.A., 2007. Motor learning: concepts and applications, eighth ed. McGraw Hill, New York.

Oslin, J., Mitchell, S., 2006. Game-centred approaches to teaching physical education. In: Kirk, D., Macdonald, D., O'Sullivan, M. (Eds.), The handbook of physical education. Sage Publications, London, pp. 627–651.

Schmidt, R.A., Bjork, R.A., 1992. New conceptualizations of practice: common principles in three paradigms suggest new concepts for training. Psychol. Sci. 3, 207–217.

Schmidt, R.A., Wriseberg, C., 2004. Motor learning and performance, third ed. Human Kinetics, Champaign, IL.

References

Abbott, A., Collins, D., 2004. Eliminating the dichotomy between theory and practice in talent identification and development: considering the role of psychology. J. Sports Sci. 22, 395–408.

Abraham, A., 2006. Star letter: why am I teaching this and why is it useful to a coaching student? Sport and Exercise Scientist 9, 26.

Abraham, A., Collins, D., 1998a. Declarative and procedural knowledge assessment in novice and intermediate coaches. J. Sports Sci. 16, 70.

Abraham, A., Collins, D., 1998b. Examining and extending research in coach development. Quest 50, 59–79.

Abraham, A., Collins, D., 2006. Problem solving and DM by athletics coaches: it wasn't me. Bell College Research Conference, Hamilton, Bell College, Hamilton, Lanarkshire.

Abraham, A., Collins, D., Martindale, R., 2006. The coaching schematic: validation through expert coach consensus. J. Sports Sci. 24, 549–564.

Anderson, J.R., 1982. Acquisition of a cognitive skill. Psychol. Rev. 89, 369–406.

Anderson, J.R., 1987. Skill acquisition: compilation of weak-method problem solutions. Psychol. Rev. 94, 192–210.

Anderson, J.R., 1990. Cognitive psychology and its implications, third ed. Freeman, New York.

Armour, K., 2004. Coaching pedagogy. In: Cassidy, T., Jones, R., Potrac, P. (Eds.), Understanding sports coaching: the social, cultural and pedagogical foundations of coaching practice. Routledge, Abingdon, Oxfordshire, pp. 84–115.

Bailey, R., Morley, D., 2006. Towards a model of talent development in physical education. Sport Education and Society 11, 211–230.

Balyi, I., 2002. Long term athlete development: the system and solutions. Faster Higher Stronger January 9–12.

Bangsbo, J., Peitersen, B., 2004. Offensive soccer tactics. Human Kinetics, Champaign, IL.

Berliner, D.C., 1991. Educational psychology and pedagogical expertise: new findings and new opportunities for thinking about training. Educational Psychologist 26, 145–155.

Biggs, J.B., Collis, K.F., 1982. Evaluating the quality of learning: the solo taxonomy (structure of the observed learning outcome). Academic Press, Sydney, New South Wales.

Bompa, T.O., 1999. Periodization: theory and methodology of training, fourth ed. Human Kinetics, Champaign, IL.

Bowes, I., Jones, R., 2006. Working at the edge of chaos. Understanding coaching as a complex interpersonal system. Sport Psychologist 20, 235–245.

Calderhead, J., 1996. Teachers: beliefs and knowledge. In: Berliner, D.C., Calfree, R. (Eds.), Handbook of educational psychology. Macmillan, New York, pp. 709–725.

Chambers, K.L., Vickers, J.N., 2006. Effects of bandwidth feedback and questioning on the performance of competitive swimmers. Sport Psychologist 20, 184–197.

Chen, A., Hancock, G.R., 2006. Conceptualizing a theoretical model for school-centered adolescent physical activity intervention research. Quest 58, 355–376.

Claxton, D.B., 1988. A systematic observation of successful and less successful high school tennis coaches. Journal of Teaching in Physical Education 7, 302–310.

Collins, D., Abraham, A., Martindale, R., 2003. Coaching research technical report. United Kingdom Sports Institute, London.

Côté, J., Salmela, J., Russell, S., 1995a. The knowledge of high performance gymnastic coaches: competition and training considerations. Sport Psychologist 9, 76–95.

Côté, J., Salmela, J., Trudel, P., et al., 1995b. The coaching model: a grounded assessment of expert gymnastic coaches' knowledge. Journal of Sport and Exercise Psychology 17, 1–17.

Côté, J., Baker, J., Abernethy, B., 2003. From play to practice: a developmental framework for the acquisition of expertise in team sports. In: Starkes, J.L., Ericsson, K.A. (Eds.), Expert performance in sports. Human Kinetics, Champaign, IL, pp. 89–135.

Côté, J., Young, B., North, J., et al., 2007. Towards a definition of excellence in sport coaching. International Journal of Coaching Science 1, 3–17.

Culver, D.M., Trudel, P., 2006. Cultivating coaches' communities of practice: developing the potential for learning through interactions. In: Jones, R. (Ed.), The sports coach as educator. Routledge, Abingdon, Oxfordshire, pp. 97–112.

Cushion, C.J., 2007. Modelling the complexity of the coaching process. International Journal of Sport Science and Coaching 2, 395–401.

Cushion, C.J., Armour, K., Jones, R., 2006. Locating the coaching process in practice: models 'for' and 'of' coaching. Physical Education and Sport Pedagogy 11, 83–99.

Davids, K., Button, C., Bennett, S., 2008. Dynamics of skill acquisition – a constraints led approach. Human Kinetics, Champaign, IL.

Davies, S.P., 1994. Knowledge restructuring and the acquisition of programming expertise. International Journal of Human-Computer Studies 40, 703–726.

Fenoglio, R., 2007. A neuro-physiological basis for developing future skilful players. Available online at: http://www.footy4kids.co.uk/developing_skilful_players.htm (accessed 17.03.09).

Gilbert, W.D., Trudel, P., 2001. Learning to coach through experience: reflection in model youth sport coaches. Journal of Teaching in Physical Education 21, 16–34.

Gilbert, W., Trudel, P., 2004a. Analysis of coaching science research published from 1970–2001. Res. Q. Exerc. Sport 75, 388–399.

Gilbert, W.D., Trudel, P., 2004b. Role of the coach: how model youth team sport coaches frame their roles. Sport Psychologist 18, 21–43.

Gilbert, W.D., Trudel, P., 2005. Learning to coach through experience: Conditions that influence reflection. Physical Educator 62, 32–43.

Haywood, K., Getchell, N., 2005. Life span motor development, fourth ed. Human Kinetics, Champaign, IL.

Hughes, M.D., Franks, I.M., 2004. Notational analysis of sport – better systems for improving coaching and performance, second ed. E & FN Spon, London.

Johnson, P.E., Duran, A., Hassebrock, F., et al., 1981. Expertise and error in diagnostic reasoning. Cogn. Sci. 5, 235–283.

Jones, R., Turner, P., 2006. Teaching coaches to coach holistically: can Problem-Based Learning (PBL) help? Physical Education and Sport Pedagogy 11, 181–202.

Jones, R., Wallace, M., 2006. The coach as 'orchestrator': more realistically managing the complex coaching context. In: Jones, R. (Ed.), The sports coach as educator: reconceptualising sports coaching. Routledge, Abingdon, Oxfordshire, pp. 51–64.

Jones, R., Armour, K., Potrac, P., 2004. Sport coaching cultures: from practice to theory. Routledge, London.

Kidman, L., Thorpe, R., Hatfield, D., 2005. Athlete-centred coaching: developing inspired and inspiring coaches. Innovative Print Communications, Christchurch, New Zealand.

Knudson, D., Morrison, C., 2002. Qualitative analysis of human movement. Human Kinetics, Champaign, IL.

Lewin, K., 1952. Field theory in social science: selected theoretical papers by Kurt Lewin. Tavistock, London.

Lyle, J., 2002. Sports coaching concepts: a framework for coaches' behaviour. Routledge, London.

McPherson, S.L., 1994. The development of sport expertise: mapping the tactical domain. Quest 46, 23–41.

Magill, R.A., 2007. Motor learning: concepts and applications, eighth ed. McGraw Hill, New York.

Martindale, A., Collins, D., 2007. Enhancing the evaluation of effectiveness with professional judgement and decision making. Sport Psychologist 21, 458–474.

Martindale, R., Collins, D., Abraham, A., 2007. Effective talent development: the elite coach perspective in UK sport. Journal of Applied Sport Psychology 19, 187–206.

Morgan, G., 2006. Coaching behaviours and players' motivation in elite youth football. Sport and Exercise Sciences. PhD Thesis, Loughborough University, Loughborough, Leicestershire.

Nash, C., Collins, D., 2006. Tacit knowledge in expert coaching: science or art? Quest 58, 464–476.

Nelson, L.J., Cushion, C.J., 2006. Coach education, reflection and learning from experience: the case of the national governing body coaching certificate. Sport Psychologist 20, 172–181.

O'Neill, P., Willis, S., Jones, A., 2002. A model of how students link problem-based learning with clinical experience through 'elaboration. Acad. Med. 77, 552–561.

Orlick, T.D., Partington, J., 1988. Mental links to excellence. Sport Psychologist 2, 105–130.

Oslin, J., Mitchell, S., 2006. Game-centred approaches to teaching physical education. In: Kirk, D., Macdonald, D., O'Sullivan, M. (Eds.), The handbook of physical education. Sage Publications, London, pp. 627–651.

Pennington, N., Nicolich, R., Rahm, J., 1995. Transfer of training between cognitive subskills: is knowledge use specific. Cogn. Psychol. 28, 175–224.

Perry, W.G., 1988. Different worlds in the same classroom. In: Ramsden, P. (Ed.), Improving learning: new perspectives. Kogan Page, London, pp. 145–161.

Potrac, P., Cassidy, T., 2006. The coach as 'a more capable other. In: Jones, R. (Ed.), The sports coach as educator. Routledge, Abingdon, Oxfordshire, pp. 39–50.

Potrac, P., Brewer, C., Jones, R., et al., 2000. Toward a holistic understanding of the coaching process. Quest 52, 186–199.

Reber, A.S., 1985. Dictionary of psychology. Penguin, Harmondsworth, Middlesex.

Reber, A.S., 1993. Implicit learning and tacit knowledge: an essay on the cognitive unconscious. Oxford University Press, New York.

Rutt-Leas, R., Chi, M.T.H., 1993. Analyzing diagnostic expertise of competitive swimming coaches. In: Starkes, J.L., Allard, F. (Eds.), Cognitive issues in motor expertise. Elsevier, Amsterdam, pp. 75–94.

Saury, J., Durand, M., 1998. Practical knowledge in expert coaches: on site study of coaching in sailing. Res. Q. Exerc. Sport 69, 254–266.

Schempp, P.G., McCullick, B., Mason, I.S., 2006. The development of expert coaching. In: Jones, R. (Ed.), The sports coach as educator: Re-conceptualising sports coaching. Routledge, London, pp. 145–161.

Schmidt, R.A., Bjork, R.A., 1992. New conceptualizations of practice: common principles in three paradigms suggest new concepts for training. Psychol. Sci. 3, 207–217.

Schmidt, R.A., Wriseberg, C., 2004. Motor learning and performance, third ed. Human Kinetics, Champaign, IL.

Smith, M., Cushion, C.J., 2006. An investigation of the in-game behaviours of professional, top-level youth soccer coaches. J. Sports Sci. 24, 355–366.

Smith, R.E., Smoll, F.L., 1996. Behavioral assessment and interventions in youth sport. Behav. Modif. 20, 3–44.

Smith, N., Bellamy, M., Collins, D., et al., 2001. A test of the processing efficiency theory in a team sport context. J. Sports Sci. 19, 321–332.

Strean, W.B., Senecal, K.L., Howlett, S.G., et al., 1997. Xs and Os and what the coach knows: improving team strategy through critical thinking. Sport Psychologist 11, 243–256.

Thompson, N., 2000. Theory and practice in human services. Open University Press, Buckingham.

Vansteenkiste, M., Sheldon, K.M., 2006. There's nothing more practical than a good theory: integrating motivational interviewing and self-determination theory. Br. J. Clin. Psychol. 45, 63–82.

Vickers, J.N., Reeves, M.A., Chambers, K.L., et al., 2004. Decision training: cognitive strategies for enhancing motor performance. In: Williams, A.M., Hodges, N.J. (Eds.), Skill acquisition in sport: research theory and practice. Routledge, London, pp. 103–120.

Vygotsky, L.S., 1978. Mind in society: the development of higher psychological processes. Harvard University Press, Cambridge, MA.

Weinberg, R.S., Gould, D., 2003. Foundations of sport and exercise psychology, third ed. Human Kinetics, Champaign, IL.

Williams, M., 2006. Whatever happened to motor behaviour? The missing ingredient for Olympic success. Sport and Exercise Scientist June, 15–16.

Williams, M., Davids, K., 1995. Declarative knowledge in sport: a by-product of experience or a characteristic of expertise? Journal of Sport and Exercise Psychology 17, 259–275.

Zeitz, C.M., Spoehr, K.T., 1989. Knowledge organization and the acquisition of procedural expertise. Applied Cognitive Psychology 3, 313–336.

Mental practice: neuroscientific support for a new approach

16

Paul Holmes* Claire Calmels†

*Institute for Performance Research, Manchester Metropolitan University, Crewe, Cheshire, UK; †Institut National du Sport, de l'Expertise et de la Performance, Paris, France

CHAPTER CONTENTS

Introduction

Mental practice techniques continue to be popular for performers in sport, exercise, dance and clinical settings. Typically, the techniques form part of a psychological skills training programme that supports physical or rehabilitative practice, the goal normally being to enhance or maintain performance of a skill or task. Mental practice techniques can take many forms and can focus on different aspects of an individual's mental profile. For example, while one athlete may feel the need to reduce pre-competition worry, others may need to improve attention and concentration skills or experience greater confidence prior to an important event. Applied sport psychology literature has always supported the inclusion of some form of mental practice regime in a performer's training programme.

One technique that persists in applied sport and exercise psychology is imagery (e.g. Morris et al 2005, Murphy et al 2008). Imagery has received considerable academic attention and, according to Short et al (2002), remains one of the most popular intervention techniques delivered by sport psychologists. It has many reported uses: visual rehearsal of a skill; skill learning; strategy development; enhancing confidence; and improving recovery from injury are just a few. Therefore, given the comprehensive research, the prevalence of its use and its perceived importance within the mental skills 'toolkit', it should be expected that there would be detailed and agreed procedures for the delivery of effective imagery interventions. Unfortunately, this does not seem to be the case. Callow & Hardy (2007) have recently provided a critical analysis of applied imagery research. In this, they report what is known, what might be known and what is not known about effective imagery interventions. The authors raise a number of important research questions from the review that suggest that there is still a considerable way to go before imagery can live up to its claim to be the central pillar of sport psychology interventions.

While many individuals attribute their performance to their structured mental practice regimes, a detailed understanding of what practice comprises during imagery remains very much an illusion. By its very nature, mental practice is covert and indefinite; the most detailed, prescriptive imagery programmes cannot predict what performers actually generate in their brains. It is not disputed that imagery and associated mental practice techniques offer benefit to performers through a number of

DOI: 10.1016/B978-0-443-06734-1.00016-X

psychological and/or psychophysiological mechanisms. Theories that have received support include: Lang's (1977) bioinformational theory, Ahsen's (1984) triple code theory, Schmidt's (1982) attention-arousal set theory, Bandura's (1977a, b) self-efficacy/self-confidence theories, Paivio's (1985) motivational theory and, more recently, Jeannerod's (1994) simulation theories. As with many theoretical debates, there are similarities across these theories and, as you would expect, there is evidence that would support all the ideas. However, 'none of the theories... have sufficient research to support them as definitive theories of imagery functioning' (Morris et al 2005, p. 55). As a consequence of these ongoing debates, some authors have suggested that imagery cannot be explained easily by one theory alone and that progress will only be made through the integration of approaches. This idea has also been advocated by Murphy et al (2008). They suggest that imagery investigations should be guided by a new comprehensive model. We would certainly support such ventures but, given the well documented methodological and operational concerns that will always remain with covert techniques, maybe the time has come to use what we know, develop what we might know and explore what we don't know with a different, more overt approach to mental training.

It is our opinion that imagery and associated mental practice techniques will continue to be useful interventions for performers but that their effectiveness will always be compromised by the brain's ability to (re)create an experience that mimics a real experience. Further, the moderators and mediators of imagery effectiveness, highlighted by Callow & Hardy (2007), remain important aspects of research in this area. They include imagery perspective, movement agency, task type, practice conditions and timing. In addition, imager skill expertise, imaging ability, skill confidence and arousal state should also be considered (the reader is referred to Callow & Hardy (2007) for further consideration of some of these variables). Without a greater understanding and control of these and other variables, predictions and applications from the imagery research should continue to be made cautiously.

In this regard, we propose that the best elements of imagery research should be retained and integrated into a new working model of observation for mental practice. We will highlight some of our fundamental concerns with imagery as a sport psychology intervention and suggest that observation-based techniques may be better positioned to meet the goals that imagery advocates. We will introduce neuroscientific research to provide an evidence base to support the development of our observation model.

Analysis of imagery for mental practice interventions

Defining imagery and observation

In order to develop the concept of observation as a valid technique that may operate alongside, or in some cases replace, conventional imagery-type interventions, it is important to define clearly what we mean by the two processes; this is not easy. Morris et al (2005) have highlighted the problems with trying to define the imagery process in a sporting context; they suggest that there is a lack of consistency in the features that constitute the process, stating 'the focus of each definition seems to vary depending on the purpose for which the imagery description is used' (Morris et al 2005, p. 14). Similar problems are evident in the more sparse definitions for observation (see McCullagh & Weiss 2001 p. 221–222). To reflect the neuroscientific focus of our paper and the underlying assumption in some theories that imagery and observation share at least some brain activity with the corresponding physical execution, it would seem appropriate to include reference to this within our working definitions.

> Imagery, in the context of performance, may be considered as the neural activation of a brain representation/neural network involving primarily top-down sensorial, perceptual and affective characteristics that are normally under the conscious control of the imager and which may occur in the absence of perceptual afference functionally equivalent to the actual physical experience.
>
> Holmes & Calmels 2008, p. 433

We contrast the definition of imagery with that of observation.

> Observation, in the context of performance, may be considered as the neural activation of a brain representation/neural network involving primarily bottom-up sensorial, perceptual and affective characteristics, that are primarily under the subconscious control of the observer and which normally occur in the presence of perceptual afference functionally equivalent to the actual physical experience.
>
> Holmes & Calmels 2008, p. 433

Imagery is, therefore, a top-down, knowledge-driven process whereas observation is a bottom up, percept-driven process. What is of interest here is how much these processes truly reflect the neural activity associated with overt behaviours, their ability to influence future behaviour, and how they can be used effectively in performance contexts.

Much of what follows in our discussions will relate to the terminology used in these definitions. We will provide evidence to support a distinction between the processes of imagery and observation in relation to the control afforded to the practitioner and the performer over some of the moderating variables identified above. In this regard, we will also propose that observation offers greater efficacy in terms of access to functional cortical and subcortical neural networks shared with overt behaviour. We do not propose that imagery and observation are in direct competition as interventions, as they too share, in part, similar brain sites. Common sense dictates that there will be times when one technique is more appropriate than another; for example, immediately prior to a performance, imagery may offer far greater flexibility of use than observation simply because the process does not require equipment (i.e. camera, screen). In contrast, during training sessions, observation delivered through portable digital media may be more effective. Therefore, we see their roles as separate although occasionally complementary if there is consideration of some important procedural concerns. Imagery and observation both have the potential to support permanent structural changes in the brain but it is the extent of the neuronal modulation offered by each approach that will be considered here.

Our investigation of brain substrates for observation will, at this stage, join the pre-reflective simulation camp and focus on shared circuits; that is, those neural networks that are common to both physical execution of an action and also the observation of the same action. These shared circuits are involved in our intuitive actions, sensations and emotions and in the perception of these behaviours in others. The concept of shared circuits may be a better term than functional equivalence for understanding the neuroscience of imagery and observation, since there is increasing evidence that neural overlap is inexact and incomplete. Given the variability in methods of delivery of the interventions, this 'sharedness' will also be variable. Functional equivalence implies a more comprehensive neuronal matching that cannot, at present, be substantiated theoretically or empirically. The term should be restricted to the matching of behaviours and environments that attempt to achieve shared circuits.

Some concerns with imagery

If observation is to provide a valid alternative to imagery for performance training, the theoretical justification to explain its effectiveness must be strong and address the methodological concerns observed for performance imagery. In a recent paper, summarized in Figure 16.1, we suggest that there are a number of procedural problems when considering imagery as an intervention. These include:

- image generation, maintenance and transformation ability (i.e. can the performer actually 'create' an image and, if so, for how long, and how well are they able to manipulate the content?);
- control of visual perspective and viewing angle (i.e. whether the imager uses a first person, third person, or combination of visual perspectives and what angle the imager takes for viewing the behaviour);
- behaviour agency (i.e. is the imaged behaviour associated with the self or another?); and
- image modalities (i.e. which senses are represented within the image, is it purely visual? are there concurrent sounds? does the imager 'feel' movements either concurrently with the visual image or independent of it?).

Furthermore, for many performers, practitioners and coaches, it is generally accepted that the practice of imagery is performed with the eyes closed while inhibiting overt movement. These actions directly compromise the shared circuit with physical performance; eye closing significantly increases alpha-band synchronization over the posterior cortex as visual information is reduced. Similarly, as a consequence of the motor inhibition associated with imagery, activity is seen in the posterior cerebellum. These neural profiles are not observed for the physical action. We have already tried to address some of these issues through the use of a mnemonic for effective mental practice usage – PETTLEP (Holmes & Collins, 2001).

However imagery is approached there will be some inherent problems, many of which cannot be addressed. The performer may be provided with extensive and detailed scripts in an attempt to direct

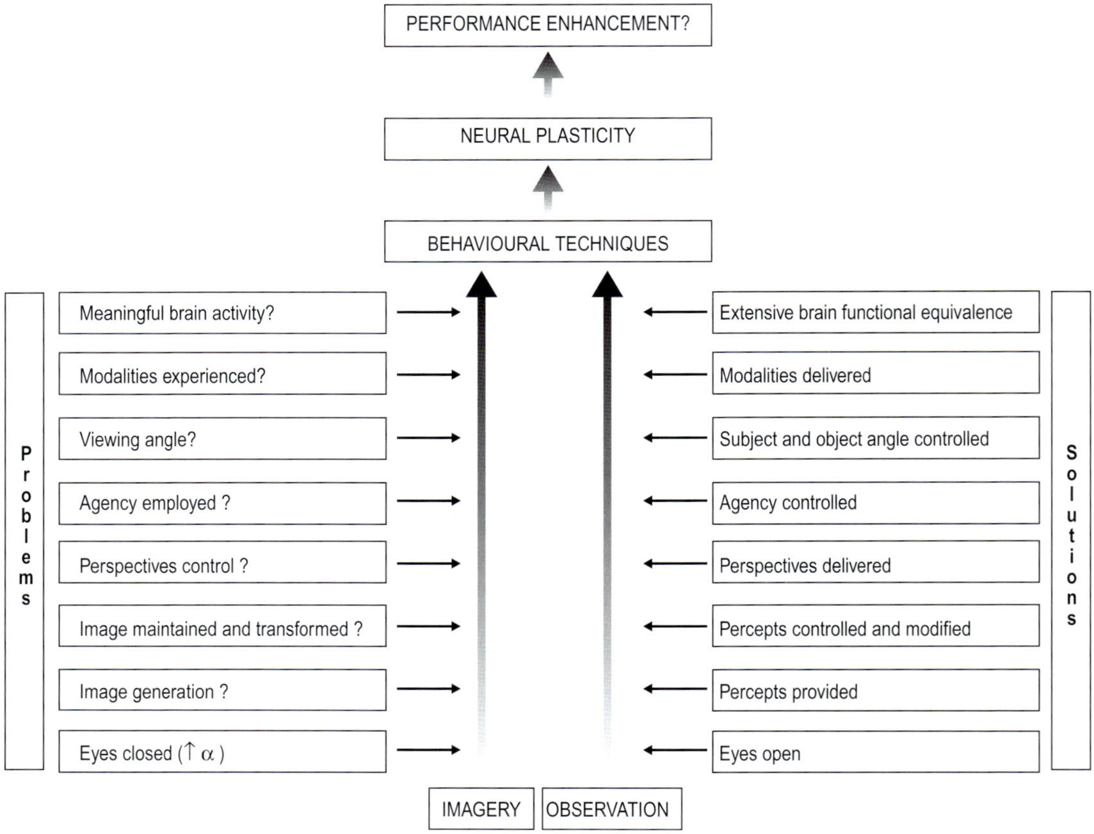

Fig. 16.1 • A schematic to represent the factors influencing the potential effectiveness of imagery and observation when used in the context of performance. From Holmes & Calmels 2008; Journal of Motor Behaviour 40(5): 441. Reprinted with permission of the Helen Dwight Reid Educational Foundation. Published by Heldref Publications, 1319 18th Street NW, Washington, DC 20036–1802, USA. Copyright © 2008.

the exact content of the image but the resultant image will always be unknown, even with comprehensive debriefs. Given this lack of control over image content, practitioners should look to more manageable interventions. Therefore, we aim to provide a neuroscientific approach to developing a working model for observation as a more valid intervention. With the modern technology available to performers and support teams, we propose that many of the concerns highlighted above can be addressed. In addition, we have also found some associated procedural benefits for observation interventions in comparison to imagery by adopting this approach; these include improved adherence to observation interventions, greater mental skills training time, improved imagery ability, and direct involvement in managing and progressing the content of the intervention.

Observation as a mental practice intervention for performance

A mechanism to support the observation process

The mechanisms that underlie the process of imagery are not fully understood; they are complicated further by the lack of control over the covert behaviours. However, the recent discovery of 'mirror neurons' has provided some evidence to begin to explain observation-based behaviours. Early work suggested that mirror neurons (MNs) may be capable of encoding not just the goal of the movement but also the characteristics and meaning behind the movement; specifically action and intention understanding. MNs have also been suggested to have an important role in imitation. While there are limits to how much these neurons can explain, and with a number of functions still limited to the primate brain, their discovery does provide an insight into a mechanism by which humans may communicate their actions, desires and feelings.

MNs were first discovered in the ventral premotor cortex of the macaque monkey with single neuron recordings (e.g. Di Pellegrino et al 1992, Rizzolatti et al 1988). These visuomotor neurons showed special characteristics. They fired when the monkey executed a goal-directed hand movement and also when it observed the same action executed by another monkey or by a human. Some evidence for the existence of similar neurons in humans has been provided by neurophysiological (i.e. electroencephalographic and magnetoencephalographic techniques) and brain imaging studies, which suggests that MNs may contribute to a shared circuit or observation–execution matching system (Calmels et al 2006a, b). This system, also known as the motor resonance system or mirror neuron system (MNS), supports the proposal that perception of an action activates a brain representation similar but not identical to that used to perform the action, in effect, a 'shared' neural circuit (Grèzes et al 2003).

Characteristics of the MNS in humans

In humans, the MNS shows differential activation depending upon the forms of observed motor behaviours. For example, viewing a grasping action performed by another human activates the MNS more than viewing the same action performed by a non-biological, robotic model. Further, the MNS shows less activity during observation of objectless actions, where movements are mimicked, compared to the identical movement that includes the object of interest. Therefore, the MNS would be expected to be more active while viewing a thumb and finger grasp of a golf ball than the replica movement without the golf ball present; an important practical consideration for demonstrators. In a similar way, observation of non-object-related actions, so-called intransitive actions, also activates the MNS.

The MNS is only minimally active when the observed action is impossible for the observer to perform and, similarly, only limited activation is seen in the MNS when the observed movements do not belong to the observer's motor repertoire. For example, strong activation of premotor cortex, parietal cortex and superior temporal sulcus (a shallow cleft at the top of the temporal area) has been recorded in the brains of experienced dancers when observing dance movements they possess the motor capabilities to perform. This brain activity contrasts with that recorded in the same dancers observing dance movements not previously performed before, even though the movements are visually familiar to them (Calvo-Merino et al 2006). The moderating influences of motor familiarity and task expertise interaction on the involvement of the MNS are of obvious importance to the development of the applied use of observation. They will be discussed in more detail throughout the chapter.

Functions of the MNS in humans

The mirror system has been linked to four main functional roles in humans: action and intention understanding, imitation and empathy (Rizzolatti 2005). Simulation theorists would suggest that the involvement of the motor system is a necessary requirement to understand fully an observed action; the perception of an action without the involvement of the motor system only providing a superficial description of the action and not allowing for its thorough comprehension. Intention understanding (i.e. why an individual is performing a particular action) has also been linked to activation of the MNS. The intention of a movement should not be confused with the movement goal. For example, one could observe a tennis player who makes a movement to pick up a ball from the court; the movement *goal*. However, the *intention* of the movement is not known at this stage; it may be to use that specific ball for the next serve, reject it or put it in a pocket for a possible second serve. Observing actions in different contexts will allow the observer to infer intentions for these actions, a concept not dissimilar to variable practice. We will discuss observation context in later sections.

MNS activation is also implied during motor imitation. Imitation of an action that belongs to the motor repertoire of the observer includes activity in the neural circuitry of superior temporal sulcus and frontal and parietal mirror areas (Iacoboni 2005). In contrast, imitation of a novel action activates the same neural circuitry and, additionally, Brodmann's area 46, an area suggested to be associated with the selection of appropriate motor acts (Buccino et al 2004).

Finally, the MNS seems to be closely associated with human empathy, the capacity to feel and understand the same emotional states experienced by another. It is well known that observing a person laughing or crying can generate a similar emotional state in the observer. In such observation situations, neural activity is present in the insula and limbic system of the observer in a similar way to actually experiencing the real emotional behaviour. Since human performance is frequently associated with emotive behaviours and environments, for example, winning and losing in front of large crowds of spectators, understanding how observation interventions can access and share neural circuitry linked to these emotive contexts to generate empathy more optimally would seem beneficial.

Factors that impact on observation

The following section will consider some of the task and observation factors and individual characteristics that can be identified from the neuroscience research that impact directly on observation modulation. These include:

- task type (form-based tasks and perceptually driven tasks) and general observation factors
- internally generated and externally triggered tasks
- specular and anatomical imitation
- live and video observation
- still and temporally altered motion
- pre-observation instructions
- observation context
- observer motor expertise; and
- observer gender.

Task type (form-based tasks and perceptually driven tasks) and general observation factors

In closed skill, form-based tasks, movement aesthetics and quality are important for successful performance (e.g. dance, gymnastics and diving). Performing these kinds of task requires a precise body segment organization. For example, gymnasts who do not reproduce an exact form of their routine have penalties imposed on their score by the judging panel. This form of task contrasts with more open, perceptually driven tasks (e.g. tennis, soccer or wrestling). For example, a tennis player will be judged on her ability to win points against an opponent and not on the form or aesthetic quality of her shot in doing so. Therefore, while it is useful to have a model for form-based tasks, and it is easy to see how observation-based interventions can provide the relevant information, perhaps it would also be useful to observe a model for perceptually driven tasks.

The imagery literature on this issue has identified that performance of closed skills may benefit more from imagery because of the predictability of the movement patterns without direct, less controllable opposition. The imagery research also proposes that task type may direct the choice of visual perspective. Adopting a third-person visual perspective, as if seeing oneself on television (the optimal viewing angle for this perspective has not been specified, and is also likely to be task-specific) has been shown to enhance performance of form-based tasks in novice athletes, probably because of the additional relative visual cues available. This contrasts with more perceptual tasks, where a first-person visual perspective (as if looking through one's own eyes) seems to be more beneficial, possibly because of the kinesthesis associated with this visual perspective for these tasks. Research is ongoing to explore further these task-perspective distinctions. For example, there seems to be a task-visual perspective/modality-motor capability interaction for imagery effectiveness. Once motoric ability for a closed-skill, form-based task has been acquired, performers are able to use third-person perspective visual imagery and kinesthesis to enhance future performance.

These findings are important and should direct the development of observation interventions. For form-based, closed skills the observed movements will, without any manipulation, provide a third-person visual perspective (e.g. viewing oneself or another performing via DVD). To extend the perspective issue, the observation intervention should provide multiple angles of the behaviour of interest. Where the observer has motoric capability, the instructions for observation should include reference to kinesthetic experiences during the viewing. For tasks that rely on perceptual information the process is more complex and requires us to expand on some of the terminology used in this field.

Three separate image characteristics have tended to be compounded: image perspective, image agency and image modality. There is now considerable evidence that these characteristics show different and separate patterns of cortical and subcortical activity both within and across variables. For example, in imagery conditions, employing a different visual perspective involves different parts of the cortex: the right inferior parietal, precuneus (posteromedial portion of the parietal lobe) and somatosensory cortex. These areas have been found to distinguish self-produced actions from those generated by others. The language used in the sport psychology literature does not help the issue: 'internal' imagery, for example, is typically a combination of a first-person visual perspective and a kinesthetic modality. It is also used synonymously for just first-person visual imagery, kinesthetic imagery and motor imagery in some literature. The ambiguity raises obvious concerns for the user and, in the case of the former definition, assumes imagery ability in two modalities. However, if the performer is less skilled in kinesthetic imagery and is instructed to use this 'internal' approach, the content of the imagery will only be visual and, therefore, hypothetically, sharing a limited circuitry with motor areas. While perspective, agency and modality factors may be related and share some neural properties, they are not the same. Their conflation can complicate the delivery of imagery for the practitioner and confuse the recipient about what s/he is required to image. Observation, therefore, may be better positioned to support perceptual tasks. Control of visual perspective, behaviour agency and modality should be effective, since observation interventions overcome the language ambiguity that currently exists in imagery. The ability to (re)create and control variable practice environments through edited filming can also address the need to provide multiple training environments for performers.

Internally generated movement versus externally triggered movements

In the neuroscience literature, it has been shown that internally generated movements (i.e. movements that can be initiated by a performer) do not involve the same cortical pathways as externally triggered movements (i.e. movements that can be imposed on a performer by some external agent). The findings of van Donkelaar et al (1999) suggest that the former engages the ganglio-thalamocortical pathway whereas the second engages the cerebello-thalamocortical pathway.

This point is of interest because in performance both movement types exist. For example, reacting to a gun to start a race or performing to a tightly choreographed piece of music contrast with self-selected movements. In imagery interventions, however, it could be argued that both types of movement become internally generated through the more reflective and conscious process. Again, observation may offer a more ecologically valid environment to address these tasks. However, the observed actions need to access the shared neuronal circuitry for the task for the intervention to be valid. Often, in anticipation–coincidence tasks, coaches and educators use internally generated movements to teach athletes externally generated movements; this is true for the physical execution condition as well as the observation condition. For example, in baseball practice, a novice performer may execute and observe internally generated movement towards a motionless ball and also movements without the ball before progressing to perform dissimilar, externally generated movements linked to a moving ball. Pedagogically, this progression may seem to be full of common sense and practical for the instructor. However, the cortical activation associated with the procedure does not concur. Although movements made without the inclusion of the object of interest seem identical, they actually require the involvement of quite different neuronal populations. Therefore, the transfer of learning from one movement style to another may not be systematic and may explain some of the performance decrements at transition phases. (This same point is well made, albeit from a different perspective, in Ch. 14.)

Specular imitation versus anatomical imitation

In the context of performance, imitation refers to 'a copying of the feature of the bodily movement of a model by an observer' (Heyes 2001, p. 254). This activity represents a fundamental part of human behaviour, is used to acquire new skills and is part of social interaction with other individuals. It has also been identified as one of the key roles of the MNS. Imitation can take different forms and two are particularly relevant for this chapter: specular imitation and anatomical imitation. Specular imitation describes a situation where the observational behaviour occurs as if looking into a mirror. For example, when the model moves the left hand, the observer moves the right hand. In contrast, anatomical imitation describes a state where the imitated movement is reproduced in the same hand as the observed model: when the observed model moves the left hand, the observer moves the left hand. Both could be adopted using a third- or first-person visual perspective.

Specular imitation may be considered a more natural behaviour than anatomical imitation and there is evidence that specular responses predominate over non-specular responses until about 10 years of age (Wapner & Cirillo 1968).

The contralateral action associated with specular observation may predominate to reduce the image rotation ability required to anatomically match the observed action. MN research has also revealed that specular imitation activates the mirror neuron system more than anatomical imitation (Koski et al 2003) and this could explain the greater frequency with which individuals imitate others' behaviours and actions in a specular way.

In applied observation settings, coaches and educators should be aware of these imitation processes. For example, when artistic gymnasts are involved in a choreographic session, often the gymnasts will be facing a large mirror displaying not only their movements but also most of the environment in which they are performing. Instructors can either face the observers or face the mirror; thereby providing both specular and anatomical perspectives. Simultaneously, gymnasts can observe themselves in the mirror with a specular configuration.

MNS activation has also been shown to be related to the physical position of the person being observed (Kilner et al 2006). When the observed person faces towards the observer, the MNS is actively involved. The authors observed, in the parietal area of the brain, a reduction in the alpha band activity during action observation. This reduction was also seen during the execution of the same action. In contrast, however, when the observed person faced away from the observer, no electroencephalographic attenuation was detected. While some of this activity may be a consequence of the facial interaction, it may be that specular observation is more effective at eliciting similar activity in the MNS.

Live observation versus video-based observation

In this section, we will discuss the use of live and video-based observations. We will also include discussion relating to observation perspectives and agency, since we believe the concepts are linked. A question that could legitimately be posed is whether the observation of videotapes or live performance benefits the performer more. The answer is not easy, as performance depends on many factors. However, what is known is that stronger primary motor cortex activation has been detected during live hand movements compared to viewing of video and that this higher activation may be due to the greater ecological validity and contextual meaning of live movements (Jarvelainen et al 2001).

In applied settings, coaches and educators frequently invite their performers to observe teammates performing live motor skills, normally to facilitate the learning or execution of motor performance. Similarly, performers spontaneously observe their teammates during training sessions, mainly to improve their own performance. We have found that elite young female gymnasts observe peers mainly to increase engagement and activation and to improve performance of technical execution by detecting and correcting technical errors performed by others.

Video sequences taken during training sessions or competitions can also be presented to individuals. Performers can observe their own behaviours and actions or teammates' performances. Just as for imagery, these records of performance can be used for many purposes: instant review, pre-performance preview and stimulated recall are just a few. Therefore, coaches and educators may find the use of video sequences more beneficial and practical than live performance. Video permits an unlimited number of viewings of edited, successful performances and allows for a decreased physical training load. The visual content can also be controlled by the coach, in terms of perspective, agency and other modalities, to a far greater extent than for imagery interventions.

Observation of live actions is frequently about actions performed by others. Observation agency through video, however, can include actions performed by oneself or by others. Agency can be differentiated by different neural correlates. Knoblich & Flach (2001) have found behavioural differences between the observation of one's own performance and the observation of others' performance. They presented participants with videos of dart-throwing actions that they had previously performed. They were also shown the same action performed by others. Unsurprisingly, the results indicated that prediction of accuracy of the observed actions was greater when participants observed their own actions. According to the shared circuit theory, observation of self-generated actions may be more informative because of the functional similarity of the neural activity to that during motor execution.

As with agency, different observational perspectives also show different neurological profiles. Using a technique known as transcranial magnetic stimulation to modulate neural activity, researchers have shown that action observation enhances corticospinal excitability; the motor evoked potential observed in a muscle associated with the observed movement is of greater amplitude. Observation of a hand movement increased functional motor output and the degree of motor evoked potential modulation was maximal when the observed action was presented from a first-person perspective. It is also known that the extrastriate body area, an area that responds to the visual appearance of the human body, distinguishes an egocentric view of the self and other people from an allocentric, third-person visual perspective; extrastriate body area activity has been found to increase significantly for allocentric relative to egocentric views in the right hemisphere.

Still and temporally altered motion

As video sequences progress, the images can be slowed, sped up or paused to allow observation of slow or temporally altered actions. While temporally incongruent observation challenges the shared circuit theory, which has both spatial and temporal characteristics, observation of still action shots should not be ruled out completely. There is strong evidence that observation of photographs and still video frames that imply motion can also activate cortical MNS areas involved in the analysis of movement sequences (Kourtzi & Kanwisher 2000). While we are aware that slow-motion video is frequently used in performance contexts, especially for technique analysis, its neural benefit remains untested. Similarly, increasing the speed of the viewed image has been proposed as a possible observation intervention to improve performance. With the technology now available to support such interventions, well designed studies would be welcome in this area.

Instructions provided prior to the observation process

The observational neural profile is also sensitive to the instructions that are provided prior to the observation process. Participants can be invited to observe a movement with the purpose of later imitation, of recognizing it or with no specific goal. Each of these instructional sets has been shown to significantly change the observational neural profile. For example, Decety et al (1997) showed that the dorsolateral prefrontal cortex and the presupplementary motor area were activated when participants were provided with instructions to observe a movement with a later requirement to imitate it. In contrast, the right parahippocampal gyrus was activated in a situation where there was a requirement to recognize the movement after its observation. Coaches and educators should be aware that clear, unambiguous instructions relating to the observation content may be important to optimize the theoretical neural equivalence with the executed profile. When we work with performers, we are very specific in asking them to observe to understand the actions, the goals of the actions, the intentions of the model and, where appropriate, to imitate the action or to empathize with the behaviour.

The observation context

Neuroscience is not purely cognitive. Where human performers are acting as agents of behaviour, the social impact will, inevitably, lead to affective reactions. Therefore, the MNS, in contextually relevant situations, is likely to also include cognitive and emotional neural systems.

An action, performed in different psychosocial contexts, can have very different meanings and intentions to the same observer. Similarly, two observers may have quite different neural responses to the same observed action.

MN areas in the inferior frontal cortex are activated more strongly when individuals observe an action embedded in a particular context compared to observation of the same action in a non-contextual environment. Neuroscience studies are beginning to explore the influence of context in observation. For example, grasping hand actions, seen in different contexts, allow an observer to infer different intentions for the actions. A grasping hand action associated with a cup embedded in a 'before tea' context and an 'after tea' context provides the observer with a different intentional understanding: to drink the contents of the cup or tidy away the cup from the table (Iacoboni et al 2005). Therefore, it will be important to develop observation interventions that have contextual meaning for the observer and actions may need to be embedded within performance contexts to increase shared circuit activity.

Contextual congruence may also need to be considered alongside the observation viewing environment; recent evidence from the imagery research suggests that this may be true. While the viewed action offers contextual relevance, it is possible that the neural response will be influenced by the context in which the observation is performed. For example,

Chatterton et al (2008) have found evidence for greater action and intention understanding, empathy and sensorimotor engagement to observation performed in training environments compared to home environments. While interesting, these findings are still at the case study stage and will require more detailed empirical research to develop the observation context debate. To be effective, observation interventions cannot just provide action viewing; they must activate social, cognitive, affective neural systems. Understanding and developing performance context will be essential to the effectiveness of the intervention.

Observer motor expertise

Using models whose motor skill expertise is similar to that of the observer has been recommended to promote more optimal motor representation access. More specifically, Calvo-Merino et al (2005) have shown stronger activation of the MNS for expert classical ballet dancers compared to novice dancers when observing professional classical dance movements. They also recorded stronger activation of the MNS when the expert ballet dancers viewed movements for which they had been trained compared to movements they had not (e.g. classical ballet vs capoiera). The modulation of the MNS as a result of motor competence may, therefore, be closely associated with visual and motor familiarity of the action. The same research group studied male and female expert classical dancers who had trained together for the same period of time, suggesting that they possessed a similar visual familiarity with the ballet moves. However, some of the moves were specific to one sex and had, therefore, not been physically trained by the other gender group. Activity in the MNS was increased only for observation of gender-specific ballet moves in contrast to familiar, but untrained ballet moves. To be optimally effective therefore, an observation session requires the observer to possess a visual and motor familiarity with the observed action; just because a coach shows a video of a double back somersault to a novice gymnast several times does not mean that the gymnast will then be able to use the (audio) visual information concerning the movement's goals and intentions to be able to perform it! The gymnast will require some motor capabilities to integrate with the visual percepts from the video. Observation should, therefore, be considered carefully alongside the maturational progression of the performer and introduced as their motor capabilities develop. Just as with some of the imagery research, there is evidence that only skilled performers are able to use the third-person visual perspective information to support concurrent kinesthetic proprioception. The sensorimotor integration of the MNS requires physical capability acquired through physical experiences for observation to be most effective in accessing a more elaborate shared circuitry. Conducting some form of observational skill analysis prior to employing observation as an intervention is certainly recommended. Imagery ability questionnaires are regularly used to assess imaging skill; the same should be done for observation.

Observer gender

Until recently, observer gender was not considered as a moderating variable of the neural profile. Recently, however, it has been shown that the MNS is sensitive to sex differences (Cheng et al 2006). There is evidence that female observers show a stronger MNS activation in the right primary motor cortex than their male counterparts when viewing sensorimotor scenes. This finding has been interpreted as a marker of greater empathy by females. The research has not been conducted in sporting or performance contexts and may, therefore, be of limited applied value at this stage.

Applied perspectives

Coaches or educators planning to use observation as a mental practice intervention should be aware that a number of factors can have an impact on observation effectiveness. Figure 16.2 displays a list of primary components to help coaches and educators when devising observation sessions. Support staff should make clear choices in the delivery of the observation factors. The choices will be dictated by the observed task characteristics, the individual observer characteristics and the functions of the observation intervention. Components of tasks and individual characteristics, except motivation, will not be developed here since they have been discussed previously.

Coaches or educators should consider the motivation of their athletes to adhere to observation interventions; athletes can observe and remember a modelled skill, they can have the physical abilities to perform that skill but, if they are not motivated, observation sessions will not be effective.

Understanding the functions of observation is also important when devising observation sessions since it helps the coaches or psychologist define appropriate

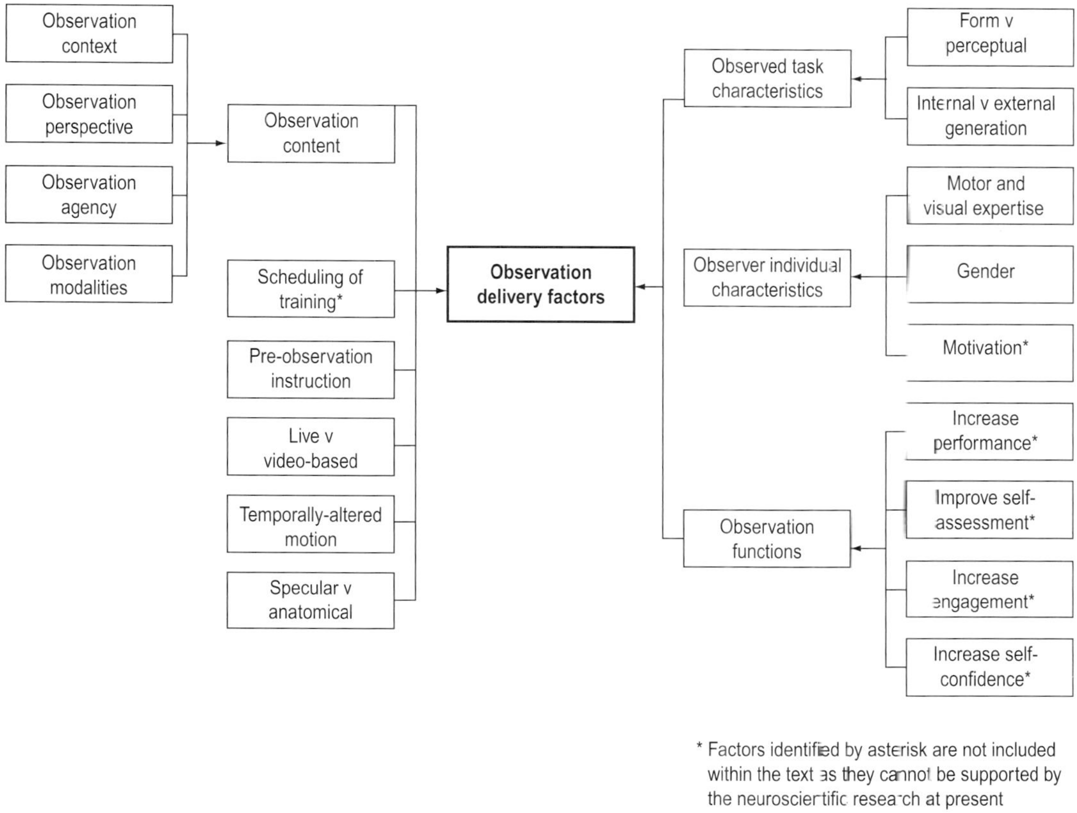

Fig. 16.2 • Schematic representation of the factors impacting on observation effectiveness. Factors identified by asterisks are not included within the text as they cannot be supported by the neuroscientific research at present.

content. There is little research that has focused on observation function. To our knowledge, only Cumming et al (2005), Hars & Calmels (2007), and Gallin-Martel et al (2007) have examined the reasons why athletes observe models. However, only Hars & Calmels (2007), and Gallin-Martel et al (2007) showed that the content of observation is linked clearly to its function. For example, observation of one portion of a complex gymnastics movement and only one part of the body resulted in the performers detecting and correcting technical errors. Whereas, when the same gymnasts observed the full movement but again for only one body part, they used the observation to check their self-assessment against the analysis of the coach. The same kind of relationship has also been highlighted by Fournier et al (2008) for mental imagery. Therefore, coaches should consider the observation function when using the technique. For example, in a form-based task, such as a floor routine in gymnastics, the observation function could be to increase performance or to increase engagement in the task. The observation content, the pre-observation instructions and the (temporally altered) motion are, therefore, likely to be different. If the observation function is to increase performance, coaches could choose a third-person visual perspective, invite the performer to observe their own behaviour at a slow rate with paused images followed by a normal rate and then ask the performer to focus their attention on a particular point of the movement. If the observation function is to increase engagement, the choices may be different. The visual perspective could still be third-person; however, the observed model may be a respected other and the video could be observed at a normal rate. Coaches should use Figure 16.2 as a reminder and individualize the observation sessions for each performer just as they would for imagery interventions.

If mental practice techniques propose to offer, at best, degraded versions of physical practice, there will always be reduced neural afference to the sensorimotor network. Therefore, one could legitimately propose that training time may be spent more effectively in physically training. In an ideal performance world, the answer is probably 'Yes, it could'. However, the world is not ideal and the mental practice techniques described here allow the performer to continue to reinforce shared circuits outside of physical practice conditions. A number of advantages are proposed. First, using observation within a learning framework to support more traditional physical training sessions could be a useful addition to the holistic training environment. Training supported in this way can remain positive and reduce physical training loads, fatigue and, potentially, injury. Second, observing third-person perspective parts of team plays, such as offensive and defensive strategies or exchange of actions between two opponents, allows athletes to anticipate the actions of others (i.e. opponents or partners) more effectively than just first-person physical training for the skill. If the MNS is concerned fundamentally with movement prediction, then where and how others move has obvious relevance for sporting interactions. Understanding others' actions in terms of movement kinematics allows performers to make predictions about their behaviour goals; performers can infer the intentions behind movements and judge whether movements are intended or not. In these cases, the mirror neuron system could be depicted as the neural substrate of our capacity to understand an action, an intention or the state of mind of others. Finally, in sports rehabilitation, athletes may recover more quickly after viewing diverse and repeated sport video sequences. Observation of relevant performance sequences could allow cortical structural changes, reorganization and reinforcement in the motor architecture to support more physically based therapies. These ideas remain to be tested empirically in sporting contexts.

Conclusion

It is our opinion that observation may offer a more valid mental practice technique than more traditional covert interventions. More specifically, the modifiers of the neural activity during imagery are better controlled through an observation process than through imagery. The MNS offers a theoretical mechanism, and the reviewed research provides some evidence, to support the application of observation-based interventions in sport and performance environments. We propose that observation affords both practitioners and researchers greater control over some of the fundamental characteristics to optimize the abstract concept of shared neural circuitry with overt behaviour. Imagery also has the potential to achieve this outcome, but with less assurance that it will be conducted in the prescribed way by the athlete.

Generating an image is no longer a problem since the visual percepts are provided by the information displayed, typically through individualized DVDs, and observed with the eyes open. Observation of still photographic action shots can also generate functional neural activity, since the percepts imply motion. Video observation controls for the imagery ability factors of clarity, vividness and image management (maintenance and rate of exposure) because they are manipulated through the filming and editing processes. Image transformations and rotations are also more effectively managed through dynamic use of camera angles. Observation, provided through digital video, is able to offer the viewer every conceivable viewing angle from either first- or third-person visual perspective and avoids the need for the performer to transform or rotate a transient image. The major benefit, however, is the 'shared' observational image that really differentiates observation from imagery; the researcher or practitioner no longer has to accept the debriefed account of the process from the imager.

There are likely to be further factors that influence neural activity during observation and imagery. Because of the limited or equivocal neuroscientific research findings, we have not considered individual differences in: age; amount and duration of observation dosage; intervention adherence strategies; motivation to undertake the intervention; outcomes goals; external encouragement; and many other psychosocial factors. As brain imaging techniques become more readily available, cognitive and social neuroscientists will provide answers to many of these issues; the future for sport and performance psychology looks exciting!

References

Ahsen, A., 1984. ISM: the triple-code model for imagery and psychophysiology. Journal of Mental Imagery 8, 15–42.

Bandura, A., 1977a. Self-efficacy: towards a unifying theory of behavioral change. Psychol. Rev. 84, 191–215.

Bandura, A., 1977b. Social learning theory. Holt, Reinhart & Winston, New York.

Buccino, G., Vogt, S., Ritzl, A., et al., 2004. Neural circuits underlying imitation learning of hand actions: an event-related fMRI study. Neuron 42, 323–334.

Callow, N., Hardy, L., 2007. A critical analysis of applied imagery research. In: Tenenbaum, G., Eklund, R.C. (Eds.), Handbook of sport psychology, third ed. John Wiley, New York, pp. 21–42.

Calmels, C., Holmes, P., Jarry, G., et al., 2006a. Variability of EEG synchronization prior to, and during, observation and execution of a sequential finger movement. Hum. Brain Mapp. 27, 251–266.

Calmels, C., Holmes, P., Jarry, G., et al., 2006b. Cortical activity prior to, and during, observation and execution of sequential finger movements. Brain Topogr. 19, 77–88.

Calvo-Merino, B., Glaser, D.E., Grèzes, J., et al., 2005. Action observation and acquired motor skills: an fMRI study with expert dancers. Cereb. Cortex 15, 1243–1249.

Calvo-Merino, B., Grèzes, J., Glaser, D. E., et al., 2006. Seeing or doing? Influence of visual and motor familiarity in action observation. Curr. Biol. 16, 1905–1910.

Chatterton, H., Ewan, L., Kinmond, K., et al., 2008. Observation of meaningful activities: a case study of a personalized intervention on post-stroke functional state. J. Neurol. Phys. Ther. 32, 52–59.

Cheng, Y.W., Tzeng, O.J.L., Decety, J., et al., 2006. Gender differences in the human mirror system: a magnetoencephalography study. Neuroreport 17, 1115–1119.

Cumming, J., Clark, S.E., Ste-Marie, D.M., et al., 2005. The functions of observational learning questionnaire (FOLQ). Psychology of Sport and Exercise 6, 517–537.

Decety, J., Grèzes, J., Costes, N., et al., 1997. Brain activity during observation of actions: influence of action content and subject's strategy. Brain 120, 1763–1777.

Di Pellegrino, G., Fadiga, L., Fogassi, L., et al., 1992. Understanding motor events: a neurophysiological study. Exp. Brain Res. 91, 176–180.

Fournier, J.F., Deremaux, S., Bernier, M., 2008. Content, characteristics and function of mental images. Psychology of Sport and Exercise 9, 734–748.

Gallin-Martel, E., Hars, M., Calmels, C., 2007. Apprentissage par observation. Etudes des activités mises en œuvre. GymTechnic 60, 2–13.

Grèzes, J., Armony, J.L., Rowe, J., et al., 2003. Activations related to 'mirror' and 'canonical' neurones in the human brain: an fMRI study. Neuroimage 18, 928–937.

Hars, M., Calmels, C., 2007. Observation of elite gymnastic performance: processes and perceived functions of observation. Psychology of Sport and Exercise 8, 337–354.

Heyes, C., 2001. Causes and consequences of imitation. Trends Cogn. Sci. 1, 253–261.

Holmes, P.S., Calmels, C., 2008. A neuroscientific review of imagery and observation use in sport. J. Mot. Behav. 40, 433–445.

Holmes, P.S., Collins, D., 2001. The PETTLEP approach to motor imagery: a functional equivalence model for sport psychologists. Journal of Applied Sport Psychology 13, 83–106.

Iacoboni, M., 2005. Neural mechanisms of imitation. Curr. Opin. Neurobiol. 15, 632–637.

Iacoboni, M., Molnar-Szakacs, I., Gallese, V., et al., 2005. Grasping the intentions of others with one's own mirror neuron system. PLoS Biol. 3 (3), e79.

Jarvelainen, J., Schurmann, M., Avikainen, S., et al., 2001. Stronger reactivity of the human primary motor cortex during observation of live rather than video motor acts. Neuroreport 12, 3493–3495.

Jeannerod, M., 1994. The representing brain. Neural correlates of motor intention and imagery. Behavioral and Brain Research 17, 187–245.

Kilner, J.M., Marchant, J.L., Frith, C.D., 2006. Modulation of the mirror system by social relevance. SCAN 1, 143–148.

Knoblich, G., Flach, R., 2001. Predicting the effects of actions: interactions of perception and action. Psychol. Sci. 12, 467–472.

Koski, L., Iacoboni, M., Dubeau, M.C., et al., 2003. Modulation of cortical activity during different imitative behaviors. J. Neurophysiol. 89, 460–471.

Kourtzi, Z., Kanwisher, N., 2000. Activation in human MT/MST by static images with implied motion. J. Cogn. Neurosci. 12, 48–55.

Lang, P.J., 1977. Imagery in therapy: an information processing analysis of fear. Behav. Ther. 8, 862–886.

McCullagh, P., Weiss, M.R., 2001. Modeling: considerations for motor skill performance and psychological responses, In: Singer, R.N., Hausenblas, H.A., Janelle, C.M. (Eds.), Handbook of sport psychology, second ed. John Wiley, New York, pp. 205–238.

Morris, T., Spittle, M., Watt, A.P., 2005. Imagery in sport. Human Kinetics, Leeds, West Yorkshire.

Murphy, S., Nordin, S., Cumming, J., 2008. Imagery in sport, exercise and dance. In: Horn, T. (Ed.), Advances in sport and exercise psychology, third ed. Human Kinetics, Champaign, IL, pp. 297–324.

Paivio, A., 1985. Cognitive and motivational functions of imagery in human performance. Can. J. Appl. Sport. Sci. 10, S22–S28.

Rizzolatti, G., 2005. The mirror neuron system and its function in humans. Anat. Embryol. (Berl.) 210, 419–421.

Rizzolatti, G., Carmada, R., Fogassi, L., et al., 1988. Functional organization of inferior area 6 in the macaque monkey: II. Area F5 and the control of distal movements. Exp. Brain Res. 71, 491–507.

Schmidt, R., 1982. Motor control and learning: A behavioral emphasis. Human Kinetics, Champaign, IL.

Short, S.E., Bruggeman, J.M., Engel, S.G., et al., 2002. The effect of imagery function and imagery direction on self-efficacy and performance on a golf-putting task. Sport Psychologist 16, 48–67.

Van Donkelaar, P., Stein, J.F., Passingham, R.E., et al., 1999. Neuronal activity in the primate motor thalamus during visually triggered and internally generated limb movement. J. Neurophysiol. 82, 934–945.

Wapner, S., Cirillo, L., 1968. Imitation of a model's hand movements: age changes in transposition of left-right relations. Child Dev. 39, 887–894.

Developing the performance brain: decision making under pressure

17

Duncan R.D. Mascarenhas* Nickolas C. Smith†

*Sport & Exercise Sciences, Glyndŵr University, Wrexham, UK;
†Department of Sport and Exercise Science, MMU Cheshire, Crewe Green, Cheshire, UK

CHAPTER CONTENTS

Introduction

The physical performance environment contains distinctive, often time-constrained conditions with uncertainties, complexities and dynamics that require participants to make decisions under intense pressure. A range of paradigms of investigation have contributed to the body of knowledge in this area: motor control, normative or classical decision making (CDM) models and naturalistic decision making (NDM). Much has been learned about the skills and processes that high-performing individuals and teams use to make effective decisions. This in turn has led to training interventions designed to advance the process of skilled decision making (DM). This chapter discusses the contribution of research from various paradigms to expertise in DM. We will highlight the theoretical underpinnings to the processes that experts engage in, how stress affects these DM processes and, finally, how they can be trained to allow physical performers such as athletes, coaches, sports officials and dancers, to make effective decisions under pressure.

The study of decision making

The study of factors affecting human DM has a long and venerable history in psychology (Von Neumann & Morgenstern 1947). Operationally, DM can be defined as the process of committing to a particular course of action. Such courses of action can range from the relatively trivial (e.g. deciding what clothes

DOI: 10.1016/B978-0-443-06734-1.00017-1

to wear to work) to life-affecting (e.g. a military combat situation deciding whether a potential target is hostile or friendly).

Two main theoretical viewpoints, CDM and NDM, have been advanced to explain the processes involved in making decisions. These two viewpoints make quite different assumptions about how DM should be studied and how 'expertise' in DM is acquired.

Classical decision-making theory

According to CDM theory (also referred to as a normative DM model), DM is a rather structured, formulaic process. CDM theorists, such as Ward Edwards (1954) tended to focus on the 'outcomes' of decisions in terms of their 'correctness' and assumed that, in all DM settings, correct decision options could be identified through a process of rational analysis. Within such an account, the most effective way to make a decision involves a clear identification of the problem, the generation of a range of alternative solutions, a criteria-based evaluation of these solutions, one against the another and, finally, the selection of the preferred option (Beach & Lipshitz 1993, Cannon-Bowers et al 1996). Within this paradigm, decisions are represented as discrete, static, unchanging and self-contained events, often separated from the context in which the decision occurs. Errors in such settings are assumed to be due to the failure to consider all the relevant information or to evaluate such information in an inappropriate manner. Errors can also occur as a result of applying inappropriate heuristics or 'rules of thumb' where the decision maker erroneously assumes a similarity between the decision problem and one previously encountered.

Such classical theories have been successfully applied to structured DM problems, often in situations where the speed of decision is not critical. For example, someone purchasing a new car might establish a need for something economical, reliable, spacious and with safety extras such as air bags and anti-lock brakes. Based on this information, the purchaser may draw up a shortlist of different vehicles that fit the individual's requirements. Comparing the relative merits of each car – e.g. one has better fuel economy but a smaller boot – will lead the individual to a 'best choice' option. This methodical 'choice-behaviour' approach may seem appealing in some decision settings. However, applying CDM theory to time-pressured, complex, ambiguous, and dynamic situations such as sport may risk misrepresenting what actually takes place in the real world (Lipshitz 1993). Perhaps the greatest limitations of the CDM approach have been the tendencies to separate characteristics of the DM task from the context in which decisions occur and also the failure to consider the expertise of the decision maker.

Interestingly, in organizational environments where there is low time pressure, when DM skills based on CDM theory have been taught to experts in business management (Isenberg 1984), financial analysis (Paquette & Kida 1988) and medical diagnosis (Alessi 1988), they rarely appear to use them (Beach & Lipshitz 1993, Means et al 1993), choosing instead to use more subjective, intuitive factors as the basis of their decisions (Dreyfus & Dreyfus 1980, Isenberg 1985, Roth 1997). Evidence also suggests that such professionals find the prescribed operations cumbersome, time-consuming and inefficient in terms of time and resources (Beach & Lipshitz 1993). So, while normative models of rational choice may have theoretical justification, they are often not used, even in situations where they may appear to present an effective solution. Consistent with these findings is evidence from studies showing that individuals often fail to consider all the available options before making a decision (Payne et al 1993). Such research has highlighted that individuals may only consider potential solutions to a point where they identify one that fulfils the minimum criteria for a desired goal to be achieved, a process that has been termed 'satisficing' (Eysenck & Keane 2005, Simon 1955). Johnson & Raab (2003) suggest that individuals are governed by a goal-driven heuristic that leads them to 'take the first option', rather than comparing between options. For example, in sport, the decision to pass or shoot (see Bennis & Pachur 2006) may be driven by the individual's belief about their role in the team, i.e. a passer or a goal scorer, and such heuristics may drive them to short-cut the decision selection process. Thus, it is unclear what circumstances actually 'prompt' the evaluation of multiple options in many DM tasks.

Payne et al (1993) have pointed out that the theoretically 'optimal' decision rule in naturalistic settings may be far from optimal when the time to decide is limited. These authors also highlight that people are capable of adjusting their DM strategies as time constraints vary. Given the apparent reluctance of experts to use rational choice strategies, one might assume that time constraints force them to use alternative methods, reflecting a form of speed–accuracy trade-off. There is some evidence that supports this view. In a series of studies examining DM in gambling, Payne et al (1988) showed that professional gamblers changed their DM strategies significantly when performing under unaccustomed time pressure. In contrast, studies of DM in chess grand masters and experienced aircraft pilots have shown declines in decision accuracy to be minimal when decision speed is increased. Calderwood et al (1988) found that the proportion of tactical errors made by chess masters, as rated by an independent grand master, showed no effect of time pressure, with error rates of 8% under regulation time (approximately 2.6 min per move) but only 7% under 'blitz' conditions (moving within 6 s). Intermediate players, on the other hand, made more mistakes with the introduction of time pressure, with performance errors increasing from 11% to 25%. Similarly, Stokes et al (1997) showed that, when asked to respond under real-time pressure to challenging situations such as abrupt changes in cockpit instrument panels, experienced pilots chose the correct answer as their first choice 71% of the time, compared to 53% correct decisions in less experienced pilots. Since the experts were deemed to have no greater cognitive advantage or reasoning ability than their less experienced colleagues (Barnett 1989), their increased performance was attributed to their access to 'aviation-specific' knowledge structures held in long-term memory (Stokes et al 1997).

All these findings have been taken to reflect the importance of experience and task-specific practice within particular domains of achievement. In turn, considerable interest has been generated in the perceptual and cognitive factors that underpin such expertise in DM. Central to this area of research has been the study of how experts appear able to make the correct decision without generating and deliberating between alternatives. In order to address such complex issues, alternative approaches to the study of DM have been developed, reflecting an important change of emphasis from normative models that stress 'making decisions correctly,' to real-world investigations that are more concerned with 'making the correct decisions' (Beach & Lipshitz 1993). Such approaches place less emphasis on prescriptive processes and greater emphasis on contextual factors within the decision environment and also the level of experience of the decision maker.

Naturalistic decision making

Given the limitations of CDM theory as previously described, researchers have recently focused their efforts on investigating the actual processes that expert decision makers engage in. Typical of this work have been investigations of expert military commanders, aviators, firefighters and astronauts on the NASA space program (see Klein 1997a). Evidence tends to confirm the view that in these environments experts generally make effective decisions without lengthy deliberation over a range of alternatives as predicted by CDM theory (Klein 1997b, Orasanu & Connolly 1993, Zsambok 1997).

Studying DM behaviours in naturalistic settings has intuitive attraction for those interested in decision processes in performance settings. Such settings often share many of the contextual characteristics of those mentioned above where performance takes place in situations of high uncertainty, under time pressure and, often, for high stakes. The growing body of research into naturalistic decision making (NDM) has led to a clearer definition of this perspective, which characterizes human DM as prone to error as a consequence of:

- ill-structured problems;
- uncertain dynamic environments;
- shifting, ill-defined or competing goals;
- multiple event–feedback loops;
- time constraints;
- high stakes;
- multiple players or team members; and
- organizational norms and goals that must be balanced against the decision maker's personal choice (Cannon-Bowers et al 1996, Zsambok 1997).

Although it has become generally accepted that only some of these factors need to be present for a decision to be considered naturalistic (Orasanu & Connolly 1993), often all these characteristics feature in performance environments. For example, goalkeepers in football or hockey have to react to a range of attacking and defensive patterns, often without formal structure. In these settings they have to decide whether to come out to challenge the attacker and risk either being chipped or the attacker passing the ball to a team-mate. They also have to be aware of their own team-mates, who may intervene, and make such decisions quickly, often under considerable pressure, in the knowledge that a mistake could cost the team a goal and potentially the game.

Consequently, in an attempt to understand the processes that experts actually go through, NDM researchers have used a variety of different and more ecologically valid techniques to examine DM in the context it occurs. Such an approach has been widely advocated within the sport science literature (e.g. Williams et al 1999).

Contrary to CDM theory, NDM findings suggest that, in time-constrained settings, expert decision makers use context dependent pattern recognition or framing, based on highly developed 'mental models' to generate potential decisions rather than the systematic evaluation of options. Seminal work investigating expert and novice differences in chess (DeGroot 1978, Simon & Chase 1973) revealed grand masters' superior abilities to recognize familiar chessboard patterns. When asked to recall complex, yet realistic board configurations, experts were more accurate in reproducing them than novices, whereas when presented with random arrays of chess pieces there were no differences between the two groups. Simon & Chase (1973) suggested that experts perceived the structured display in terms of highly familiar patterns made up of meaningful chunks of information.

The research into this structuring of information has elicited an array of terminology to describe the advantages in recognition performance shown by experts, from *chunking* (Means et al 1993) into a decision *type* (Cannon-Bowers & Bell 1997) based on shared characteristics or highly familiar patterns, to *framing* (Tversky & Kahneman 1981), which suggests experts are better able to parse cues rapidly through the processes of *pattern recognition* (Means et al 1993) and *pattern matching* (Klein 1997b) into *templates* (Cannon-Bowers & Bell 1997).

Despite the potential loss of context-specific details when making decisions that are based on a series of template accounts of the situation (Tolcott et al 1989), researchers sanction it as an effective way of organizing information when time pressure is inherent. Leaving aside the idiosyncrasies of terminology, there has been consistent evidence in the sport psychology literature of experts' superior pattern recognition of key features within structured displays (Janelle & Hillman 2003). While differences in pattern recognition may reliably distinguish between skilled and less skilled performers, recognition advantages appear to provide a necessary but not sufficient overall account of expert behaviour. Such expert behaviour also appears to rely on a more complex interplay of perceptual/attentional factors and underlying knowledge structures.

What supports effective decision making?

Underpinning most NDM theories is the assumption that experts possess highly developed, domain-specific knowledge acquired from extended practice in relevant contexts. Such knowledge is organized in a fashion that enables rapid access and retrieval to help guide decisions made in time-constrained and stressful settings (Tenenbaum 2003). The organization of such knowledge in memory is argued to enable expert performers to represent problems and generate potential solutions in a manner that allows them to circumvent the normal limitations of information processing (e.g. attentional and working memory limitations).

Knowledge structures and their support for decision making

Attempts to more clearly identify the characteristics of the knowledge structures that underpin expert performance have highlighted some important conceptual distinctions. Anderson (1995) suggests that knowledge can be categorized as either declarative or procedural in nature. Procedural knowledge supports the 'how to' aspects of task performance and is manifest in the performance of motor actions and sequences. Such knowledge is often closed to introspection (i.e. performers cannot always verbalize the processes involved) and has been examined using a range of measurement approaches that employ both cognitive–behavioural measures (e.g. recognition paradigms and eye movement behaviours (McLennan & Omodei 1996)) and verbal reports (e.g. 'think aloud' protocols (Schraagen 1997)).

By contrast, declarative knowledge represents the 'what and whys' that support task performance. Declarative knowledge involves knowing that something is the case (e.g. that it is illegal for a back row player to make an attack hit in volleyball from within the front court playing area) and relies on access to both episodic and semantic memory. Episodic memory is a form of long-term memory that involves personal memory of experiences that have occurred in particular places and times. Such memory is also important in recalling recent events and the strategies performers used to achieve important goals (i.e. events that are active in working memory). Semantic memory consists of more general knowledge about the world and the relationships that exist within it (Eysenck & Keane 2005).

By way of illustration, in the straightforward task of going for a walk, declarative knowledge will tell us that we need to put our shoes on because it is wet outside. The procedural knowledge holds information to ensure that we put the shoes on the correct feet and know how to tie our laces. In the performance environment, taking refereeing as an example, declarative knowledge represents the official's knowledge and understanding of the laws, players and the environment, and the nuances on the day (i.e. both episodic and semantic memory). Procedural knowledge is seen in the officiating behaviours the referee uses, such as their use of the whistle, voice and body language. Therefore, the relationship between such knowledge and demonstrated expertise in DM is of central importance in understanding superior performance across a range of achievement settings.

Relationship between knowledge and expertise in decision making

While it seems clear that expertise cannot wholly be accounted for by differences in task-related knowledge between skilled and less skilled performers, strong support exists that this proposition is partially correct. Salthouse (1991) has argued that expert–novice differences in performance can largely be accounted for by differences in knowledge between such individuals. Unlike expert performers, novices' lack of knowledge means they are less able to predict events, less sure about what information sources to attend to, what course of action to take and when to take it, and finally, less knowledgeable about the relationships that exist between performance-related variables. A similar view has been expressed more recently by Ste-Marie (2003), who found that differences in expertise between skilled and less skilled judges and referees could largely be explained by variations in task-related knowledge.

More direct evidence of differences between skilled and less skilled performers in their underlying knowledge structures and the importance of these to expert performance comes from the work of McPherson & Kernodle (2007). These authors studied the verbal reports of advanced beginners and entry-level professional tennis players obtained during actual play to compare differences between the groups in knowledge and problem representation. Previous findings using similar methods (French & McPherson 1999) support the view that superior performance shown by experts is the result of increased elaboration and flexibility of 'action plan' and 'current event' profiles that experts hold in long-term memory and that are accessed rapidly during play. Action plan profiles are rule-governed representations (i.e. stored in prototypical form) that are used to link characteristics of the current environment to stored visual events or motor actions. In the tennis context, these profiles may represent characteristics of an opponent's court position and shot selection, or information on the coordination pattern shown by opponents during shot execution. Current event profiles refer to structures in memory that are used to monitor and guide more global tactical and strategic aspects of play. These draw on information from both past experience and current events to form a developing 'script' that supports performers' ongoing tactical behaviours.

McPherson & Kernodle (2007) used interview data taken from participants during breaks in play that was used to compare the immediate recall of the two groups regarding events from the previous point (i.e. a recall interview) and the problem representations players showed for the subsequent point (i.e. a planning interview). Although we must be conscious of the limitations of self-reports of performance (for a review, see Nisbett & Wilson 1977), McPherson & Kernodle showed that advanced beginners had relatively poorly developed action plans compared to entry-level professionals. They were also less able to strategically plan for the subsequent point, based on well developed current event profiles. In contrast, entry-level professionals showed elaborate tactical and strategic representations of their own and their opponent's behaviours in both their action plans and current event profiles. These findings support the view that sport expertise and the advantages shown by experts in sport-specific DM tasks are dependent on highly elaborate knowledge structures held in long-term memory that guide tactical and strategic behaviours.

How is such knowledge developed? Practice implications

Research suggests that quite specific features of the practice undertaken by experts may account for their superior DM skills. The term 'deliberate practice' has been used extensively in recent years to describe the form and types of activity that seem important to the eventual development of expert status (Ericsson et al 1993, Starkes & Ericsson 2003). Deliberate practice is defined as being effortful in nature, with the main goal of personal improvement of performance rather than enjoyment, and is often performed without immediate reward. Interestingly for those seeking to understand the relationship between knowledge development and expert performance, Ericsson et al argue that experts continually strive to make practice environments progressively more challenging and non-routine in nature. As a consequence, practice activities are seldom, if ever, characterized by mere replication or repetition of movement patterns or drills without a progressively more challenging goal in mind. Such orientation to practice helps them resist or delay the automaticity that accompanies the more routine practice of cognitive and motor skills. In so doing, this enables the generation of increasingly elaborate and complex mental representations of tasks, factors that appear important foundations of subsequent expertise.

The findings that experts use practice strategies that help them remain at the cognitive stage of learning (see Chs 13, 14 and 15) has considerable relevance to recent research interest in the development of metacognitive skills (Barnett & Ceri 2002). Metacognitive skills are those processes used by the learner to monitor and control the learning process itself (i.e. skills that help learners manage their own learning). Learning strategies that encourage the development of such skills have close association with 'mastery-orientated' learning environments in which the learner's goal is to focus their attention on activities related to the skill acquisition process (e.g. self-monitoring of learning attempts) rather than performance outcomes (Kozlowski 1998). Studies of learning activities that encourage the development of metacognitive skills suggest that two key consequences result. First, the learner develops a range of self-regulatory skills that are important to eventual expert performance. These self-regulatory skills include both learning-related (e.g. self-reflection) and motivation/affect-related (e.g. the regulation of emotions) outcomes. Second, as a result of metacognitive skill development, performers often demonstrate higher self-efficacy or task-related competence, an attribute that has been associated with persistence in challenging practice environments and resilience in the face of setbacks (Kozlowski 1998).

The development of mental models

Despite the general consensus that skilled decision makers possess highly elaborate knowledge structures that support DM and expert performance, there is less agreement about how such knowledge structures develop. Perhaps the most cited theoretical account, which has also received considerable support outside the NDM literature, suggests that experts use mental models to help individual and team coordination by forming accurate and meaningful expectations and explanations of events (Cannon-Bowers et al 1990, Norman 1983). In this regard, Rouse et al (1992) suggest that mental models provide knowledge of the situation to direct attention, classify information and form an understanding of its meaning. More recently, Endsley (1997) has argued that mental models also create expectations regarding future events and provide a link between recognition processes and typical actions. Thus, they are not only capable of directing attention to incoming information but also priming potential solutions, through constructive processing (Klein 2000, McLennan & Omodei 1996). Consequently, this negates the need for deliberation amongst alternatives as prescribed by CDM. The purpose of mental models is to aid interpretive processes, helping to screen out information in order to prevent overload, a factor that seems crucial when individuals are performing complex tasks under time pressure. Holyoak (1984, p. 193) defines mental models as 'a psychological representation of the environment and its expected behaviour' that helps individuals make sense of their surroundings (Klimoski & Mohammed 1994). Such models are used to both represent and organize knowledge by simulating the important characteristics of situations that are to be cognitively mastered and they do so in such a fashion that complex phenomena become manageable (Seel et al 2000).

Thus mental models provide a conceptual framework for describing, explaining and predicting future system states (Rouse & Morris 1986). Such skilled behaviours have also been argued to form the foundation of 'situation awareness'. Situation awareness involves three levels of awareness: (1) perceptual, (2) comprehension and (3) prediction, which direct the decision maker to an appropriate decision point (Endsley 1997). It is the third level of awareness (prediction) that allows individuals to anticipate the actions of others and adjust their performance accordingly.

The shared nature of knowledge between team members represents an important area of study since both independent and interdependent understanding is critical to effective DM in team settings. Thus, although mental models have been examined more extensively at the level of the individual, recently there have been considerable efforts to explore these phenomena at the team or group level (Webber et al 2000).

The development of shared mental models

NDM postulates that, when team members have accurate and equally detailed conceptualizations of the problem and the requirements of team functioning necessary to solve it (i.e. common declarative and procedural knowledge), they have developed shared mental models (Cannon-Bowers et al 1990, Noble et al 1987). The earliest reference to the existence of a shared mental-model was in Torrance's (1953) report on Second World War military units downed behind enemy lines. In this account, the unit leader took responsibility for communicating information to develop a shared understanding of the situation. More recently, and perhaps more appropriately, this has been termed a shared situation-model (see Rouse & Morris 1986), mirroring theories on problem framing and typing, as previously discussed, which subsequently drives the construction of appropriate mental models (cf. Tversky & Kahneman 1974, 1981).

Conceptualizing problems through explicit and timely interactions has been identified as a key factor in reduced error rates amongst commercial airline cockpit crews (Means et al 1993). Expert crews have been shown to communicate their shared goals and adapt to environmental demands through monitoring, feeding back and carrying out backup behaviours (Salas & Morgan 1989). Cockpit crews with lower error rates were shown to spend more time framing problems, justifying their decisions, contingency planning and managing their shared resources, actions that led to the formulation of a shared mental model (Orasanu 1990).

Shared mental models provide the organization of experiences that allow the individual to discriminate between similar and non-similar experiences, thus providing the link to appropriate (and shared) responses. They provide team members with the necessary knowledge to predict both future events and the likely needs of other team members. This allows inferences to be drawn in order to anticipate team members' actions and make adjustments to maintain overall team coordination (Johnson-Laird 1983, Rouse et al 1992). Shared mental models guide the evolution of 'same expectations' and 'same patterns of thinking' that lead team members to respond in a similar manner (Cannon-Bowers et al 1990). Furthermore, they reflect the shared knowledge, attitudes and behaviours that help to form a common understanding of a situation. When two or more individuals share this level of understanding based on the recognition of the situation, comprehension of the problem and prediction of future events, it often leads to the same decision processes and coordinated actions (Cannon-Bowers et al 1990).

Such coordinated responses and actions that take place without the need for lengthy communication have been referred to as team coherence (Mascarenhas 2005). Thus, shared knowledge of task components and the relationships that exist amongst them provided by a shared mental model often leads to coherent DM (Rouse & Morris 1986, Rumelhart & Ortony 1977). In the sporting domain, this can lead to flawless acts of coordination, where team-mates are able to anticipate each others' movements and work fluidly together. Similarly, for elite sports officials, shared mental models and the collective situational understanding they foster, appear to provide the platform for different decision makers to independently judge situations in a coherent manner. Thus, the effective development of collective mental models of the situation (Lipshitz & Ben Shaul 1997) is one solution to achieving effective team performance.

However, team coherence in sport is not always achieved through shared mental models. In fact, as identified by Brehmer (1992), three types of DM style exist:

- **Command-based**, where each decision is made centrally and relayed to the other team-mates
- **By plan**, often referred to in the military as 'standard operating procedures (SOPs)', where team members act in a predetermined manner without the need to communicate or change the course of action in response to evolving situation factors
- **By shared mental model**, where team-mates are empowered to respond based on their previous experiences of the situation and the decisions made by other team members.

An example of command-based DM in sport is the quarterback in American football, who calls the play to his team members, who then carry out their roles accordingly. A free-throw in basketball exemplifies a plan-based, SOP DM style, where each defender lining up along the free-throw lane 'boxes-out' the player next to them (i.e. puts their body in front of the attacker to prevent them from rebounding the ball), and the defender at the top of the key boxes-out the shooter. In this example, there is no need for communication as this is simply the standard operating procedure when a free throw is taken. Finally, shared-mental-model-based DM is built upon detailed knowledge of the task, the team and the environment (Kraiger & Wenzel 1997) that allows team members to function synchronously. This can often be seen in open team sports such as soccer, when players are able to anticipate the movements and actions of team-mates and adjust accordingly, resulting in fluid and implicit interactions that lead to faultless passages of play (Riley 1993).

All three styles of DM present potential solutions for coping with the time-pressured and often stressful performance environment. SOPs are typically deep-rooted plans that circumvent the need for additional cognitive processes. The command-based style similarly reduces the need for multiple players to develop action plans, with one individual typically 'calling the shots'. However, these solutions to developing team coherence are limited to a finite range of situations. For example, in the complex and dynamic open team sports environment events are often completely unpredictable. This may render the team member responsible for 'making the call' with insufficient time to either develop a plan or communicate it. So perhaps the most appealing is the shared mental model style. Although we have mentioned some evidence for shared mental models' resilience to fatigue, we must first consider the sources and characteristics of stress in the performance environment before exploring appropriate decision-training methods.

Stress and decision-making performance

No consideration of the factors affecting DM in sport would be complete without mention of how the speed and accuracy of such decisions are affected by emotions and other sources of stress. Similarly, as one's susceptibility to the negative effects of stress on DM are linked to individual difference factors such as trait anxiety and neuroticism (Muris et al 2004), some consideration of these factors is also warranted.

This section reviews the research that has examined sources of stress in DM environments and the performance effects that are typically observed. The principles of stress exposure training are then described. The role of individual differences in moderating the effects of stress on performance is also considered. Subsequently, the cognitive mechanisms that appear to be affected by negative emotional states such as anxiety and the pattern of performance disruption that occurs are described. Finally, the section presents an overview of two influential accounts of how performance is affected by anxiety in the form of processing efficiency theory (PET) (Eysenck & Calvo 1992) and its theoretical extension in attention control theory (ACT) (Eysenck et al 2007).

Sources of stress in decision-making environments

Numerous attempts have been made in the literature to define the nature of stress (Cassidy 1999). While many important nuances exist between such definitions, most emphasize that stress is the consequence of an appraisal process where a situation of high demand is judged to exceed the performer's ability to cope (Nicholls & Polman 2007). Additionally, these situations normally hold high significance for the performer (i.e. the outcomes are perceived as highly important), often with considerable uncertainty surrounding the outcome. The psychological significance of such situations is frequently heightened by the presence of others (e.g. opponents, judges or an audience) or by a genuine threat (e.g. extreme sports). Unsurprisingly perhaps, these settings have the potential to generate performance-related concerns and worry, alongside physical and behavioural symptoms of distress (Kerr 1997), and to disrupt performance.

In DM environments a distinction is often made between 'task related' sources of stress (e.g. time pressure, the requirement to monitor multiple information sources) and 'psychobiological' sources of stress (e.g. fatigue, worry based on ego-related threat or the risk of physical harm). Task-related stressors are variables that are intrinsic to task performance, whereas psychobiological stressors can vary depending on a range of dispositional and situational factors. The effectiveness of DM in stressful environments will, to a large extent, depend on the degree of practice individuals have in managing the stress sources in simulated practice conditions. The term 'stress exposure training' (Driskell & Johnson 1998) has been used to describe a form of training that aims specifically to help performers maintain effective performance in stressful conditions. Surprisingly, many practice environments in sport often fail to provide performers with the cognitive skills needed to perform effectively under pressure, or even the experience for them to evolve their own. This is perhaps based on the assumption held by many coaches that well-structured practice of the technical and tactical skills of the sport alone is sufficient to equip performers with the necessary mental skills to cope with the stresses encountered in the cauldron of competition (Smith et al 2001b). The simple message is clear: don't just expose performers to stressful challenge and leave them to sort it out; rather, teach skills and systems explicitly to provide the basic skills on which they can build. Accordingly, a number of 'brand name' approaches, usually combinations of theories and/or techniques, have been developed.

Stress exposure training (SET) is based on three underlying principles (Driskell & Johnson 1998). The first is the notion that benefit can be gained by becoming knowledgeable about the sources of stress performers will face and their likely effects on performance. These include knowledge of the typical physiological, cognitive and behavioural reactions that accompany stressful encounters. In addition, knowledge is developed about the typical pattern of performance disruption that occurs when under stress. Such knowledge often enhances feelings of predictability in these settings and heightens feelings of personal control. It is also argued that, by acquiring knowledge of potential sources of stress, performers are less likely to be distracted by them if and when they are encountered. Finally, by familiarization with the typical effects of stress on performance, individuals are assumed to be better able to self-monitor and correct errors as they occur.

The second principle of SET assumes that individuals should practise regulatory skills highly specific to those eventually required in stressful settings. For example, if a performer has to make effective decisions when physically fatigued, facing hostile opponents and dealing with multiple sources of information of varying priority, quite specific simulated practice is required during training periods to replicate these demands (see also Ch. 14). Emphasis is particularly placed on cognitive control strategies during this stage of SET linked to overlearning of the physical techniques involved. These cognitive strategies aim to help performers control dysfunctional thoughts and emotions that are likely to impair performance and focus available resources on the task at hand.

The final principle of SET is related to the earlier discussions on mastery-orientated practice environments (see Chs 13, 14 and 15) and the development of metacognitive skills. Individuals who are exposed to such environments during SET and who are trained to develop metacognitive skills typically show greater confidence in their ability to perform under pressure. They also develop greater 'trust' in both their own and their team-mates' ability to perform effectively under stress.

Stress, anxiety and performance

Susceptibility to the negative performance effects of stress has been found to vary between individuals. Evidence suggests that this is the result of both dispositional and situational factors. As a consequence, anxiety in both its dispositional (i.e. trait anxiety) and situational (i.e. state anxiety) forms has become the most widely studied psychological factor affecting performance in sport (Craft et al 2003). Trait anxiety is a construct reflected in most models of personality and refers to a relatively stable disposition within the individual to judge a wide range of environmental events as potentially threatening. Situational stressors prompt increases in state anxiety in the form of worry and concern over performance that are often, but not always, accompanied by heightened physiological activation (e.g. increased heart rate and muscle tension). These increases in physiological activation can themselves lead to further performance concerns if athletes interpret such bodily symptoms as threatening.

Individuals high in trait anxiety typically view the world as a threatening place, believing that sources of stress will be frequently encountered and, as a consequence, react to situational stressors with higher state anxiety reactions than those low in trait anxiety (Weinberg & Gould 2007). Thus, the level of experienced anxiety is determined interactively by trait anxiety and perceived situational threat. The threatening feelings and cognitions commonly felt by anxious individuals often reflect a strong 'future focus' with worry over the potential adverse consequences of failure and harm tending to predominate. Low trait anxious individuals on the other hand, tend to judge events in a more benign manner, normally seeing little threat in a wide range of social and achievement settings (Weinberg & Gould 2007). In addition to more stable personality-linked factors, situational factors in sport that increase context-specific perceptions of threat (i.e. the level of state anxiety) include such factors as outcome uncertainty and the potential threat of negative evaluation by others.

Anxiety is typically considered a multidimensional emotion with both somatic (i.e. physical sensations) and cognitive (e.g. worrying thoughts) components. While these two components share some degree of variance, they appear to have different antecedents (Lane et al 1995) and effects on performance (Craft et al 2003). Factors that elevate the cognitive component of anxiety are normally ego-related concerns (e.g. fear of failure and negative evaluation by others), while somatic anxiety appears to increase when individuals encounter environmental stimuli that are present in the performance environment (e.g. the sights and sounds of the actual setting) or anticipate physical harm.

In performance terms, cognitive and somatic anxiety seem to affect performance rather differently (Butt et al 2003). High levels of somatic anxiety have been associated with increases in processing speed on simple, reactive tasks (e.g. a start in a 100 m sprint (Parfitt et al 1995), but see also the example discussed in Ch. 14). However, this gain in speed is often at the expense of decision accuracy (i.e. more errors or 'false-positive' responses are made, e.g. a 100 m runner leaving the blocks before the gun). Also, motor actions that require the simple coordination of large muscle groups, particularly those requiring maximal strength or power output, have been shown to improve in some cases when individuals experience heightened somatic anxiety (Parfitt et al 1995). While the exact cause of these performance changes is still the focus of debate, it seems likely that they are mediated by changes in physiological factors that affect neuromuscular function.

Performance changes that accompany increases in cognitive anxiety appear more diverse and complex in nature. In studies that have examined the effects of cognitive anxiety on speed and accuracy of DM, anxiety has generally been found to slow processing speed on a wide range of cognitive tasks (Richards et al 2000). Such tasks include verbal and spatial reasoning, tasks that require the sustaining and switching of attention and those that place high demand on working memory (Eysenck et al 2007).

Why do these changes in performance occur when individuals become anxious? Early views on this question argued that cognitive anxiety in the form of worry had two inter-related effects. Firstly, worrisome thoughts about failure and the adverse consequences of poor performance serve as a source of distraction that disrupts DM processes. Anxious individuals have been consistently shown to be more easily distracted from tasks and they also experience heightened feelings of self-consciousness (Keogh et al 2004). This in turn is reflected in a strong self-focus that makes anxious individuals appear preoccupied with self-concerns rather than dealing with the task in hand.

What is clear from individual accounts of athletes' experiences of cognitive anxiety is that it seems very difficult to 'disengage' from worry once it begins to preoccupy one's thoughts (Hatzigeorgiadis & Biddle 2000). In this sense, worry appears to have a distinctive 'cyclical' quality that serves to represent negative thoughts to individuals' consciousness while also making them particularly vigilant for sources of threat in the environment (Eysenck, 1997).

The second related effect of cognitive anxiety is that it also 'consumes' processing resources that are required for performance itself. The performance consequences of this effect become more apparent as the complexity of tasks increase. Research has provided consistent support for the proposition that the adverse effects of anxiety on performance become much more apparent as tasks increase in complexity (Eysenck et al 2007). This suggests that, on relatively simple decision tasks that require few mental resources, individuals are able to compensate for the negative effects of cognitive anxiety, when motivated to do so, by devoting more processing resources to the task. As task complexity increases, however, and more information sources have to be attended to, a point is reached where no further compensatory resources are available to offset the influence of worry and performance consequently declines.

Decision making in threatening settings

More recent accounts of the way cognitive anxiety affects performance have both refined these early ideas and helped to clarify the specific psychological mechanisms involved (Eysenck et al 2007). With specific reference to tasks involving DM, it may be useful to return briefly to the topic of situation awareness that was discussed earlier in this chapter. We argued that situation awareness was an important attribute that contributes to effective DM in both individuals and team settings. Situation awareness was assumed to involve three key processes: perceptual skills, comprehension and an ability to predict the likely outcome of a developing situation. Importantly, research suggests that each of these three key contributors appears to be affected by anxiety. To understand how this occurs, it may be useful to briefly consider the actual function of an emotion such as anxiety.

The main function of anxiety appears to be the detection of sources of threat in our environment. Many centuries ago this may have served a very useful evolutionary purpose as the detection, and hopefully avoidance, of physical threats may have been vital for our predecessors' survival. Fast-forward many generations and we find that most environments we encounter hold little physical threat to our wellbeing. The things that stimulate anxiety most commonly in 21st century life are often of a more abstract, psychological nature than the threat posed by dangerous wild animals. These include situations in which social evaluation is a common feature and in which ego-threat is heightened. Not surprisingly, as an example of such a situation, competitive sport holds the potential to be perceived as a highly attractive or highly threatening arena, depending on the situation and the performer's disposition.

Given that the main evolutionary function of anxiety is the detection of threat, anxious individuals are predicted to be particularly vigilant for sources of threat in their environment when they appear. As one of the main components of situation awareness is perceptual skill, factors that disrupt perceptual processes are of particular interest. Considerable research evidence shows that anxious individuals are prone to distraction (Eysenck 1997). This performance effect is generally found with a wide range of distracting stimuli but is particularly marked with stimuli of a threatening nature (Keogh & French 2001). Anxiety therefore appears to reduce the focus on the task at hand by affecting the individual's control of the allocation of attention. Thus, in DM tasks where the effective monitoring of a complex set of environmental events is crucial to eventual performance, anxious individuals are particularly prone to errors because of vigilance for, and preferential processing of, threatening cues (Mogg et al 2000).

Returning to the function of anxiety as an emotion responsible for priming the detection of threat, it is perhaps understandable that anxious individuals appear particularly alert to sources of threat when they appear. Thus, in threatening situations it may be appropriate for anxious individuals to allocate attentional resources quite widely in an attempt to best identify threatening events when they occur (Wilson & MacLeod 2003).

Such an explanation of the attentional effects of anxiety is in direct opposition to the arousal-based 'cue utilization' theory proposed by Easterbrook (1959). This theory presents an account of how arousal affects the range of cues attended to and the performance consequences that arise. According to Easterbrook's theory, increases in arousal are directly associated with an involuntary narrowing of attention, which leads to a narrow, but stable focus on relatively few task features. High levels of arousal are predicted to lead to a decline in performance due to important task-related cues being 'missed'. This effect is predicted to become more apparent in complex DM tasks as they are assumed to have a greater number of task relevant cues to attend to. Easterbrook's theory has become a widely advanced 'explanation' of the effect of arousal on performance. This appears to be largely due to the theory's apparent alignment with predictions based on Yerkes & Dodson's (1908) inverted-U model of arousal and performance.

Despite the evidence that appears to support Easterbrook's attentional narrowing account, closer scrutiny of the research reveals a number of problematic findings for the theory. Firstly, extensive support is available that shows anxious individuals are easily distracted from the task at hand (Janelle et al 1999, Keogh et al 2004). According to Easterbrook's account, anxious individuals, assuming they are experiencing high arousal, should exhibit a narrow, but stable focus of attention and thus be *less* susceptible to distraction. Secondly, much of the research that has examined Easterbrook's theory has used variants of the dual-task paradigm in which a central or main task is performed, normally continuously, alongside a secondary task that is presented periodically, often in the periphery of the visual field. Typically the secondary task involves some form of target-detection or probe reaction time task, with the latency of detection or the number of event omissions being the measured variables. In the majority of sport-related studies, arousal has normally been manipulated by a combination of ego-relevant instructions and competition. The main prediction based on Easterbrook's account is that, as arousal increases, performance on the secondary task should be impaired to a greater extent than performance on the main task.

The general pattern of findings from dual-task studies supports the prediction that secondary task performance is impaired under high arousal when the main task being performed is cognitively demanding and when the secondary task is low in salience (Staal 2004). Problems with Easterbrook's account arise, however, when the secondary task is perceived by the performer as equally important. In such situations, when secondary tasks are perceived to be of equal salience or, as in the case of anxious individuals, potentially threatening, the available evidence shows that secondary task performance actually improves under high arousal (see Eysenck et al 2007 for a fuller discussion). These findings are clearly at odds with Easterbrook's predictions and highlight the importance of taking into account the nature of distracting stimuli and how processing priorities change when anxious individuals encounter distractors that signal threat. Taken together, current evidence supports the view that the attentional characteristics of anxious individuals reflect a 'hyper-vigilant' rather than a narrow attentional state as would be predicted by Easterbrook's theory.

Working memory, attention control and decision making

The two other main attributes of situation awareness are comprehension (or situational understanding) and prediction. In both instances there is evidence to implicate anxiety as a disruptive influence. As well as biasing perceptual processes towards threat, anxiety also exerts a strong influence on attentional control. Recent accounts of the effects of anxiety on performance have highlighted the influence of anxiety on attentional control and in particular the central executive of working memory. According to Baddeley (2001), working memory comprises four components, of which the most important is a limited capacity storage system referred to as the central executive (Fig. 17.1).

Within Baddeley's conception of working memory, the central executive serves a number of functions crucial to DM. Its major functions have much in common with those of human attention. It serves as a control system for the planning, regulation and deployment of attentional resources between task

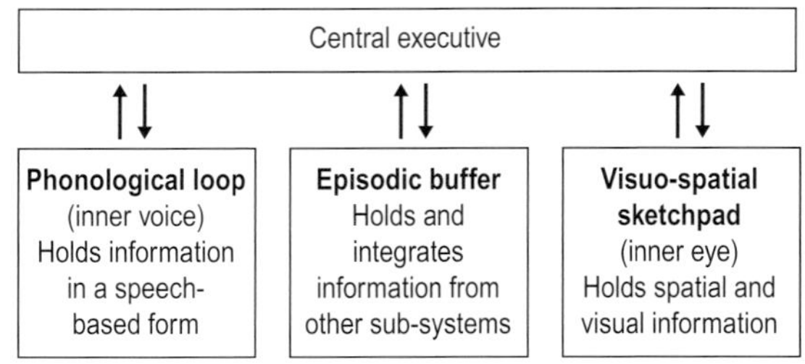

Fig. 17.1 • The main components of Baddeley's model of working memory. Adapted from Baddeley 2001.

components. As such, it serves a 'switching' function of resources between task elements as task demands change. It also regulates attentional resources in tasks that require selective attention and those where an inhibitory function is needed to block irrelevant or distracting information from entering awareness. The central executive also serves a goal-directed, planning and updating role that requires periodic checking of the two major support systems (the articulatory loop and the visuospatial sketchpad). Finally, it has responsibility for coding representations in memory according to time and place of appearance, a role that is crucial to the memory of event sequences.

Supporting the central executive are two main slave systems that have been termed the 'inner voice' and the 'inner eye' (Eysenck & Keane 2005). These two systems are responsible for the temporary holding of speech based and visuospatial information respectively. The final component of the working memory model is an episodic buffer, which holds the integrated information from the central executive in a unitary form.

Three functions of the central executive of working memory have particular relevance to DM (Miyake et al 2000). First, the central executive is responsible for the control of attention necessary to inhibit the disruptive influence of task-irrelevant stimuli and thoughts. Second, the central executive shifts processing resources between task components when performance requires the effective balancing of multiple task demands or operations. Finally, the central executive is responsible for the monitoring and updating of working memory based on the activities of its two main 'slave' systems (the phonological loop and the visuospatial sketchpad). Since situation comprehension and the ability to predict future events as they unfold rely strongly on the operations of the central executive of working memory, it is unsurprising that anxiety has the potential to exert such a strong negative effect on DM performance.

Recent attempts to account for anxiety-induced changes in cognitive performance have identified the disruption of attentional processes as the main mechanism involved. Given this view, it is unsurprising that the central executive of working memory has become a particular focus for research into the disruptive effects of anxiety. Two influential theories that have elaborated on the processes involved are processing efficiency theory (Eysenck & Calvo 1992) and attentional control theory (Eysenck et al 2007).

Processing efficiency theory

Processing efficiency theory (PET; Eysenck & Calvo 1992) seeks to account for the influence of state anxiety on performance from a cognitive/motivational perspective. The theory is most applicable to tasks that place high cognitive demands on performers and is therefore particularly applicable to complex DM tasks. The theory is of additional interest to sport performers as it emphasizes the importance of coping behaviours in potentially aversive settings where evaluation and social comparisons form part of the performance environment. While the theory places greater emphasis on the influence of state anxiety on performance, dispositional factors (i.e. trait anxiety) are also important as, along with situational threat, they interactively determine the level of state anxiety experienced.

PET makes an important distinction between performance effectiveness and processing efficiency. Performance effectiveness refers to the quality of performance in terms of its speed and accuracy. Processing efficiency is defined as performance effectiveness divided by the processing resources invested in the task. Thus processing efficiency declines in situations where performers maintain performance levels by investing additional resources in the task. This distinction is central to the theory, as it argues that anxiety affects processing efficiency more often than performance effectiveness.

Why is this distinction between processing effectiveness and efficiency important? Despite the generally held view that cognitive anxiety in the form of worry exerts a negative effect on performance, findings to support this view have been inconsistent (Eysenck et al 2007). Indeed, some of the more recently developed multidimensional models of the anxiety–performance relationship that have been applied to sport (e.g. Catastrophe theory; Hardy & Fazey 1987) make explicit predictions that, under certain conditions, increases in cognitive anxiety can have beneficial effects on performance (Hardy et al 1996).

PET explains this by highlighting that cognitive activity in the form of worry has two main effects. First, worry takes up processing and storage resources in working memory and as a mental activity it 'competes' with task-relevant thoughts for the available resources. Secondly, worry also serves a strong 'motivation' function, with anxious individuals generally being motivated to avoid the adverse consequences of the threatening situation in which they find themselves. One strategic response to such situations is to allocate more processing resources to performance by increases in effort. Increases in effort aim to maintain performance effectiveness, thus helping to avoid the potential adverse consequences of failure.

Anxiety-induced changes in effort deployment in sport have been indexed using a range of measurement approaches. These include self-report methods (Smith et al 2001a, in a study involving elite volleyball players; Wilson & Smith 2007, in a field-hockey study involving international standard players), psychophysiological measures (Hardy & Hutchinson 2007, in a study of skilled rock climbers) and dual-task performance (Wilson et al 2006, in a simulated rally driving task).

Smith et al (2001a) conducted a season-long study of anxiety and performance in English National League volleyball players. Anxiety ratings were taken from players both before and during matches along with ratings of mental effort. Performance was analysed from video records using a computer-based volleyball analysis system. Consistent with PET predictions, the authors found that high anxious individuals reported higher levels of effort than low anxious performers during matches when their performance levels were comparable. A second prediction of PET relates to the impact of motivational factors on the performance of high and low anxious individuals. PET argues that, because high anxious performers typically exert greater effort during performance, motivational incentives designed to increase effort will have less effect on the performance of high compared to low anxious individuals. The Smith et al (2001a) study examined this prediction in games where the 'criticality' of sets varied across the course of the match. The authors analysed mental effort and performance effectiveness in sets where the point-spread between the two teams differed, reflecting the criticality (or closeness) of play. Low critical sets were those in which more than six points separated the teams, moderately critical sets were those in which between three and six points separated the teams, finally, high critical sets were those in which the margin between the teams was two points (i.e. the minimum point margin). Smith et al argued that these variations in criticality could be argued to reflect playing conditions in which the motivation to exert greater effort (in order to eventually win the set) would also vary. Consistent both with this view and the predictions of PET, less anxious performers showed greater variation in mental effort across sets of varying criticality than did highly anxious players. Of particular importance was the finding that, in highly critical sets, dispositionally low anxiety performers continued to improve their performance as they exerted greater efforts, while the performance of highly anxious individuals declined significantly despite increases in effort.

These initial findings have recently been extended in a study of simulated rally driving (Wilson et al 2006) and an ecologically valid study of field hockey conducted during international competition (Wilson & Smith 2007). In the Wilson & Smith (2007) hockey study, highly critical matches were associated with higher state anxiety and effort in high anxiety compared to low anxiety individuals. Highly anxious individuals also reported higher levels of effort than their less anxious counterparts during matches when their performance levels were comparable.

Taken together, the findings from sport-related research that have tested the predications of PET provide testimony to its usefulness as a theoretical framework for studying the effects of anxiety on performance. Recent research findings into the phenomenon of 'choking' in pressure situations also suggests that PET has greater explanatory power than other, self-focus explanations of performance disruption (Wilson et al 2007). Therefore, while PET may appear to have greater relevance to cognitive rather than motor aspects of performance (particularly attentional factors), the theory offers continued promise as an appropriate framework for studying anxiety-induced changes in DM effectiveness.

Attentional control theory

Despite the usefulness of PET in advancing our understanding of the effects of anxiety on performance, a number of problems existed with the theory. Recently, Eysenck et al (2007) have presented an extension of the original theory that has addressed many of these concerns (for a more complete discussion of PET's limitations see Eysenck et al 2007). Attention control theory (ACT) attempts to refine and extend the scope of PET by making more explicit predictions regarding the functions of the central executive of working memory that are disrupted by anxiety. The theory also takes account of recent developments in neuroscience that have begun to identify the neural basis of the mechanisms involved in the control of attention (Miller & Cohen 2001). These developments provide support for the view that at least two key attentional systems can be isolated that perform different functions during attention-demanding tasks (Corbetta & Shulman 2002, Duncan 2006). A goal-directed system is responsible for the 'top-down' control of attention based on current goals and expectations. Located in the prefrontal cortex of the brain, this system interacts closely with the anterior cingulate cortex to monitor and regulate the attentional requirements of goal-directed behaviour. A second system, described as the stimulus-driven attentional system, is responsible for the 'bottom-up' control of attention. This system is particularly responsive to behaviourally relevant sensory cues that are salient at the time. This system is located in the right hemisphere of the brain including the temporoparietal and ventral frontal cortex.

ACT argues that anxiety disrupts the coordination of these two attentional systems with top-down influences being attenuated in anxious individuals, resulting in less on-line goal direction, with heightened processing priority being given to salient sensory events. The consequence of this disruption of coordination is the prioritizing of the processing of threatening cues observed in anxious individuals because of the increased activity of the stimulus-driven system. While it is still in the early stages of development, the revised theory mostly focuses on two distinct executive functions that appear particularly affected. These are described in the theory as the 'inhibition' and 'shifting' functions of attention. These two main functions have considerable significance for DM performance. The inhibitory function of the central executive describes attempts to deliberately avoid or inhibit the production of highly automated or dominant responses that can disrupt performance. As such, inhibition involves the use of attention to resist the disruptive influence of task-irrelevant stimuli. This function of the central executive appears particularly sensitive to disruption by anxiety, as a considerable body of evidence shows that performance is affected by both neutral and, particularly, threatening distracters. ACT predicts that this occurs as a result of anxiety directly impairing the efficiency of the inhibition function of the central executive of working memory. Thus, anxious individuals are less able to inhibit the allocation of attention to potential threats, which in turn leads to the diverting away from the task of essential processing resources.

The second function considered by ACT is the shifting function of the central executive. Shifting refers to the ability of performers to allocate attentional resources flexibly between multiple tasks (or changing task demands) that are being performed concurrently. Again, ACT predicts that anxiety impairs the shifting function of the central executive and that negative performance effects are likely to be observed when the demands of working memory are high (e.g. when information load or complexity is high). While the basic predictions of ACT are in the early stages of being scrutinized experimentally, the theory holds considerable promise as a framework that will allow a clearer understanding of how anxiety disrupts attentional factors central to DM performance. Perhaps one of the most intriguing avenues of research is the potential within the theory for attentional 'retraining programmes' to be developed that may enable anxiety's disruptive effects on attentional processes to be avoided (see Chs 14 and 23). This would provide important evidence to supplement the following ideas on training high-performance DM.

The application and training of decision making: current thinking

Introduction to naturalistic training approaches

Until recently, in high-performance domains, it was assumed that the accumulation of many years of hands-on experience was necessary to develop elite performance levels. For example, it took nearly 3 years to develop the minimum competencies necessary to become an air traffic controller (Means et al 1993). Similarly, in sports officiating, there was little formal DM training for referees outside of amassing experience in match officiating (Mascarenhas et al 2005). However, such amassing of experience does not necessarily lead to expert-level performance (Williams & Davids 1995). The performance environment alone may not provide a sufficient number of varied and challenging scenarios in close succession to develop expertise (Means et al 1993). Thus, since effective teams need a number of accurate mental models to form an understanding and generate predictions about events (Salas et al 1997), presenting 'typical scenarios' to trainees alongside expert accounts of the factors to consider when reaching decisions may present an alternative to on-the-job learning (Ericsson & Lehman 1996, Stokes et al 1997). Such forms of training may hasten the development of pattern recognition skills and more effectively promote the development of shared mental models of typical 'representative' situations characteristic of the specific performance domain (see Cannon-Bowers & Bell 1997, Cohen et al 1997). Additionally, such training may also help individuals develop both the procedural and declarative knowledge required for effective problem solving in situations not previously encountered (Seel et al 2000).

Through such naturalistic training, trainees learn not only the cognitive skills required to make rapid and accurate assessments of situations through an understanding of the significance of certain cues, but also the metacognitive skills relating to the effective allocation of their mental resources. Evidence in support of this view comes from the sporting domain, where research has shown that novice squash players who received structured and knowledge-based video training improved their anticipatory skills more than a group who just engaged in physical practice (Abernethy et al 1999; see also Ch. 14). Of relevance, such perceptual and cognitive skills have been shown to discriminate elite and sub-elite association football players as early as age 9 (Ward & Williams 2003).

In order to train high-performance DM, less experienced performers need to recognize what elite performers look at (situation awareness – level 1), what this means and how they weigh this information in a variety of different situations (situation awareness – level 2), and the most appropriate solution or action to undertake given likely future events (situation awareness – level 3). Training exercises should be developed that challenge performers to provide accounts of the factors they considered in reaching decisions (i.e. the underpinning reasons for specific decisions) rather than relying exclusively on outcome measures (Brannick & Prince 1997, Klinger 2000, Langan-Fox et al 2000, Mascarenhas et al 2002).

Situation awareness level 1: visual perception skills

A range of studies has used event occlusion methods combined with eye movement or gaze behaviour to identify the critical cues that experts attend to when viewing structured displays (Mann et al 2007). Findings from such studies, in turn, have been used to help develop training methods that attempt to enable less skilled performers to emulate the gaze behaviour of experts (Adolphe et al 1997).

Much of this research has explored single actor scenarios performing relatively simple skills, i.e. participants attending to only one performer, such as a penalty kicker in soccer (e.g. Williams et al 1994) or a badminton player performing an overhead shot (e.g. Abernethy & Russell 1987). Frequently in team sport environments, dynamic situations have to be monitored, often with simultaneous events occurring on different parts of the field.

Interestingly, early findings suggest that, even in a relatively simple skill like a football penalty kick, blanking out different areas of the penalty kicker led to experts using compensatory strategies that proved to be equally successful (Williams et al 1994). In fact, expert sports officials such as rugby union referees are able to make accurate decisions even when partially unsighted or presented with ambiguous information (Bettman & Sujan 1987, Mascarenhas 2005). These findings have been taken as evidence that experts have a better sense of the criteria against which a set of options should be evaluated than do novices (see Sanbonmatsu et al 1992).

Furthermore, as conceded by Abernethy & Russell (1987), while visual fixation data may provide useful information on the point of gaze, the fixation point in a task that has widespread cues may only reflect a pivot point for peripheral rather than centrally orientated perception. Thus, developing an understanding of the information to be gleaned from such visual search strategies, as presented in literature on judgments, may be more important than studying gaze behaviour alone.

Situation awareness level 2: judgement and comprehension

Recognizing the relative significance of the objects and the events in the environment, known as 'weighting', is crucial to coordinated performance (Endsley 1997). For example, imagine a doubles pair in badminton, where one's weighting scale is dominated by her regard for maintaining consistency and the other's is more centred on aggressive attacking play. When presented with the same situation they are unlikely to respond in the same fashion. This weighting represents a priority system, which Rasmussen (1985) refers to as hierarchical task analysis, guiding one to the expert's consensus of what are the most important elements of the situation.

However, there is not always a 'gold standard' in the weighting scale that represents the ideal option in a DM task. For example, a sports player who is transferred from one team to another would bring the previously established weighting scale of their old team. As a consequence, when asked to make a decision, particularly under the time pressure associated with elite sport, they are likely to use their previous team's more established weighting scale, which may not match the new team's weighting. For example, a player from a team who were very offensively orientated who moves to a more defensively minded team may well act in a way that disrupts the flow and synergy of the new team.

Furthermore, in addition to differences based on team nuances, the situation itself might present the need for different weighting scales to be applied. For example, a defensively orientated team trailing by three goals might alter their weighting scales to become more attack-orientated. Therefore, training should focus on developing the declarative knowledge of both the team and the situation to ensure coherent thinking and DM.

Situation awareness level 3: prediction and coordination skills

Cannon-Bowers et al (1990) point out that mental models also include inter-positional knowledge of roles, allowing team members to anticipate behaviour and the information needs of each other more consistently. Such knowledge is dynamic and provides information on the likely DM behaviours of other team members, enabling individuals to respond in accordance with these predicted actions and to develop backup plans if preliminary solutions fail (Stout et al 1996).

Consistent with this view, Converse & Kahler (1992) suggest that mental models are constructed of a declarative mental model that provides information about the concepts in the domain and relationships between them, a procedural mental model that provides knowledge of how to respond in order to complete the task, and a strategic mental model that includes 'knowledge of the context and relationships between team members, actions to be taken if the proposed solution fails, and how to respond if necessary information is absent' (Stout et al 1996).

As there is a shortage of research that has specifically attempted to train DM in expert players, the following section will draw upon interventions that have been developed to train more effective situation awareness skills in elite rugby union officials, and show how similar strategies might be used to develop player performance.

Training high performance sports officials

Referees are often presented with complex, partially structured displays in which players move at high speeds and in which game flow and player control issues have to be balanced. In these settings, decisions are made not in isolation but embedded in evolving patterns of play. Referees are expected to reach decisions quickly, often under intense media scrutiny, while simultaneously processing input relevant to their DM from other officials. Additionally, they also have to balance their interpretation of the laws with variations in cultural context that guide the ways laws are interpreted. Given these complex and potentially conflicting demands, such settings present an ideal setting in which to explore how DM may best be trained.

Developing decision making in rugby union refereeing

In Mascarenhas et al's (2002) study, a group of English Rugby Football Union national panel referees, divided into a control group ($n = 15$) and an experimental group ($n = 41$), made a series of decisions on video-presented scenarios before and after a 6-week training programme aimed at developing DM skills. During the 6-week training period the experimental group studied training tapes consisting of five sets of five tackles, in each case with an expert providing a declaratively and procedurally rich interpretation of the technical, declarative and procedural knowledge underpinning correct DM. The control group was further subdivided into a group who watched the same video scenarios as the experimental group but without the expert's interpretation ($n = 7$) and a group who neither viewed the video scenarios nor heard the expert's commentary ($n = 8$).

Each video scenario was filmed from the referee's perspective and was taken from real game situations in order to maintain fidelity in accordance with NDM theory. The lowest ranked referees in the experimental group (those ranked from 48th to 65th on the national panel) significantly improved their percentage of correct decisions, becoming 17.43% more accurate in their decisions post-test. No changes in decision accuracy were found in the control group. Qualitative feedback from the training such as 'it's given me an insight into the thinking of a top referee' and 'I really have a clear understanding of my priorities now' suggested that this group, whose original decisions showed widespread inter-official variability, had developed mental models that were more coherent and in close alignment with the expert.

Since this study, video reviews of tackles (and other pertinent areas of rugby union refereeing) involving elaborate discussions of declarative and procedural information have become commonplace among Rugby Football Union referees and are seen as a crucial mechanism for developing a shared vocabulary (Mascarenhas et al 2001), which can aid the development of shared mental models through problem framing (Orasanu 1990). Similarly, findings have emerged from studies that have used cross-training methods in which team members are asked to perform another person's role to help develop interpositional knowledge. The results from such studies illustrate how cross-training methods can be used effectively to enhance coherence in DM within teams (Volpe et al 1996).

Building on this research, Mascarenhas used the same principles to train DM in elite rugby league and netball referees (Mascarenhas 2006). Results from these studies showed that coherent DM between officials and across sports relied on the development of a shared mental model reflecting three key characteristics.

- **Decision outcome** – who the penalty was awarded to
- **Reason** – the point of law (or the rule) that has been infringed
- **Explanation** – the characteristics of the event that determined the prescribed sanction.

As mentioned previously, there is a dearth of research that has specifically focused on training aspects of DM skills in team sport performers (Williams & Ward 2003). However, there are some notable exceptions.

Video-based decision-making training with high-performance sports teams

Christina et al (1990) used video-based training scenarios to develop pattern recognition and DM skills in American football. A 16-day video training programme was used where an experienced linebacker was asked to move a joystick to indicate his choice of defensive actions in response to a video presenting the movement of a defensive line. The results of the training programme showed daily improvements in the number of correct decisions from 25% on day 2 to over 90% on day 6, as judged by the linebacker's ability to track the tight-end's movement. Tentatively interpreted, such findings suggest that benefits from such decision-training regimes can be gained that are of relevance to performance settings. More research in this area with both larger sample sizes and appropriate transfer conditions remains a priority.

Mascarenhas and colleagues argue that principles used in training referee DM can be effectively applied to sport performers. They highlight that the development of shared mental models between team players, and the mutual understanding and coordinated actions that result, can best be achieved by the following:

1. Recording a range of typical scenarios from the performance domain, ideally from the same perspective that the performer will typically encounter. This could involve the use of a head mounted camera (see Omodei et al 1998) for increased visual fidelity
2. These high fidelity video or DVD recordings should be presented to the trainees, together with rich descriptions of an expert's declarative, procedural and strategic mental model. This will include information on all three levels of situation awareness, identifying the important cues in the event, what they mean, the corresponding appropriate actions based on the expert's predictions of future events and the possible interactions with other team members. Such exposure of the expert's weighting scale can be extracted via a 'think-aloud' process where they verbalize their thoughts, either during or after the event
3. If trainees undertake the training as a group they should be encouraged to discuss the scenarios in order to develop a shared vocabulary. Exposure to a wide range of archetype situations that are regularly encountered will help to develop implicit DM skills, so that trainees are able to respond automatically
4. Finally, to ensure transfer to the actual performance environment trainees should be asked to participate in small-sided games to develop problem solving skills, as well as combination training, which intersperses physically demanding skills with cognitively demanding skills (see Ch. 24).

The use of high-fidelity video scenarios in decision-making training

Video scenarios can be used to provide officials with realistic and experience-dependent practice opportunities in DM. Used in conjunction with expert commentary, they also provide a vehicle for presenting clear and timely feedback on DM effectiveness closely aligned to the event itself. Such a method of training has advantages over post-match debriefing sessions, which often take place sometime after the incident under scrutiny has occurred (Means et al 1993, Williams & Ward 2003).

Video has been used to assess DM performance (McLennan & Omodei 1996), with structured video training providing a useful adjunct to 'in-game' training (Starkes & Lindley 1994). Although Starkes & Lindley failed to show any conclusive evidence of such training affecting game performance, other researchers have suggested that such transfer will be evident when transfer-appropriate processing occurs (Bransford et al 1979). Specifically, transfer will occur when the presented scenario and subsequent response demands the same cognitive processes that are required in the real task (Starkes & Allard 1993). In addition, the fidelity of the video (e.g. the observational perspective from which the video is filmed and the level of detail presented) is important to ensure transfer, particularly when training elite performers (Alessi 1988).

Conclusion

The aim of this chapter was to present a review of factors that influence the effectiveness of DM in pressure situations. We highlighted the importance of naturalistic paradigms when studying DM in real-world settings, given the complexity and

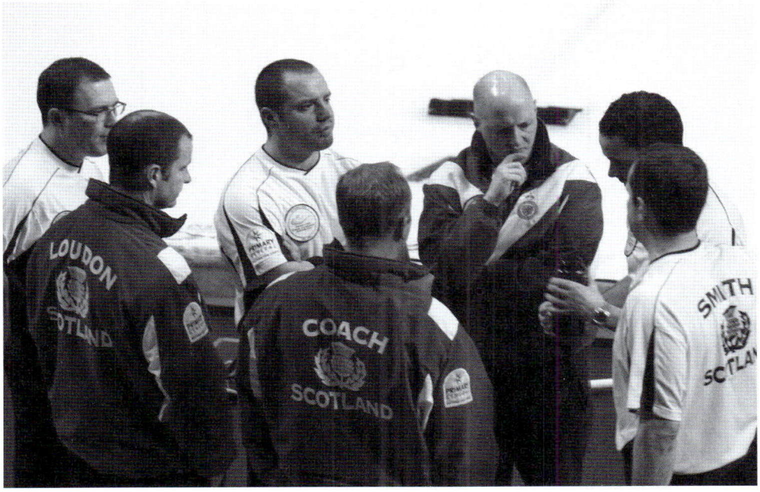

Fig. 17.2 • Even when decision making isn't time pressured, a shared mental moment helps confidence.
(c) Lesley-Ingram Brown. Reprinted with kind permission.

time pressures associated with many performance environments. Effective DM was argued to rely on the development of highly elaborate knowledge structures with both declarative and procedural elements, and expert behaviour can often be discriminated on the basis of differences in such knowledge. We showed that deliberate practice helps to develop this knowledge, together with other metacognitive and self-regulatory skills important for peak performance. It was argued that knowledge structures guide the development of mental models and the importance of developing coherent shared mental models in team situations was highlighted (Fig. 17.2). Such shared models hold information at three levels, each of relevance to the development of situational awareness; visual perception (SA 1), comprehension (SA 2) and prediction (SA 3).

Evidence that DM performance is affected by situational stress and emotion was considered and the principles of stress exposure training were explained. The importance of recognizing individual differences in anxiety and threat processing was noted, as these factors exert strong influences on DM performance. Current thinking would argue that anxiety states are characterized by a hypervigilant rather than a narrow attentional style that prioritizes the processing of threatening information. The underlying psychological mechanism responsible for performance disruption when individuals are anxious is the control of attention, particularly the inhibition and shifting functions of working memory, as explained by attention control theory. Also, in reviewing research into sports officiating we offered some ideas for improving team DM through the use of high-fidelity video training scenarios that focus on all levels of situation awareness. Finally, it was noted that while there is a large body of research that has studied DM across a range of settings, few studies have concerned themselves with how best to train this key aspect of performance. In particular, more research is needed on how best to train coordinated team performance in sport.

References

Abernethy, B., Russell, D.G., 1987. The relationship between expertise and visual search strategy in a racquet sport. Hum. Mov. Sci. 6, 283–319.

Abernethy, B., Wood, J.M., Parks, S., 1999. Can the anticaptory skills of experts be learned by novices? Res. Q. Exerc. Sport 70, 313–318.

Adolphe, R.M., Vickers, J.N., LaPlante, G., 1997. The effects of training visual attention on gaze behaviour and accuracy: a pilot study. International Journal of Sports Vision 4, 28–33.

Alessi, S.M., 1988. Fidelity in the design of instructional simulations. Journal of Computer-Based Instruction 15, 40–47.

Anderson, J.R., 1995 Cognitive psychology and its implications, fourth ed. Freeman, New York.

Baddeley, A.D., 2001. Is working memory still working? Am. Psychol. 56, 851–864.

Barnett, B., 1989. Modeling information processing components and structural knowledge representations in pilot judgment. PhD thesis, University of Illinois, Champaign, IL.

Barnett, S.M., Ceri, S.J., 2002. When and where do we apply what we learn? a taxonomy for far transfer. Psychol. Bull. 128, 612–637.

Beach, L.R., Lipshitz, R., 1993. Why classical decision theory is an inappropriate standard for evaluating and aiding most human decision making. In: Klein, G.A., Orasanu, J., Calderwood, R., Zsambok, C.E. (Eds.), Decision making in action: models and methods. Ablex, Norwood, NJ, pp. 21–35.

Bennis, W.M., Pachur, T., 2006. Fast and frugal heuristics in sports. Psychology of Sport and Exercise 7, 611–629.

Bettman, J.R., Sujan, M., 1987. Effects of framing on evaluation of comparable and noncomparable alternatives by expert and novice consumers. Journal of Consumer Research 14, 141–154.

Brannick, M.T., Prince, C., 1997. An overview of team performance measurement. In: Brannick, M.T., Salas, E., Prince, C. (Eds.), Team performance assessment and measurement: theory, methods, and applications. Lawrence Erlbaum Associates, Hillsdale, NJ, pp. 3–16.

Bransford, J.D., Franks, J.J., Morris, C.D., et al., 1979. Some general constraints on learning and memory research. In: Cermak, L.S., Craik, F.I.M. (Eds.), Levels of processing in human memory. Lawrence Erlbaum Associates, Hillsdale, NJ, pp. 331–354.

Brehmer, B., 1992. Dynamic decision making: human control of complex systems. Acta Psychol. 81, 211–241.

Butt, J., Weinberg, R.S., Horn, T., 2003. The intensity and directional interpretation of anxiety: fluctuations throughout competition and relationships to performance. Sports Psychologist 17, 35–54.

Calderwood, R., Klein, G.A., Crandall, B.W., 1988. Time pressure, skill and move quality in chess. Am. J. Psychol. 101, 481–493.

Cannon-Bowers, J.A., Bell, H.H., 1997. Training decision-makers for complex environments: Implications of the naturalistic decision-making perspective. In: Zsambok, C.E., Klein, G.A. (Eds.), Naturalistic decision making. Lawrence Erlbaum Associates, Hillsdale, NJ, pp. 99–110.

Cannon-Bowers, J.A., Salas, E., Converse, S.A., 1990. Cognitive psychology and team training: Shared mental models in complex systems. Human Factors Society Bulletin 33 (12), 1–4.

Cannon-Bowers, J.A., Salas, E., Pruitt, J.S., 1996. Establishing the boundaries of a paradigm for decision making research. Hum. Factors 38, 193–205.

Cassidy, T., 1999. Stress, cognition and health. Routledge, London.

Christina, R.W., Barresi, J.V., Shaffner, P., 1990. The development of response selection accuracy in a football linebacker using video training. Sport Psychologist 4, 11–17.

Cohen, M.S., Freeman, J.T., Thompson, B.B., 1997. Training the naturalistic decision maker. In: Zsambok, C.E., Klein, G.A. (Eds.), Naturalistic decision making. Lawrence Erlbaum Associates, Hillsdale, NJ, pp. 257–268.

Converse, S.A., Kahler, S.E., 1992. Knowledge acquisition and the measurement of shared mental models. Unpublished manuscript, Naval Training Systems Center, Orlando, FL.

Corbetta, M., Shulman, G.L., 2002. Control of goal-directed and stimulus-driven attention in the brain. Nat. Rev. Neurosci. 3, 201–215.

Craft, L.L., Magyar, T.M., Becker, B.J., et al., 2003. The relationship between the competitive state anxiety inventory-2 and sport performance: a meta-analysis. Journal of Sport and Exercise Psychology 25, 44–65.

DeGroot, A.D., 1978. Thought and choice in chess, second ed. Mouton, New York [Original published work 1946].

Dreyfus, S.E., Dreyfus, H.L., 1980. A five-stage model of the mental activities involved in directed skill acquisition. Operations Research Center (ORC-80-2), University of California, Berkeley, CA.

Driskell, J.E., Johnson, J.H., 1998. Stress exposure training. In: Cannon-Bowers, J.A., Salas, E. (Eds.), Making decisions under stress: implications for individual and team training. American Psychological Association, Washington, DC, pp. 191–217.

Duncan, J., 2006. EPS Mid-Career Award 2004: brain mechanisms of attention. Q. J. Exp. Psychol. 59, 2–27.

Easterbrook, J.A., 1959. The effect of emotion on cue utilization and the organization of behavior. Psychol. Rev. 66, 183–201.

Edwards, W., 1954. The theory of decision making. Psychol. Bull. 51, 380–417.

Endsley, M.R., 1997. The role of situation assessment in naturalistic decision making. In: Zsambok, C.E., Klein, G.A. (Eds.), Naturalistic decision making. Lawrence Erlbaum Associates, Hillsdale, NJ, pp. 269–283.

Ericsson, K.A., Lehmann, A.C., 1996. Expert and exceptional performance: evidence for maximal adaptions on task constraints. Annu. Rev. Psychol. 47, 273–305.

Ericsson, K.A., Krampe, R.T., Tesch-Römer, C., 1993. The role of deliberate practice in the acquisition of expert performance. Psychol. Rev. 100, 363–406.

Eysenck, M.W., 1997. Anxiety and cognition: a unified theory. Psychology Press, Hove, West Sussex.

Eysenck, M.W., Calvo, M.G., 1992. Anxiety and performance: the Processing Efficiency Theory. Cognition and Emotion 6, 409–434.

Eysenck, M.W., Keane, M.T., 2005. Cognitive psychology: a student's handbook. Psychology Press, Hove, West Sussex.

Eysenck, M.W., Derakshan, N., Santos, R., et al., 2007. Anxiety and cognitive performance: attentional control theory. Emotion 7, 336–353.

French, K.E., McPherson, S.L., 1999. Adaptions in response selection processes used during sport competition with increasing age and expertise. International Journal of Sport Psychology 30, 173–193.

Hardy, L., Fazey, J., 1987. The Inverted-U hypothesis: a catastrophe for sport psychology?, Paper Presented at the Annual Conference of the North American Society for the Psychology of Sport and Physical Activity, Vancouver, BC.

Hardy, L., Hutchinson, A., 2007. Effects of performance anxiety on effort and performance in rock climbing: a test of processing efficiency theory. Anxiety, Stress and Coping 20, 147–161.

Hardy, L., Jones, G., Gould, D., 1996. Understanding psychological preparation for sport. John Wiley, Chichester, West Sussex.

Hatzigeorgiadis, A., Biddle, S.J.H., 2000. Assessing cognitive interference in sport: development of the Thought Occurrence Questionnaire for Sport. Anxiety, Stress and Coping 13, 65–86.

Holyoak, K.J., 1984. Mental models in problem solving. In: Anderson, J.R., Kosslyn, S.M. (Eds.), Tutorials in learning and memory. Freeman, New York, pp. 103–218.

Isenberg, D.J., 1984. How senior managers think. Harv. Bus. Rev. (November), 81–90.

Isenberg, D.J., 1985. Some hows and whats of managerial thinking: implications for future army leaders. In: Hunt, J.G., Blair, J. (Eds.), Military leadership in the future battlefield. Pergamon Press, New York.

Janelle, C.M., Singer, R.N., Williams, A. M., 1999. External distraction and attentional narrowing: visual search evidence. Journal of Sport and Exercise Psychology 21, 70–91.

Janelle, C.M., Hillman, C.H., 2003. Expert performance in sport: current perspectives and critical issues. In: Starkes, J.L., Ericsson, K.A. (Eds.), Expert performance in sports: advances in research on sport expertise. Human Kinetics, Champaign IL, pp. 19–47.

Johnson, J.G., Raab, M., 2003. Take the first: option-generation and resulting choices. Organ. Behav. Hum. Decis. Process. 91, 215–229.

Johnson-Laird, P.N. (Ed.), 1983. Mental models. Lawrence Erlbaum Associates, Hillsdale, NJ.

Keogh, E., French, C.C., 2001. Test anxiety, evaluative stress, and susceptibility to distraction from threat. European Journal of Personality 15, 123–141.

Keogh, E., Bond, F.W., French, C.C., et al., 2004. Test anxiety, susceptibility to distraction and examination performance. Anxiety, Stress and Coping 17, 241–252.

Kerr, J.H., 1997. Motivation and emotion in sport. Psychology Press, Hove, West Sussex.

Klein, G.A., 1997a. Naturalistic decision making: Where are we going. In: Zsambok, C.E., Klein, G.A. (Eds.), Naturalistic decision making. Lawrence Erlbaum Associates, Hillsdale, NJ, pp. 383–397.

Klein, G.A., 1997b. An overview of naturalistic decision making applications. In: Zsambok, C.E., Klein, G.A. (Eds.), Naturalistic decision making. Lawrence Erlbaum Associates, Hillsdale, NJ, pp. 49–59.

Klein, G., 2000. Sources of power. MIT Press, Cambridge, MA.

Klimoski, R., Mohammed, S., 1994. Team mental model: construct or metaphor. Journal of Management 20, 403–437.

Klinger, D., 2000. Observing teams in natural settings: a helpful tool to aid in team observation and feedback, Paper presented at the 5th Conference on Naturalistic Decision Making, Tammsvik, Sweden, 26–28 May 2000.

Kozlowski, S.W.J., 1998. Training and developing adaptive teams: theory, principles and research. In: Cannon-Bowers, J.A., Salas, E. (Eds.), Making decisions under stress: implications for individual and team training. American Psychological Association, Washington, DC, pp. 115–153.

Kraiger, K., Wenzel, L., 1997. Conceptual development and empirical evaluation of measures of shared mental models as indicators of team effectiveness. In: Brannick, M. T., Salas, E., Prince, C. (Eds.), Team performance assessment and measurement: theory, methods, and applications. Lawrence Erlbaum Associates, Hillsdale, NJ, pp. 63–84.

Lane, A., Terry, P., Karageorghis, C., 1995. Antecedents of multidimensional competitive state anxiety and self-confidence in duathletes. Percept. Mot. Skills 80, 911–919.

Langan-Fox, J., Code, S., Langfield-Smith, K., 2000. Team mental models: techniques, methods and analytic approaches. Hum. Factors 42, 242–271.

Lipshitz, R., 1993. Decision making as argument-driven action. In: Klein, G. A., Orasanu, J., Calderwood, R., Zsambok, C.E. (Eds.), Decision making in action: models and methods. Ablex, Norwood, NJ, pp. 172–181.

Lipshitz, R., Ben Shaul, O., 1997. Schemata and mental models in recognition-primed decision making. In: Zsambok, C.E., Klein, G.A. (Eds.), Naturalistic decision making. Lawrence Erlbaum Associates, Hillsdale, NJ, pp. 293–303.

McLennan, J., Omodei, M.M., 1996. The role of prepriming in recognition-primed decision making. Percept. Mot. Skills 82, 1059–1069.

McPherson, S.L., Kernodle, M., 2007. Mapping two points on the tennis expertise continuum: tactical skills of adult advanced beginners and entry-level professionals during competition. J. Sports Sci. 25, 945–959.

Mann, D.T.Y., Williams, A.M., Ward, P., et al., 2007. Perceptual-cognitive expertise in sport: a meta-analysis. Journal of Sport and Exercise Psychology 29, 457–478.

Mascarenhas, D.R.D., 2005. Helping the man in the middle: assessing and training referee performance. PhD Thesis, University of Edinburgh.

Mascarenhas, D.R.D., 2006. Coherence training for elite netball umpires, Paper presented at the Netball New Zealand Coach and Umpire Development Conference, Christchurch, New Zealand.

Mascarenhas, D.R.D., Mortimer, P., Collins, D., 2001. Helping the man in the middle: coherence re-test data. Technical Report to the RFU Referees. PESLS Department, University of Edinburgh, Edinburgh.

Mascarenhas, D.R.D., Collins, D., Mortimer, P., 2002. The art of reason versus the exactness of science in elite refereeing: comments on Plessner and Betsch (2001) Journal of Sport and Exercise Psychology 24, 328–333.

Mascarenhas, D.R.D., Collins, D., Mortimer, P., et al., 2005. Training accurate and coherent decision making in rugby union referees. Sport Psychologist 19, 131–147.

Means, B., Salas, E., Crandall, B., et al., 1993. Training decision makers for the real world In Klein, G.A., Orasanu, J., Calderwood, R., Zsambok, C.E. (Eds.), Decision making in action: models and methods. Ablex, Norwood, NJ, pp. 306–326.

Miller, E.K., Cohen, J.D., 2001. An integrative theory of prefrontal cortex function. Annu. Rev. Neurosci. 24, 167–202.

Miyake, A., Friedman, N.P., Emerson, M.J., et al., 2000. The unity and diversity of executive functions and their contributions to complex 'frontal lobe' tasks: a latent variable analysis. Cogn. Psychol. 41, 49–100.

Mogg, K., Bradley, B.P., Dixon, C., et al., 2000. Trait anxiety, defensiveness and selective processing of threat: an investigation using two measures of attentional bias. Personality Individ. Differ. 28, 1063–1077.

Muris, P., De Jong, P.J., Engelen, S., 2004. Relationships between neuroticism, attentional control, and anxiety disorders' symptoms in non-clinical children. Personality Individ. Differ. 37, 789–797.

Nicholls, A.R., Polman, R.C.J., 2007. Coping in sport: a systematic review. J. Sports Sci. 25, 11–31.

Nisbett, R.E., Wilson, T.D., 1977. Telling more than we can know: verbal reports on mental processes. J. Soc. Psychol. 138, 495–504.

Noble, D., Boehm-Davis, D., Grosz, C.G., 1987. Rules schema and decision making. Engineering Research Associates, Vienna, VA.

Norman, D.A., 1983. Some observations on mental models. In: Gentner, D., Stevens, A.L. (Eds.), Mental models. Lawrence Erlbaum Associates, Hillsdale, NJ, pp. 7–14.

Omodei, M.M., McLennan, J., Whitford, P., 1998. Using a head-mounted video camera and two-stage replay to enhance orienteering performance. International Journal of Sport Psychology 29, 115–131.

Orasanu, J.M., 1990. Shared mental models and crew decision making. Technical Report for Princeton University 46, 19.

Orasanu, J., Connolly, T., 1993. The reinvention of decision-making. In: Klein, G.A., Orasanu, J., Calderwood, R., Zsambok, C.E. (Eds.), Decision making in action: models and methods. Ablex, Norwood, NJ, pp. 3–20.

Paquette, L., Kida, T., 1988. The effect of decision strategy and task complexity on decision performance. Organ. Behav. Hum. Decis. Process. 41, 128–142.

Parfitt, C.G., Hardy, L., Pates, J., 1995. Somatic anxiety and physiological arousal: their effects upon a high anaerobic, low memory demand task. International Journal of Sports Psychology 26, 196–213.

Payne, J.W., Bettman, J.R., Johnson, E.J., 1988. Adaptive strategy selection in decision making. J. Exp. Psychol. Learn. Mem. Cogn. 14, 534–552.

Payne, J.W., Bettman, J.R., Johnson, E.J., 1993. The adaptive decision maker. Cambridge University Press, New York.

Rasmussen, J., 1985. The role of hierarchical knowledge representations in decision making and system management. IEEE Trans. Syst. Man. Cybern. SMC-15, 234–243.

Richards, A., French, C.C., Keogh, E., et al., 2000. Test anxiety, inferential reasoning and working memory load. Anxiety, Stress and Coping 13, 87–109.

Riley, P., 1993. The winner within: a life plan for team players. Putnam, New York.

Roth, E.M., 1997. Analysis of decision making in nuclear power plant emergencies: an investigation of aided decision making. In: Zsambok, C.E., Klein, G.A. (Eds.), Naturalistic decision making. Lawrence Erlbaum Associates, Hillsdale, NJ, pp. 175–182.

Rouse, W.B., Morris, N.M., 1986. On looking into the black box: prospects and limits in the search for mental-models. Psychol. Bull. 100, 349–363.

Rouse, W.B., Cannon-Bowers, J.A., Salas, E., 1992. The role of mental models in team performance in complex systems. IEEE Trans. Syst. Man. Cybern. 22, 1296–1308.

Rumelhart, D.D., Ortony, A., 1977. The representations of knowledge in memory. In: Anderson, R.C., Spiro, R.J. (Eds.), Schooling and the acquisition of knowledge. Lawrence Erlbaum Associates, Hillsdale, NJ, pp. 99–135.

Ste-Marie, D., 2003. Expertise in sport judges and referees. In: Starkes, J., Ericsson, K.A. (Eds.), Expert performance in sports: advances in research on sport expertise. Human Kinetics, Champaign, IL, pp. 169–189.

Salas, E., Morgan, B.B., 1989. Role of teamwork in the development of effective work groups, Paper presented at the Annual Meeting of the American Psychological Association, New Orleans, LA, August.

Salas, E., Cannon-Bowers, J.A., Johnston, J.H., 1997. How can you turn a team of experts into an expert team?: Emerging training strategies. In: Zsambok, C.E., Klein, G.A. (Eds.), Naturalistic decision making. Lawrence Erlbaum Associates, Hillsdale, NJ, pp. 359–370.

Salthouse, T.A., 1991. Expertise as the circumvention of human processing limitations. In: Ericsson, K.A., Smith, J. (Eds.), Towards a general theory of expertise: Prospects and limits. Cambridge University Press, Cambridge, pp. 286–300.

Sanbonmatsu, D.M., Kardes, F.R., Herr, P.M., 1992. The role of prior knowledge and missing information in multiattribute evaluation. Organ. Behav. Hum. Decis. Process. 51, 76–91.

Schraagen, J.M., 1997. Discovering requirements for a naval damage control decision support system. In: Zsambok, C.E., Klein, G.A. (Eds.), Naturalistic decision making. Lawrence Erlbaum Associates, Hillsdale, NJ, pp. 227–232.

Seel, N.M., Al-Diban, S., Blumschein, P., 2000. Mental models and instructional planning. In: Spector, M., Anderson, T.M. (Eds.), Integrated and holistic perspectives on learning, instruction and technology: understanding complexity. Kluwer, Amsterdam, pp. 129–158.

Simon, H.A., 1955. A behavioral model of rational choice. Quantitative Journal of Economics 69, 99–118.

Simon, H.A., Chase, W.G., 1973. Skill in chess. Am. Sci. 61, 393–403.

Smith, N.C., Bellamy, M., Collins, D.J., et al., 2001a. A test of processing efficiency theory in a team sport context. J. Sports Sci. 19, 321–332.

Smith, N.C., Jones, B., Roach, N.K., 2001b. Competitive stress and coping in young sport performers. In: Maffulli, N., Chan, K.M., MacDonald, R. et al., Sports medicine for specific ages and abilities. Churchill Livingstone, Edinburgh, pp. 109–117.

Staal, M.A., 2004. Stress, cognition, and human performance: a literature review and conceptual framework. NASA, Hanover, MD.

Starkes, J.L., Allard, F., 1993. Cognitive issues in motor expertise. Elsevier, Amsterdam.

Starkes, J.L., Ericsson, K.A. (Eds.), 2003. Expert performance in sports:

advances in research on expertise. Human Kinetics, Champaign, IL.

Starkes, J.L., Lindley, S., 1994. Can we hasten expertise by video simulations? Quest 46, 211–222.

Stokes, A.F., Kemper, K., Kite, K., 1997. Aeronautical decision making, cue recognition, and expertise under time pressure. In: Zsambok, C.E., Klein, G.A. (Eds.), Naturalistic decision making. Lawrence Erlbaum Associates, Hillsdale, NJ, pp. 183–196.

Stout, R.J., Cannon-Bowers, J.A., Salas, E., 1996. The role of shared mental models in developing team situational awareness: implications for training. Training Research Journal 2, 85–116.

Tenenbaum, G., 2003. Expert athletes: an integrated approach to decision making. In: Starkes, J., Ericsson, K.A. (Eds.), Expert performance in sports: advances in research on sport expertise. Human Kinetics, Champaign, IL, pp. 191–218.

Tolcott, M.A., Marvin, F.F., Bresnick, T.A., 1989. The confirmation bias in military situation assessment. Decision Science Consortium, Reston, VA.

Torrance, E.P., 1953. The behaviour of small groups under the stress conditions of 'survival'. Am. Sociol. Rev. 19, 751–755.

Tversky, A., Kahneman, D., 1974. Judgment under uncertainty: heuristics and biases. Science 185, 1124–1131.

Tversky, A., Kahneman, D., 1981. The framing of decisions and the psychology of choice. Science 211, 453–458.

Volpe, C.E., Cannon-Bowers, J.A., Salas, E., Spector, P.E., 1996. The impact of cross training on team functioning: an empirical investigation. Hum. Factors 38, 87–100.

Von Neumann, J., Morgenstern, O., 1947. Theory of games and economic behaviour, second ed. Princeton University Press, Princeton, NJ.

Ward, P., Williams, A.M., 2003. Perceptual and cognitive skill development in soccer: the multidimensional nature of expert performance. Journal of Sport and Exercise Psychology 25, 93–111.

Webber, S.S., Chen, G., Payne, S.C., et al., 2000. Enhancing team mental model measurement with performance appraisal practices. Organizational Research Methods 3, 307–322.

Weinberg, R.S., Gould, D., 2007. Foundations of sport and exercise psychology. Human Kinetics, Champaign, IL.

Williams, A.M., Davids, K., 1995. Declarative knowledge in sport: a by-product of experience or a characteristic of expertise. Journal of Sport and Exercise Psychology 17, 259–273.

Williams, A.M., Ward, P., 2003. Perceptual expertise. In: Starkes, J., Ericsson, K.A. (Eds.), Expert performance in sports: advances in research on sport expertise. Human Kinetics, Champaign, IL, pp. 219–249.

Williams, A.M., Davids, K., Burwitz, L., Williams, J.G., 1994. Visual search strategies of experienced and inexperienced soccer players. Res. Q. Exerc. Sport 65, 127–135.

Williams, A.M., Davids, K., Williams, J.G. 1999. Visual perception and action in sport. E & FN Spon, London.

Wilson, E., MacLeod, C., 2003. Contrasting two accounts of anxiety-linked attentional bias: selective attention to varying levels of stimulus threat intensity. J. Abnorm. Psychol. 112, 212–218.

Wilson, M., Smith, N.C., 2007. A test of the predictions of processing efficiency theory during elite team competition using the Thought Occurrence Questionnaire for Sport. International Journal of Sport Psychology 38, 245–262.

Wilson, M., Smith, N.C., Chattington, M. et al., 2006. The role of effort in moderating the anxiety performance relationship: testing the predictions of processing efficiency theory in simulated rally driving. J. Sports Sci. 24, 1223–1233.

Wilson, M., Chattington, M., Marple-Horvat, D.E., et al., 2007. A comparison of self-focus versus attentional explanations of choking. Journal of Sport and Exercise Psychology 29, 439–456.

Yerkes, R.M., Dodson, J.D., 1908. The relationship of strength of stimulus to rapidity of habit-formation. Journal of Comparative Neurology and Psychology 18, 459–482.

Zsambok, C.E., 1997. Naturalistic decision making: Where are we now? In: Zsambok, C.E., Klein, G.A. (Eds.), Naturalistic decision making. Lawrence Erlbaum Associates, Hillsdale, NJ, pp. 3–16.

Practical dimensions of developing skill – views from the performer's panel

18

Dave Collins

Grey Matters/UCLan

CHAPTER CONTENTS

Introduction

Section 3 provides yet more material, drawn once again from a fairly 'broad church' of approaches, that is far from typical of mental skills heavy performance psychology texts to date. Hopefully, this section, like the previous two, offers a firm and well structured research rationale for the constructs used and approaches espoused. I suggest that your best approach, irrespective of whether you are a performer, coach or psychology practitioner, is to carefully weigh up the ideas presented against your current practice. There is a lot to take in but, as I highlight later in this chapter, several 'core concepts' appear in multiple chapters, albeit from subtly different perspectives but with a common core implication.

Reflecting these considerations, the PP picked up on some of these themes, pursuing applications across the section rather than chapter by chapter.

Key practical issues

The application of modern concepts in motor learning was one such theme. Several members of the PP noted ideas that were counterintuitive, or at least in contradiction to their own experiences. One such idea was 'error-free learning', which was presented by Chris, Clare and Rich in Chapter 13. Poolton et al (2005) specifically confirmed the presence of this phenomenon in a brief initial period of errorless learning in golf putting. This idea, that (if I may paraphrase) a brief period of 'just getting on with the task', with practice conditions carefully structured to keep the repetitions error-free, can set an important trend for subsequent development, is a fascinating one, with big implications for how we introduce new skills to learners. The idea is that, if early learning avoids a dependence on overly detailed verbal instruction, then learners will not turn to an overly complex, verbal analysis when things go wrong. This advice, together with the use of analogies rather than explicit instruction, is worthy of consideration by all concerned with performance.

Interestingly, all PP members needed some clarification of this, feeling that it stood at odds with several features of their own practice, for example the importance of making and learning from errors. In this regard, the educationalist John Holt (1967) said that people learnt most from 'good errors', which he defined as errors that were recognized as

DOI: 10.1016/B978-0-443-06734-1.00018-3

such, where the solution or way to remedy the error was known and where the learner had the confidence to carry on trying. All these factors were picked up by the PP. For example, both SB and RR felt that they learned most from sessions where they made mistakes; the process of sorting things out and seeking new ways of doing things was seen as essential for progress. KB pointed out the contradiction in coaching when performers are encouraged to have 'zero tolerance' of mistakes but are often concurrently told to have 'no fear' in trying new things. Juxtapose this conundrum with the 'too much telling' explicit coaching referred to in Chapter 13 and things get very unproductive. In simple terms, encouraging and equipping the learner to sort out their own challenges will almost always be more positive than taking charge and telling them what to do.

Of course, one problem is that many learners, especially adults, often rate the quality of their coaching by the volume (quantity not loudness) of instruction provided. However, the ideas presented across the section suggest that other, less autocratic and coach-controlled methods may be more effective, at least in the long term. Under this approach, the coach is seen far more as the 'organizer' or 'shaper' of a learning or practice environment, with the performer left almost to their own devices to experience and meet the various challenges presented. KB was certainly supportive of this approach, eschewing the use of 'drills' as choreography (no dig at the dancers here!) rather than 'game-like practices' that developed players holistically. As presented later in this chapter, this approach is clearly the best way forwards, but performers' personal preferences and expectations can often make them uncomfortable with such an open approach.

The theme of 'thinking how performers learn best' was continued in the next two chapters. While coming at the issue from slightly different stances, both Chapter 14 and Chapter 15 present a compelling case for the application of motor learning principles to coaching environments. Joan Vickers in Chapter 14 provides a typically well supported and thoroughly academic consideration of the advantages to be gained from these methods. The weight of evidence is overwhelming that long-term retention, real-life application and transfer of skills are enhanced by, as she puts it, 'apparently paradoxical' approaches that seem to result in slower development but actually generate genuine learning. In the next chapter, Andy and I come at many of the same issues, but from the coach rather than the performer perspective.

Yet again, however, the client-learner may raise some concerns. Under the traditional, coach direction-heavy environment, learners are used to having things 'made easier' for them, with new ideas carefully and gradually presented in bite-size chunks. The PP pointed out that giving these new methods 'time to work' may well need some selling up front to ensure learner buy-in. This was certainly my experience when working with one youth squad in a racket sport. After two sessions of a more randomized and challenging practice regimen, the athletes appealed for a return to the old ways. 'We don't think it's good to make so many mistakes in training' was the basis of their argument. This is an important argument to win with your own performers. The methods presented in this section, especially in this context within Chapters 12–14, are specifically designed to best match the ways in which humans learn. Furthermore, they are almost always more 'ecologically valid'; that is, they more faithfully match or reproduce the challenges involved in actual performance than a simplified, almost sanitized version thereof.

Our solution to this problem was threefold. Firstly, we revisited the logic of the methods with both coaches and players, taking time to secure their understanding and allowing for debate about why one method may be advantageous over another. Secondly, we used error counts (a very common approach from naturalistic decision-making (NDM; see Ch. 17)) to show the performers that their practice results were almost identical to those achieved in match play; in short, they were practising like they played, which was surely what was needed. Finally, we used video and performance analysis to demonstrate to each player how the new approaches gave them the chance to work on their specific weaknesses. The use of this three-way presentation got the players on-side long enough for us to secure performance data that showed clear signs of accelerated progress.

You should learn from our mistakes here, and do a better 'selling' job up front. In fact, even more sensibly, you wouldn't be there as your young performers would always have been training this way. Of course, this takes a major and carefully executed coach education initiative (see Section 2 for some ideas on effective culture change), probably best in tandem with some education for significant other opinion influencers. Senior and past players, parents and other support practitioners (less enlightened and informed than yourself!) are suitable cases for treatment: getting these guys on board will prevent a lot of the challenging and distracting 'noises off' that often hamper innovation.

This challenge – getting coaches and performers to work in new and proven more effective ways – is a key practical issue for the effective application of this section, and indeed a good argument for the sections selected for this book. The culture change and leadership techniques described in Section 2 should be considered against some of the ideas for specific behaviour change, the coach development methods presented in Chapter 15, for example.

As a final exemplar 'practical issue', consider the development of decision making (DM) skills covered in Chapter 17. DM, or at least in-performance DM, is less pertinent for some performance domains; 100 m sprint athletes have few decisions to make, in the race at any rate. For the majority, however, it is 'front and centre' as one of the most crucial concerns. Once again, the excellent advice offered should be considered against other naturally occurring 'pressures', which can influence both development and execution of these DM skills. In fact, both Joan (in Chapter 14) and Duncan and Nick (in Chapter 17) allude to some of these, many of which emanate from the social setting or interaction. In team sports, for example, a player's decisions may often be more influenced by presentational concerns (i.e. what s/he thinks *they* want to see) than all the good stuff preached and practised by the coaches. To counter this, ideas on role clarity from the previous section (see also Ch. 25) can be used to (once again) sell the message and ensure consistent encouragement from all aspects of the environment to 'do the right thing'.

Extreme sports offer a different but related challenge to DM, especially in slower-time, planning decisions. Instructors in these activities, almost always high-level performers themselves, can suffer from a distorted 'weighting scale' (see NDM) on what they feel is an appropriate challenge for their less talented (and often very gripped) group members. Similar social pressures will lead performers in this world to take silly risks, or even to attend insufficiently in apparently 'simple' situations. The number of climbers killed on easy descent routes or mucking about on low-grade stuff is disturbingly high. Accordingly, one aspect of the training environment in these sports, for both performers and coaches, should attend to the establishment, maintenance and effective deployment of a suitable DM weighting scale.

Things to think about

As an inevitable consequence of pushing the boundaries, chapters within this section may, at first read, seem somewhat contradictory. For example, contrast the 'quiet eye' ideas in Chapter 14 with the ideas presented in Chapter 17, viz.: 'the fixation point in a task that has widespread cues may only reflect a pivot point for peripheral rather than centrally orientated perception. Thus, developing an understanding of the information to be gleaned from such visual search strategies, as presented in literature on judgments, may be more important than studying gaze behaviour alone'. No contradiction, however. You will note that tools such as eye tracking are often used in 'triangulation'; in other words, the phenomenon is examined by use of three or more related measures and the consistency of answers yielded across the measures offers a consequently stronger or weaker interpretation, depending on the level of agreement or lack thereof. Thus, the quote above suggests the combination (triangulation) of gaze data with debriefs of performers ('what are you looking at when...') and coaches ('what should they be looking at when...' – 'what would *XXXX* mean?'). This method is very powerful and the PP reported several examples of ways in which this same approach has been used.

In similar fashion, what about the relatively light treatment of imagery in Chapter 16? Paul and Clare provide a lot of 'food for thought' in their very technical but 'application-rich' chapter. Does the lack of emphasis on imagery as a tool for mental practice contradict the central role presented for imagery in, for example, Chapter 4? Not at all, it's actually a question of which tool is best used where. The internal neurological systems necessary to employ imagery-stimulated mental practice or observation-stimulated mental practice are actually quite overlapping; the use of observation (especially on one's self) may be more effective in some environments. In fact, for many activities, Paul and Clare provide strong evidence for equal if not predominant use of observation (especially self-observation) over traditional imagery approaches. As they observe (no pun intended), observation will be particularly powerful in form-based tasks (e.g. dance, kata in martial arts, gymnastics and diving), and SM was very supportive of using 'watch and try' digital cameras in training sessions. Certainly, even one viewing of a performance can have benefits for motivated learners (Ram et al 2007), so it is difficult to see why an 'externally viewed and evaluated' activity, such as dance, would not use this tool at every stage of development.

Furthermore, improved technologies in video, including head cams as well as the increased use of individualized records of execution, mean that practitioners should read through Paul and Claire's unashamedly technical chapter with care. Once again, there is a lot of food for thought here, most notably on why video images (or of course, other technologies) may be used in different circumstances, with different performers or groups of performers for different purposes. For example, technical development in dance is a long process, some would say lifelong, and performers can sometimes lose motivation when they perceive themselves to be in a slump and not making progress. Access to individual records, held on video, can demonstrate the amount of progress made since the last benchmark and assist the slump-busting process.

In considering the ultimate mindset for expert performance, I would also want to highlight the often unconscious nature of learning (if this is possible under the current definition) or, at the very least, the evidence for genuine behaviour change at a subconscious level. Certainly, as a javelin thrower, SB's mantra for learning new refinements was 'see it – feel it – trust it', the last stage reflecting the move getting internalized and almost screened from subsequent thought. This idea is strongly supported by Chris, Clare and Rich, and should encourage the use of external constraints (e.g. a metronome to keep movements in the correct rhythm) in learning environments rather than too much coach talk. The use of rhythm as such an 'unconscious' teaching cue is well supported by research (MacPherson et al 2009) and such ideas are already commonly deployed in many performance domains. The use of different pitch sizes (Davids et al 2007) or surfaces (see Chapter 13) are other examples of ways in which the practice environment can be 'shaped' or constrained to generate learning without explicit instruction. Getting trainee weightlifters to squat facing a wall (stops them leaning forwards and overusing the back) is another traditional method built on these same ideas. In all these approaches, the learner feels less 'busy' and with less to think about they (and more importantly, their body) can work out the best ways to achieve the skill challenge.

So what should you do?

Consideration of this chapter, let alone the rest of the section, will show the potential complexity of optimizing learning and training environments.

Use more constraints than verbal instruction in your coaching

Conventional coaching wisdom used to push the old adage 'a picture is worth a thousand words', and for years coaches have employed a variety of visual stimuli such as demonstrations, film loops of elite performers, photos and the like. We have moved on from this, and modern approaches stress far more the 'doing' of the skill than watching, albeit this is still very useful at the right time and in the right way (see Chapter 16). Similar arguments should apply to coach instruction, however. Doing is even better than listening, so coaches should be encouraged to explore ways in which detailed explanations and complex guidelines can be minimized. The use of analogy and constraints is explored well in Chapter 13. Using such structures saves time in the coaching process and facilitates the 'non-verbal exploration' essential to optimum learning. At higher levels, these approaches let performers come up with their own solutions, often more creative than the coaches and usually with better buy-in!

Use 'decision-training'/toolbox approaches to focus on genuine learning

These two ideas (decision training, see Table 14.1; toolbox, see Fig. 15.5) cover much of the same approach. In both cases, however, one important point to emerge should be that there is not one best method available to meet the challenges and goals of a particular coaching situation. Consequently, any solution set of behaviours and actions (a.k.a. the plan) will be made up of numerous 'best-fit' options. As such, the question 'Well, how did that session go?' should always be responded to with 'Well, what were your aims?'

The other crucial feature to note is the dichotomy between different 'sets' of learning approaches, which have been summarized as 'quick learning' versus 'retention/transfer'. I have highlighted earlier in this chapter the concern over whether the first should even be seen as learning at all, especially when learning is seen as a 'permanent change in behaviour'. I also explored the selling job that may often be necessary when apparent progress is sacrificed for longer-term development. Once again, use of the methods discussed earlier is the best on-the-ground solution. Managers, administrators or sports leaders may like to consider the extent to which these approaches are both espoused and supported by higher orders, or even considered within coach education schemes.

The use of devices such as the toolbox can also enable greater self-reflection by the coach. They offer a vocabulary through which coaches can think through, by themselves or with their peers, how well their performers are learning. Unfortunately, research suggests that many coaches are particularly weak at this element of their skill set (pedagogy – the study of how people learn and can best be taught), so the use of tools that raise awareness and facilitate debate can make a significant contribution. Both KB and SM talked about the need for coaches to reflect carefully on the methods they use. In dance, SM endorsed the idea of 'peer supervision' (an idea borrowed from clinical psych practice), where teachers pair up for scheduled observation and feedback on their sessions. Changing partners at intervals helps to keep the stimulus fresh, while the use of common vocabulary (easy for dance teachers talking about dance, less easy about pedagogy) facilitates mutual growth. KB stressed the need for this reflection process to also take place during, as well as after, the session so that the coach becomes aware and can counter any performer difficulties in 'getting the message'.

Use observation as a key coaching tool

Chapter 16 presents a compelling and scientifically rigorous case for observation as a key tool – back to the picture/thousand words perspective. The point here is that watching yourself (or perhaps a similar-level performer) in execution generates all sorts of useful thoughts and other mental processes, so long as care is taken. This care should extend to use with the right level of performer (better with those who already have a good internalized picture and 'feel' for the movements), the right sort of model (see my earlier comments – you need to ensure that the watcher can both cognitively appreciate and imagine the feel of what the model is doing – see the final block on combining technical training with the development of other skills) and the setting conditions, literally what the watcher is set up to watch and with what aims, coupled with the follow through in terms of practices and feedback.

Develop decision making by means of naturalistic decision-making approaches

In order to train high-performance DM, less experienced performers need to recognize what elite performers look at (situation awareness – level 1), what this means and how they weigh this information in a variety of different situations (situation awareness – level 2), and the most appropriate solution or action to undertake given likely future events (situation awareness level 3). Systematic attention to these factors can generate improvement at any level. For example, recent research has generated improvements in the perceptual skills of 60-year-old very experienced tennis players (Caserta et al 2007). As such, and of course as DM is so crucial to certain domains, performers should include this sort of work at every stage of their development, even on the way down!

Chapter 17 contains several practical suggestions on how to do this. Most practitioners would agree that such training can come in a variety of forms, including situation-specific drills, 'stop the action and talk' sessions, team/performer meetings, explicit ('look at *this*') and implicit ('watch and tell me what you see') use of performance video and team meetings. At present, we have no evidence as to which factors, or more likely combination of factors, are most effective in developing DM at expert levels. What clearly emerges from both literature and practice is the need to promote a common understanding across the team/group as to what the critical factors are, together with a common vocabulary (set of constructs) with which to discuss them (Richards et al 2009). As such, informal/impromptu discussion between team members should be added to the list above as important tools in the coach's box. Interestingly, and in keeping with many of the ideas in this section, DM may best be developed by coaches' informal manipulation of the environment than by formal coach-directed activity. Generating a team setting where performers 'talk about their work' is an important marker on the road to excellence.

Combine skill training with challenges to develop mental skills for learning and performance

Obviously, the development of mental skills and strategies for performance is the focus of the next section. However, all members of the PP stressed that these skills should not be considered in isolation from skill development but rather worked on 'in tandem' wherever possible. For example, the skill of being able to lift and/or adjust your skill in an event was emphasized by both SB and RR. SB talked about the need to lift performance by choice, within the boundaries of a particular session. Thus, in a fairly 'mediocre' session (for him around the 70 m mark), SB would decide 'the next one is having it' and lift performance to 72–75 m. In a better (80 m average) session, the 'having it' target went up to 84 m, and so on. The discipline of being able to focus to lift performance offered a useful training stimulus and check for SB.

From a learning perspective, both SB and SM talked about how skilled performers used observation to evolve new skills. Reflecting the ideas on 'mirror neurons' presented in Chapter 16, both talked about the process of observing others and trying to translate what was seen into 'feel'; literally, the consequences of the movement if they did it themselves. Once this was accomplished, a new 'hybrid' version of the skill could be created, tried and refined. For both these PP members, the ability to translate observation into feel was important (intersensory integration – Connolly & Jones 1970). SB stressed the use of feel as a bridge for 'converting cues to consequence'; this is an important learning skill which can be developed 'in parallel' to technical practice. SM talked about the application of 'what you observe' to develop kinesthetic consequences to direct 'what you do'; the capacity to manipulate and combine 'feeling images' to generate sensory consequences for novel combinations of movements (see Calvo-Merino et al 2005, Orgs et al 2008, Ramenzoni et al 2008). In short, skill practice is an (other) important learning environment for skills needed across the range of component tasks for a high-level performer.

Conclusion

Hopefully, this section has provided much food for thought. For practitioners, coaches and the like, many of the ideas may challenge. Accept and enjoy this, thinking through the wherefores but most importantly the whys of the points made. For psychologists, particularly those without a motor control/skills acquisition base, once again the points made should be considered critically against current practice in your working environment. Integration of these ideas with more 'conventional' mental skills should yield some significant benefits.

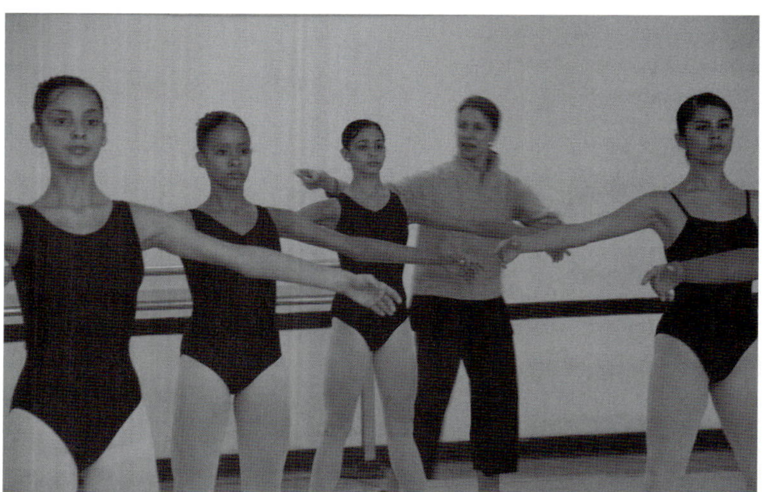

Performance Panel member Sara Matthews teaching young dancers in Cuba

References

Calvo-Merino, B., Glaser, D.E., Grezes, J., et al., 2005. Action observation and acquired motor skills: An fMRI study with expert dancers. Cereb. Cortex 15, 1243–1249.

Caserta, R., Young, J., Janelle, C., 2007. Old dogs, new tricks: training the perceptual skills of senior tennis players. Journal of Sport and Exercise Psychology 29, 479–497.

Connolly, K., Jones, B., 1970. A developmental study of afferent-reafferent integration. Br. J. Psychol. 61, 259–266.

Davids, K., Button, C., Bennett, S., 2007. Dynamics of skill acquisition – a constraints led approach. Human Kinetics, Champaign, IL.

Holt, J., 1967. How children learn. Pitman, New York.

MacPherson, A., Collins, D., Obhi, S., 2009. The importance of temporal structure and rhythm for the optimum performance of motor skills: a new focus for practitioners of sport psychology. Journal of Applied Sport Psychology 21, S48–S61.

Orgs, G., Dombrowski, J.H., Heil, M., et al., 2008. Expertise in dance modulates alpha/beta event-related desynchronization during action observation. Eur. J. Neurosci. 27, 3380–3384.

Poolton, J.M., Masters, R.S.W., Maxwell, J.P., 2005. The relationship between initial errorless learning conditions and subsequent performance. Hum. Mov. Sci. 24, 362–378.

Ram, N., Riggs, S.M., Skaling, S., et al., 2007. A comparison of modelling and imagery in the acquisition and retention of motor skills. J. Sports Sci. 25, 587–597.

Ramenzoni, V.C., Riley, M.A., Shockley, K., et al., 2008. An information-based approach to action understanding. Cognition 106, 1059–1070.

Richards, P., Mascarenhas, D.R.D., Collins, D., 2009. Implementing reflective practice approaches with elite team athletes: parameters of success. Reflective Practice: International and Multidisciplinary Perspectives 11, 353–363.

Section 4

Performance

Introduction: performing on the day

19

Dave Collins

Grey Matters/UCLan

So after selecting the right people, setting up a superb organization around them and training them to a razor-sharp pitch, THE day has arrived. However you are involved in performance, as performer, coach/teacher, significant other or 'just' interested spectator, the performance is the moment of truth. This is where, for most of the uninformed, progress is measured. As a consequence, if your head isn't right on the day, the whole preparation can get slagged off right royally as a waste of time and money. The pressures of this demand are apparent in many ways, not least in the game of musical chairs that seems to characterize most football management. The fact is that, irrespective of the quality and comprehensiveness of the preparation, performers often 'commit suicide' in pressure situations. Performance can collapse for so many reasons, with a variety of consequences on a continuum from dire downwards. The aim of the performance psychologist, coach/teacher and performer is to gain sufficient control of the chaotic influences while maintaining sufficient confidence, calm and enjoyment (yes, even at that level) to fully realize or even exceed potential.

Of course, there is a lot of truth in this emphasis; the training and preparation are there against producing a performance on one occasion, or finite set of occasions. That's part of the fun! We would also commend a longer-term view, however, where criticism takes account of process efficacy as much as outcome. To this end, and of course to be able to influence the performer's state of mind, gaining a deeper understanding of the interconnecting constructs that can accentuate the positives and minimize or even eliminate the negatives. In seeking this Holy Grail, several concerns are evident, not least ensuring that all are agreed – and correct – on what these positives and negatives are!

How about the content of these chapters? Well we can't even begin to suggest that they offer a complete and total coverage of the Preparation topic. There are whole books, even more wordy than this one, about specific issues raised in the chapters, while many others offer (or purport to offer) the whole answer through a sole focus on mental strategies. These strategies or skills are the psychologist's stock in trade and certainly play an important role; accordingly, you will find a range of approaches from sport-specific 'twists or tweaks' to whole method imports from mainstream psychology, such as cognitive behaviour therapy (CBT). Hopefully, however, careful consideration of this book will have shown you that there is a lot more to performance, and therefore of course to performance psychology, than a box of mental tricks! So consider the use of the techniques offered (the presentation is comprehensive if not complete), but as a feature of an integrated programme that addresses all the components from each of the four sections.

So to the Section. In Chapter 20, Hugh Richards considers the coping process: methods of handling the pressure that is an almost inevitable consequence of placing yourself in an elite performance challenge. In fact, the coping process is often necessary because focus has wavered. Reflecting this interaction, Aidan Moran considers the allocation of attention in Chapter 22, offering some practical ways to train focus. In Chapter 21, two very experienced performance psychologists, Sheelagh Rodgers and Britt Tajet-Foxall, consider the performance challenges posed by emotion and the application of

DOI: 10.1016/B978-0-443-06734-1.00019-5

CBT to do something about it. Sheelagh's considerable experience in performance and in clinical psychology offers an informed opinion on what can be done and what should be passed on to other better qualified individuals. The section concludes with two chapters focused on the practical methods of enhancing performance in individual (Chapter 23 by Mark Wilson and Hugh Richards) and team/group (Chapter 24 by my daughter Judy and me) settings. Section 4 concludes with the usual consideration of practical implications offered by the Performers Panel.

Coping and mental toughness

20

Hugh Richards

University of Edinburgh, Edinburgh, UK

CHAPTER CONTENTS

Introduction

Almost every person involved in high performance either as performer, director, coach, psychologist or any support professional acknowledges the importance of coping and mental toughness to attain highest-level performance. This relates to both the long periods of 'getting there' – including preparation and training, and the shorter intense periods of 'being there' – performance. Coping and mental toughness are thought to offset the chronic and often relentless demands of preparation and training phases, and the high intensity of in-event performance experiences, in which factors such as anxiety and distraction can easily impair performance. Throughout this chapter I would like you to keep in mind that coping, and being mentally tough, are continual requirements for performers. It is not just on the 'big stage' where these factors count, it is just the case that it is at these times that other people notice it most. But performers must first earn the opportunity to get on to the big stage and they do this over a long period of time, and in the process endure cold, lonely training, injury, curtailed social life, failed relationships, low earnings and constantly pushing to do things never previously done, so that failure is a common friend. Thus the ideas and suggestions in this chapter are intended to be used and developed regularly, in the performers' day-to-day activity, and deployed more specifically when the demands escalate.

Coping is an established topic with a long track record as both a research focus and area of applied practice. This is mirrored in publications related to physical, systematic reviews (Nichols & Polman 2007) and book chapters (Richards 2004). In this chapter, I summarize the leading approaches to coping and focus specifically on the way in which the evidence base supports coping interventions to develop performers. In contrast to coping, the concept of mental toughness has received a sudden upsurge in interest from around 2002, with book chapters (Clough et al 2002) and peer-reviewed articles (Bull et al 2005, Jones et al 2002). These efforts

DOI: 10.1016/B978-0-443-06734-1.00020-1

have spawned a raft of self-help books extolling the virtue of mental toughness for performance professionals in other domains, notably business (e.g. Bull 2006, Jones & Moorhouse 2008). In this chapter, I also examine the evidence for this construct and how it can contribute to our understanding of the psychological factors associated with successful performance. Finally, this chapter considers the applied implications for other constructs within psychology that are aligned with the general concepts of coping and mental toughness and have clear relevance for supporting performers in physical performance situations.

Coping

What is coping?

Within psychology, two approaches to studying coping have developed, which can essentially be divided on the basis of permanence. One approach, following in the tradition of trait psychology, assumes that individuals have a coping style that is relatively fixed and stable across time and place (Carver et al 1989). In this approach, coping style is considered in terms of a fixed individual difference. In terms of utility, this approach to coping has limitations because it assumes individuals have predispositions to respond that may be relatively unaffected by any intervention. Thus, this work might be able to predict how people might respond, which could be used to channel those responses to maximum benefit (or least disadvantage) or alternatively select the most appropriate individuals for the situation and demands. While this selection idea might seem appealing, the complex, multifaceted nature of most physical performance situations means that it is highly unlikely that the data will ever strongly support selection based on this feature alone.

The second approach to coping is based on the work of Lazarus & Folkman (1984, p. 141) who described coping as 'constantly changing cognitive and behavioural efforts to manage specific external and/or internal demands'. They subsequently produced evidence of coping changing over time, confirming that it was not fixed and stable as the style approach would suggest (Folkman & Lazarus 1985). The coping process approach has dominated the bulk of research efforts in coping and performance, although interest in the style approach still continues. Some authors have found evidence of both stability and change (Crocker & Issak 1997) and several authors support the need to coordinate these views so that they are not conceived of as mutually exclusive opposites (Lazarus 1993). This reconciliation might be achieved by adopting a cognitive–affective model of personality (Mischel & Shoda 1995) to identify conditions under which stable patterns of coping response might occur (Richards 2004, Smith 2006). However the process approach remains the dominant perspective (Nichols & Polman 2007) and this is understandable, in part, because it assumes that it is possible to intervene with, and enhance performers' abilities to cope. The remainder of this chapter discusses coping in relation to this dominant process perspective.

Coping: categories and emotion

Analysis of how individuals cope with the demands of performance has, in keeping with the main psychology literature base, used large categories to group the specific coping thoughts and actions reported by performers. For example, Giacobbi et al (2004) suggested that golfers' reports of drinking beer, not riding in the same cart as opponents and talking to friends could all be categorized under a group title of Avoidance coping. Similarly, performance artists coping responses to 'let go' and view the 'art as bigger than me' were both ascribed to the category Appraisal focused (Poczwardowski & Conroy 2002). Within the literature, several forms of category labels have emerged, the most frequently used including problem-focused & emotion-focused (Lazarus & Folkman 1984), appraisal (Cox & Ferguson 1991) and avoidance (Endler & Parker 1990).

Problem-orientated coping is coping designed to deliberately address the cause of an issue, whereas emotion-orientated coping focuses on managing and changing the internal response that the problem has caused. Clearly, if the cause remains unchanged then there is perpetual demand to cope using emotion-orientated coping and this is one of the reasons why this style of coping is less recommended. Appraisal coping refers to changing the initial thinking processes that stimulated perception of challenge or threat. Appraisal is described in terms of questions that are asked about an event. Primary appraisal asks if the event or situation is important, and if there is a significant chance of threat, challenge loss or harm that might be experienced. If the answer to these is yes, then secondary appraisal is reflected in the question whether abilities and coping resources are sufficient to meet the demands. The answer to these appraisal questions will then trigger coping responses. However, reappraisal can be used as coping so that an event that was initially appraised as relevant, threatening and to which resources were inadequate can be reappraised as irrelevant and therefore not threatening, nor requiring coping. Reappraisal can work very quickly but can often be associated with relinquishing goals. The cost–benefit analysis of this type of coping needs to be considered in relation to the exact event and performance demands. The final type of coping, avoidance, can occur through behavioural or mental activity. Avoidance is usually considered to be a weak coping strategy. However, for physical performers many issues to do with performance, for example worry before the start, dissipate very quickly once performance commences. Performers may be able to utilize avoidance effectively, in contrast to the general perception, if they can avoid the issue, which will disappear once the performance is done.

This approach to creating larger category groupings, either by inductively grouping similar responses and labelling them or deductively assigning responses to existing category labels, allows conclusions to be made in a simplified fashion. For example, males have been reported to use more Approach coping than females (Anshell et al 1998), elites to use more Problem-focused coping than non-elite (Yoo 2001) and sports performers from the USA to respond directly to the issue of an opponent cheating – approach coping – whereas Australian counterparts avoid the issue (Anshell et al 1997). These category labels seem initially to offer a sensible means of summarizing general differences. However, there would appear to be a flaw in this thinking, in that coping responses are often utilized by performers to have more than one outcome and so grouping coping responses risks making categorical errors in analysis. Furthermore, the same response might be utilized to achieve different outcomes in different situations (Gould et al 1993). Cox & Ferguson (1991) suggest that the relationship between types of coping should be reconfigured to account for the fact that, ultimately, all coping serves a single function, which is to address the emotion-driven state of the performer. Therefore, rather than being mutually exclusive, all categories of coping should be subordinate to emotion-focused coping (Richards 2004). This central role for emotion is important to recognize and is addressed in much more detail in the following chapter. The key point to remember is that performers are not driven to cope, for example by establishing a clear plan, just because they enjoy the process. It is the fact that being organized and prepared makes them feel confident, reassured and less anxious that provides the motivation to do it. The motivation for all coping responses therefore stems from an emotion-based origin and this places emotion at the heart of performance concerns.

Measuring coping

In order to investigate coping, researchers have developed several different approaches to assess it. While this chapter is not designed to prepare readers for research in coping, the measurement tools and approaches are very important in relation to designing and monitoring training and so they have strong applied relevance. It is therefore valuable to consider examples of these different approaches together with their relative limitations to determine how to use these in an applied context.

In the definition of coping provided earlier, Lazarus & Folkman (1984) emphasize that coping consists of cognitive and behavioural aspects. This definition means that accessing thought content is essential to determine coping – observation alone cannot be used to assess coping. Accessing thoughts means that we have to get performers to tell us what they are thinking and various types of self-report – questionnaire, interview, think aloud and diary – can be used to achieve this. One of the most widely used questionnaires, designed for general use, is the COPE scale (Carver et al 1989), which assesses 12 different coping responses (Table 20.1). In their development, Carver and colleagues also went so far as to suggest which of these categories they believed were beneficial and which were not, although there remained some (humour, alcohol and drugs) that they did not comment on.

When the list is considered in detail it is perhaps surprising to see responses such as acceptance identified as a maladaptive coping response. For a physical performer, accepting an injury might prove very functional if they reduce the load on the injured area and adhere to rehabilitation and treatment schedules. In a similar vein, recent research in a non-competitive, ultra-endurance environment has shown how much performers use mental disengagement to their benefit (Richards & Collins 2005). 'Switching off' and holding out when you have been running for 3 hours, there are 5 hours more to go, the sun is up and it is 35°C is quite functional coping. These issues reflect the fact that it is difficult to

Table 20.1 Coping responses measured by the COPE questionnaire (Carver et al 1989)

Coping responses	Proposed effect
Active coping Planning Positive reframing	Adaptive
Emotional support Religion	May be adaptive
Acceptance Mental disengagement Venting emotions Behavioural disengagement Denial	Maladaptive
Alcohol and drugs Humour	Not considered

determine whether a coping response might be useful or not, and this is an important issue in measuring coping. This problem is about determining not what the coping response is but what effect it has. Although Carver et al designed the COPE for general use, its origins, like much of our knowledge on coping, came from medical settings and people coping with illness and disease and so the views on adaptiveness were context-specific. I will come back to the issue of effectiveness shortly. However, the point to take from this is that coping responses usually have some consequence or effect but are not inherently good or bad. In short, do not judge or exclude responses based on a principle or personal preference until they have been accurately judged in relation to the specific person, situation and intended goal.

There is a general recommendation that measures of constructs that relate to the performance domain should be made specific to that domain. So, for example, questionnaires for a sports population should be designed with reference to sport settings and terminology (Marsh 1997). Several sports-specific questionnaires have been developed or been modified from other questionnaires for this purpose, for example the M-COPE (Crocker & Graham 1995) a modified version of COPE, and the CICS (Gaudreau & Blondin 2002). These are likely to have significant potential for transfer to use in other physical performance domains. However, the application must be done with care so respondents feel the questionnaire is relevant to them but also so that the validated properties of the scale are not lost. In theory, any modification to change the domain context should be revalidated with a sample of the new population. Questionnaires provide a quick, comparable means of assessing coping but the quality of information relies on them being comprehensive. For example, the M-COPE does not include mental disengagement (removed as part of the modification for sport) even though, as I have discussed above, mental disengagement (dissociation) is known to be commonly used as a strategy by endurance performers. Questionnaires will only measure what they ask about and will not pick up unexpected or unusual responses. As a consequence, they might miss a significant type of coping, or be so long in order to capture everything that they become unwieldy to use.

An alternative measurement approach and one which circumvents this problem is to use verbal reports from performers about what they did to cope. This can be done with an interview (debrief), through written accounts, possibly in the form of a diary, or through video or audio recording. In all cases, the degree of structure put on this process can be adapted according to what is required. Interviews can have set questions, be more free-flowing or combine elements of these. Diaries can have boxes and sections to complete or be blank, and recording can be made about specific preordained categories of information or left to the performers' choice. Self-report is all about how a performer has responded but, when it is applied retrospectively to performance, is susceptible to being influenced by the outcome. For example, a successful performance gives a glossy veneer to the memories and people typically report less of the hardship and recall fewer responses, especially those that did not work. If the performance went well, then coping responses are usually given little attention, while the reverse is true if the performance has not gone well. The alternative to retrospective measurement is to assess coping in the event. For example, following the think aloud protocol of Schomer (1986), we used small digital voice recorders to assess coping of endurance performers. They reported information in categories listed on a prompt card during short water breaks or on easy declines sections (Richards & Collins 2005) of a multiday, hill-running marathon. Although this technique is good because it accesses thoughts without being influenced by outcome, it is also clearly limited by the practicalities and access opportunities.

Coping can also be assessed through the impact it has either on the performer or performance. Since most coping is meant to reduce stress, changes in physiological variables associated with stress response can be used. Heart rate is probably the easiest of these but heart rate variability, blood pressure, cortisol, adrenaline (epinephrine) and pupil dilation have all been used as indirect indices of reduced anxiety. None of these should be used on its own as an index of coping; after all, if your leader has a racing heart but feels fine and produces an outstanding performance, who cares what the heart rate trace says? Coping for physical performance frequently demands something other than the mainstay of coping utilized in clinical settings – namely, relaxation. That is not to say that relaxation cannot be used in the right time and place but, if it is the only response offered to alleviate pressure and assist performers to produce high-level performances, then it is time to look for alternatives.

It is also possible to measure coping through changes in behaviour and performance. Both of these have the advantage of being accessible by others, often during performance. If a performer plans to cope by adopting a pre-performance routine, for example a climber pausing, mentally rehearsing and chalking up before the crux move (see Ch. 23 for more detail on this), then this can be observed by others. Furthermore, if the targeted elements of performance can be measured, this outcome can also be used as evidence of coping. So, if a rugby player wants to reduce the number of penalties they commit as result of losing their temper, this can be easily monitored.

In summary, coping can be measured in several ways and, to help performers effectively, we need to know what they currently do and to track any changes as a result of their efforts and any intervention. As with any skill acquisition process, feedback is very useful and so this section on measurement is essential to underpin practical help for performers – without measurement of some kind there is no feedback. Good measurement would combine more than one of the approaches discussed above, where possible, and attempt to balance the application with what is possible in the situation while avoiding the known limitations of the approach.

Coping effectiveness

It is very important to determine whether coping is effective, particularly in relation to developing coping training with performers. In the previous sections of this chapter, I have emphasized that attempts to label coping responses as maladaptive or adaptive fail to recognize the interaction between person, situation and their goal. This interaction is the starting point for effective coping training, in order to give it a clear direction. If a performer wants to keep performance level up but avoid being physically sick beforehand, then this is clear. But an intervention that just tries to help the performer 'cope better' lacks the same clarity. People differ vastly, too, and this needs to be recognized in the intervention. In the high-testosterone, chest-beating, ego-charged atmosphere of sprinting it is possible to find performers who do not do, or like, this element. Sitting in a confined holding room before the big event can be hugely stressful for such individuals (Do I stare at the others? Do I look away? Do I shut my eyes?). In this real case, when we hit upon the solution – a cheap pair of wraparound mirror sunglasses that could be discarded as the athlete walked on to the track – as the performance psychologist, I remember almost feeling deflated. There was no training intervention, no known psychological technique, no theory explaining the effect. But the solution was a perfect match; performer, situation and immediate goal (avoiding involvement in the ego-wars). In addition to emphasizing the need to carefully unpick the needs of the performer, analyse the situation and identify the goals, this example also helps to illustrate the importance of not forgetting to look for easy, practical and effective solutions, wherever and in whatever guise they may occur.

Working out what is effective coping is of great importance for practitioners and the ideas that have been established in the coping literature offer some general guidance of where to begin to formulate plans for helping performers cope. For example, the goodness-of-fit model (Folkman 1992) would suggest a bias towards problem-orientated responses if the situation is appraised as controllable, and emotion-orientated coping if it is uncontrollable. As a general rule this is fine (and logical!) but it is worth remembering that any coping efforts will have some cost to the performer. Cost may not just be time but also in terms of psychological resources. In this regard, Baumeister and colleagues have proposed that coping efforts deplete resources and this inevitably means there is less available until these are recovered (Baumeister et al 1999, Muraven et al 1998). This resource depletion makes intuitive sense; for example, it is harder to ignore being the focus of a joke when anxious before an important performance. It is worth noting that performers who are using humour to cope themselves may easily be depleting valuable resources of fellow performers and team members and possibly create an argument or conflict at the most damaging time.

So the goodness-of-fit model is only right if the issue is controllable and very important to address. Reappraisal may offer a much less depleting coping response and is certainly achieved more quickly. Choosing carefully what battles to fight is an important caveat to the 'controllable – use problem-orientated' versus 'no control– use emotion-orientated' guidance that some see as gospel. It is also interesting to recognize that perceptions of control are not determined universally the same way. Personal experience of working with performers from an eastern culture with a strong Buddhist influence revealed that perceptions of control were intermeshed with responsibility. A potential problem that was not the responsibility of the performer was not considered something that required action, even though they had the potential to exert some control. This passive response did not seem to exacerbate any perceived stress and whatever the eventual outcome turned out to be was just accommodated. This observation is in line with the findings of Yoo (2001), who reported on transcendental coping in Korean athletes, outlining the Korean concept of *han* – a positive acceptance of reality that is, in the performance context at least, often unfortunate. Views of coping in the literature may be heavily biased by the cultural backdrop and personal philosophy of researchers. Westernized cultural values seem particularly focused on control, approach/problem-orientated coping and attempts to dominate the situation. This may be exacerbated by a performance culture that continually drives towards the 'perfect' performance. Perfection may cause performers to believe that every aspect must conform to a preordained ideal and their attempt to control all the minutiae is a considerable burden. The cost–benefit analysis of falling into this way of thinking deserves some carefully scrutiny.

Training coping skills

Training of coping skills has been long established in counselling and clinical psychology but, among performers and professionals in physical performance situations, opinions can vary widely on whether such training has any benefit. For example, some people believe that changing the way they think is not possible. This is addressed in more detail later in relation to learned optimism and again in Chapter 21. For the moment, and reflecting such beliefs, it is absolutely essential that time is spent on explaining the impact of intervention work and the evidence in support of it so that those involved in training understand what is involved and the potential value to them and can commit accordingly.

The development of coping training can be divided into three elements which we will consider in turn:

- **Content** – the different skills and strategies
- **Learning** – how learning skills takes place and can be enhanced
- **Format** – scheduling and timing.

Content of coping training

The content of training can comprise many different coping skills and strategies. In some cases, performers might want to train for specific instances: for example, a dancer returning from rehabilitation completing the move that caused injury, a hockey player who regularly takes penalties, or a climber who struggles with a particular kind of problem (Fig. 20.1). In each of these cases the focus is very specific but the exact content must be selected to specifically suit the individual, situation and goals. Anshell et al (2001) emphasize that standardized, 'canned' programmes are significantly limited by their failure to take individual and situational features into account. Coping training can also be approached more

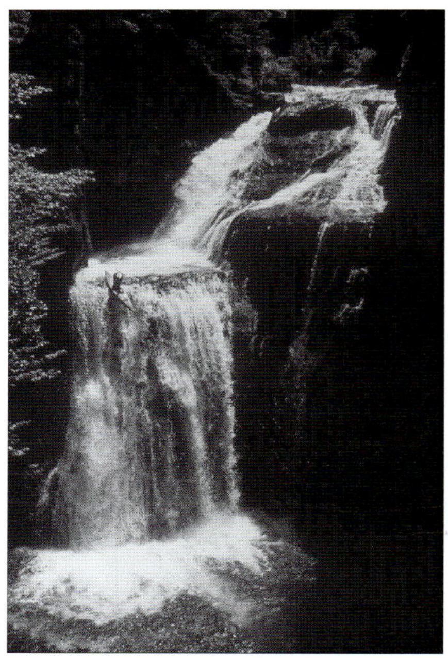

Fig. 20.1 • Coping powers in full application as Ray Rowe completes another first descent.

globally so that performers learn a range of coping skills and how to apply them to different situations and in different ways. This approach helps them to prepare for unexpected occurrences and should, if completed correctly, provide a good response framework for the performer (Smith 1999). Several types of commonly used coping skills and training techniques are summarized in Table 20.2. Many of these are covered in depth elsewhere in the book and these are identified in the table, along with brief descriptions of the others. The interested reader may also find useful descriptions of some of these coping skills, in Lascelles et al (1989) and Anshell (1990).

Coping training programmes need to include a range of skills and strategies covering both those that are task-orientated and those concerned with how the performers feel. Coping training also needs to deliberately expand the repertoire of performers in the areas where they are less well skilled. There is a natural tendency to work more on the things that are already done reasonably well at the outset but widening the range of coping skills is the optimum goal.

Learning coping skills

Understanding and applying the process of learning skills is also important to coping training. It is remarkable how frequently programmes billed as training are actually just educational programmes. The distinction is simple – if a performer attends a workshop but does not actually repeatedly do the skill, then it is an educational workshop. Educational workshops are fine, but they are not training. If training is required then three critical factors need to be present; instruction (educational style perhaps) in the beginning, then repeated cycles of practice and feedback, and finally deployment and evaluation in the heat of battle/event itself. Physical performers are well experienced in learning physical skills and a review of the evidence suggests that cognitive skills can be acquired in the same way (Rosenbaum et al 2001, 2006). Furthermore, the acquisition of cognitive skills is also positively influenced by the same practice manipulations used to learn physical skills (e.g. spaced and random practice produce better learning than massed practice; Schmidt & Bork 1992; see also Ch. 15).

Coping is usually most necessary when the demands are high and it is essential that performers are able to produce the correct coping responses under extreme pressure (Fig. 20.2). Therefore, training coping programmes need to explicitly address the problem that the environment in which the skills are learned and practice is not as hard or demanding as the performance environment. Military trainers refer to this problem as the 'training gap'. One well used technique to address this is to combine practice of the skill with progressive exposure to more stressful situations. Using this concept of progressive exposure is the hallmark of stress inoculation training (Meichenbaum 1977), designed originally as a psychotherapeutic procedure but which has successfully been applied to physical performance (Mace & Carroll 1985).

In addition to practice under progressive exposure, trainers should also consider the need to provide suitable simulation of the performance environment. This can at times be very difficult and requires considerable ingenuity, time and effort, but the return in terms of effectively closing the training gap is highly significant. Even attempts to mirror some of the conditions can help. So, for example, if you know auditory communication will not be possible because of the volume of noise at the time of performance, then practice coping with events without any verbal communication or even with loud taped noise from a similar event. Performers may also benefit from using imagery, following the PETTLEP approach (Holmes & Collins 2001), to internally simulate the performance environment. However, this may be restricted to those who have sufficient experience of the performance environment to recreate an appropriately realistic, detailed and vivid image. Simulation can also be achieved in part by simulating the factors that characterize the performer's physical and mental state during real performance. So if performers have to operate quickly and without warning, or when they are fatigued, tired, distracted by other concerns, have a high heart rate or are under evaluation, then any or all of these can be manipulated within a training programme. Integrating physical and psychological coping training can help to achieve this (e.g. 'combination training', discussed in Ch. 25). This is also very efficient for the performer who is able to complete both aspects in one well organized session.

One final issue in coping training is the use of modelling. In physical skills, this is a very common technique but it can be used for cognitive skills too. Experienced performers can pass on information to other performers as a part of the training programme. Systematic debriefs, identifying the coping responses taken, and why, provides a model to emulate. Importantly, if the figure has credibility with those being

Table 20.2 Example content of coping skills training

Coping	Comment
Self instruction	See 'Self-talk' section in Chapter 23
Practice simulation	See below, Learning coping skills
Planning	See Planning section in Chapter 23 (and Ch. 10)
Familiarization	Performers benefit from reduced uncertainty addressed by increased familiarity. Knowing the environment and conditions, sticking to routines, having experienced the timing and structure of performance for real or in dress rehearsal can all assist. Even briefings from those with relevant experience or knowledge as performers will have some value in this regard
Imagery	See section in Chapter 23, and Chapter 16 (Holmes & Collins 2001)
Distractions	Performers often have to work hard to fill the time. Feeling aimless can produce feelings of lethargy and being disconnected, so being able to decide on something to occupy time and attention is a good coping skill. Films, books, puzzles, games, going for a walk, meals, shopping, emails, work/study, phone calls, sightseeing, light exercise are all examples of items for a repertoire. Performers should be guided to recognize and think around conflicting factors in advance. Will they get lost, be late back, get too tired, be exposed in the heat, worry the director/coach by their absence? These can mostly all be effectively countered
Cognitive restructure	See Chapter 21
Attention control	See Chapter 22 and section on routines in Chapter 23
Problem solving	Problem solving is a common feature of coping training for general psychology yet its features are still very relevant to physical performers. This can take the form of scenario 'what if'-style training ('Your travel has been delayed/you have missed the scheduled transport and you are late – what do you do?'). In addition, the broad principles of problem solving can be taught, illustrated and then practised. These might include a step-based approach such as problem identification (key issues), identify two or more solutions, test for viability, select best alternative (costs/effectiveness), check it (what can go wrong?), act
Thought stopping	Using an attention grabbing action/thought to stop chain of irrelevant unhelpful thoughts. Typically people are taught to say 'STOP!' Out loud this technique can be awkward to apply and internally the covert verbalization might lack impact. A behaviour can help here instead: closing eyes or changing visual field can also benefit. Stopping thoughts should be followed immediately by further coping such as self-instruction. Nature abhors a vacuum and the voracious ability of worry to occupy any available 'head space' means thought stopping alone will often have little effect
Assertiveness/ communication skills	Assertiveness training is widely misunderstood as help for 'wallflowers'! In reality the training is quite simply teaching people how to communicate in ways that more effectively get them what they want. For example, the best way to make requests of other people, how to say no and exit strategies from conversations that are unhelpful. Given the fact that performers often report support team and team mates as a significant source of stress (Scanlan et al 1991) input into more effectively managing this social stress represents an important element of widening the repertoire
Diaries	Diaries can provide a good means of organizing thoughts and completing self-reflection, which might help performers to keep a balanced perspective. Ethnotherapy has received some recent interest as an intervention tool. Be careful about the focus of diary entries. Borkovec et al (1983) suggested that a daily worry period (in which worries are identified and addressed) reduces overall daily worry and frequency of intrusion. However, more recently Duncan & Sheffield (2004) suggested that writing down worries increased anxiety. The solution might be to enter factual information and only to include solutions to problems and plans of actions and avoid free-form diaries that might allow lists of worries to emerge

Table 20.2 Example content of coping skills training—Cont'd

Coping	Comment
Physical exercise/routines	Light jogging, static bike, stretching or swimming. Be careful not to do something that is not usually in your activity and that might compromise physical condition. Sudden availability of a machine in a hotel gym does not mean it is a good time to give it a go. Doing your back in rowing and injuring a wrist falling off a hired mountain bike are examples of what can go wrong and should have been avoided
Humour	This can be an excellent antidote to high-pressure situations and the famed black humour of emergency services, medical and military personnel is perhaps evidence of its benefit. But performers must be self-aware enough to know where, when and with whom, to avoid fall out. A simple example (and personal favourite) is the acronym 'DILLIGAFF' a quick, innocent-sounding expression which can be said to oneself or exchanged between team mates. It stands for 'Do I look like I give a flying ****?' and has found favour with several performers (and colleagues!) over the years!
Relaxation	In performance, see section on breath control in Chapter 23. Outside or removed in time from the performance environment, more global physical relaxation is fine used carefully at the right time (LeScanff & Taugis 2002). Progressive muscular relaxation (tensing and relaxing body parts in sequence, usually head to toe or vice versa) can be learned quite easily using a tape/CD product.

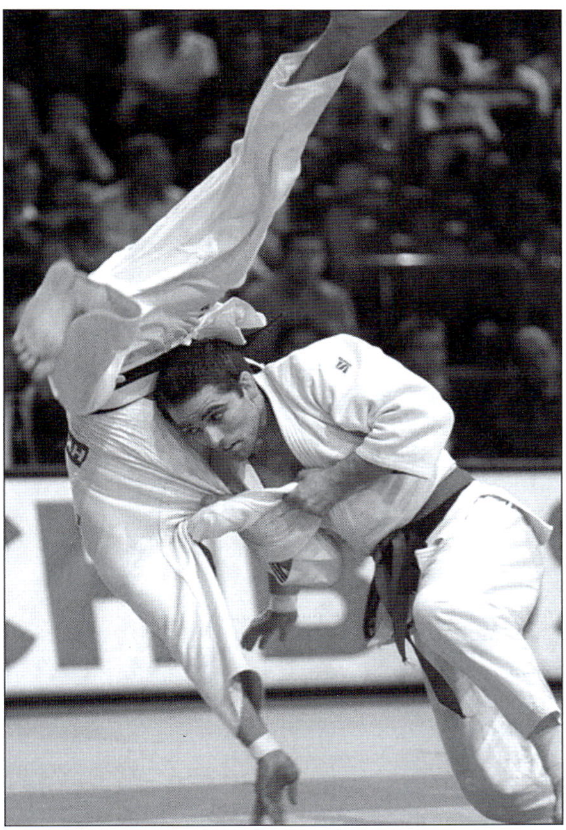

Fig. 20.2 • Once the event has started you HAVE to cope. Graeme Randall applies the pressure at the 1997 World Championships. Photo © judophotos.com and David Finch Photos, with thanks.

trained, the model also provides an important motivational boost to apply effort to the coping training. The systematic debrief is more than just a cosy chat and should be organized and facilitated to meet specific training needs. It is a common practice in emergency services, medical and military environments but, surprisingly, is not well used across all physical performance domains. Holding debriefs closer in time to the event and using techniques such as playing video footage of the performance to stimulate accurate and detailed recall (Gilbert et al 1994) will increase the effectiveness.

Taken together, the chapter so far has formulated a picture of developing coping skills in performers that can be illustrated by the model shown in Figure 20.3. In this model, information or action involving the performer is contained in ovals and the basic building blocks of content or guidance from the psychology are illustrated through boxes. The basic coping skills and strategies are the basis of training but can and frequently are delivered in educational workshops. This gives performers the

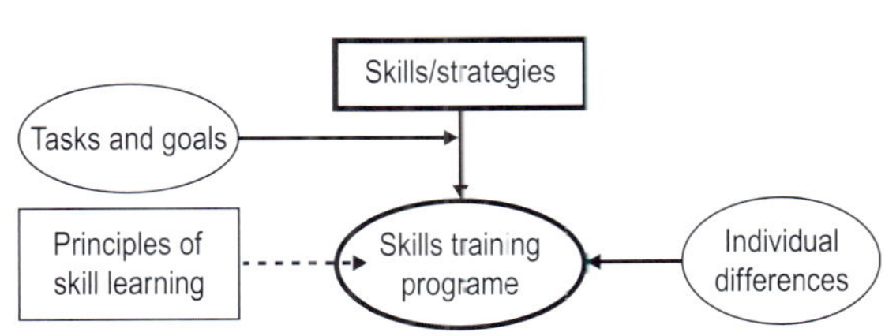

Fig. 20.3 • Components of effective coping skills training.

declarative knowledge about these. The procedural knowledge, how to use these skills, is only developed through training distinguished from educational programmes by repeated practice and feedback.

In order to be effective, training programmes must also reflect the individual differences and preferences of performers together with the situational context of the performance task and the specific goals of the individual. Finally, the training programme can be further enhanced by the application of principles of learning that have been discussed in this section. Together these components represent the elements required for effective coping training.

Format of coping training

The format of coping training needs to allow time for practice and learning to occur so it cannot happen in just one or two sessions. The literature offers some examples of programmes that can be used as guidance but inevitably the practicalities of time, cost and availability will set parameters on the programme. Usually, coping training involves several stages or phases, commencing with brief educational/awareness sessions before moving on to specific practice and application (Fenz 1988, Mace & Carroll 1985, Prapavessis et al 1992). For comparison, Anshell (1990) used a format of six 1-hour sessions twice a week for 3 weeks whereas Prapavessis et al (1992) used 12 sessions over 6 weeks. For a much more specific programme (reducing anxiety to a high abseil), 2 weeks with seven 45-minute sessions was sufficient to produce a beneficial effect (Mace & Carroll 1985). While these formats are not described here to be replicated exactly, they give some indication of the format and time likely to be needed to deliver effective training. They also demonstrate that more global coping training involving different coping responses is inevitably a longer process than specific training. One final guideline on the timing of training and formats is a suggestion emanating from coping training with snake phobics. In a study assessing changes using a stress inoculation procedure, Wiedenfeld et al (1990) found that rapid mastery, or specifically the speed at which efficacy in the situation was achieved, was associated with enhanced responses in psychophysiological markers (immune function). Although this has not been tested in training physical performers, it does hint at the possibility that getting quick changes and providing feedback to this effect, in order to build confidence of performers in their ability to cope, may have additional benefits.

Anshell also specifically recommends the use of homework, a common feature of training in clinical settings, and this helps to promote independent learning and increases the speed at which learners can acquire coping skills. Homework does need to be followed up, however, and a completed diary with discussion can achieve this effectively. Decisions about format also need to consider the use of group or individual sessions. With unlimited resources the ideal would be individual sessions, whereas a training format at the other end of the spectrum, group sessions only, will struggle to achieve the individual tailoring required for effective programmes. Using a composite model of some group sessions plus individual sessions, in the role of psychological coaching, may provide a midpoint to meet the twin aims of effectiveness and efficiency. It is also worth recognizing some benefits of group work: performers may learn from the experiences of others, buddy support can assist in the learning process and importantly remain active after training has ended, helping to increase the impact, and also performers who interact with other during performance may be active in triggering and supporting coping at the most critical time: learning together enables this to take effect.

It is strongly recommended that, where possible, follow-up sessions in the months following training are included as part of the complete programme, to support the new skills, to assist in transferring them from practice to performance and to help performers make adaptations as required. In situations with repeated performances, these sessions can be placed strategically around the performance schedule. These follow-up sessions also permit a thorough evaluation of the intervention to take place. The measures of coping discussed earlier in this chapter can be used for this purpose. So, too, can debriefs and ratings by other professionals and performers who have seen the performer in action. In Chapter 23 we elaborate on evaluation techniques that can be used for performers, and adding coping-related issues to normal performance evaluation allows this extra element to be 'picked up' conveniently.

Mental toughness

It is clear that knowledge of coping skills and training that enables performers to implement coping efficiently, under significant challenge and pressure, are important for performance. However, there remains a sense that there is something more than just this that characterizes the performance of individuals who can maintain and even increase levels of performance under extraordinary circumstances. The search for this extra ingredient has, recently, focused on the concept of mental toughness.

What is this thing called mental toughness?

In 2002, Jones and colleagues published an article entitled 'What is this thing called mental toughness? An investigation of elite sport performers'. This was a well timed article for two reasons. First, it occurred at the time that several other researchers were conducting work on the same construct (Bull et al 2005, Clough et al 2002, Fourie & Potgeiter 2001, Golby et al 2003, Middleton et al 2004). Second, it was well timed because none of these pieces of research shared or established the same definition of the construct under investigation. Jones and colleagues identified 12 key attributes of mental toughness (Table 20.3) from interview/focus groups with ten elite sports performers (which they defined as national representation at Olympic or Commonwealth games). They defined mental toughness as generally coping better than opponents, being more consistent at remaining determined, focused, confident and in control under pressure. In summary, the research produced a multilayered definition and a construct with 12 attributes.

Table 20.3 Key attributes of mental toughness (Jones et al 2002)

1	Unshakeable belief in ability
2	Unshakeable belief in possessing unique qualities and abilities
3	Insatiable desire, internalized motives to succeed
4	Bouncing back from performance setbacks
5	Thriving on pressure
6	Accepting competition anxiety is knowing you can cope with it
7	Not being adversely affected by others' performances
8	Remaining fully focused in face of life distractions
9	Switching focus on and off as required
10	Remaining fully focused on task in face of performance distractions
11	Pushing back boundaries of emotional and physical pain
12	Regaining psychological control after unexpected, uncontrollable events

Reprinted with permission from Jones, G., Hanton, S., Connaughton, D. (2002). What is this thing called mental toughness? An investigation of elite sports performers. Journal of Applied Sport Psychology 14: 205–218

The qualitative inductive study by Jones et al (2002) has limitations. For example, basing a working definition solely on input from ten participants and without subsequent follow-up means the support for this definition is weak. Of course, as an initial study this could be combined with other studies; however, only Thelwell et al (2005) have strongly supported this (although this might be expected since their aim was to 'confirm the findings' (p. 330) of Jones et al). The work of Bull et al (2005) found some similarities. The general approach adopted by inductive, bottom-up research intended to develop a definition relies on the selected performers knowing something about the construct they are being asked about. Indeed, several of the studies assume that the level of performance achieved by the selected participants means that they must be mentally tough. Questions remain over whether this assumption is correct and also in relation to determining what constitutes elite or high level of performance. Research might be better focused if participants were selected on the basis of being rated as exhibiting mental toughness by individuals who are knowledgeable about the performer and informed about the construct (Thelwell et al 2005). Furthermore, mentally tough performers may be unaware of their own personal characteristics or unable to access them in a way that can be collected by researchers in verbal form.

Although the Jones et al study was one of the first of the recent surge in interest, the original work on mental toughness came from Loehr (1986). He described the outcome of his own investigation into athletic performance, from which he identified **consistency** as the hallmark of mental toughness, predicated on control. However, the picture was not that simple and Loehr described a 'roadmap' to mental toughness, achieved by identifying and controlling an ideal performance state characterized by 12 characteristics. Although 12 characteristics were found by Loehr, and by Jones et al (2002) and also by Fourie & Potgeiter (2001), this seems a 'happy coincidence' as, in every case, the lists differ. A few factors did emerge in all cases, such as confidence and, inevitably, the use of coping skills, but there were many factors that only appeared from one study (e.g. religious convictions and ethics (Fourie & Potgeiter 2001), imagery and energy control (Loehr 1986), and enduring emotional and physical pain and remaining unaffected by others' performances (Jones et al 2002)). More recently, Jones et al (2007) have confirmed their earlier definition but extended the characteristics to 30 attributes relevant to different time periods of performance (e.g. training, competition, postcompetition). In summary, it seems that, while attractive to consumers, much of this work remains at the anecdotal/descriptive level.

Alternative research perspectives to mental toughness

Another approach to studying mental toughness has focused on the development and subsequent application of measures of mental toughness. One such approach has capitalized on the concept of hardiness (Kobasa 1979), which incorporates challenge, control and commitment. Golby & Sheard (2004), using the established hardiness measure, found that elite performers in rugby league scored more highly on all three elements than performers at lower levels. They also measured mental toughness using a measure from Loehr (1986) and found differences in two of seven subscales. This study suggests that hardiness can discriminate performers at different levels more effectively than the mental toughness measure.

A related development focusing on measuring the construct is the work of Clough and colleagues (2002), who developed a questionnaire based on the three subcomponents of hardiness (control, challenge and commitment) with the addition of confidence (a recurring attribute from the studies above). They called this scale the Mental Toughness Questionnaire (MTQ48). This is a little confusing because it measures the entire hardiness construct, with just one quarter of it measuring something beyond this. Nevertheless, the scale seems to have been welcomed by researchers, who have employed it at face value to describe differences and relationships (Horsburgh et al 2009, Levy et al 2006, Nichols et al 2008, 2009). None of these researchers has scrutinized or evaluated the properties of the scale.

A difficulty with the conceptual approach of this line of research is that hardiness and the MTQ48 seem to assume that the construct being measured is stable and trait-like and that performers would exhibit it across domains (cf. my earlier comments on the trait versus process conceptualizations of coping). At the same time, the researchers are interested in the construct in order to intervene and assist performers to become more mentally tough. In fact, the company website that markets the MTQ48 questionnaire advertises development courses. This inconsistency is puzzling and casts some doubt on the approach. If a construct can be readily measured by one administration of a questionnaire, this suggests it is measuring something dispositional (permanent) but if it can be influenced through a training programme then the construct is much more malleable and this raises some questions about the questionnaire's ability to measure mental toughness.

Aside from several lines of enquiry that have developed different questionnaires, one final approach to mental toughness deserves mention. Dienstbier (1989) investigated toughness from a physiological response perspective and suggested that the hormonal response to stress was indicative of a level of toughness. Specifically, cortisol, a catecholamine from arousal of the hypothalamus–pituitary–adrenal axis, was associated with a lack of appropriate responses. Conversely, increasing control and positive interpretation – challenge rather than threat – was associated with reduced cortisol levels. While there are complexities involved in measuring cortisol, which are only made worse by attempting this with performers whose physical activity levels disturb hormonal activity, such investigations are possible. Eubank and colleagues (1997) found responses consistent with Dienstbier's conceptualization in canoeists, based on appraisal-related differences. Crust (2008) identifies this approach in some detail in reviewing mental toughness, but consideration of this theoretical basis for toughness, with associated measurement opportunity, is notable by its absence in the bulk of the literature. This may yet prove to be the best approach in order to make significant and meaningful advances in this area.

Why do we love mental toughness so much?

It is clear from the points raised above that there are inconsistencies and problems associated with defining this thing called mental toughness. In fact, in answering the question posed by Jones et al (2002) 'What is mental toughness?', we still have no definitive answer. Researching the area for this chapter has also led me to realize that there is another side to the story of mental toughness that has been influential in the lack of development of knowledge. The first point is that mental toughness as a general, not scientific, term is something we all think we know and recognize. In reality, the bottom-up research shows that this understanding does not produce a consensus definition. But our belief that there is something there causes persistence with the idea. It is almost as if we are mentally tough about mental toughness and keep at it, believing in it, despite the setbacks (cf. ideas on prediction in Ch. 10).

The second point relates to the perceptions of elite physical performers who are widely admired for the qualities that they possess. In attempting to understand the achievements of elite performers, we look for explanations, and one obvious feature is the mental qualities they possess. However, for everyday conversations, complex explanations are no good – we need a single concept, like mental toughness, that encapsulates everything about the performers' characteristics. The concept of mental toughness is perhaps borne out of convenience and natural conversations and explanations. This oversimplification makes the feats more understandable and allows straightforward explanations that the elite champions as more mentally tough than the others. A more complicated explanation that isolated all the individual factors is just not easy enough.

Finally, mental toughness is attractive because it offers the idea of a potential panacea. In other words, if we know what this thing is we can develop it to develop elite performers. We can also use it in other areas such as business and this makes the idea manageable and marketable. The concept of mental toughness may be perpetuated in part because it sells and has commodity value. There are at least four different measures of hardiness and mental toughness that can be bought on the internet. Many of the authors researching in the area are also producing self-help books for business people, acting as consultants and running toughness training course. One website even offers to teach the 177 secrets of mental toughness during an 11-week course! On inspection this looks like a good test of mental toughness itself.

The verdict on mental toughness

At the present moment the picture of mental toughness is disjointed. Qualitative descriptions and the attempts by other research to organize measurement approaches with a theoretical basis are not working in a concerted fashion and so knowledge development has not progressed very far. A recent review (Crust 2008), although it does not agree exactly with the position I have adopted here, highlights significant gaps in developing a coherent body of knowledge on the construct. For example, Jones et al (2007) suggests different forms of mental toughness for different times/phases of performance.

Crust extends this idea and suggests that different types of performance, for example snooker and mountaineering, might involve quite different types of mental toughness (Crust 2008). This seems quite plausible: for example, an article on a blind Everest mountaineer describes mental toughness as 'the ability to withstand tremendous amounts of cold, discomfort, physical pain, boredom, bad food, insomnia and tedious conversation when you're snowed into a pup tent for a week on 3-ft wide ice shelf at 20 000 ft' (Greenfeld 2001). In comparison, a mentally tough performer who believed they possessed 'unique qualities and abilities' and 'an insatiable desire for success' (mental toughness characteristics from Jones et al 2002) would seem like a very difficult tent-mate in such circumstances. Other issues also can be raised about the effectiveness of mental toughness across domains. The well documented Everest disaster in 1996 was, in part, caused by poor decision making on the part of the climbing teams, perhaps due to a single focus on the summit and a belief that things would be OK for them (and again, note the comparisons with ideas in Ch. 10). This begs the question whether associated mental toughness characteristics might negatively impact on effective decision making, especially when that entails relinquishing a long-term goal.

The bottom line is that the lack of weight of evidence does not support the application of this construct to aid and enhance performance, at this time. In other words, psychology can contribute significantly to coping skills and development but efforts organized and directed to a mental toughness idea are not supported by the current literature. The research needs to be able to provide a supported definition and explanatory theory, and have validated measurement capacity and an evidence-based track record in the efficacy of applying the construct to performers.

To avoid creating a new unwieldy multidimensional construct it may be more effective and logical to consider whether existing psychological constructs, either individually or in combination, can fulfil all the requirements that the general concept of mental toughness was focused on achieving. One obvious contender to consider in this regard is self-regulation. An additional benefit of this approach is that established constructs have conceived ways in which they can be explicitly measured and developed, offering a means for performance psychologists to apply this knowledge to enhance performance. This final point, 'So what can psychologists do?' is not well addressed by the recent descriptive work on mental toughness or measures based on a stable (trait-like) construct. In the next section we examine the evidence for applying self-regulation and consider other relevant constructs in relation to supporting performers.

Self-regulation

What is self-regulation?

Self-regulation refers to the process by which individuals monitor, manage and control their behaviours, thoughts, emotions and interactions with the environment, including task performance but also including social interactions. With such a wholesale remit, self-regulation offers the opportunity to understand how responses can be orchestrated across the wide range of different coping skills and strategies discussed earlier in the chapter. In addition to those discussed as possible content for coping training, the broad focus of self-regulation helps understand the loss of control that might be associated with an angry outburst, a night's heavy drinking after a setback, or other negative behaviours that are not uncommon in different performance situations. Adopting a self-regulatory approach to developing coping may therefore make it possible to avoid these lapses becoming significant negative influences.

Self regulation is defined as; 'actions occurring during the actual performance of a cognitive task that allow an individual to control or direct his own activity through self-imposed rules or regulations that better adapt his performance to different circumstances or surroundings' (Chen & Singer 1992). Furthermore, self-regulation can be considered as comprising three connected functions. The primary one of the three functions is the ability to think meta-strategically. What this means literally is thinking about what you are thinking. For example, a rally driver crashes on a stage and the car becomes stuck. As the driver gets out, thoughts are based around getting the car going again and the potential danger of following cars on the 'live' stage. As he takes in the information and makes a decision, meta-strategic processes running simultaneously allow him to check how this is going. For example, suppose the codriver has offered an alternative option. The driver's 'ideal' concept of how he should operate in these situations includes consultation and consideration of alternatives. Meta-strategic thinking flags up a mismatch, effectively telling the driver that current practice (a decision without consideration of alternatives) deviates from his ideal. He is then able to quickly change his actions, consider the alternative (matching the ideal) and proceed to make a decision. Carver & Scheier (1981) referred to this system as a negative feedback loop, in which the current situation (in this case the decision-making process) was compared to what the performer ought to be doing, and the mismatch became a stimulus for action.

This meta-strategic function can be broken down into different activities and Table 20.4 illustrates how these operate.

The second component of self-regulation is positive motivation (confidence and optimism) for the task. It may be worth considering also that, if performers are being trained or expected to self-regulate, then confidence in the ability to perform this cognitive skill effectively too will also play an important part in them choosing and persisting with adopting this approach. It is noteworthy because of its importance, rather than being unexpected, to see such a strong reoccurrence of confidence (self-belief) as a theme important for performers under the mental toughness construct and self-regulation. This serves as a constant reminder in training people to cope and self-regulate the need to develop and maintain positive motivation. Teaching performers to use process goals rather than outcome goals is one key aspect to achieve this. The final component in

Table 20.4 Meta-strategic functions – a component of self-regulation

Monitoring	How am I doing? Do I feel how I want to feel before performance?
Plan and select responses	I feel a bit tense. I need to go for a walk/do some light stretches
Organize and execute response	I'll go for a 15-minute walk and do some stretches using the usual stretch routine I use before a light training session
Evaluate consequences	I feel fine now but a bit thirsty (this last comment would trigger further monitoring against what the performer would like as an ideal)
Learning	I might think about putting this into my plan for performance

self-regulation is behavioural management. The idea of behavioural management can be extended to include the ability to manage the environment (including others) effectively. While emotional intelligence has been suggested as a component important for performers (e.g. Zizzi & Deaner 2003), the concept of self-regulation already recognizes the important function of this activity. In other words, while we might consider this an important factor for performers we do not need to add something to the self-regulation construct in order to reflect this. Earlier in this chapter I highlighted the role of problem solving and assertiveness training as potential features of coping training content. Ensuring that performers have the behavioural management capability (including social skills) to effectively organize the environment would be an important element of self-regulatory training.

Self-regulation, learning and expertise

Another important point about self-regulation is that the term refers to regulation by the self, not just of the self (Vohs & Baumeister 2004). This point emphasizes the personal volitional control that is at the core of self-regulation and equally central to what I believe is an effective model of psychological support and development for performers. This perspective guides interactions with performers. Outlining a philosophical approach to intervention with performers is a recommended procedure. While this can be interpreted as meaning that you adopt and apply an approach such as cognitive–behavioural to your work (see Chapter 21, which explains this approach), my suggestion is to outline philosophy more in terms of the ideal outcome of support. So I explain my approach in terms of what I do (cognitive–behavioural) and what I want to achieve.

Although I often find myself referring to 'coping training', what I should really be saying is that I attempt to train people how to learn to cope. This is not just about playing with words but rather attempts to outline to them a stance that should govern our work together. It is important when working with developing self-regulation to make this absolutely explicit to performers. In other words, the fundamental changes that I believe occur as someone learns how to cope take place over a much longer duration than might typically occur on a training course (see above on the format of coping training for a guide to this). Performers need to understand this from the outset, although true recognition by them of what the changes might mean may take considerably longer. In one case, a performer with whom I worked for 4 years retired after an Olympic Games. Several months later we met and inevitably reflected on the work we had done together. Then, for the first time, he acknowledged that he saw the big picture and wide potential impact of the work we had done. It had changed from developing and practising separate elements such as routines, planning, strategy, attention control and self-talk to recognizing a holistic change in his approach that was characterized by autonomous, flexible, self-regulated performance.

Several years ago, a charity organization advertised its approach using a slogan along the lines of 'give a person some fish and they will not be hungry for the week but teach them how to fish and they will not go hungry again'. My suggestion that the focus should be on developing and training a performer's self-regulatory capacity is analogous to this idea. The idea is too simple, though: if I was given a net I would fully expect to be dead with hunger before I learnt to fish properly! So performers do need input right away and grand plans with distant payoffs will not sustain performance in the here and now. This means that we do not focus only on self-regulation but also provide necessary basic coping mental skills as required. However, the focus on self-regulatory development is blended with more traditional skill development. Over time this blend may change in concentration as progress is made and in response to immediate demands of performance schedules.

The aim is for performers to be able to learn from, and make adaptations to, performance independent of outside input. It is totally impractical to assume that a scientific practitioner/psychologist can support a performer fully through their career because they will not be there for all the crucial moments, it would be prohibitively expensive to fund this level of support and ultimately the performer's dependence on support would be strengthened rather than diminished. So it is necessary to train performers how to learn to cope and models of self-regulation explain how we can set about developing performers to achieve this (Cleary & Zimmerman 2001).

Specifically, the learning model of self-regulation has performance, self-reflection and forethought phases organized in a cycle. During performance phases, performers follow through on the preconceived plan using skills such as task strategies, imagery and self talk, while simultaneously they monitor how well they are keeping to the plan and how effective the plan appears to be for the task – making adjustments accordingly. In the self-reflection phase, performers self-generate feedback and determine the perceived cause of the outcome – this is called attributing (e.g. Why did I miss my entrance? Because others had missed a section of the performance). Finally, this information feeds into an emotional response that might be rewarding, or one designed to increase effort of persistence such as feeling disappointed. The third phase – forethought – plans the next performance, utilizing information from previous attempts to set goals and reflecting the attributions that have been made in terms of confidence and emotional responses that stimulate motivations.

Using this model, it is possible to deliberately develop performers' skill in self-regulating. Remember that training requires instruction, practice and feedback. So telling performers about the process (instruction), asking them to use it while completing physical training (practice) and getting them to describe thoughts under each phase so that you can give feedback, constitutes training self-regulatory skills. The specific content for each stage can be further elaborated with the detailed model provided by Zimmerman (2006). Furthermore, he summarizes several studies that have tested the effects of increased self-regulation (achieved by teaching one, two or three stages of the cycle) and found superior learning and physical performance for those with most training. In testing the model, the method employed also effectively outlines the basics of training interventions to achieve adaptive changes in self-regulatory ability. Zimmerman (2006) strongly advocates the value of self-regulation in relation to learning in order to complete deliberate practice and through this move towards acquiring expertise (Ericsson 2006).

Self-regulation training

Although we have already discussed training aspects in the previous section, this short section is intended to briefly summarize training self-regulation and link it with the coping training section above. Coping training, as depicted in Figure 20.3, can be considered as analogous to developing declarative and procedural knowledge (see Ch. 13). However, the coping training does not necessarily equip a performer with the conditional knowledge required to cope effectively. Conditional knowledge content can be considered to be related to questions such 'When should I start using a coping strategy?' and 'What is the most effective coping response in this situation and context?' The answer to these, as the tabulated operations of meta-strategic thinking show, is determined by having accurate information about the current state and the environment and also an idea of what it should ideally be. If monitoring is not effective, the message to cope might be missed or too late. Equally problematic is not having a realistic comparison model of how things should be (the ideal). The self-recording process of self-regulation that takes place in the performance phase (Cleary & Zimmerman 2001) is critical in developing an effective comparison. In Chapter 21, the approach developed by Hanin and colleagues known as individualized zone of optimal functioning will be discussed. In essence, the process of determining this 'zone' is a directly equivalent process to the self-monitoring, self-recording activity needed to develop a comparison.

Self regulation can be considered in relation to coping in the way shown in Figure 20.4. Coping skills are therefore a subset of self-regulation, as the intervention studies described by Zimmerman (2006) illustrate; for example, by discussing developing process rather than outcome goal setting. But it is important to recognize that traditional mental skills training is not all that comprises self-regulation (notwithstanding several published papers with self-regulation in the title but no reference to the construct). The features of self-regulation that do not fall inside

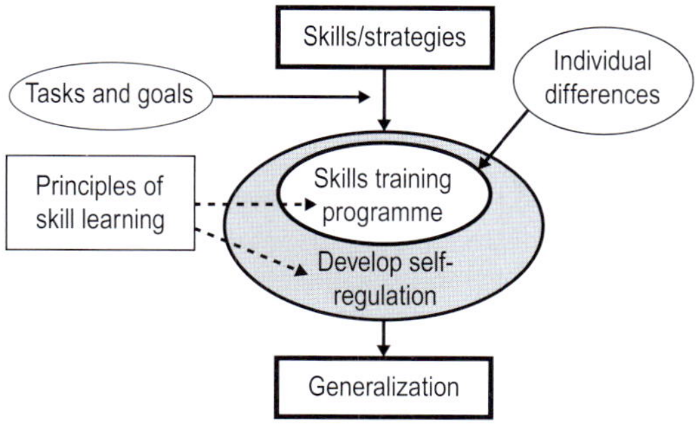

Fig. 20.4 • Self-regulation and coping.

coping training are the self-monitoring, self-recording, self-evaluation, attribution making and self reaction.

In Figure 20.3 you will see that the principle of skill learning that we discussed as relevant to coping skills training is equally applicable to those specific self-regulatory processes. The cluster of self-processes listed above, and positive motivation and behavioural management, must all be isolated and trained in the same way (instruction, practice and feedback) as any other skill. Chen & Singer (1992) highlight a number of features that they recommend in order to help develop self-regulation, which are summarized below.

1. **Explicit focus of training**. The self-regulation construct and processes will need to be described and illustrated to performers through example and analogy
2. **Develop basic coping skills**. These are an inherent facet of self-regulation so must be included
3. **Exposure to challenge, rapid and unexpected**. Self-regulation requires these conditions to be effectively practised and so these should be engineered into training programmes
4. **Simulation and progression**, as with (3) above, helps performers build up to more realistic practice and bridge the training gap
5. **Benefits demonstrated** – this has links to the development of motivation
6. **Model using 'think aloud'**. People only learn to think in particular ways by observing (hearing) how other do it. The same method can be used to see if those in training are operating correctly. Cleary & Zimmerman (2001) used a microanalytical method to access self-regulation in their studies that could offer options here
7. **Debriefs** – to review performance on self-regulation and apply learning to future plans for self-regulating
8. **Develop awareness of self-regulatory process through errors**. When self-regulation doesn't operate smoothly then tracing through the process helps identify more specifically the source of errors and remedial action.

The final aspect of self-regulation training is the suggestion, illustrated in Figure 20.4, that training performers to self-regulate is the critical key to achieving skill generalization (Smith 1999). Generalization refers to the ability to take a skill learned in one place and reapply it elsewhere. Basic coping training may not address the development of conditional knowledge. Because of this, the understanding required to evaluate the conditions and make adjustments for using a skill differently or in a different context or domain is then not available to aid the generalization.

Conclusion

In this chapter, I have carefully examined coping and described the content, format and process of training individuals to cope. An important feature emphasized here is the use of general principles of learning and distinguishing educational from genuine training programmes, if only by virtue of the use of repeated practice with feedback. The chapter then examined the construct of mental toughness, which has achieved some recent popularity in research and non-academic publications. Although in concept mental toughness and coping seem aligned, the evidence from the work on mental toughness is disorganized, without clear definition and characterized by two broad approaches: bottom-up inductive descriptions and top-down comparison studies using several different measurement tools. Significantly, none of the questionnaires appears to have been subjected to independent evaluation of psychometric properties. As a consequence, my conclusion is that mental toughness is not sufficiently coherent nor has sufficient weight of evidence to justify it as the basis of interventions to develop physical performers. Finally, the chapter described the construct of self-regulation, an established construct that does offer an organizing structure for the use of coping skills by performers in real, unexpected performance environments. Furthermore, self-regulation provides a learning framework that should help sustain performers through their careers to become self-sufficient and constantly developing, as well as facilitating the generalization of skills across context and domain.

References

Anshell, M.H., 1990. Towards validation of a model for coping with acute stress in sport. Int. J. Sport Psychol. 21, 58–83.

Anshell, M.H., Williams, L.R.T., Hodge, K., 1997. Cross-cultural and gender differences on coping style in sport. Int. J. Sport Psychol. 28, 141–156.

Anshell, M.H., Porter, A., Quek, J.J., 1998. Coping with acute stress in sport as a function of gender: an exploratory study. J. Sports Behav. 21, 363–376.

Anshell, M.H., Kim, K.W., Kim, B.H., et al., 2001. A model for coping with stressful events in sport: theory application and future directions. Int. J. Sport Psychol. 32, 43–75.

Baumeister, R.F., Faber, J.E., Wallace, H.M., 1999. Coping and ego depletion: recovery after the coping process. In: Snyder, C.R. (Ed.), Coping: The psychology of what works. Oxford University Press, New York.

Borkovec, T.D., Wilkinson, L., Folensbee, R., Lerman, C., 1983. Stimulus control applications to the treatment of worry. Behav. Res. Ther. 21, 247–251.

Bull, S., 2006. The game plan: Your guide to mental toughness at work. Capstone Publishing, Oxford.

Bull, S.J., Shambrook, C.J., James, W., et al., 2005. Towards an understanding of mental toughness in English cricketers. J. Appl. Sport Psychol. 17, 209–227.

Carver, C.S., Scheier, M.F., 1981. Attention and self-regulation: a control theory approach to human behaviour. Springer, New York.

Carver, C.S., Scheier, M.F., Weintraub, J.K., 1989. Assessing coping strategies: a theoretically based approach. J. Pers. Soc. Psychol. 56, 267–283.

Chen, D., Singer, R.N., 1992. Self-regulation and cognitive strategies in sport participation. Int. J. Sport Psychol. 23, 277–300.

Cleary, T.J., Zimmerman, B.J., 2001. Self-regulation differences during athletic practice by experts, non-experts and novices. J. Appl. Sport Psychol. 13, 185–206.

Clough, P., Earle, K., Sewell, D., 2002. Mental toughness: the concept and its measurement. In: Cockeril, I. (Ed.), Solutions in sport psychology. Thomson, London, pp. 32–45.

Connaughton, D., Wadey, R., Hanton, S., et al., 2008. The development and maintenance of mental toughness: Perceptions of elite performers. J. Sports Sci. 26, 83–95.

Cox, T., Ferguson, E., 1991. Individual differences, stress and coping. In: Cooper, C.L., Payne, L. (Eds.), Personality and stress: individual differences in the stress process. John Wiley, Chichester, West Sussex, pp. 7–30.

Crocker, P.R.E., Graham, T.R., 1995. Coping by competitive athletes with performance stress: Gender differences and relationships with affect. Sport Psychologist 9, 325–338.

Crocker, P.R.E., Isaak, K., 1997. Coping during competition and training sessions: are youth swimmers consistent? Int. J. Sport Psychol. 28, 355–369.

Crust, L., 2008. A review and conceptual re-examination of mental toughness: implications for future researchers. Personality Individ. Differ. 45, 576–583.

Dienstbier, R.A., 1989. Arousal and physiological toughness: implications for mental and physical health. Psychol. Rev. 96, 84–100.

Duncan, E., Sheffield, D., 2004. Report of presentation to the Division of Health Psychology Annual Conference, Edinburgh. Psychologist 17, 557.

Endler, N., Parker, J., 1990. Multi-dimensional assessment of coping: a critical review. J. Pers. Soc. Psychol. 58, 844–854.

Ericsson, K.A., 2006. The Influence of experience and deliberate practice on the development of superior expert performance. In: Ericsson, K.A., Charness, N., Feltovich, P.J. et al., The Cambridge handbook of expertise and expert performance. Cambridge University Press, New York, pp. 683–703.

Eubank, M., Collins, D., Lovell, G., et al., 1997. Individual temporal differences in pre-competition anxiety and hormonal concentration. Personality Individ. Differ. 23, 1031–1039.

Folkman, S., 1992. Making the case for coping. In: Carpenter, B.N. (Ed.), Personal coping: theory research and application. Praeger, Westport, CT, pp. 31–46.

Folkman, S., Lazarus, R.S., 1985. If it changes it must be a process: a study of emotion and coping during three stages of a college examination. J. Pers. Soc. Psychol. 48, 150–170.

Fourie, S., Potgieter, J.R., 2001. The nature of mental toughness in sport. South African Journal for Research in Sport, Physical Education and Recreation 23, 63–72.

Gaudreau, P., Blondin, J.P., 2002. Development of a questionnaire for the assessment of coping strategies employed by athletes in competitive sports settings. Psychol. Sport and Exerc. 3, 1–34.

Giacobbi, P., Foore, B., Weinberg, R.S., 2004. Broken clubs and expletives: the sources of stress and coping responses of skilled and moderately skilled golfers. J. Appl. Sport Psychol. 16, 166–182.

Gilbert, W., Trudel, P., Bloom, G., 1994. Simulated recall interviews as a data collection technique, Paper presented at the Association for the Advancement of Applied Sport Psychology, Lake Tahoe, CA.

Golby, J., Sheard, M., 2004. Mental toughness and hardiness at different levels of rugby league. Personality Individ. Differ. 37, 933–942.

Golby, J., Sheard, M., Lavallee, D., 2003. A cognitive-behavioural analysis of mental toughness on national rugby league football teams. Percept. Mot. Skills 96, 455–462.

Gould, D., Eklund, R.C., Jackson, S.A., 1993. Coping strategies used by US Olympic wrestlers. Res. Q. Exerc. Sport 64, 83–93.

Greenfeld, K.T., 2001. Adventure: Blind to failure. Time Magazine 18 June. Available online at: http://www.time.com/time/magazine/article/0,1971,1000120-1,00.html (accessed 20.11.09).

Heyneman, N., Fremouw, W.J., Gano, D., et al., 1990. Individual differences and the effectiveness of different coping strategies for pain. Cog. Ther. Res. 14, 63–77.

Holmes, P.S., Collins, D., 2001. The PETTLEP approach to motor imagery: a functional equivalence model for sport psychologists. J. Appl. Sport Psychol. 13, 83–106.

Horsburgh, V.A., Schermer, J.A., Veselka, L., et al., 2009. A behavioural genetic study of mental toughness and personality. Personality Individ. Differ. 46, 100–105.

Jones, G., Moorhouse, A., 2008. Developing mental toughness: gold medal strategies for transforming your business performance. Spring Hill, Oxford.

Jones, G., Hanton, S., Connaughton, D., 2002. What is this thing called mental toughness? An investigation of elite sports performers. J. Appl. Sport Psychol. 14, 205–218.

Jones, G., Hanton, S., Connaughton, D., 2007. A framework of mental toughness in the world's best performers. Sport Psychologist 21, 243–264.

Kobasa, S.C., 1979. Stressful life events, personality and health: an enquiry into hardiness. J. Pers. Soc. Psychol. 37, 1–11.

Lascelles, M.A., Cunningham, S.J., McGrath, P., et al., 1989. Teaching coping strategies to adolescents with migraine. J. Pain Symptom Manage. 4, 135–145.

Lazarus, R.S., 1993. Coping theory and research: past, present and future. Psychosom. Med. 55, 234–247.

Lazarus, R.S., Folkman, S., 1984. Stress appraisal and coping. Springer, New York.

Le Scanff, C., Taugis, J., 2002. Stress management for police special forces. J. Appl. Sport Psychol. 14, 330–343.

Levy, A.R., Polman, R.C.J., Clough, P.J., et al., 2006. Mental toughness as a determinant of beliefs, pain and adherence in sport injury rehabilitation. J. Sport Rehabil. 15, 246–254.

Loehr, J.E., 1986. Mental toughness training for sports: achieving athletic excellence. Stephen Green, Lexington, MA.

Mace, R.D., Carroll, D., 1985. The control of anxiety in sport: stress inoculation training prior to abseiling. Int. J. Sport Psychol. 16, 165–175.

Marsh, H.W., 1997. The measurement of physical self-concept: a construct validation approach. In: Fox, K. (Ed.), The physical self: from motivation to well being. Human Kinetics, Champaign, IL, pp. 27–58.

Meichenbaum, D., 1977. Cognitive behaviour modification: an integrative approach. Plenum Press, New York.

Middleton, S.C., Marsh, H.W., Martin, A.J., et al., 2004. Discovering mental toughness: a qualitative study of mental toughness in elite athletes. Self Research Centre Biannual Conference, Berlin.

Mischel, W., Schoda, Y., 1995. A cognitive-affective system theory of personality: reconceptualizing situations, dispositions, dynamics, and invariance in personality structure. Psychol. Rev. 102, 246–268.

Muraven, M., Tice, D.M., Baumeister, R.F., 1998. Self-control as limited resource: regulatory depletion patterns. J. Pers. Soc. Psychol. 74, 774–789.

Nichols, A.R., Polman, R.C.J., 2007. Coping in sport: a systematic review. J. Sports Sci. 25, 11–31.

Nichols, A.R., Holt, N.L., Polman, R.C.J., 2005. A phenomenological analysis of coping effectiveness in golf. Sport Psychologist 19, 111–130.

Nichols, A.R., Polman, R.C.J., Levy, A.R., et al., 2008. Mental toughness, optimism, pessimism and coping among athletes. Personality Individ. Differ. 44, 1182–1192.

Nichols, A.R., Polman, R.C.J., Levy, A.R., et al., 2009. Mental toughness in sport: achievement level, gender, age experience and sport type differences. Personality Individ. Differ. 47, 73–75.

Poczwardowski, A., Conroy, D.E., 2002. Coping responses to failure and success among elite athletes and performing artists. J. Appl. Sport Psychol. 14, 313–329.

Prapavessis, H., Grove, J.R., McNair, P.J., et al., 1992. Self-regulation training, state anxiety and sport performance: a psychophysiological case study. Sport Psychologist 6, 213–229.

Richards, H., 2004. Coping in sport. In: Lavallee, D., Thatcher, J., Jones, M. (Eds.), Coping and Emotion in Sport. Nova Science Publishers, New York, pp. 27–50.

Richards, H., Collins, D., 2005. Coping and extreme physical performance. 26th International Conference of the Stress and Anxiety Research Society, Halle, Germany, 21st–23rd July.

Rosenbaum, D.A., Carlson, R.A., Gilmore, R.O., 2001. Acquisition of intellectual and perceptual-motor skills. Annu. Rev. Psychol. 52, 453–470.

Rosenbaum, D.A., Augustyn, J.S., Cohen, R.G., et al., 2006. Perceptual-motor expertise. In: Ericsson, K.A., Charness, N., Feltovich, P.J. et al. (Eds.), The Cambridge handbook of expertise and expert performance. Cambridge University Press, New York, pp. 505–520.

Scanlan, T.K., Stein, G.L., Ravizza, K., 1991. An in-depth study of former elite figure skaters: III. Sources of stress. J. Sport and Exerc. Psychol. 13, 103–120.

Schmidt, R.A., Bork, R.A., 1992. New conceptualization of practice: common principles in three paradigms suggest new concepts for training. Psychol. Sci. 3, 207–214.

Schomer, H., 1986. Mental strategies and the perception of effort of marathon runners. Int. J. Sport Psychol. 17, 41–59.

Smith, R.E., 1999. Generalization effects in coping skills training. J. Sport and Exerc. Psychol. 21, 189–204.

Smith, R.E., 2006. Understanding sport behaviour: a cognitive affective processing systems approach. J. Appl. Sport Psychol. 18, 1–27.

Thelwell, R., Weston, N., Greenlees, I., 2005. Defining and understanding mental toughness within soccer. J. Appl. Sport Psychol. 17, 326–332.

Vohs, K.D., Baumeister, R.F., 2004. Understanding self-regulation. In: Baumeister, R.F., Vohs, K.D. (Eds.), Handbook of self-regulation. Guilford Press, New York, pp. 1–9.

Wiedenfeld, S.A., O'Leary, A., Bandura, A., et al., 1990. Impact of perceived self-efficacy in coping with stressors on component of the immune system. J. Pers. Soc. Psychol. 59, 1082–1094.

Yoo, J., 2001. Coping profile of Korean competitive athletes. Int. J. Sport Psychol. 32, 290–303.

Zimmerman, B.J., 2006. Development and adaptation of expertise: the role of self-regulatory processes and beliefs. In: Ericsson, K.A., Charness, N., Feltovich, P.J. et al. (Eds.), The Cambridge handbook of expertise and expert performance. Cambridge University Press, New York, pp. 705–722.

Zizzi, S.J., Deaner, H.R., 2003. The relationship between emotional intelligence and performance among college baseball players. J. Appl. Sport Psychol. 15, 262–269.

21

Emotional issues of peak performance: managing mood

Sheelagh Rodgers* Britt Tajet-Foxell†

*NHS Highland, Inverness, UK; †The Royal Ballet, London, UK and Olympiatoppen, The Olympic High Performance Centre, Oslo, Norway

CHAPTER CONTENTS

Introducing emotions – what they do and how they do it

Thinking not feeling?

Standard undergraduate textbooks of sports psychology usually contain a chapter or some reference to mood, usually anxiety, and its role in performance. Many references to mood are made in the context of research, with authors commenting on measurement of mood, how moods affect performance and sometimes how athletes might recognize mood.

Performance is emotional. In competitive sport, from the football terraces to test cricket, world cup rugby to Wimbledon, the great sporting tournaments are awash with emotions. Dealing with the crowds is only one of the problems faced by many sports people. Most people can call to mind John McEnroe at tennis tournaments and his outbursts, or Daley Thompson's reaction to his gold medal. In extreme sports, there is a common acknowledgement of the role played by 'peak' experience and 'flow' as a key motivation for taking part (Csikszentmihalyi 1990). Finally, in aesthetic sports and dance, the effective presentation and communication of emotion is arguably the distinguishing characteristic between good and poor performance (Hanna 1983). Consequently, optimally dealing with and employing emotion can separate the elite from the mediocre.

DOI: 10.1016/B978-0-443-06734-1.00021-3

In many domains, performance is big business and the hope of an Olympic medal or place in a particular company is the lifetime goal for many. Few make it to the very top, but what separates the elite from the rest is undoubtedly psychological attitude. In short, managing moods is essential, and recognizing and coping with moods can be the difference between winning and losing, success and failure. Most psychology texts fall short of describing interventions that might assist athletes in managing their moods. In fairness, some texts speak about relaxation techniques for anxiety, but rarely do they discuss the very individual factors that can underlie a person's mood, or even how the impact of this mood may operate, or be ameliorated, in influencing behaviour.

Thoughts, emotions and behaviour

The point is that these three important constructs (what Dave refers to later in Ch. 25 as 'the triad') are inextricably linked. Unfortunately, for a number of reasons, sport psychology was lured up what was a 'dark alley' (for us at any rate) in an overly restrictive focus on anxiety. There is no doubt that anxiety is a common emotion in performance, nor that it can influence performance level. The point here is that each individual is subject to a range of emotions, usually several at any one time, which provide a plethora of often competing influences. These emotions can generate cognitions, be generated by cognitions, or act in a cyclical, almost spiral-like manner. Throw in the interactions with behaviour and the permutations can get very complex indeed.

For just these reasons, the individuality and complexity of the interactions, we favour theoretical approaches that consider intraindividual differences between good and not so good performances, as opposed to the very impressive, statistically rigorous but group-based studies that dominated sport psychology for so many years (cf. the purposes underpinning performance science discussed in the Introduction to this book). The leader in this field is Yuri Hanin, whose work on the Zone of Optimal Functioning (ZOF – also sometimes referred to as the Individual Zone of Optimal Functioning or IZOF; Hanin 2000, 2007) has spanned a wide variety of performance applications, including team, individual, combat, extreme and aesthetic sports. The approach is descriptive/ideographic, in that an individual's perceptions on levels of a variety of emotions are collected prior to performances. By a process of comparison, the individual's ZOF is identified by consideration of the emotion descriptors that precede better performances. The approach has received a lot of support, although generally in studies involving Hanin and his colleagues. For example, a meta-analysis showed that (perhaps unsurprisingly, given how the ZOF is derived) comparisons show that performances are significantly better for in-zone athletes than for those out of the zone (Jokela & Hanin, 1999). While others have criticized the approach, citing, for example, its lack of consistency with other more nomothetic constructs (e.g. Davis & Cox 2002), there is little doubting ZOF's applicability to practical settings. The idea that each individual has an optimum state is both face valid and appealing, and represents a pretty good start in seeking control as the precursor for performance enhancement.

A recent extension of the ZOF concepts has really strengthened its potential for understanding the interplay between emotions, cognitions and behaviour. Already mentioned by Hugh in the previous chapter, the qualitative technique of composite sequence analysis (CSA; Miles & Huberman 1994) offers a way to understand the chronological interplay between the triad as the performer copes (or doesn't) with the challenge. Two examples, taken from an international sailor's experiences of good and bad races, are shown in Figures 21.1 and 21.2 (Nieuwenhuys et al 2008). The horizontal lines split the race into meaningful phases, while the arrows show the directional/chronological flow of ideas to actions and vice versa.

The figures make use of a coping process sequence developed by Hanin and colleagues that they call the Triple-A (Awareness–Acceptance–Action) model. These ideas are covered in more depth in Chapter 20. For our present purpose, however, the CSA approach takes us one more step towards understanding the impact of emotions on cognition and thence coping. The use of structured narrative (almost literally story telling by the performer) is shown as a very useful technique for practitioners, a way to access what Hanin (2007) calls the 'meta-experiences' of the situation, what you felt and tried to do about what happened. Crucially, however, even this process is still descriptive. What is really needed is a way to control the emotions and their impact.

Understanding emotions and moods

Before considering how emotions might be challenged and managed, it is important to define what is meant by an emotion and how it can affect behaviour in the performance context. Defining emotions

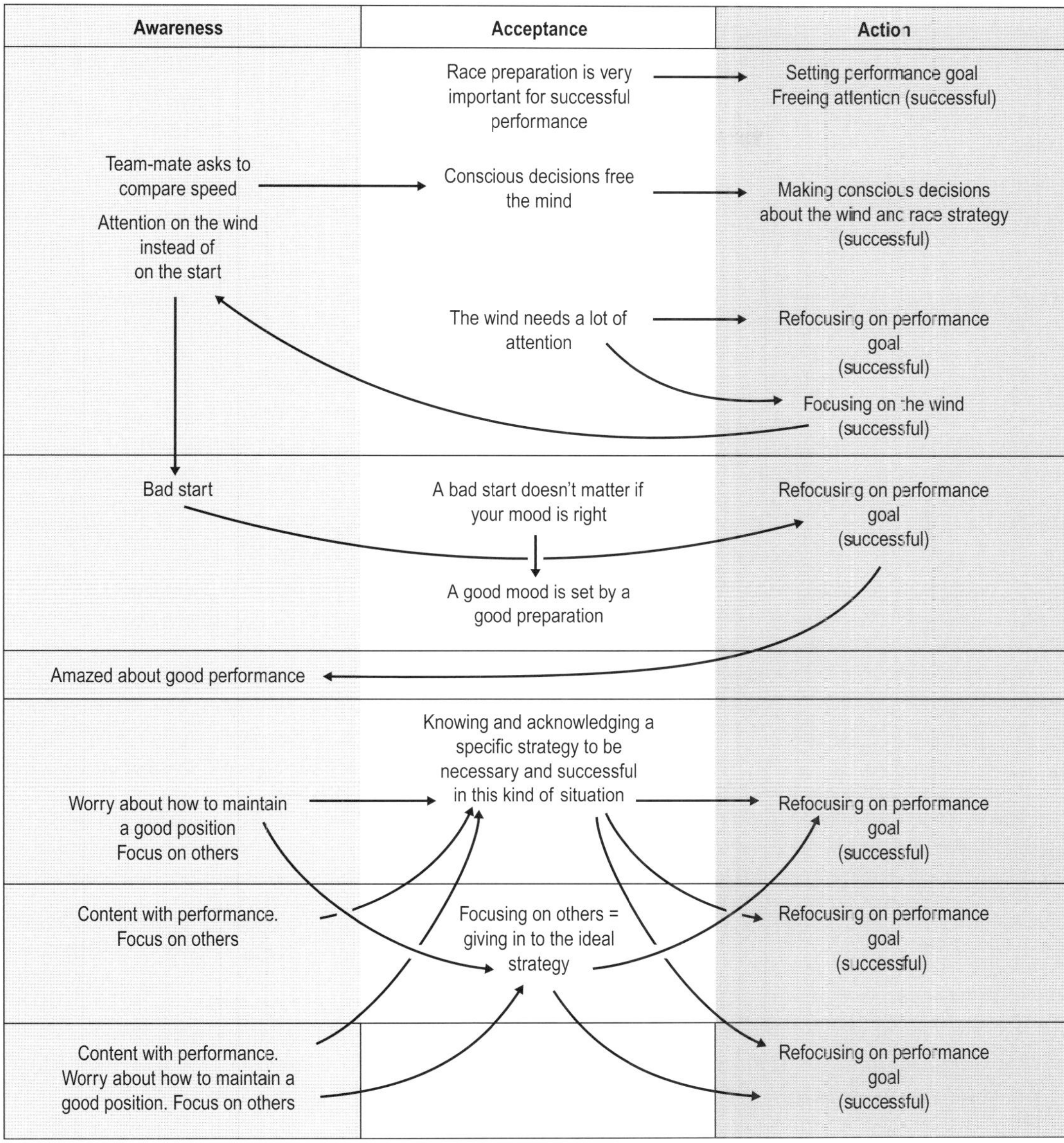

Fig. 21.1 • CSA of experiences and coping in different parts of a good race. Reprinted from Psychology of Sport and Exercise, 9, 61-76, Nieuwenhuys A., HaninY., Bakker F., Performance-related experiences and coping during races: a case of an elite sailor, 2008, with permission from Elsevier.

can be difficult in that anger, happiness and anxiety and fear are multifaceted. Physical sensations may be strong and thinking patterns can come into play and this can result in behavioural changes. Jones & Uphill (2004) comment on how they view the difference between emotions and moods, but state that emotions are believed to be more transient and intense in comparison to moods (Jones et al 2000).

A useful definition of emotion as applied to sport is offered by Vallerand and colleagues (Butler 2000, Vallerand 1983, 1989, Vallerand & Blanchard 2000):

> An emotion is viewed as a reaction to a stimulus event (either real or imagined); it involves changes in the viscera and musculature of the person, is experienced by the person subjectively in characteristic ways, and is expressed through such means as facial changes and action tendencies which may mediate and energize subsequent behaviours.

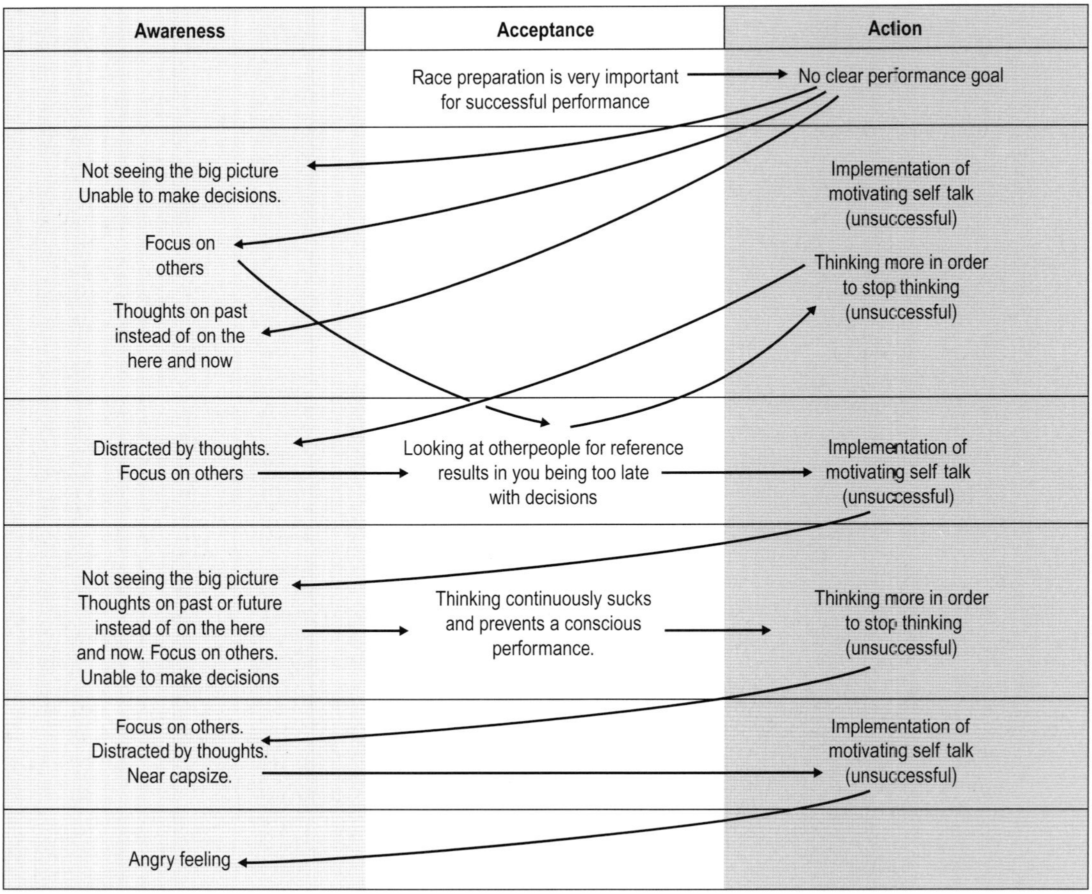

Fig. 21.2 • CSA of experiences and coping in different parts of a bad race. Reprinted from Psychology of Sport and Exercise, 9, 61-76, Nieuwenhuys A., HaninY., Bakker F., Performance-related experiences and coping during races: a case of an elite sailor, 2008, with permission from Elsevier.

Understanding emotions can help an individual make sense of what is happening in their performance (cf. the CSA approach in the earlier figures). Crucially, however, controlling the emotions and challenging the thinking underlying the emotion can help an athlete attain a better state for performance. Several theoretical perspectives have investigated how emotions arise in performance, including attributionally based approaches (Vallerand 1989, Weiner 1986), reversal theory (Apter 1989) and cognitive–motivational relational theory (Lazarus 1991, 2000). Given our emerging focus of understanding and controlling emotion, however, the rest of this chapter will mainly draw on the work of Beck (1976) and others such as Greenberger & Padesky (1995) and Williams (2001). The latter approaches have investigated how emotions affect thinking and how, through challenging and changing thoughts and beliefs, emotions can be altered. We will consider how we can draw from this work in primarily clinical areas of our work with performers.

It is also worth considering the longer-term impact of emotions, which has traditionally been examined by the measurement of mood. In this respect, mood is seen as the more enduring manifestation of emotions (see the definition above). The Profile of Moods Scale (POMS), as first developed by McNair et al (1971) was designed to provide a 'rapid, economical measure of identifying and assessing transient, fluctuating affective states'. The POMS questionnaire is normally presented as a 65-item checklist that measures six facets of emotion – tension, depression, fatigue, confusion, anger and vigour. It has a rich history in sport psychology. For example, Morgan (1979) was able to demonstrate that a particular set of scores on the POMS (high in Vigour and low on other items, known as the 'Iceberg' profile) predicted success in Olympic qualification. POMS continued to stand as a strong predictor of athletic success, despite questions about its reliability and validity in the sports arena. Yet again, however, it provided information about the state of the athlete but no plan as to how mood states might be altered.

In another application, Morgan and colleagues (1987) discovered that the POMS was sensitive to emotional changes as the intensity of training varies. Accordingly, the scale has been used as a means of monitoring overtraining, fatigue and staleness (see also considerations of this application in Ch. 10). However, the scale remains long, although there have been attempts to shorten it. For example, Butler (2000) discusses a 'Feelings Scale' developed from personal construct theory, which consists of a 20-item scale where the adjectives describing the mood are generated by the athlete themselves. However, how the mood is described and rated is the first step towards the challenge of altering the mood and hence the performance. Reflecting this, Table 21.1 presents some of the adjectives that people commonly use to describe how they are feeling; what their moods or emotions are at a given time. If a performer has trouble describing a mood, they may be able to recognize changes in the body. For example, tight shoulders may indicate that you are afraid or tense; heaviness in the body may suggest tiredness or depression.

Finally, Terry and colleagues have made broad use of the POMS as a means of predicting performance level (e.g. Beedie et al 2000). Unfortunately, while intellectually and academically interesting, this approach again offers little in the way of practical implication, unless clear and consistent individual mood profiles emerge that precede good performances. In this regard, the IZOF seems to offer a great deal more potential for understanding the pre-performance state but, as we have already shown, still not enough on what can be done about it. The key 'missing element' for much of this work is how moods can be monitored and challenged so that performance can be improved. It is through identifying the thoughts that a person is having, we suggest, that we can help alter the mood and ultimately, with practice of monitoring these thoughts and challenging them, that an individual can learn to deal with emotions and improve performance.

Doing something about it – the cognitive–behavioural therapy approach

Relaxation and imagery are standard sports psychology methods to deal with excess anxiety. Yet cognitive therapists have long realized that a relaxation tape handed to a client offers little to most people. Performers, like clinical patients, need an individual, tailored intervention to help them understand and cope with the emotions they experience in the sporting situations that they encounter. We suggest that the field of cognitive therapy has plenty to offer, but this approach is generally not available to athletes as sports psychologists are not experienced or trained in delivering cognitive therapy.

In this chapter, we advocate and explain change using evidence-based therapy, namely cognitive–behavioural therapy (CBT), and employ case studies to demonstrate how clients and psychologists can work towards recognizing emotions/moods/feelings. These terms are used interchangeably, but need to be differentiated from 'thinking'. I feel' is often used when 'I think' or 'I believe' would be more accurate. We believe that it is through changing the thinking processes that we can genuinely access (as opposed to just passively experience) the mood state and assist the athlete in changing their emotions.

Table 21.1 The mood checklist

Sad	Anxious	Angry	Depressed	Excited
Frightened	Panicky	Frustrated	Irritated	Disappointed
Ashamed	Mad	Happy	Nervous	Proud
Powerful	Confident	Tired	Restless	Dejected

From Richard J. Butler, Sports Psychology in Action, 2000. Reproduced by permission of Edward Arnold (Publishers) Ltd.

CBT is the psychological treatment of choice for a wide number of psychological problems (Hollon & Beck 2004, Salkovskis 1991), and is probably the best researched and validated psychotherapeutic approach. Reading about CBT can be daunting, and a newcomer may struggle with the concepts offered. We are trained, experienced and supervised practitioners of CBT and believe that it is a model that has much to offer the performance world and some of the problems and difficulties experienced by athletes, dancers and participants.

One criticism of our (CBT) approach might be that CBT has developed its evidence base largely from the world of clinical psychology. However, more recently Williams (2001) has developed a CBT skills approach that allows people to be trained in a CBT model in a shorter period of time. This development means that CBT is not only a model used by experienced and highly trained therapists but has grown into a set of skills that can deliver a CBT approach to clients who have a mild–moderate range of problems after undertaking a shortened training course. The model has been used as a self-help approach where workers deliver interventions for a few sessions only, and the clients learn to help themselves and become their own therapists. We would still advocate that all practitioners of CBT skills receive supervision for their work, but here is a technique that can assist an athlete in recognizing a model and changing it through challenging their own thought processes.

The CBT skills approach involves clients in having active involvement in their own care and provides them with tools (techniques) to prevent relapse. A structured approach is used with an emphasis on current problems rather than just past history, and it allows the client to gain an understanding about what is happening to themselves and why, as well as learning techniques that they can use to tackle the problem and move on. Through the self-help approach, Williams (2001) has promoted the use of CBT skills for a population that has largely been ignored, as their problems were not considered serious or severe. Now people with a mild level of anxiety or depression can be helped quickly and effectively. Most performers do not experience severe mental health problems, so this approach is appropriate. Of course, if they do, they should be referred to clinical psychologists or psychiatrists, or even CBT therapists, all of whom have experience of complex and challenging mental health issues (see Conclusion, at the end of the book).

Next, we look at what a basic CBT model consists of and how by challenging thinking we can alter moods. Through case studies we then explore the moods and emotions that performers may experience, attempting to define the thinking processes, challenge 'thinking errors' and follow through to the outcomes of the sessions undertaken.

Exploring the thinking: 'It's the thought that counts'

Understanding the emotion is just one part of the picture that needs to be built up from our interviews with performers. The cognitive–behavioural model offers the idea of formulation (assessment) of all factors that might play a part in the total problem. This framework allows us to define the thinking, emotion, physical symptoms and behaviours that occur in a given situation. The model considers the environmental factors (life situations) that surround the individual and what part past experiences might have played and how they relate and are relevant to the present difficulties.

Greenberger & Padesky (1995) use the concept of the 'cognitive hot-cross bun', as shown in Figure 21.3. All areas can interact with each other, forming the cross pattern seen on the top of a hot-cross bun. Williams (2001), in the cognitive–behavioural skills approach, refers to these areas as the 'Five areas approach'. This modification is presented in Figure 21.4.

Both the Padesky and Greenberger and the Williams models present areas that can be explored with the individual when assessing mood and thinking and the effects they have on performance. Building from these ideas, a CBT assessment consists of:

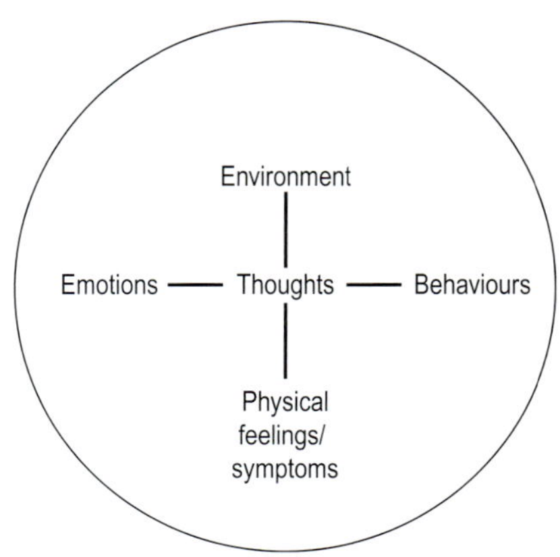

Fig. 21.3 • The cognitive hot-cross bun. After Greenberger & Padesky 1995.

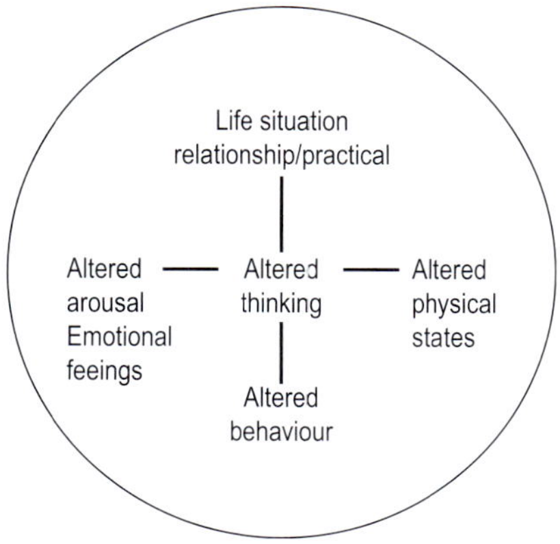

Fig. 21.4 • The Diamond Model. From Williams C, Overcoming depression: a five areas approach (2001). Reproduced by permission of Edward Arnold (Publishers) Ltd.

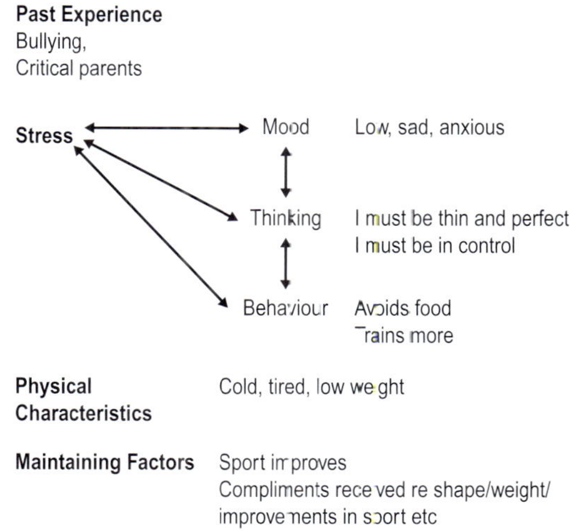

Fig. 21.5 • A structured approach to understanding – a case study in disordered eating.

- A full description of the presenting problem
- A detailed analysis of mood, thinking, physical feelings and behaviours
- An understanding of how past factors and current events contribute to the presenting problem
- An understanding of what factors help maintain the problem.

The primary focus is on the factors that maintain the current difficulties. This is usually explored through thought diaries, where thinking is dissected and challenged, underlying beliefs and assumptions held by the person are explored and finally an altered thinking pattern emerges.

The past and present can interact to produce an individual picture of the presenting problem. It is important not just to view the athlete as anxious or worried, for example, but to look at why and how the problem has built up into its current state. Assessment is not just about providing a diagnosis that attaches a label to the problem, but can provide a method of helping the athlete understand the onset, development and maintenance of the problem. It can also help to develop an insight into an individual's subjective understanding of their problem. Let us consider an exemplar case study to demonstrate these processes.

Case example: an athlete with disordered eating

Building up a picture of an individual's difficulty can provide the psychologist with a unique understanding of that individual (Fig. 21.5). Without a thorough formulation of the problem, only the low mood may be detected/addressed and the eating behaviours ignored. By using an approach such as Williams's Five areas, an individual's thinking, behaviour and physical symptoms can be discussed. This can lead to an understanding of what triggers the mood and what might help the individual change the problem. Past experiences can be relevant to the current issues, as old behaviours and past ways of coping may be reverted to, even when these are not particularly adaptive, because they are habitual and known to the individual. This picture can help a performer understand what is happening to them and can aid them in challenging the thoughts and exploring the thinking errors that might exist. An exemplar Thought Diary, which would form part of the monitoring and therapeutic process, is presented in Table 21.2.

Thinking can undermine a person's ability to perform a task or their belief in their ability. Doubts may be normal for an individual in a challenging environment but powerful negative thoughts can impede, overwhelm and destroy their performance. Cognitive therapy is not just about changing negative thoughts, it is about helping the person to recognize what a thought is. Thoughts can arise in less than a second; we may be unaware of a lot of our thinking, but learning to recognize the automatic thoughts that arise in any situation is the start to learning about the way we think and behave in stressful situations. Thinking errors can arise (Burns 2000). In recognizing the patterns that individuals can slip into and keep returning to, we can help the athlete become

Table 21.2 An exemplar thoughts diary

Situation	Negative automatic thoughts	Emotions	Alternative and balanced thoughts	How do you feel now?
Describe clearly and concisely	Rate believability 0–100%		Rate believability 0–100%	

more aware of the whole cognitive process. Burns refers to the negative thinking patterns as 'cognitive distortions' The cognitive distortions are set out below:

- **All or nothing thinking**: Events are seen in absolutes as black or white
- **Over-generalization**: Negative events are seen as a never-ending pattern of defeat
- **Mental filter**: You dwell on the negative and ignore the positive
- **Discounting the positives**: You believe your achievements or positive qualities 'don't count' or they are seen as 'lucky'
- **Jumping to conclusions**:
  - *Mind reading* – you assume people are reacting negatively to you when there is no evidence for this
  - *Fortune telling* – you predict things will turn out badly
- **Magnification or minimalization**: You blow things out of proportion or shrink their importance inappropriately
- **Emotional reasoning**: You resort from how you feel – 'I feel stupid' – to 'I really must be stupid'
- **Should statements**: You criticize yourself or others with *shoulds* or *should nots*. *Musts, oughts and have tos* have the same effect
- **Labelling**: you identify with your shortcomings – instead of saying 'I made a mistake' you tell yourself 'I'm an idiot'
- **Personalization and blame**: You blame yourself for things you were not responsible for, or you blame others and overlook the way your own attitudes and behaviour might contribute to a problem.

In addressing these distortions, a useful first step is to develop a set of constructs that characterize them but also offer some indication of the negative influence they can generate. In attempting this, Butler (2000) emphasizes the importance of clear thinking. He notes that the first step in dealing with this is to identify the negative thoughts. Importantly, though, Butler recognizes that this might be difficult for the individual performer to do, but that an outside observer who is not enmeshed in the training/performance environment might be able to point out the thinking styles that are emerging. A suggestion that might make the individual more aware of this thinking is to audiotape the discussion, leaving them to subsequently listen to the tape and recognize for themselves the habits and patterns they resort to.

Negative thinking, as described by Butler, consists of seven different ways of expressing the thoughts and beliefs held.

- **The don'ts**: This includes *should not, would not* and anything that includes a not! Such statements only serve to tell an athlete what not to do, the 'not' being ignored. So 'don't drop the shoulder in a throw' will be interpreted as 'drop the shoulder' (cf. the ideas presented in Chs 13 and 23)
- **Limitations**: These are self-imposed barriers to performance. The statements may use the words *can't* or *never* e.g. 'I can't run well on this track' Using such thinking styles will define what an athlete expects to do, not what they might be capable of achieving
- **Put-downs**: Such statements relate to perceived weaknesses e.g. 'My run up is too slow'. Such thinking can dominate a performance and can become self-fulfilling. This can be seen when an athlete overcompensates for being slow, and this confirms their belief in the technique. An athlete may expect to act in this way and this will reinforce the belief of their behaviour
- **What ifs**: These describe a negative loop. The worry is made in the form of a question to which there is no answer, so the performer repeatedly poses the question to himself 'What if I am not selected?'
- **Self-doubt**: Expressions of doubt as to ability to perform well may reflect concern over physical fitness or psychological readiness. This again can become self-fulfilling, becoming the source of information on which performers evaluate themselves, and thus perpetuates the doubt

- **Letting others down**: These are concerns about how others might be seen to have judged the performance
- **Preoccupations**: These relate to problems outside the performance world, such as personal problems, money difficulties, etc. and they can impinge on performance and cause distraction.

Cognitive therapy is not just about thinking being irrational or rational. Of course, many thoughts can be considered irrational: for example, it is irrational to be scared of snakes in the UK as the majority of people are unlikely to meet an adder. Yet many people suffer from a genuine snake phobia. Rather more, cognitive therapy aims to analyse the thinking and look at the underlying beliefs behind the thinking. CBT has provided a constructionist approach to dealing with thinking and emotions. It attempts to look at why the fears have arisen and takes into account past experiences and unpacks the thinking around the fear of snakes. Unfortunately, just telling someone it is irrational to be frightened of snakes does not go very far towards helping them overcome their fear.

Using the concept of thinking errors

Thinking errors can affect mood and behaviour, as has been shown in the 'Hot-cross bun' and 'Five areas' approaches. The different types of cognitive distortion or thinking error have been discussed and we will now look at how performers in particular may use these thinking practices in maladaptive ways.

- **Misfocus**: Because of mental filters and discounting the positives, the performer may attend only to the negative thoughts
- **Self-fulfilment**: Jumping to conclusions, such as mind reading and fortune telling, and hence performing in the way the mindset expects you to perform
- **Perpetuation of thinking**: Overgeneralization and 'magnification and minimization', where thoughts are repeatedly gone over, and through emotional reasoning you resort from feelings to actual statements 'I feel stupid' becomes 'I am stupid'
- **Playing not to lose**: Where the individual allows their thinking to influence their behaviour to take the easiest route; consequently, performance can be mediocre as the individual plays safe and avoids risk
- **Trying to please others** (incorporates personalization and blame): Thinking is about others and their views and requirements rather than about focusing and thinking about one's own performance
- **Becoming tense**: Thinking leads to physical reactions and physiological responses, which in turn affect mood so that performance is affected
- **Reduced confidence**: Again, the individual discounts the positives. Using 'should' statements and labelling the shortcomings are all forms of distorted thinking, which can lower self-belief, and thinking can then affect the actual performance (behaviour).

Identifying moods and thoughts

The preceding sections have shown that there are many skills based in the CBT model that can help an individual identify their moods, create a desired behaviour change and challenge the thinking that interferes with them moving on. These challenges and changes can be summarized using the daily thought records and an example is presented in Table 21.3 below.

Briefly, in its therapeutic application the diary provides for the following:

- **Situation**: The performer needs to identify the situation in which the emotion occurs. This is important as often the performer will report it as occurring all the time, but it can usually be narrowed down to a specific time or place
- **Thinking**: The performer needs to find the thought or image they have in a given situation and rate their belief in that thought
- **Emotion**: The performer identifies how they feel and how intense this feeling is
- **Alternative view**: The performer looks for another view of the situation. For example, they may collect evidence from past experiences to challenge the original thought. As another alternative, they may critically consider the usefulness of the thought, thus enabling its dismissal as self-limiting
- **Changed mood**: Changing and challenging the thinking should produce a change in the mood.

This process of 'cognitive restructuring' is commonly presented in textbooks. Unfortunately, however, the associated complexities and mechanisms receive much less coverage. Consideration of genuine case studies can serve to demonstrate the complex interactions that can be associated with these dysfunctional thoughts, another factor that emphasizes the need for training.

Table 21.3 An exemplar thoughts diary entry for a high-board diver

Situation	Thoughts & rate belief 0–100%	Emotions Intensity 0–100%	Alternative/balanced thoughts Rate belief 0–100%	Altered feelings 0–100%
Standing on a 10 m diving board	I can't do this I will hurt myself 100%	Anxiety/ fear 100%	I have done this many times before with success 90%	Anxiety 20% Fear 10%
			I know what to do 100%	
			I believe I am a good diver 99%	

Case studies: using CBT with performers to enable them to change their moods through challenging and changing their thinking processes

The following examples are taken from our work with clients who have been referred to us for help with their performance. Instead of looking at how their performances could be altered by use of other performance psychology techniques, we have focused on the use of CBT methods, as discussed in the preceding sections. The case studies have been altered to ensure that the performers remain anonymous.

When reading these case studies, it is important to bear in mind the often lengthy process of exploring, identifying, testing and challenging the performers' thought processes/thought problems that will have been undertaken by the psychologists. Things are certainly not as simple as just handing over a thought diary – but you might be surprised how many people believe that they are!

A relatively short description of the thoughts and accompanying feelings of the performer, as presented here, may be the outcome of a lengthy session between the psychologist and the client. If an athlete lives abroad or in a different part of the UK, for practical and geographical reasons the athlete may only be able to access the psychologist once. In such a case, the session may only offer a couple of hours or more in order to explore, identify and develop alternative thinking patterns. We believe that the CBT model does offer a set of techniques to work with a performer, provides a framework for interpreting the problems and provides the individual athlete with a set of 'tools' to use independently of the psychologist.

Case 1: Athlete A

Athlete A was recovering from a long-term injury. He had been operated on, and had been in rehabilitation for some considerable time. Working back to a full training programme he reported he had lost 'the edge' to his performance, and found it hard to integrate into the GB squad. However, he felt comfortable training and working at club level.

He was acutely aware that it was rapidly approaching competition time, and he was keen to regain his sharpness in training and preparations towards the World Cup season. His physiotherapist confirmed that he was fully recovered from the surgery, and the psychologist was working with the athlete exploring his thoughts around the forthcoming season. The thoughts read:

- 'I enjoy club training' *but*...
- 'I don't enjoy GB team training camps'
- 'I don't enjoy endurance training, but I should do it'
- 'I don't want to be at this GB camp: I want it to be over.'

The feelings he experienced were described as 'sinking', 'apprehension' and 'a loss of control'. The underlying meanings underpinning his thought processes about his reluctance to join the GB camp were: 'They are all much better than me. I am not good enough to be here. I can't find 'the edge', I'll never make it!'

When the athlete was asked to value the mental representation of his performance by imagining it (the performance), he rated it 5/10.

The work undertaken with the athlete was based on challenging the negative thinking patterns in order to develop a more positive mindset when challenged. The assumption 'I'll never make it' was too global. The athlete would need to break it down to more specific assumptions, exploring the thought's exact meaning.

When identifying and exploring his past experiences with GB training camps, which the athlete had attended in the past, he found that there were numerous examples of him getting benefits from the camp training. He was made aware of his motivational attitude and physical and technical skills. His talent became obvious and he recognized that he did indeed want to go to the Olympic Games, with a passion that had been lacking before. The negative thought processes were turned into alternatives: 'I have come back from injury before. It's normal to find it hard to integrate back into the team. But I can do it again- I can do it by taking SMART steps – small steps that I have control over'.

By introducing the alternative mindset, the mood became more positive. The athlete felt challenged rather than overawed. He felt back in control and excited about being back in the thick of championship preparations. In viewing the same mental video of his performance, he rated it 9/10 compared to the previous 5/10 rating.

The more rational thinking mindset resulted in overall improved mood and this gave the athlete a sense of mastery over the task, and he felt confident that he could cope with the squad training camp. Cognitive distortions of *overgeneralization*, *magnification* and *mental filtering* existed in the original thinking patterns. By challenging the threatening thoughts and looking for a more functional alternative, the athlete was able to change the way he was feeling about the training camp and could use the new patterns of thinking to cope with the forthcoming tasks and demands.

Case 2: Athlete B

Athlete B was a university student as well as a GB team member for her sport. She was preparing for the youth Olympics and feeling apprehension, doubt and anxiety at the tasks facing her. She had been working hard at her studies and had just completed a period of demanding exams.

Her thoughts read: 'Compared to everyone else in the team, I am at a real disadvantage. They have been able to train more than me, and they must be much better prepared.'

The reinforcing thought read: 'Because of my being at university and doing a demanding subject, I have not been able to train as much as the others. Therefore, I am not as well prepared as them (team-mates). I expect I won't be performing as well, so I'll probably do badly'.

These negative thoughts made her feel vulnerable and at a disadvantage.

In discussion, the evidence behind these thoughts was explored. *Refocusing* involved working on the evidence that she was extremely hard working, self-motivated and committed; she had been able to keep up an excellent training regime despite her study demands. This athlete was completely professional in her approach both to her studies and her training/performance preparations.

The *alternative thinking* described the reality of her situation, which painted a picture of resilience and of someone who never took any short cuts:

- 'I have worked really hard for this, both by keeping on top of my studies and fitting in my training programmes'
- 'This is a really good opportunity to compare where I am at, performance-wise, with my competitions'
- 'I am well prepared and determined to make the most of the games.'

She felt excited about the possibility of competing and began to see the competition as a measure of her present skill level and ability. This helped her feel on top of the situation. She felt comfortable and in control rather than apprehensive and frightened.

This athlete went on to win her competition. This further proved to her that her training was not lacking in any respect. She had concrete measurable evidence that she was on track despite having to divide her attention and focus between training and studies. The thinking errors seen in this case fell within the category of *overgeneralization*, *jumping to conclusions* and *magnification*.

Case 3: Athlete C

Athlete C was an athlete whose sport covered several disciplines. He had been injured for a long time but had fully recovered and already in the early part of the season achieved personal bests.

However, he felt he was at a standstill with one of his disciplines. He was struggling to perform and the media was starting to highlight his difficulties. The athlete was beginning to worry that his poor performance in this one discipline would lead to problems in other areas. He was anxious that these other disciplines could be contaminated by his poor performance in *X*.

He had received a full medical and physical assessment and was told that he could train fully and that there was no trace of the old injury. The athlete had in the past been plagued by injuries, which had specifically affected discipline X, and he was beginning to think of it as a curse.

The athlete was afraid to commit fully to his performance, as he was anxious about the possibility of the injury recurring. He was afraid to train and afraid to compete, experiencing a high level of anxiety and physical tension when he thought about it. His thoughts read:

- 'I may get hurt again'
- 'I may reinjure myself.'

The increased physical tension accompanying this mindset made it difficult to perform the technical routine of the moves clearly and sharply. His mental image was described as blurred compared to the clear, sharp mental images of the other disciplines, which made up his sport. By examining the fear surrounding the movement and exploring the thoughts underpinning this fear, a host of negative thinking was exposed and identified. From 'I may get hurt again' the athlete's identified thoughts read: 'I probably will get injured again. . .' and became: 'I am going to injure myself if I do this.'

This type of error thinking falls into the category of *fortune telling*, leading into *catastrophizing*. When looking for evidence for these thoughts, no evidence whatsoever was found. However, 'C' believed these thoughts to be 100% true, and the fact for him was that he was going to reinjure himself when performing this specific routine. In trying to challenge his assumptions, the psychologist moved the athlete out of the problem discipline and into the disciplines in which he was successful and where he felt confident. His thoughts then read:

- 'I have the recipe for success, I have already proved to be successful, and I already have an Olympic medal to prove it'
- 'I have lots and lots and lots of experience'
- 'I am resilient'
- 'I am generally stronger and fitter than before'
- 'I have a lot of great experiences'
- 'I am totally committed to my work'
- 'I am a true professional'
- 'I have much more insight with my programme now'
- 'I am robust mentally and I am professionally tough'
- 'I am a fighter'
- 'I have a very good physio(therapist) who knows me well and I have always been able to trust him and my support team'
- 'If I don't trust his professional judgement I am insulting his clinical expertise, and I can trust him.'

When rating his belief in these statements, which were generated in collaboration with the psychologist, the athlete noticed that he could indeed trust himself. It also helped him feel confident that he could put his trust in the physio and the rest of his support team.

This modified thought pattern based on strong measurable evidence made him feel safe. The athlete moved from being fearful and tense about performing certain moves towards being confident and relaxed. Feeling safe helped him feel prepared and ready to fully commit himself to training. He could again focus with confidence on every discipline of his sport.

Case 4: Athlete D

This was an athlete who was anxious and worried about the selection procedures, a recurrent theme when working with elites. This athlete also described herself as feeling small, insignificant and unimportant in comparison to the others in the team. She felt insecure and uncertain about how the coaches rated her performance. Her thoughts read:

- 'They don't believe in me'
- 'They don't think I can do it, they back *X* and obviously prefer her to me'
- 'They will make sure she gets the place'
- 'I will not get selected and I will fail!'

The coaching staff had taken on an enormous dimension in her mind, while she saw herself shrink to insignificance. She became tense, she felt stressed and she could not relax. She constantly compared herself to others and always unfavourably. Her focus was directed to how well everyone else was doing, and how pleased the coach was with their progress.

In the session with the psychologist, the athlete explored the role of the coach and how her support system worked. She agreed that, although the coaches may seem to have favourites, at the end of the day they were judged on how well their athletes performed. It was important, even crucial, for them to produce results. The training programmes and support systems were there to enable the athletes to fulfil their potentials. Funding rested on results. The alternative thinking read:

- 'They are there to help me become the best'
- 'They do want me to succeed'
- 'My succeeding reflects well on their coaching abilities'
- 'Their success reflects on the whole support system.'

By challenging the original thinking patterns, the athlete was able to learn how she might produce a more functional mindset that she could use to underpin her performance. Her main thought then became: 'They want me to succeed and they are here to help me realize my full potential, to achieve my goals of becoming a world champion.'

The level of tension and stress diminished and she was able to trust the support staff, *her* support staff. She felt she was able to relax and focus on her own progress rather than on how her team-mates were doing. When looking at herself compared to the others she viewed herself as being of normal size and equal to the rest of the team. The tiny being she had originally been had gone!

In this case relaxation techniques might have helped this athlete, but relaxation alone would not tackle the underlying thinking processes and the assumptions made. By exploring her thought processes and challenging them, the athlete could begin to understand what was happening to her. This knowledge and introspection enabled her to take stock, then move on.

Case 5: Dancer E

In the world of dance, as in the world of sport, there is a lot of anxiety around the selection procedures and about performing consistently well. This young dance student described being frightened, and felt extremely anxious and self-conscious in ballet class. Ballet dancers all begin the day with 1¾ hours of exercise class, going through the traditional classic ballet movements to prepare for the day's rehearsals and performance on stage.

The dancer would never stand in the front of the class. She did not feel confident, her self-esteem was low and she believed the teacher would criticize her verbally in front of the other students. When she got anxious the dancer became tense and found it very difficult to pick up on the corrections she needed to make. She dreaded the possibility of the teacher 'rolling her eyes to heaven' if she made a mistake in a dance sequence. Her thoughts associated with these feelings of dread were:

- 'I am scared; I cannot do it'
- 'The teacher will humiliate me in front of the class'
- 'I can't remember the corrections'
- 'I will never get into the/a ballet company.'

Along with the feelings of dread and anxiety were a strong sense of frustration as well as one of shame and embarrassment. The student wanted to leave and to give up dancing. She was convinced her dancing was substandard and that she had no talent.

After formulating the problem with the psychologist and looking back for evidence of how far she had already come in her training, the dancer came slowly to realize that she was in fact doing well. She had a strong tendency towards being a perfectionist and obsessing about always having to get it right. She admitted she was disciplined, always worked hard and tried to be professional. She had been accepted into the ballet school through very stringent criteria and tough competition. Her grades were above average and her stage presence exceptional. She had what is often called 'star quality'. Most importantly, she was passionate about ballet and she loved to dance. The alternative thoughts agreed became:

- 'I am still a student, and I am here to learn and develop'
- 'It's OK not to be perfect all the time'
- 'The teacher is trying to correct me to help me improve, it does not mean she is criticizing me as a person'
- 'I always do my best, and I am striving for excellence'

With the change in thinking style came increased confidence. She began to believe she could make it into the company. She had lots of evidence to draw on and to support her progress. She became much less fearful, and persuaded herself she would be fine placing herself up front in the class. Having stood up front once, it became easier to do so again.

Challenging the thinking processes became a routine practice for this young, talented dancer. She came to believe that challenging her thinking was important to becoming a mature dancer, and important for developing physically, technically and artistically to her full potential. The thoughts she reported became: 'I can do this! I am in the right place and I have earned my place by working hard to improve.'

The young ballet dancer moved from feelings of total hopelessness and of being a failure into recognizing that she was still training to become a dancer and that no one was expecting her to be perfect. Challenging her negative thinking patterns led her to become a better dancer and a fine artist. She was given a place in the ballet company and is developing into a mature dancer and an exciting performer.

Case 6: Athlete F

This athlete was seen by the psychologist while recovering from a stress fracture. He sought help because he felt frustrated and impatient. He was beginning to doubt if he did have a future in sport. This athlete felt anxious and depressed for 80–90% of the time. The depression was beginning to wear him down and it was hard to be able to map out a journey ahead. His thoughts read:

- 'I am not healing quickly enough'
- 'This does not feel natural, and I will never get back at this rate'
- 'I'm falling further and further behind'
- 'I won't make it – it's not gonna work!'
- 'I'll never get back!'

These thoughts were another example of *catastrophizing* and *fortune telling*. The evidence behind this type of thinking was that the athlete was indeed badly injured and there were some undisputed reasons why full recovery might take some time.

In working with the psychologist, the athlete looked at how other athletes who had suffered similar injuries had learnt to cope and had gone on to achieve great success. He recognized that he was in excellent hands. His physiotherapist and medical team were of the highest quality, and all had a great deal of experience working with fractures. Stress fractures are fairly common in athletes and statistically people recover well. The athlete began to realize that the word 'never' made him feel nervous but when challenged did not always represent the truth. 'Never say never' became a more hopeful phrase. Admitting he was in a difficult place for an athlete to find himself, he came up with the thoughts:

- 'This is really tough, BUT, I am young and strong and at the beginning of my career'
- 'It's OK and normal to feel frustrated, but I will heal and improve'
- 'I am in the best hands for getting back to full functioning'
- 'Looking back to when I first got injured, I have come a long way.'

The athlete began to feel more in control of the rehab and recovery process. He began to measure his progress in terms of small, SMART steps rather than huge global statements of gloom and disaster. The athlete did get back to training and performing, with the help of an excellent rehabilitation team.

The therapy process with the psychologist took much longer. The athlete's anxiety and depression were at a clinical level and, to prevent relapse, he needed to develop tools for recognizing negative automatic thought patterns. In cognitive therapy one of the goals is to develop relapse prevention. The athlete needed to learn how to apply this even when old thinking patterns come into play. Thoughts around the assumption 'I'll never make it' required him to collect fresh evidence for the thought as it came back, and challenge the original thought with the relevant evidence. Challenging thinking around the cycle of feeling inadequate, helpless and depressed helped the athlete to notice his signs of relapse and use his cognitive therapy tools to combat these feelings.

Conclusion

Emotions. . .

The chapter started by focusing on emotions as a key component in the causes of performance, both good and bad. In contrast to the insights offered by Hanin's ideographic approach, many performers fail to cash in on the benefits of, or are helpless victims of the problems caused by, emotion. This 'blindness' seems, at least in part, to be a feature of the traditions or mores of particular performance domains.

Dancers and aesthetic sports athletes (e.g. figure skating or rhythmic gymnastics) are well aware of the need to be 'set up' emotionally for a performance; these components of preparation lift the execution from being just a series of moves to a genuine performance. In short, there is a general recognition that failure to engage emotionally with the character portrayed will generate a rather wooden and substandard display (Fig. 21.6).

Surprisingly, perhaps, emotional setting is also part of the preparation routine for boxers and rugby players, the opposite end of almost any continuum you care to mention! By contrast, however, many sports fail to cater for emotional setting as a feature of warm-up, leaving pervading and usually negative anxieties and self-doubt to fill the void. The message of the first section to the chapter is clear. Take the trouble to evaluate and genuinely *know* what sets of emotions are best for you; don't just go with the flow that predominates in your domain. Not *all* rugby players perform best from a macho anger generated by running on the spot and counting to ten. Elite performers usually acknowledge this, and cater for it through using a combination of self-talk, music and images in the run-up to an event. For some, this emotional setting ('getting the competition head on') can take several days.

. . .and controlling them

The bulk of this chapter focused on ways to take control of emotion; as we have shown, it is a perfidious and powerful factor. In this regard, we believe that CBT has a crucial role to play in helping individuals change their mood and improve their performance. We believe that it is through the challenging of thought processes and the development of alternative ways of thinking that performers can become aware of their moods and the way in which their thinking can alter these emotions. To realize these benefits, each individual needs a thorough assessment of their difficulties and an individual formulation of their problem. Too frequently, sports psychologists work with athletes without undertaking this formulation (see Martindale & Collins 2005, 2007 and Conclusion) and are often very quick to apply techniques such as relaxation without looking to the source of the problem. This is just about acceptable in an intervention focused solely on performance enhancement, but to get stuck in without at least checking for limiting issues seems to us to be both careless and unprofessional, resources notwithstanding. In short, a bespoke and individualized intervention is *always* going to be better than the provision of group educational sessions, despite the fact that the latter approach is still all too common in performance environments.

Frequently, with a performer who is unused to the CBT model, the psychologist will have to spend time explaining the process of recognizing thoughts and feelings before they can be challenged and altered. For some individuals, their awareness is focused on performance and 'doing'. Thinking about thinking can be difficult for any individual – but to realize that thoughts are not facts and can have alternative meanings can be a powerful tool for the athlete to have in

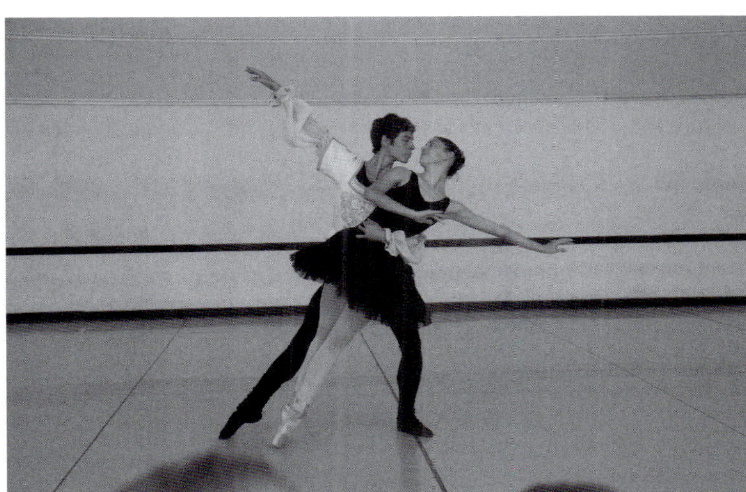

Fig. 21.6 • Dance is the ultimate, all-body expression of emotion. Photo © Sara Matthews.

their toolbox. If an individual can grasp the CBT model, there can be very powerful changes to mood and thinking, which in turn will go on to affect and improve performance.

Unfortunately, the training of many performance psychologists does not equip them to offer CBT either at a skills level or at the therapy level. Their work concentrates on performance enhancement or the teaching of a limited range of mental skills and strategies, not necessarily on an understanding of the individual's problem. The training of CBT has been developed so that it can now be applied to those with mild–moderate levels of problems such as anxiety and depression. This level of problem is frequently seen among individuals who are experiencing a transient issue (e.g. injured) or stuck in their views of their performance. The CBT skills model has been taught to workers who do not have a professional background in mental health work. Some problems may need to be referred on, and will in fact require more time to develop the strategies to work with the athlete's moods and thinking. In developing these CBT skills, it is important to have a qualified supervisor who can help the psychologist develop and understand the applications of the model, as well as providing a sounding board to test out ideas and theories. Some performers, like many members of the public, will struggle with the CBT model. Some people do not like the idea of a collaborative therapy, wanting only to state their problem and get direct advice. Some people struggle with accessing their thoughts, or challenging them and looking for alternatives. At times the depth of their feelings overwhelms many people, and it can be difficult to think about thoughts when physical sensations can be very strong.

The need for training in, and considered development of, CBT skills is paramount. Cognitive therapy can often be viewed by novice practitioners as a menu of techniques that can be applied – after *A*, do *B* then C and so on. This process offers nothing, however: many clients are told to relax or given a relaxation tape, 'therapy' appears to go nowhere and working with the psychologist is seen as a waste of time. The important parts of any consultation are building an effective relationship, history taking and the individual's view of the problem they are experiencing. Identifying thoughts and feelings is important but it is also necessary to identify past experiences (have they had this before, what worked and what didn't help) and what is currently going on in the performer's life. Having financial problems is going to affect behaviour no matter what therapy is applied!

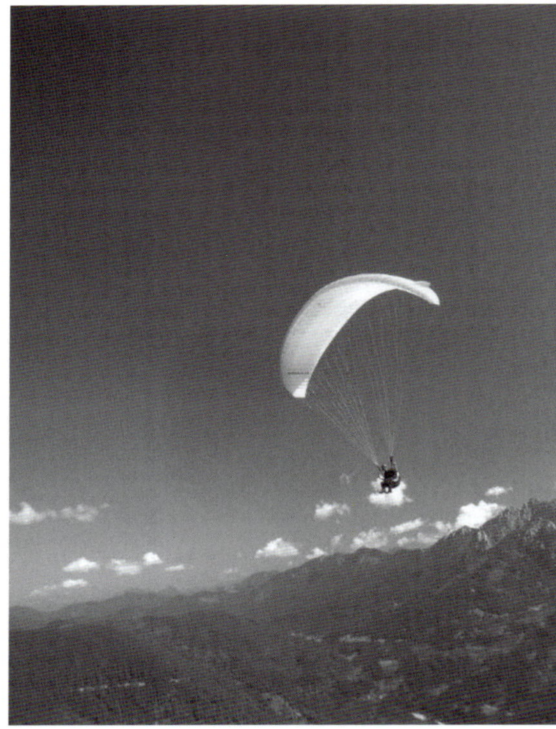

An emotional 'high'. Extreme sports offer much in the way of emotional enforcement. Thanks to Martin Colclough for the photo.

Although performance at an elite level takes over the greater part of an individual's life, they experience the same ups and downs as non-participants. They all have relationship issues at times, and money can be in short supply. Considering these factors is important. When performers are experiencing clinical problems of anxiety and depression they should be referred to a clinical psychologist or psychiatrist. CBT has an excellent evidence base for these clinical problems, and is almost as effective as antidepressants in some clinical trials. It is also, of course, a lot more useful in teaching people how to change their lives.

Enfin

We hope that this chapter has provided those working with performers who are experiencing problems with their emotions a new way of conceptualizing and approaching the problems. Rather than applying questionnaires offering a numerical score on whether someone has problems with moods/

emotions, we suggest CBT offers a way to assist performers in changing these moods through altering their thinking. Of course, there are other approaches that are commonly used, and these may offer good outcomes, based on the effectiveness of the therapeutic relationship developed between therapist and client. These advantages notwithstanding, however, the nature of physical performance challenges is ideally suited to CBT and we commend its use.

References

Apter, M.J., 1989. Reversal theory: motivation, emotion and personality. Routledge, London.

Beck, A.T., 1976. Cognitive therapy and the emotional disorders. International Universities Press, New York.

Beedie, C.J., Terry, P.C., Lane, A.M., 2000. The profile of mood states and athletic performance: two meta-analyses. J. Appl. Sport Psychol. 12, 49–68.

Burns, D.D., 2000. The feeling good handbook, second ed. Plume Books, New York.

Butler, R.J., 2000. Sports psychology in action. Arnold, London.

Csikszentmihalyi, M., 1990. Flow: the psychology of optimal experience. Harper & Row, New York.

Davis, J.E., Cox, R.H., 2002. Interpreting direction of anxiety within Hanin's Individual Zone of Optimal Functioning. J. Appl. Sport Psychol. 14, 43–52.

Greenberger, D., Padesky, C.A., 1995. Mind over mood. Guilford Press, New York.

Hanin, Y.L. (Ed.), 2000. Emotions in sport. Human Kinetics, Champaign, IL.

Hanin, Y.L., 2007. Emotions in sport: current issues and perspectives. In: Tenenbaum, G., Eklund, R. (Eds.), Handbook of sport psychology, third ed. Wiley, Hoboken, NJ, pp. 31–58.

Hanna, J.L., 1983. The performer-audience connection: emotion to metaphor in dance and society. University of Texas Press, Austin, TX.

Hollon, S., Beck, A.T., 2004. Cognitive and cognitive behavioural therapies. In: Lambert, M.J. (Ed.), Bergin & Garfield's handbook of psychotherapy and behaviour change, fifth ed. Wiley, New York.

Jokela, M., Hanin, Y.L., 1999. Does the individual zones of optimal functioning model discriminate between successful and less successful athletes? A meta-analysis. J. Sports Sci. 17, 873–887.

Jones, M.V., Mace, R.D., Williams, S., 2000. Relationship between emotional state & performance. J. Appl. Sports Psychol. 12, 16–33.

Jones, M.V., Uphill, M.A., 2004. Emotion in sport: antecedents and performance consequences. In: Lavallee, D., Thatcher, J., Jones, M.V. (Eds.), Coping and emotion in sport. Nova Science Publishers, Hauppauge, NY, pp. 9–28.

Lazarus, R.S., 1991. Emotion and adaptation. Oxford University Press, Oxford.

Lazarus, R.S., 2000. How emotions influence performance in competitive sports. Sport Psychologist 14, 229–254.

Martindale, A., Collins, D., 2005. Professional judgment and decision making: the role of intention for impact. Sport Psychologist 19, 303–317.

Martindale, A., Collins, D., 2007. Enhancing the evaluation of effectiveness with professional judgement and decision making. Sport Psychologist 21, 458–474.

McNair, D.M., Lorr, M., Droppelman, L.F., 1971. Profile of mood states manual. Educational and Industrial Testing Services, San Diego, CA.

Miles, M.B., Huberman, A.M., 1994. Qualitative data analysis: an expanded sourcebook, second ed. Sage Publishers, Thousand Oaks, CA, pp. 172–205.

Morgan, W.P., 1979. Prediction of performance. In: Klavora, P., Daniel, J.D. (Eds.), Coach, athlete and the sport psychologist. Human Kinetics, Champaign, IL.

Morgan, W.P., Brown, D.R., Raglin, J.S., et al., 1987. Psychological monitoring of over training and staleness. Br. J. Sports Med. 21, 107–114.

Nieuwenhuys, A. Hanin, Y., Bakker, F.C., 2008. Performance-related experiences and coping during races: a case of an elite sailor. Psychol. Sport and Exerc. 9, 61–76.

Salkovskis, P.M., 1991. The importance of behaviour in the maintenance of anxiety and panic a cognitive account. Behavioural Psychotherapy 19, 5–19.

Vallerand, R.J., 1983. On emotion in sport: theoretical and social psychological perspectives. J. Sports Psychol. 5, 197–215.

Vallerand, R.J., 1989. Antecedents of self related affects in sport: preliminary evidence on the intuitive reflective appraisal model. J. Sports Psychol. 9, 161–182.

Vallerand, R.J., Blanchard, C.M., 2000. The study of emotion in sport and exercise: historical definitional and conceptual perspectives. In: Hanin, Y.L. (Ed.), Emotions in sport. Human Kinetics, Champaign, IL.

Weiner, B., 1986. An attributional theory of motivation and emotion. Springer Verlag, New York.

Williams, C.J., 2001. Overcoming depression: a five areas approach. Arnold, London.

Attention

22

Aidan Moran

University College, Dublin, Ireland

CHAPTER CONTENTS

You are creating something within the stage, and the concentration has to be total, on what you're doing, all the way through. You can't let up for a minute.

The late Moira Shearer, ballerina and actress, cited in Roland 1997, p. 32

On the days we're doing gigs, I'd visualize the venue all through the day; see myself sitting on the stage. That's the whole focus of the day, the gig. . .. It's important to focus, to have a sense of occasion about performing.

Martin Hayes, Irish traditional musician, cited in Boland 1999, p. 6

Everything is about concentration and that's what I've learnt this season. We have a great team and we're always on the attack so our opponents get maybe one or two chances in the game. Sometimes it can be one chance in 90 minutes and it's difficult to be concentrated for the right moment.

Petr Cech, goalkeeper of Chelsea who set a record for goalkeepers by keeping 24 'clean sheets' in the Premiership, cited in Szczepanik 2005, p. 100

Introduction

As the above quotations illustrate, the ability to focus effectively is a crucial prerequisite of highly skilled performance in any field such as dance, music or sport. But what happens in our minds when we pay attention to something and how can we improve our focusing

DOI: 10.1016/B978-0-443-06734-1.00022-5

skills? Since the cognitive revolution of the 1950s, the mind has been regarded as a limited-capacity information processing system. Given this cognitive limitation, how can we prevent ourselves from being overwhelmed by the enormous amount of stimulation that is available to us at any given moment from our senses, our memories and our imagination? 'Attention' is the cognitive system that facilitates the selection of some information for further processing while inhibiting other information from receiving further processing (Smith & Kosslyn 2007). One aspect of this system is 'concentration' or the ability to focus effectively on the task at hand while ignoring distractions. But what exactly should people focus on in order to produce their best performances?

A possible answer to this question comes from a recent review of research on attentional processes in motor learning (Wulf 2007). This review shows that the accuracy and quality of skilled actions depends significantly on what the performer focuses on while executing the skill. More precisely, evidence is accumulating to show that an *external* focus of attention (i.e. one in which the performers concentrate on the effects of their movements on the environment) is usually superior to an *internal* focus of attention (where performers focus on their own body or on the mechanics of the skill in question) in both skill-learning and skilled performance. According to Wulf (2007), this principle is remarkably consistent across a variety of skills (e.g. balance tasks, jumping, golf, American football), levels of experience (i.e. whether the performers are experts or novices) and participant populations (including those with motor impairments). Outside the scientific literature, at an anecdotal level, this conclusion seems to make intuitive sense. To illustrate, consider the different types of attentional focus revealed by two experts as they prepared for important performances in their field – the former ballerina Deborah Bull and the golfer Paul McGinley. According to Bull, 'nerves from breakfast onwards' (quoted in Brooks 2001, p. 7) was the main reason for her retirement as a professional dancer in 2001. Apparently, a fear of making mistakes increasingly dominated her thinking before a performance – an example of an internal focus of attention. By contrast, when McGinley faced a putt to win the 2002 Ryder Cup match for Europe against the USA in the Belfry, he deliberately adopted an external focus of attention:

> At no time did I even consider the mechanics of the stroke. Of course, I knew what the putt meant and what it was for, but I became absorbed in the line of the putt. I could see it exactly from beginning to end. My only job at that moment in time was to set the ball off on the line that I had chosen. That was the only thing I could control.
>
> quoted in Clarke & Morris 2005, p. 63.

McGinley's quotation is broadly in line with Wulf's (2007) research findings and reveals two practical concentration tips for elite performers in any field. First, a performer needs to focus on a clear external target (in McGinley's case, the line of the putt). In addition, optimal concentration requires focusing only on actions that are under one's own control. Of course, it is not always easy to concentrate on the right target in any performance situation because, although motor skills can become automatic through practice, a performer's train of thoughts (and hence, attentional focus) can be derailed rather easily. For example, the pianist Louis Lortie explained how occasional attentional lapses impaired his performance on stage: 'It could happen in the middle of a phrase. You have a silly thought, or you feel the instrument is not responding exactly as you'd like. Memory slips may result' (quoted in Blau 1998, p. 17).

Against this background of insights into attentional processes from researchers and skilled performers, a number of important questions arise. Firstly, what exactly is 'concentration' and how is it related to the broader construct of attention? Secondly, what can we learn from cognitive metaphors and theoretical models of attentional processes? Third, why do skilled performers 'lose' their concentration in certain situations? Fourth, what are the practical building blocks of effective concentration for any performer? Fifth, how does anxiety affect concentration and skilled performance? Finally, what practical psychological techniques can help performers to achieve and maintain an optimal focus? The purpose of this chapter is to answer these questions using the principles and findings of cognitive psychology – a discipline that studies mental activity in an effort to understand how the mind works (Smith & Kosslyn 2007).

Attention and concentration: nature and characteristics

Research on attention is one of the fastest-growing fields in cognitive psychology and cognitive neuroscience. It explores the mechanisms by which 'voluntary control and subjective experience arise from and regulate our behaviour' (Posner & Rothbart 2007, p. 1).

But what exactly is 'attention'? For psychologists, this term is paradoxical because it is familiar yet mysterious. It is familiar because it is used frequently in everyday discourse – as happens, for example, when a dance teacher asks her students to 'pay attention' to something important that she is about to say or demonstrate in her class. Indeed, based on such apparent familiarity, William James (1890, pp. 403–404) remarked famously that 'Everyone knows what attention is. It is the taking possession by the mind, in clear and vivid form, of one of what may seem several simultaneously possible objects or trains of thought. Focalization, concentration, of consciousness are of its essence. It implies withdrawal from some things in order to deal effectively with others.'

Attention is also mysterious because it refers to many different types and levels of psychological process ranging from biological arousal or alertness to high-level conscious awareness. Not surprisingly, therefore, James's 'folk-psychology' approach to attention (i.e. one based on unsystematic but compelling insights drawn from everyday life; Pashler 1999) has been criticized for its limited scope. And so, despite more than a century of research in the field, there is still a great deal of confusion concerning the nature of attention and the mechanisms underlying it. For example, Ashcraft (2006) identified six different meanings of this term. Commenting on the multiplicity of approaches and definitions in this field, Pashler (1999, p. 1) subverted James's quotation by observing that perhaps 'no one knows what attention is, and … there may not even be an "it" to be known about'. Of course, brain scanning techniques can establish whether or not there is an 'it' in attention. So, undaunted by Pashler's somewhat pessimistic conclusion, we can see that a great deal of progress has been made in attentional research in recent years. For example, most theorists in the field accept that the hallmark of attention is the concentration of mental activity (Matlin 2005). In addition, neuroscientific studies have identified a number of different brain regions activated during attentional processing. For example, Corbetta & Shulman (2002) concluded that the task of searching for your friend in a crowded room involves activation of frontal and dorsal parietal brain regions. By contrast, redirecting your attention to an unexpected stimulus (e.g. the sound of breaking glass) involves the activation of the ventral frontal cortex (see also Smith & Kosslyn 2007). Thirdly, researchers agree on the multidimensional nature of this construct and can distinguish between at least three different types or dimensions of attention (Moran 2004).

The first dimension is called 'concentration' and refers to a person's deliberate decision to invest mental effort on what is most important in any given situation. For example, before the opening night of a play, actors will listen intently to the director for advice or instructions about what is required from the cast. By contrast, an actor's mind may wander during unstructured rehearsals. The second dimension of attention is 'selective attention' – the perceptual ability to 'zoom in' on task-relevant information while ignoring potential distractions. This dimension refers to the ability to discriminate relevant stimuli (targets) from irrelevant stimuli (distractors) that compete for our attention. To test your skill in this area, can you focus only on the vocals of a song on the radio, disregarding the instrumental backing? Interestingly, research suggests that one way of capturing people's attention is through the use of sudden-onset stimuli and movement (Strayer & Drews 2007). For example, the blinking cursor on a computer monitor makes it stand out from the static display of text that the user is typing on the screen. Internet 'pop-up' advertising exploits this perceptual principle by trying to 'steal' computer users' attention. The third dimension involves 'divided attention' and refers to a form of mental time-sharing ability whereby performers learn, as a result of extensive practice, to perform two or more concurrent actions equally well. For example, whereas inexperienced motorists cannot drive and talk at the same time, experienced drivers have no such difficulty in doing so. But even experienced motorists have trouble in dividing their attention successfully between driving and using their mobile phone. To illustrate, Strayer et al (2003) discovered that drivers who had held conversations using their mobile phone either missed or had poor recall of billboard signs along their routes. In summary, the construct of attention refers to at least three different cognitive processes – concentration or effortful awareness, selectivity of perception and/or the ability to coordinate two or more actions at the same time.

Explaining attention: metaphors and theories

In their attempt to understand how the mind works, psychology researchers use metaphors to explain the unknown in terms of the known. Fernandez-Duque & Johnson (1999) have reviewed a variety of metaphors of attention postulated by cognitive psychologists since the 1950s. These metaphors are important because they influence the way in which attention has been conceptualized and studied by psychologists. The earliest metaphors of attention ('filter' approaches) were largely auditory in nature but as a greater range of experimental procedures emerged, attention metaphors became mainly visual. More recently, resource metaphors have dominated cognitive research on attention. Let us explore this evolution of metaphors in more detail now.

The filter metaphor

The first modern theory of attention, proposed by Broadbent (1958), was based on a series of laboratory experiments on selective listening tasks. A key assumption of this theory was the idea that people are limited in their ability to process information and that there must be a mechanism that facilitates the selection of some information while inhibiting the selection of competing information. To explain this mechanism Broadbent drew an analogy between attention and a filtering device or bottleneck that screens and restricts the flow of information into the mind in accordance with a set of early perceptual or later semantic criteria. Put simply, just as the neck of a bottle restricts the flow of liquid, a hypothetical filter limits the quantity of information to which we can pay attention at any given time. Broadbent's model suggested that, although multiple channels of information reach the filter, only one channel is permitted to pass through to the perceptual analysis stage of information processing. Selection by this filtering mechanism was believed to occur on the basis of physical characteristics such as the pitch or loudness of the message being processed.

Although Broadbent's model was initially influential, it soon encountered many conceptual and methodological criticisms. For example, subsequent researchers failed to agree on either the location or timing of the filter. Another challenge to Broadbent's filter theory came from an everyday experience of attentional processing called the 'cocktail party phenomenon' – an auditory perceptual effect associated with research by Cherry (1953). Imagine that you are at a noisy party and trying to pay attention to a conversation. Suddenly, you hear your name being mentioned in another conversation somewhere else in the room. How can Broadbent's theory explain the fact that you recognized your name? Clearly, if you heard your name being mentioned, then it could not have been blocked by the filter. Put differently, if your brain had previously selected the first conversation on the basis of the physical features of the speaker's voice, how did it manage to process another set of sounds to which you had not been trying to pay attention? Interestingly, filter theory was incapable of accounting for the flexibility and sophistication of human attention and so attention researchers abandoned signal-blocking filters in favour of other metaphors. Another factor that hastened the demise of filter theory was the switch from an auditory to a visual methodological paradigm in attention research. This switch occurred mainly because experimenters found it easier to measure the presentation times of visual stimuli than their auditory equivalents. Taken together, these developments paved the way for visual metaphors of attention such as the 'spotlight' and 'zoom lens' approaches.

The spotlight metaphor

According to the spotlight metaphor (e.g. Posner 1980), selective attention resembles a mental beam that illuminates a circumscribed part of the visual field and information lying outside the illuminated region is ignored. Spotlight theorists also suggested that the attentional beam can be redirected voluntarily to other locations in space. Another popular visual metaphor of attention is the 'zoom lens' (Eriksen & St. James 1986). This metaphor proposed that attentional focus could be increased or decreased at will, as if it was like adjusting the zoom lens of a camera. For psychologists, coaches and performers, these visual metaphors have several advantages. For example, they show us that our mental beam of concentration is never truly 'lost' but can be directed at the 'wrong' target – something that is irrelevant to the task at hand, outside one's control or located too far in the future. We shall return to this idea later in the chapter when we summarize some key principles of an effective focus for optimal performance. Incidentally, this idea of specifying a target for one's attentional spotlight is important because there are relatively few studies on the question of what exactly performers should focus on when they are exhorted to 'concentrate' by their instructors (e.g. Castaneda & Gray 2007).

A second benefit of visual metaphors of attention is that they remind us that performers have control over where they 'shine' their concentration beam at all times. For example, at any given moment, when you shine your mental spotlight at a target in the world around you (e.g. as you look at your teammates before the start of a match), you have picked an *external* focus of attention. However, when you concentrate on your own feelings or bodily processes (e.g. in listening to your heart pounding with excitement before kick off), you have switched to an *internal* focus of attention. In collective activities, an external focus of attention is required when you try to synchronize your movements with those of others (e.g. when rehearsing a dance formation). By contrast, an internal focus of attention is needed whenever you rehearse a skill in your mind's eye before performing it.

Indeed, the assumption that one can control one's visual attention forms the basis of Nideffer's (1976) theory that expert performers in any field are adept at knowing which of four different types of attentional focus is required for a given task – 'broad external', 'narrow external', 'broad internal' and 'narrow internal'. These different types of focus can be illustrated using the following examples. A 'broad external' focus is required whenever a skilled performer has to assess a situation quickly to ascertain what options are available. For example, an ambulance driver called out to a motor accident needs to be able to scan the emergency scene rapidly before deciding whether or not to seek to additional medical help. A 'narrow external' focus involves a performer to 'lock on' to a specific physical target in the immediate environment. For example, a novice actor struggling to overcome self-consciousness on stage may be advised to look over the audience's heads at a specific spot on the wall at the back of the theatre. A 'broad internal' focus occurs whenever a performer (e.g. a dancer) goes through a sequence of movements in his or her imagination before actually executing them. For example, a ballerina may rehearse her dance movements in her 'mind's eye' while sitting on a sofa before actually performing them on stage later that evening. Finally, a 'narrow internal' focus involves concentrating on a single thought or image – as shown by our earlier example (see the beginning of this chapter) of the musician Martin Hayes' habit of visualizing his stage performance in advance of the event itself.

Of course, skilled performers in any field usually manage to switch between these different attentional foci as the situation requires. For example, a learner driver who is doing a driving test must be able to alternate effectively between going through the route in his or her mind (broad internal focus), scanning the environment for potential traffic hazards (broad external focus), looking in the rear-view mirror (narrow external focus) and trying to stay calm (narrow internal focus). Interestingly, the question of whether or not one's focus is *appropriate* for the skill that one is performing is a very important issue. Thus, as we learned from Wulf's (2007) literature review and Paul McGinley's quotation earlier, thinking too technically about your skills while competing in sport is rarely helpful. Likewise, shining your spotlight on yourself is not a good idea as it makes you self-conscious and worried about making mistakes.

Although the spotlight metaphor of attention has been helpful in applied settings, it is plagued by at least five conceptual and empirical problems. First, spotlight theorists have not adequately explained the mechanisms by which executive control of attentional focus is achieved. Put simply what processes govern *direction* of the spotlight? This question is difficult to answer without postulating some kind of homunculus – which invalidates the theory scientifically. A second problem is that the spotlight model assumes that our attentional beam sweeps through space en route to its target However, if that were true, then one might expect that, if an obstacle were encountered during the sweep, attention would be hampered or delayed. But research shows that 'attention is not influenced by the presence of spatially intervening information' (Smith & Kosslyn 2007, p. 131). The third problem is that the spotlight metaphor neglects the issue of what lies outside the beam of our concentration. In other words, it ignores the possibility that unconscious factors such as 'ironic' or counter-intentional processes (Wegner 1994; see below for further discussion) can affect people's attentional processes. Interestingly, such factors have attracted increasing scrutiny from cognitive scientists in recent years (e.g. Bargh & Morsella 2008, Velmans & Schneider 2007). Indeed, Nadel & Piattelli-Palmarini (2002, p. xxvi) remarked that, although cognitive science began with the assumption that cognition was limited to conscious processes, 'much of the domain is now concerned with phenomena that lie behind the veil of consciousness'.

The fourth problem of the spotlight model of attention is that it has been concerned mainly with external targets, not internal ones. The fifth weakness of the spotlight metaphor is that it neglects emotional influences on attentional processes. We shall return to this issue later when we summarize some key principles of effective concentration. For example, it seems that anxiety can narrow one's mental spotlight and encourage performers to shine it inwards. The effects of anxiety on cognition and performance, which we will address specifically later in the chapter, are accounted for in the recent 'attentional control theory' developed by Eysenck et al (2007).

The capacity metaphor

So far, we have examined two influential metaphors of attention – the filter (or bottleneck) approach, which emphasizes the auditory modality, and the spotlight approach, which is grounded in visual perception. Let us now consider a third metaphor of attention – one that is not linked to any specific sensory modality.

The 'resource' or 'capacity' metaphor of attention (Kahneman 1973) was developed in an effort to explain the mechanisms underlying divided attention or people's ability to perform two or more tasks at the same time. It suggested that attention resembles a pool of undifferentiated mental energy that can be allocated to concurrent tasks depending on various strategic principles – such as the influence of the performer's arousal level. Specifically, people have a greater amount of attentional capacity available when they are fully alert than when they are sleepy. Another strategic principle arises from the effects of task practice. For example, tasks that are highly practised require less mental effort than novel ones and hence 'free up' attentional resources (or spare mental capacity) to be devoted to other things. According to Kahneman (1973), the way in which a performer allocates their attentional capacity is determined by a combination of factors such as 'momentary intentions' (i.e. factors that are deemed important at the time, like the decision to pay attention to whoever is speaking to you at a party) and 'enduring dispositions' (i.e. factors that are always important to you, like the sound of your own name). Most resource theorists (e.g. Baddeley 1986) believe that divided attentional performance is regulated by a limited central capacity system such as the 'central executive' of the working memory model (Baddeley 2003). The extent to which two tasks can be performed concurrently depends on their combined demands on available attentional resources.

What are the strengths and weaknesses of capacity or resource models of attention for performance psychologists? Perhaps the biggest strength is the proposal that, although dual-task performance is constrained by available mental resources, extensive practice can reduce the attentional demands of any task. Unfortunately, the resource metaphor of divided attention is somewhat simplistic. For example, Navon & Gopher (1979) have argued that people may have multiple attentional resources rather than a single pool of undifferentiated mental energy. Each of these multiple pools may have its own functions and limits. For example, Schmidt & Lee (1999) discovered that the attentional resources required for a motor skill such as selecting a finger movement may be separate from those that regulate a verbal skill such as the pronunciation of a word. This idea casts doubt on the possibility of a single definition of attention. Thus Luck & Vecera (2002) suggested that 'the term attention applies to many separable processes, each of which operates within a different cognitive subsystem' (p. 261). Although intuitively appealing, however, multiple resource theories of attention have been criticized for being 'inherently untestable' (Palmeri 2002, p. 298). This is so because of the difficulty of specifying when a task has been 'automatized'. At present, the only estimate of a task's level of automaticity comes after the extent of its interference effects have been observed. For example, dual-task performance without interference is 'explained' by the fact that at least one of the tasks involved is automatic. But this inability to specify in advance the degree of automaticity of a task raises questions about the validity of capacity theories of attention.

In summary, we have explored three different metaphors of attention – the filter, spotlight and resource approaches. Whereas filter theories of attention were concerned mainly with identifying how and where selective attention occurred in the auditory information processing system, resource theories explored divided attention through dual-task interference methodology. Perhaps most persuasively, however, the spotlight metaphor has highlighted the way in which people control and focus their visual attention in everyday cognitive situations.

Evaluating cognitive theories of attention

In general, recent cognitive models of attention, whether based on spotlight or resource metaphors, have two major limitations. First, they have dealt mainly with external (or environmental) determinants of attention and have largely overlooked internal factors (e.g. thoughts and feelings). Interestingly, Posner & Rothbart (2007, p. 9) acknowledged this gap in the research literature on attention when they concluded that people 'differ in their ability to concentrate for long periods on internal trains of thought'. Of course, performers' insights into their own mental processes are not always reliable or valid from a researcher's perspective. The second weakness of cognitive models of attention is that they ignore the influence of emotional states. This neglect of the affective dimension of behaviour is lamentable because it is widely known in performance psychology that anxiety is associated with attentional narrowing. Thus Easterbrook (1959) proposed that the breadth of our attentional spotlight decreases as our level of anxiety increases. Not surprisingly, anxiety also impairs skilled performance. This was demonstrated in a study by Baddeley & Idzikowski (1985), who found that the manual dexterity skills of divers were hampered significantly by anticipatory anxiety at the prospect of an open-sea dive. For a more detailed account of the role of emotional factors in skilled performance, see Hanin 2000 and Eysenck et al 2007.

Having considered some gaps in cognitive models of attention, let us now turn to the more practical question of why skilled performers suffer lapses in attention.

Why do skilled performers 'lose' their concentration?

Have you ever discovered that you have been reading the same sentence in a book over and over again without any comprehension because your mind was 'miles away'? If so, then you have first-hand experience of losing your concentration. But is concentration ever really lost? Instead, what probably happened was that you *distracted yourself* by allowing a thought, daydream or feeling to become the focus of your attention. These could be classified as internal distractions and psychologists generally differentiate these from more objective external distractions that divert attention away from a task relevant focus (Moran 1996, 2004). As we learned in our discussion of the spotlight metaphor, performers do not really 'lose' their concentration at all. Instead, their attentional beam focuses on factors that are irrelevant to the job at hand, out of their control or too far in the future.

Typically, external distractions tend to be auditory or visual and examples might include crowd movements, flash photography and audience noise. Furthermore, in some performance contexts opponents may deliberately obscure, disguise or overload visual information. Internal distractions could include a vast array of thoughts, such as wondering what might happen in the future, regretting what has happened in the past or worrying about what other people might think, say or do. Internal distractions may also be feelings (upset, angry) and/or bodily sensations (pain and fatigue) that impede efforts to concentrate on the job at hand.

A classic example of a costly internal distraction occurred in the case of the golfer Doug Sanders, who missed a putt of less than 3 feet (1 m) that prevented him winning the 1970 Open golf championship in St. Andrews, Scotland, his first major tournament, and also deprived him of millions of pounds in prize-money, tournament invitations and advertising endorsements. Remarkably, Sanders's attentional lapse was precipitated mainly by thinking too far ahead and years later, he revealed what had happened: 'I had the victory speech prepared before the battle was over .... I would give up every victory I had to have won that title. It's amazing how many different things to my normal routine I did on the 18th' (quoted in Moran 2005, p. 21).

Unfortunately, despite the vivid testimonies of skilled performers like Sanders who have suffered dramatic attentional lapses, little research has been conducted to date on the phenomenology of internal distractibility – although a recent paper by Gouju et al (2007) explored athletes' attentional experiences in a hurdle race. Specifically, these researchers investigated hurdlers' awareness of, and thoughts about, factors such as the presence of opponents (e.g. 'I can feel him/her come closer', p. 181–182). Such thoughts can distract performers. The neglect of self-generated distractibility in psychology research is attributable to two main problems – one theoretical and the other methodological. The theoretical problem dated back to the multistore model of memory (Atkinson & Shiffrin 1968), based on which cognitive researchers assumed falsely that information flows into the mind in only one direction – from the outside world inwards. However this assumption ignored the possibility that information (and hence potentially distracting thoughts and feelings) could travel in the opposite direction – from long-term memory into the short-term/working memory system or current awareness.

A second reason for the neglect of internal distractions in psychology stems from a methodological bias. Specifically, researchers focused on external distractions simply because they were easier to measure than self-generated distractions. As a result of this bias, the theoretical mechanisms by which internal distractions disrupt concentration were largely unknown until recently. Fortunately, Wegner (1994) developed a model that rectifies this oversight by attempting to explain why attentional lapses occur ironically – or precisely at the most inopportune moment for the person involved.

Wegner's (1994) theory proposed that the mind wanders *because* we try to control it. In other words, when we are anxious or tired, trying not to think about something may paradoxically increase its prominence in our consciousness. For example, if you try to make yourself fall asleep on the night before you are scheduled to take an early-morning flight, you will probably achieve only a prolonged state of wakefulness! Similarly, if you attempt to block a certain thought from entering your mind, you may end up becoming more preoccupied with it. This tendency for a suppressed thought to come to mind more readily than a thought that is the focus of intentional concentration is called 'hyperaccessibility' and is especially likely to occur under conditions of mental load. Clearly, there are many situations in skilled performance in which such ironic self-regulation failures occur and Wegner proposes theoretical mechanisms to account for this phenomenon.

According to Wegner (1994), when people try to suppress a thought, they engage in a controlled (conscious) search for thoughts that are different from the unwanted thought. At the same time, however, our minds conduct an automatic (unconscious) search for any signs of the unwanted thought. In other words, the intention to suppress a thought activates an automatic search for that very thought in an effort to monitor whether or not the act of suppression has been successful. Normally, the conscious intentional system dominates the unconscious monitoring system. Under certain circumstances (e.g. when our working memories are overloaded or when our attentional resources are depleted by fatigue or stress), however, the unconscious monitoring system prevails and an ironic intrusion of the unwanted thought occurs. Wegner attributes this rebound effect to the excessive cognitive load. While this load is believed to disrupt the conscious mechanism of thought control, it does not interfere with the automatic (and ironic) monitoring system. Thus Wegner (1994, p. 7) proposed that 'the intention to concentrate creates conditions under which mental load enhances monitoring of irrelevancies'. To summarize, Wegner's (1994) research helps us to understand why performers may find it difficult to suppress unwanted or irrelevant thoughts when they are tired or anxious. Perhaps not surprisingly, Wegner (2002) has investigated ironies of action as well as those of thought. For example, consider what happens when people who are asked not to overshoot the hole in a golf putt are given tasks that impose a heavy mental load on them. In such situations, the unwanted action (overshooting the hole) is exactly what happens.

Principles of effective concentration

Having explored what concentration is and why we experience attentional lapses, let us now consider some principles governing effective concentration or a focused state of mind.

At least five theoretical principles of effective concentration in skilled performance may be identified from reviews of relevant research (e.g. Abernethy 2001, Abernethy et al 2007, Moran 1996; Fig. 22.1). Three of them concern the establishment of an optimal focus whereas the other two describe how it may be disrupted.

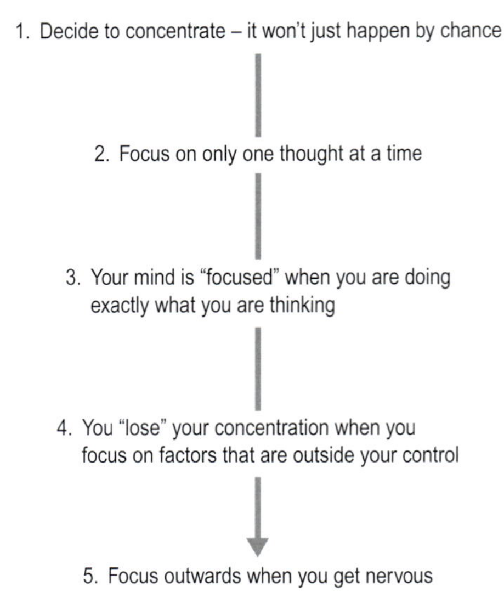

Fig. 22.1 • Concentration principles. Based on Moran 1996. The psychology of concentration in sport performers: a cognitive analysis, page 114. Psychology Press, Hove, East Sussex.

Decide to concentrate – it won't just happen by chance

The first building block of effective concentration results from a deliberate decision to invest mental effort in performance. It is essential that a performer prepares to concentrate rather than simply hope that it will happen by chance. Interestingly, this link between deciding to concentrate and subsequently performing to your full potential is well known in sport. For example, Ronan O'Gara, the Irish and British Lions rugby out-half, admitted that:

> I have to be focused. I have to do my mental preparation. I have to feel that I'm ready. I don't want to be putting myself out there for credit but I have a big impact on how Munster perform. When it's coming up to a big match, rugby is the only thing in my head. Driving around, I visualize certain scenarios, different positions on the pitch, different times when the ball is coming to me.
>
> Quoted in English 2006, p. 70

In sport, many athletes establish imaginary 'switch on' and 'switch off' zones for their performance. For example, entering the locker room before a game reminds them to turn on their concentration switch. Likewise, some athletes associate 'switching off' their concentration with stepping into the shower afterwards. This idea of learning to turn one's concentration on and off as required was proposed by Garry Sobers, the famous cricketer, when he said: 'Concentration's like a shower. You don't turn it on until you want to bathe .... You don't walk out of the shower and leave it running. You turn it off, you turn it on .... It has to be fresh and ready when you need it' (quoted in White 2002, p. 20).

Focus on only one thought at a time

A second building block of effective concentration is the 'one thought' principle – the idea that you can focus consciously on only one thing at a time. This idea is supported by research on the 'bandwidth' of attention or the number of items in working memory on which one can focus effectively. Specifically, Garavan (1998) and McElree (1998) tested people's ability to perform counting and retrieval tasks in working memory and concluded that the focus of attention is limited largely to just one item. Of course, as we mentioned earlier in our discussion of divided attention, people can perform several actions simultaneously – as long as one or more of these skills has been practised to the point where it no longer requires conscious control (hence achieving a state of automaticity).

Given the fragility and brevity of our attentional focus, it seems plausible that the ideal thought for a performer should be a single word triggering the appropriate feeling or tempo of the action to be executed (e.g. 'smooth' or 'flow') rather than a complex technical instruction (e.g. 'bend your knees and go from low to high'). Evidence to support this idea comes from research by Hardy et al (2005), which showed that athletes' 'self-talk' (what they say to themselves before or during their performance) tends to be abbreviated (e.g. 'head' instead of 'keep your head steady'). Interestingly, such cognitive single-mindedness is sometimes prompted by the challenge of facing an opponent in competition. Thus Retief Goosen, who won the 2004 US Open golf championship in New York, revealed that he plays his best when pressure situations force him to concentrate on what he has to do: 'I've reached a point where I feel like I can only play my best golf when I'm really under the cosh. When you're under pressure, it's a sort of "must"' thing. You must focus and you must make the putt. That's what I feel' (quoted in Mair 2004, p. S10).

Do exactly what you're thinking

A third principle of good concentration is the idea that your mind is truly focused when there is no difference between what you are thinking about and what you are doing. For example, after Roger Bannister had run the first sub-4-minute mile in May 1954 in Oxford, he said: 'There was no pain, only a great unity of movement and aim' (Bannister 2004, p. 12). To ensure a match between thought and action the content of thoughts should be restricted to those that are highly relevant and positively phrased.

Focus only on factors within your control

Fourth, as we indicated earlier, performers' concentration will wander when their focus 'shines' on factors outside their control, irrelevant to the job at hand or located too far in the future. A dramatic example of this problem in horse racing occurred in 2005 when a young Irish jockey, Roger Loughran, finished third in a race that he should have won.

Leading with a short distance to go and perhaps focusing on the thought of winning rather than riding, he misperceived a stick on the finishing straight as the winning post and began to celebrate his success prematurely. Punching the air in elation, he suddenly noticed two other riders passing him to claim first and second place (Muscat 2005)!

Focus outwards when you get nervous

The final building block of effective concentration is the idea that a performer experiencing anxiety should focus outwards on actions – not inwards on doubts. This outward focus is necessary because anxiety tends to make people self-critical and 'hypervigilant' (i.e. primed to detect any sign of what they may fear). As we explained at the beginning of this chapter, such advice is consistent with Wulf's (2007) review of research on the optimal attentional focus for skilled performance. Some performers have become so good at focusing outwards that they become totally immersed in the present moment – a form of 'mindfulness' (or present-centred attention) that is beginning to receive research attention in neuroscience (e.g. Jha et al 2007). For example, a story (perhaps apocryphal) tells of the time that Jack Nicklaus, the famous golf champion, was one hole down with one to play in a match. Having hit a bad drive, he produced an amazing recovery shot to win the hole and draw the match. When asked afterwards how he had managed to concentrate under such pressure, he allegedly uttered the immortal words: 'The ball doesn't know the score!' (quoted in Moran 1998).

Anxiety, concentration and skilled performance

As we indicated earlier, cognitive researchers have traditionally ignored the influence of emotional factors on task performance – due mainly to the primacy of rational computational models that did not take account of the affective side of mental life. As Smith & Kosslyn (2007, p. 326) observed, 'emotion was not considered an appropriate domain of inquiry within the study of cognition until very recently'. Fortunately, this oversight has been corrected and over the past two decades, the phenomenon of 'choking under pressure' has attracted considerable interest from cognitive as well as sport psychologists (e.g. Beilock & Carr 2001, Gucciardi & Dimmock 2008).

The term 'choking under pressure' refers to the failure of normally expert skills under pressure (Masters 1992). What makes this phenomenon intriguing for researchers and performers alike is that it seems to involve a motivational paradox. Specifically, the more effort the performer expends in trying to do well, the worse they get. In other words, choking is a form of 'paradoxical performance' (Gucciardi & Dimmock 2008) because it happens in situations where people try too hard to perform well.

In general, choking is regarded as an anxiety-based attentional problem rather than a personality trait. This insight is important because it suggests that *anyone* can choke under certain circumstances, not just performers who have a nervous disposition. In other words, all performers – regardless of their ability or experience –can choke if they focus on the 'wrong' target such as the importance of the occasion or the mechanics of the skill or movement being executed.

Two main attentional models have been postulated to account for the debilitative effects of anxiety on skilled performance. On the one hand, the 'self-consciousness' approach (Baumeister 1984) proposes that when people experience pressure to perform well, they tend to think more about themselves and the importance of the skill that they are performing than they would normally. This excessive self-consciousness causes people to try to exert conscious control over skills that had previously been automatic – hence leading to an unraveling process known commonly as 'paralysis by analysis'. An alternative approach is 'processing efficiency' theory (Eysenck & Calvo 1992, see Ch. 17 in this book) which distinguishes between processing 'effectiveness' (the quality of task performance) and processing 'efficiency' (the relationship between the effectiveness of performance and the effort or resources spent in task performance). Processing efficiency theory postulates that anxiety impairs the processing efficiency of the central executive component of working memory (Baddeley 2003). At the same time anxiety acts as a prompt to performers to try and maintain their level of performance by investing additional effort in it. Despite increased investment of effort, which may sustain performance levels initially, ultimately processing becomes so inefficient that decrements to performance occur. An interesting feature of processing efficiency theory is its assumption that the effects of anxiety on performance are mediated by the central executive component of working memory (Baddeley 2003). Although the theory did not specify which aspect of this memory system was involved, a recent theory called 'attentional control' theory – a revised version of the processing efficiency approach (Eysenck et al 2007) – is more specific. It suggests that anxiety impairs the inhibition function of the central executive, thereby hampering the performer's ability to resist distractions.

Concentration training exercises and techniques

Research psychologists have developed a variety of practical strategies that purport to improve concentration skills in performers (Greenlees & Moran, 2003). In keeping with the building blocks above (especially the third principle), the purpose of these strategies is to help performers to achieve a focused state of mind in which there is no difference between what they are thinking about and what they are doing. When this happens for an individual, the performer's mind is 'cleared of irrelevant thoughts, the body is cleared of irrelevant tensions and the focus is centred only on what is important at that moment for executing the skill to perfection' (Orlick 1990, p. 18). These practical strategies can be divided into concentration training exercises (those used during training and preparation) and concentration techniques (designed for use during the performance itself; Moran 1996, 2003).

Among the plethora of concentration exercises recommended by performance psychologists are activities such as the 'concentration grid' – a visual search task endorsed by Schmid & Peper (1998) in which the participant is required to scan as many digits as possible within a given time limit. Unfortunately, few of these activities are supported either by a coherent theoretical rationale or by adequate evidence of empirical validity. For example, no references were cited by Weinberg & Gould (1999) to support their claim that the concentration grid exercise was used 'extensively in Eastern Europe as a pre-competition screening device' (p. 347) or that it 'will help you learn to focus your attention and scan the environment for relevant cues' (*ibid.*). Despite the absence of such evidence, the grid is recommended unreservedly by Schmid & Peper (1998, p. 324) as a 'training exercise for practising focusing ability' and also by Weinberg & Gould (2007). Interestingly, Greenlees et al (2006) recently tested the validity of the grid as a concentration exercise over a 9-week period with a sample of collegiate soccer players. Results showed no significant effects of the grid on the athletes' concentration skills relative to a control group. Therefore, these authors concluded that the grid 'lacks the efficacy that has been ascribed to it in previous literature and anecdotal accounts' (Greenlees et al 2006, p. 36).

To summarize, there appears to be little empirical justification for the use of generic visual search and/or vigilance tasks in an effort to improve performers' concentration skills. By contrast with the concentration grid, 'simulation training' (Orlick 1990) appears to have a satisfactory theoretical rationale. This latter exercise, which is also known as 'dress rehearsal' (Schmid & Peper 1998), 'simulated practice' (Hodge & McKenzie 1999) and 'distraction training' (Maynard 1998), proposes that performers can learn to concentrate more effectively in real-life pressure situations by simulating them in practice conditions.

Interestingly, a number of anecdotal testimonials to the value of this practice have emerged in sport psychology in recent years. To illustrate, the late Earl Woods, father and initial coach of Tiger Woods, used such methods on him when he was a boy. Indeed, Woods senior claimed that 'all the strategies and tactics of distraction I'd learned I threw at that kid and he would just grit his teeth and play . . . and if anyone tries pulling a trick on him these days he just smiles and says "my dad used to do that years ago"' (quoted in Evening Herald 2001, p. 61). Similarly, Javier Aguirre, the coach of the 2002 Mexican national soccer team, instructed his players to practise penalty-taking after every friendly match in the year leading up to the 2002 World Cup in an effort to prepare for the possibility of penalty-shootouts in that competition. As he explained: 'there will always be noise and that is the best way to practise' (quoted in Smith 2002, p. S3).

Unfortunately, despite its intuitive appeal, simulation training has received little or no empirical scrutiny as a concentration strategy. Nevertheless, some support for its theoretical rationale may be found in cognitive psychology. For example, research on the 'encoding specificity' principle of learning shows that people's recall of information is facilitated by conditions that resemble those in which the original encoding occurred. Based on this principle, the simulation of competitive situations in practice should lead to positive transfer effects to the competition itself.

In addition, adversity training may counteract the tendency for novel or unexpected stimuli to distract performers in competition. The experience of these factors in simulation training should reduce their attention-capturing qualities subsequently. To summarize, there is some theoretical justification for the belief that simulation training could enhance performers' concentration skills. Nevertheless, this conclusion is tentative, for one important reason. Specifically, even the most ingenious simulations cannot replicate completely the *actual* arousal experienced by performers in competitive situations. For example, Ronan O'Gara, the Ireland and Lions rugby out-half, admitted that, although he can practise taking penalty kicks in training 'it's completely different in a match where my heartbeat is probably 115 beats a minute whereas in training it's about 90–100' (quoted in Fanning 2002, p. 6). Clearly, it is difficult to simulate accurately the emotional aspects of competitive action.

Concentration techniques

Having reviewed some popular concentration exercises, let us now turn to the second type of attentional skills intervention used in performance psychology – namely, concentration techniques.

Specifying performance goals

Psychologists commonly distinguish between outcome goals (e.g. successful audition or competition victory, which are usually linked with comparisons to others) and performance goals (achieving specific levels of performance that lie within the performer's control). Based on this distinction, it seems likely that the act of specifying performance goals can improve performers' concentration skills. For example, tennis players could improve their concentration on court by focusing solely on such performance goals as seeking 100% accuracy on their first serves. This suggestion seems theoretically valid because performance goals encourage performers to focus on task-relevant information and on controllable actions. Additional support for this idea stems from studies on the correlates of people's best and worst athletic performances. For example, Jackson & Roberts (1992) found that collegiate performers performed worst when they were preoccupied by result goals. Conversely, their best displays coincided with an explicit focus on performance goals. In summary, there seems to be some support for the idea that performance goals can facilitate concentration skills in performers.

Pre-performance routines

Most top-class performers display characteristic sequences of preparatory actions before they perform key skills. For example, dancers may go through the same physical stretching before going on stage. Similarly, rugby place-kickers like to go through a systematic series of steps before striking the ball. These preferred action sequences and/or repetitive behaviours are called 'pre-performance routines' and are typically performed prior to the execution of self-paced skills (i.e. actions that are carried out largely at one's own speed and without interference from other people).

At least three types of routines are common in physical performance situations. First, pre-event routines are preferred sequences of actions in the run-up to competitive events. Included here are stable preferences for what to do on the night before, and on the morning of, the performance itself. Second, pre-performance routines are characteristic sequences of thoughts and actions that performers adhere to prior to skill-execution – as in the examples above. Finally, postmistake routines are action sequences that may help performers to leave their errors in the past so that they can refocus on the task at hand. For example, a golfer may 'shadow' the correct swing of a shot that had led to an error.

Support for the value of pre-performance routines as concentration techniques comes from both theoretical and empirical sources. Theoretically, pre-performance routines may improve concentration for several reasons. First, they are intended to encourage performers to develop an appropriate mental set for skill execution by helping them to focus on task-relevant information. For example, many soccer goalkeepers follow pre-kick routines in an effort to block out any jeering that is directed at them by supporters of opposing teams. Second, such routines may enable performers to concentrate on the present moment rather than on past events or on possible future outcomes. Finally, pre-performance routines may prevent performers from devoting too much attention to the mechanics of their well learned skills – a habit that can unravel automaticity (Beilock & Carr 2001). Thus, routines may help to suppress the type of inappropriate conscious control that often occurs in pressure situations. A useful five-step pre-performance routine for self-paced skills is described by Singer (2002) (see Ch. 23 of this book).

Interestingly, the routines of expert performers are not as consistent as they have been portrayed. For example, Jackson & Baker (2001) analysed the pre-strike routine of the prolific former Welsh international and Lions rugby kicker, Neil Jenkins, who scored 1049 points in 87 games for his country. As expected, he reported using a variety of concentration techniques (such as thought-stopping and mental imagery) as part of his pre-kick routine. But surprisingly, these researchers discovered that Jenkins varied the timing of his pre-kick behaviour as a function of the difficulty of the kick he faced. This finding shows that routines are not as rigid or stereotyped as was originally believed. More recently, in another case-study, Shaw (2002) reported that a professional golfer experienced some attentional benefits arising from the use of a pre-shot routine. Although this evidence is anecdotal, the golfer reported that 'the new routine had made him more focused for each shot and therefore less distracted by irrelevancies' (Shaw 2002, p. 117).

Both these cases may be explained by the level of expertise of the participants who were studied. Thus, for an experienced kicker, different distances are, genuinely, different kicks requiring different pre-performance routines. Thus, as the performer improves, the challenges offered by different components of the performance become ever more discrete and the level of detail in preparation becomes ever more detailed.

It is possible that pre-performance routines may lead to superstitious rituals on the part of the performer. The consistent sequences of thoughts and behaviour displayed by performers as they use routines to prepare to execute key skills may appear to be an almost compulsive behaviour. However, it is important to differentiate routine from superstition and for practitioners to ensure that performers' routines maintain the key characteristics that keep routines separate.

A 'superstition' can be defined as the belief that, despite evidence to the contrary, certain behaviour is causally related to certain outcomes. Research shows that athletes are notoriously superstitious – perhaps because of the capricious nature of success in their field (Vyse 1997). For example, the South African golfer Ernie Els never plays with a ball marked with the number two because he associates it with bad luck (Laurence 1998, p. 23). Likewise, during the 2007 Open Championship the Irish golfer Padraig Harrington apparently chose a ball with 4 on it the first day, 3 the second day, 2 the third day and 1 the final day of the tournament (Gilleece 2007).

Despite their superficial similarity, routines and superstitious behaviour differ on two key criteria – control and purpose. The essence of superstitious behaviour is the belief that one's fate is governed by factors that lie outside one's control. But the virtue of a routine is that it allows the player to exert complete control over their preparation. Indeed, players often shorten their pre-performance routines in adverse circumstances (e.g. under unfavourable weather conditions). Unfortunately, the converse is true for superstitions. Thus they tend to grow longer over time as performers 'chain together' more and more illogical links between behaviour and outcome. The second criterion that may be used to distinguish between routines and rituals concerns the technical role of each behavioural step followed. To explain: whereas each part of a routine should have a rational basis, the components of a superstitious ritual may not be justifiable objectively. Despite these neat conceptual distinctions, the pre-shot routines of many performers are often invested with magical thinking and superstitious qualities.

Identifying these differences between routines and superstitions suggests that in developing routines performers should be encouraged to develop a routine that provides them with a sense of control over performance. They should also be instructed to practise varying their routine so it can be used flexibly. Finally, regular review and revision of routines will help to reduce the likelihood of them forming the basis for superstition.

Regular review and revision also assists with the second problem, which is that a routine become so old and familiar that it becomes automatic. If a performer maintained the same pre-performance routines indefinitely, their mind may begin to wander as a consequence of tuning out. Clearly, an important challenge for applied sport psychologists is to help performers to attain an appropriate level of conscious control over their actions before skill execution.

'Trigger words' as cues to concentrate

It has long been known that skilled performers talk to themselves, either overtly or silently, before and during important action sequences. This 'self-talk' is used both for motivational and instructional purposes (Hardy et al 2005). To illustrate, during the 2002 Wimbledon ladies' singles tennis final between the Williams sisters, Serena Williams (who defeated Venus 7–6, 6–3) was observed by millions of viewers to be reading something as she sat down during the change-overs between games. Afterwards, she explained that she had been reading notes that she had written to herself as trigger words or instructional cues to remind her to 'hit in front' or 'stay low' (Williams 2002, p. 6). Interestingly, she used a similar strategy in 2007 in Wimbledon when she defeated Daniela Hantuchova in the fourth round of the tournament. On this occasion, she used phrases like 'get low', 'add spin' and 'move up' (Martin 2007). In a similar vein, many skilled performers talk to themselves either silently or out loud when they compete – usually in an effort to motivate themselves. This covert self-talk can involve instructional ('Swing slowly') or motivational ('You can do this!') content and both types of content can be phrased positively or negatively. With regard to motivational influence it should be noted that the impact on performance may vary between different performers so that negatively phrased motivational self-talk ('Don't let him beat you') may be as effective for a performer as purely positive phrasing. As a cognitive self-regulatory strategy, self-talk may enhance concentration skills (Williams & Leffingwell 2002). In particular, Landin & Herbert (1999) discovered that tennis players who had been trained to use instructional cues or trigger words (such as 'split, turn') attributed their improved performance to enhanced concentration on court.

Although few studies have examined the role of self-talk on performers' concentration, Hatzigeorgiadis et al (2004) investigated how instructional self-talk influenced water-polo players' ball-throwing accuracy. Results showed that self-talk such as 'ball, target', decreased the prevalence of intrusive thoughts among water-polo players and improved their ball-throwing proficiency. Arising from such evidence, it seems likely that positive and/or instructional self-talk could enhance attentional skills by reminding performers what to focus on in a given situation (Fig. 22.2). For example, novice golfers may miss the ball completely on the fairway in the early stages of learning to swing the club properly. In an effort to overcome this problem, golf instructors may advise learners to concentrate on sweeping the grass rather than hitting the ball. This trigger phrase ensures that learners stay 'down' on the ball instead of looking up to see where it went. Ideally, trigger words should be short, vivid and positively phrased to yield maximum benefits.

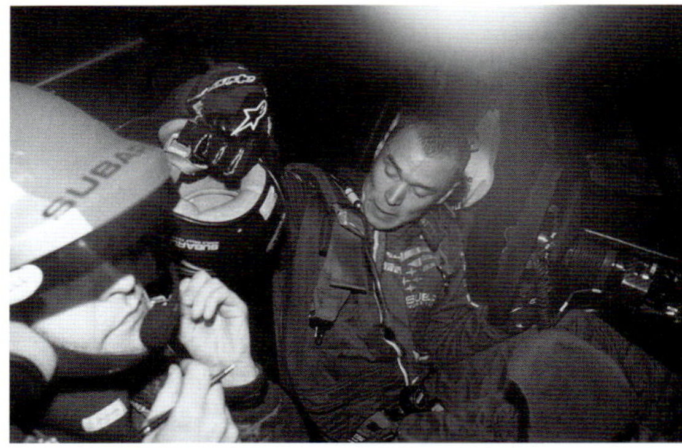

Fig. 22.2 • Switching attention. At the end of a stage, WRC Champions Richard Burns and Robert Reid prepare for the media scrum. © McKlein. With thanks to the Royal Automobile Motor Sport Association.

Mental practice

The term mental practice or 'visualization' refers to the systematic use of mental imagery in order to rehearse physical actions (see also Chs 2, 4, 16 and 23 in this book). It involves 'seeing' and 'feeling' a skill in one's imagination before actually executing it (Driskell et al 1994). Although there is considerable empirical evidence that mental imagery (Weinberg 2008) and mental practice facilitate skill learning and performance, their use as a concentration tool remains uncertain. Anecdotally, however, mental imagery is used widely by performers for the purpose of focusing. Thus Mike Atherton, the former England cricket captain, used to prepare mentally for test matches by actually going to the match venue and visualizing ' who's going to bowl, how they are going to bowl ... so that nothing can come as a surprise' (quoted in Selvey 1998, p. 2). From this quote, it seems that imagery helps performers to prepare for various hypothetical scenarios, thereby ensuring that they will not be distracted by unexpected events. However, this hypothesis has not been tested empirically to date. Therefore, despite the fact that mental imagery is known to improve athletic performance, its status as a concentration technique is uncertain.

In summary, we have reviewed four psychological techniques that are used regularly in an effort to improve performers' concentration skills. Unfortunately, few studies have evaluated the efficacy of these techniques in enhancing concentration skills. Despite the absence of such evidence, these four concentration techniques appear to be both plausible and useful in sport settings.

Conclusion

'Attention', or the concentration of mental activity on the task in hand, is a crucial prerequisite of success in any field of skilled performance (Fig. 22.3). Not surprisingly, considerable research has been conducted in psychology on the nature and improvement of attentional processes. The purpose of this chapter was to review such research and to identify relevant theoretical and practical implications. To begin with, I distinguished between three different cognitive dimensions of attention – 'concentration' or effortful awareness, selective perception, and divided attention or the ability to coordinate two or more actions at the same time. Then, I reviewed the strengths and weaknesses of three cognitive metaphors of attention; the filter approach, the spotlight theory and the capacity or resource model. The question of why skilled performers seem to 'lose' their concentration so easily was explained as a result of external (i.e. environmental) and internal (i.e. self-generated thoughts and feelings) distractions. Following on from an examination of attention based on the theoretical and empirical literature, I identified five key building blocks of effective concentration that should underpin practical work with performers. The relationship between anxiety, concentration and skilled performance that it is critical to understand to work effectively in performance situations was examined in relation to the most recent theoretical developments. In the final section of the chapter, I outlined and illustrated a range of concentration training exercises and techniques – practical tools for helping skilled performers to achieve and maintain an optimal focus of attention.

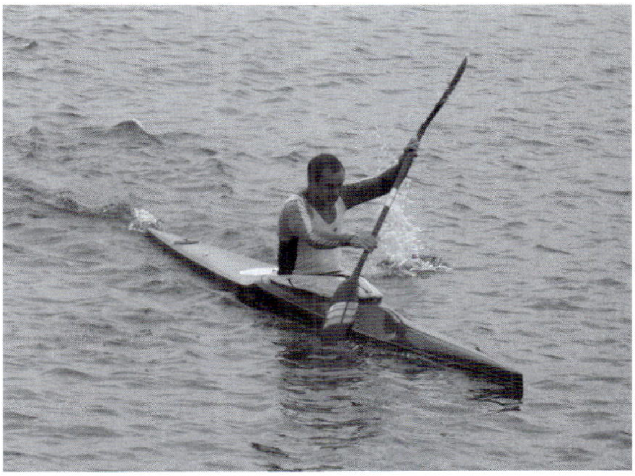

Fig. 22.3 • Focused on the finish. Performance Panel member Ray Rowe finishes a race in fine form.

References

Abernethy, B., 2001. Attention. In: Singer, R.N., Hausenblas, H.A., Janelle, C.M. (Eds.), Handbook of sport psychology, second ed. John Wiley, New York, pp. 53–85.

Abernethy, B., Maxwell, J.P., Masters, R.S., et al., 2007. Attentional processes, skill learning and expert performance. In: Tenenbaum, G., Eklund, R.C. (Eds.), Handbook of sport psychology, third ed. John Wiley, New York, pp. 245–263.

Ashcraft, M., 2006. Cognition, fourth ed. Prentice Hall, Upper Saddle River, NJ.

Atkinson, R.C., Shiffrin, R.M., 1968. Human memory: a proposed system and its control processes. In: Spence, K.W. (Ed.), The psychology of learning and motivation: advances in research and theory. Academic Press, New York, pp. 89–195.

Baddeley, A.D., 1986. Working memory. Clarendon Press, Oxford.

Baddeley, A., 2003. Working memory: looking back and looking forward. Nat. Rev. Neurosci. 4, 829–839.

Baddeley, A., Idzikowski, C., 1985. Anxiety, manual dexterity and diver performance. Ergonomics 28, 1475–1482.

Bannister, R., 2004. Fear of failure haunted me right to the last second. The Guardian 1 May, pp. 12–13.

Bargh, J.A., Morsella, E., 2008. The unconscious mind. Perspec. Psycholog. Science 3, 73–79.

Baumeister, R.F., 1984. Choking under pressure: self-consciousness and the paradoxical effects of incentives on skilled performance. J. Pers. Soc. Psychol. 46, 610–620.

Beilock, S.L., Carr, T.H., 2001. On the fragility of skilled performance: what governs choking under pressure? J. Exp. Psychol. Gen. 130, 701–725.

Blau, E., 1998. Nervous issues. The Guardian 2 October, pp. 16–17.

Boland, R., 1999. Making magic. Irish Times (Supplement) 4 December, p. 6.

Broadbent, D.E., 1958. Perception and communication. Pergamon Press, London.

Brooks, R., 2001. Nerves force ballet star Bull to quit dancing. Sunday Times 10 June, p. 7.

Castaneda, B., Gray, R., 2007. Effects of focus of attention on baseball performance in players of differing skill levels. J. Sport and Exerc. Psychol. 29, 60–77.

Cherry, E.C., 1953. Some experiments on the recognition of speech with one and two ears. J. Acoust. Soc. Am. 25, 975–979.

Clarke, D., Morris, K., 2005. Golf – the mind factor. Hodder & Stoughton, London.

Corbetta, M., Shulman, G.L., 2002. Control of goal-directed and stimulus-driven attention in the brain. Nat. Rev. Neurosci. 3, 201–215.

Driskell, J.E., Copper, C., Moran, A., 1994. Does mental practice enhance performance? J. Appl. Psychol. 79, 481–492.

Easterbrook, J.A., 1959. The effect of emotion on cue utilization and organization of behaviour. Psychol. Rev. 66, 183–201.

English, A., 2006. Munster: our road to glory. Penguin, Dublin.

Eriksen, C.W., St James, J.D., 1986. Visual attention within and around the field of local attention: a zoom lens model. Percept. Psychophys. 40, 225–240.

Evening Herald, 2001. One Tiger that will never crouch. Evening Herald 9 April, p. 61.

Eysenck, M.W., Calvo, M., 1992. Anxiety and performance: the processing efficiency theory. Cognition and Emotion 6, 409–434.

Eysenck, M.W., Derakshan, N., Santos, R., et al., 2007. Anxiety and cognitive performance: attentional control theory. Emotion 7, 336–353.

Fanning, D., 2002. Coping with a stress factor. Sunday Independent 6 October, p. 6.

Fernandez-Duque, D., Johnson, M.L., 1999. Attention metaphors: how metaphors guide the cognitive psychology of attention. Cogn. Science 23, 83–116.

Garavan, H., 1998. Serial attention in working memory. Memory and Cognition 26, 263–276.

Gilleece, D., 2007. Mind games. Sunday Independent 12 August, p. 12.

Gouju, J.L., Vermersch, P., Bouthier, D., 2007. A psycho-phenomenological approach to sport psychology: the presence of the opponents in hurdle races. J. Appl. Sport Psychol. 19, 173–186.

Greenlees, I., Moran, A., 2003. Concentration skills training in sport. British Psychological Society, Sport and Exercise Psychology Division, Leicester.

Greenlees, I., Thelwell, R., Holder, T., 2006. Examining the efficacy of the concentration grid exercise as a concentration enhancement exercise. Psychol. Sport and Exerc. 7, 29–39.

Gucciardi, D.F., Dimmock, J.A., 2008. Choking under pressure in sensorimotor skills: conscious processing or depleted attentional resources? Psychol. Sport and Exerc. 9, 45–59.

Hanin, Y., 2000. Emotions in sport. Human Kinetics, Champaign, IL.

Hardy, J., Hall, C.R., Hardy, L., 2005. Quantifying athlete self-talk. J. Sports Sci. 23, 905–917.

Hatzigeorgiadis, A., Theodorakis, Y., Zourbanos, N., 2004. Self-talk in the swimming pool: the effects of self-talk on thought content and performance on water-polo tasks. J. Appl. Sport Psychol. 16, 138–150.

Hodge, K., McKenzie, A., 1999. Thinking rugby: training your mind for peak performance. Reed, Auckland, New Zealand.

Jackson, R.C., Baker, J.S., 2001. Routines, rituals, and rugby: case study of a world class goal kicker. Sport Psychologist 15, 48–65.

Jackson, R.C., Roberts, G.C., 1992. Positive performance states of athletes: toward a conceptual understanding of peak performance. Sport Psychologist 6, 156–171.

James, W., 1890. Principles of psychology. Holt, Rinehart & Winston, New York.

Jha, A.P., Krompinger, J., Baime, M.J., 2007. Mindfulness training modifies subsystems of attention. Cogn. Affect. Behav. Neurosci. 7, 109–119.

Kahneman, D., 1973. Attention and effort. Prentice-Hall, Englewood Cliffs, New Jersey.

Landin, D., Herbert, E.P., 1999. The influence of self-talk on the performance of skilled female tennis players. J. Appl. Sport Psychol. 11, 263–282.

Laurence, J., 1998. A saunter for champs. Irish Independent 1 July, p. 23.

Luck, S.J., Vecera, S.P., 2002. Attention. In: Pashler, H. (Ed.), Stevens' handbook of experimental psychology, third ed, vol. 1. John Wiley, New York, pp. 235–286.

McElree, B., 1998. Attended and nonattended states in working memory: accessing categorized structures. J. Memory Lang. 38, 225–252.

Mair, L., 2004. Cool Goosen rides the storm. Daily Telegraph 22 June, p. S10.

Martin, A., 2007. More than words: Book of Serena, the answer to Williams' prayers. The Guardian 3 July, p. 5.

Masters, R.S.W., 1992. Knowledge, 'knerves' and know-how: the role of explicit versus implicit knowledge in the breakdown of complex motor skill under pressure. Br. J. Psychol. 83, 343–358.

Matlin, M., 2005. Cognition, sixth ed. Holt, Rinehart & Winston, New York.

Maynard, I., 1998. Improving concentration. The National Coaching Foundation, Headingley, Leeds.

Moran, A.P., 1996. The psychology of concentration in sport performers: a cognitive analysis. Psychology Press, Hove, East Sussex.

Moran, A.P., 1998. The pressure putt: doing your best when it matters most in golf (audiotape). Tutorial Services (UK) Ltd, Aldergrove, County Antrim.

Moran, A.P., 2003. The state of concentration skills training in applied sport psychology. In: Greenlees, I., Moran, A. (Eds.), Concentration skills training in sport. British Psychological Society (Division of Sport and Exercise Psychology), Leicester, pp. 7–19.

Moran, A.P., 2004. Sport and exercise psychology: a critical introduction. Psychology Press/ Routledge, London.

Moran, G., 2005. Oh dear, so near but yet so far away. Irish Times 12 July, p. 21.

Muscat, J., 2005. House of horrors torments Loughran. The Times 28 December, p. 55.

Nadel, L., Piattelli-Palmarini, M., 2002. What is cognitive science? In: Nadel, L. (Ed.), Encyclopaedia of cognitive science, vol. 1. Nature Publishing Group, London, pp. xiii–xxli.

Navon, D., Gopher, D., 1979. On the economy of the human-processing system. Psychol. Rev. 86, 214–255.

Nideffer, R., 1976. Test of Attentional and Interpersonal Style. J. Pers. Soc. Psychol. 34, 394–404.

Orlick, T., 1990. In pursuit of excellence. Leisure Press, Champaign, IL.

Palmeri, T.J., 2002. Automaticity. In: Nadel, L. (Ed.), Encyclopaedia of cognitive science, vol. 1. Nature Publishing Group, London, pp. 290–301.

Pashler, H., 1999. The psychology of attention. MIT Press, Cambridge, MA.

Posner, M.I., 1980. Orienting of attention: the VIIth Sir Frederic Bartlett lecture. Q. J. Exp. Psychol. 32 (A), 3–25.

Posner, M.I., Rothbart, M.K., 2007. Research on attention networks as a model for the integration of a psychological science. Annu. Rev. Psychol. 58, 1–23.

Roland, D., 1997. The confident performer. Nick Hern, London.

Schmid, A., Peper, E., 1998. Strategies for training concentration. In: Williams, J.M. (Ed.), Applied sport psychology: personal growth to peak performance. Mayfield, Mountain View, CA, pp. 316–328.

Schmidt, R.A., Lee, T.D., 1999. Motor control and learning: a behavioural emphasis, third ed. Human Kinetics, Champaign, IL.

Selvey, M., 1998. Getting up for the Ashes. The Guardian 20 November, p. 2.

Shaw, D., 2002. Confidence and the pre-shot routine in golf: A case-study. In: Cockerill, I. (Ed.), Solutions in sport psychology. Thomson, London, pp. 108–119.

Singer, R.N., 2002. Preperformance state, routines, and automaticity: what does it take to realize expertise in self-paced tasks? J. Sport and Exerc. Psychol. 24, 359–375.

Smith, M., 2002. Practice makes perfect. Daily Telegraph 15 February, p. 3.

Smith, E.E., Kosslyn, S.M., 2007. Cognitive psychology: mind and brain. Pearson/Prentice-Hall, Upper Saddle River, NJ.

Strayer, D.L., Drews, F.A., 2007. Attention. In: Durso, F.T., Nickerson, R.S., Dumais, S.T., et al. (Eds.), Handbook of applied cognition, second ed. Wiley, Chichester, West Sussex, pp. 29–54.

Strayer, D.L., Drews, F.A., Johnston, W.A., 2003. Cell-phone induced failures of visual attention during simulated driving. J. Exp. Psychol. Appl. 9, 23–32.

Szczepanik, N., 2005. Focused Cech puts records low on his list of priorities. The Times April 30, p. 100.

Velmans, M., Schneider, S., 2007. The Blackwell companion to consciousness. Blackwell, Oxford.

Vyse, S., 1997. Believing in magic: The psychology of superstition. Oxford University Press, New York.

Wegner, D.M., 1994. Ironic processes of mental control. Psychol. Rev. 101, 34–52.

Wegner, D.M., 2002. Thought suppression and mental control. In: Nadel, L. (Ed.), Encyclopaedia of cognitive science, vol. 4. Nature Publishing Group, London, pp. 395–397.

Weinberg, R., 2008. Does imagery work? Effects on performance and mental skills. J. Imag. Res. Sport and Phys. Activ. 3, 1–21.

Weinberg, R.S., Gould, D., 1999. Foundations of sport and exercise psychology, second ed. Human Kinetics, Champaign, IL.

Weinberg, R.S., Gould, D., 2007. Foundations of sport and exercise psychology, fourth ed. Human Kinetics, Champaign, IL.

White, J., 2002. Interview: Garry Sobers. The Guardian 10 June, pp. 20–21.

Williams, R., 2002. Sublime Serena celebrates the crucial difference. The Guardian 8 July, p. 6.

Williams, J.M., Leffingwell, T.R., 2002. Cognitive strategies in sport and exercise psychology. In: Van Raalte, J., Brewer, B.W. (Eds.), Exploring sport and exercise psychology, second ed. American Psychological Association, Washington, DC, pp. 75–98.

Wulf, G., 2007. Attentional focus and motor learning: a review of 10 years of research. Bewegung und Training 1–11. Available on line at: http://www.ejournal-but.de/doks/wulf_2007.pdf

Putting it together: skills for pressure performance

23

Mark R. Wilson* Hugh Richards†

*University of Exeter, Exeter, UK; †University of Edinburgh, Edinburgh, UK

CHAPTER CONTENTS

Introduction

When the time comes to perform at the highest level there is no margin for error and there may be no second chance. Years of training, effort, money and personal sacrifice can be condensed into a few brief moments in which aspirations can be reached or dashed. For performers, aspiring to be the best means that the odds are always against them. In an Olympic sprint final seven people will fail to cross the line as gold medallist; many more climbers attempt Everest and turn back than summit out; a dance company has a single lead. The reality is that more performers fail to attain the ultimate goal than succeed in their aspirations. Most performers recognize this challenge, which is reflected in the detail and effort spent on physical conditioning, but simply being in the physical condition to perform is just one facet of preparation towards producing the performance levels necessary at the right times. This chapter begins with a focus on the critical need for thorough mental preparation and planning that should be completed prior to performance. As Michael Johnson (1996, p. 25), holder of five Olympic and nine World Championship gold medals, noted, 'commitment and preparation are all that mark the differences among an arena full of perfect physical specimens'.

DOI: 10.1016/B978-0-443-06734-1.00023-7

Most physical performers tend to practise and train more than they perform and in some cases the training:performing ratio can be very high. For example, between September and December a swimmer completed high-volume training for 16 weeks, up to 20 separate sessions per week (pool- and land-based) and had just one competition at the end. While this example may be extreme (a training: performance ratio, in days, of 112:1), this trend – mostly practice compared to full performance – is typical across most physical performance domains. The consequence of this is that performers are focused on getting physically and mentally able to perform at the highest level, but mostly within training and practice environments and contexts. Crucially, they are not as used to performance itself. Equally significant is that for many performers the real pinnacle challenge or major event is in an unfamiliar environment and may involve travel, time away from home and changes to diet, accommodation, time zone and climate. There is a lot of opportunity in these circumstances for disruptions to occur and for the hard work and effort of performers to be undone by issues that might be categorized as practical logistics, best addressed through careful and thorough performance planning.

While thorough planning and preparation focus on attempting to control the controllable, equally important is ensuring that performers are competent and trained in adapting to the uncontrollable. Elite performers often have to find a way to maintain good levels of performance even when things are not going right. Niggling injuries, adverse conditions, distractions and demands of a life outside performance, and plain bad luck, will be encountered by most performers in their careers. But being able to sustain performance levels despite these factors is critical. To achieve this, performers need to be able to cope, be mentally tough and control attention and emotion. Thus the content discussed in detail in the preceding chapters needs to flexibly applied, in combination and in response to the changing performance environment and perceived demands. Furthermore, successful use of the techniques and skills outlined in this chapter can only be achieved if they are well learned and practised long before they are really needed to support and maintain performance in truly demanding circumstances.

This chapter concentrates on the performer at an individual level but many performers operate as members of an interacting team, so the specific approaches that can be used to enhance team performance are explored in Chapter 24. The overall focus of the chapter is to illustrate and explain the ways in which psychology, psychological techniques, practical strategies and common sense can be combined to allow performers to perform at the highest level and against the odds. At the players' entrance to Centre Court at Wimbledon two lines of poetry encourage tennis players to prepare to meet either triumph or disaster. However, in relation to the focus of this chapter the opening words of the same poem (Rudyard Kipling's 'If' (Kipling 1924)) capture the challenge to performers, psychologists and practitioners: 'If you can keep your head when all about you Are losing theirs'.

Planning and preparation

Planning and preparation are essential to ensure that key tasks are completed and everything is in place and to avoid events that might disrupt the performer and performance itself. It might appear almost impossible to imagine that an athlete might arrive at the Olympic stadium without their running spikes, that a performer selected for a prestigious international tour might fail to bring their passport to the airport or that a performer might drink, 'by accident', 2 litres of fluid in the hour immediately before their important performance, leaving them feeling heavy and bloated. However, all of these events really did occur with mature, experienced performers and aptly demonstrate the need to attend to detailed planning and preparation. Even factors that have never gone wrong, been forgotten or caused problems in the past should be considered in planning, as these are still susceptible to failure or error with the increased pressure, challenge and tempo of high-level performance environments.

Good preparation not only avoids pitfalls but is an important factor in enhancing self-confidence and reducing the potential for cognitive anxiety (Jones et al 1990). Thus, thorough and detailed planning and preparation will help to ensure that performers are in the optimum mental state in the period leading up to their performance. Performers also often mistakenly assume that planning and preparation is only concerned with the time up to the start of their performance. However, performers will benefit from thinking through the elements of their performance and the possible permutations that might occur and plan their strategic and tactical response to these. The fastest athlete in the world may sprint 100 m in under 10 seconds but they will have completed several races over 2 days to qualify for the final. In this time they might have taken strategic decisions to put in performances to worry opponents or to conserve themselves, or a combination of these, and may well have contended with a false start that would alter the potential risk of being disqualified and consequently influence their tactics. They should have prepared and planned for all these circumstances. Even an event of less than 10 seconds duration demands high-level planning if high-level performance is the goal. The critical relationship of planning to performance was exemplified by Michael Johnson (1996, p. 212), who explained his own attention to planning: 'Earlier in the day of competition I have met with my coach and we've gone over every outstanding detail. Where will I go between races? Will I stay in the stadium or return to the warm-up track? When will I begin my final warm-up? I want every detail considered and planned.'

Expert opinion, research and common sense all converge on the need to plan and organize preparation carefully. But common sense is often not common practice and some of the key issues that prevent planning taking place are that performers do not know how to plan, what content should be included or what time periods the plan should cover. In this section we will explain the way in which planning can be undertaken, ranging from simple analytical frameworks to structure the process and performance segmentation through to 'what if' sessions and contingency planning. In the process we will also discuss the content of planning. However, it is self-evident that for all physical performers the essential cornerstones of food, fluid and sleep remain fundamental considerations to being well prepared and should feature in the content of all planning. Planning should be explicitly addressed long in advance of performance, with increasing detail and modifications nearer the time as the precise details and schedules become known. Physical performers often find that planning is not intrinsically motivating and there is a role for performance psychologists to ensure that this is done and, if necessary, to facilitate and cajole until it is. For planning, two heads are better than one and performers, plus any of performance managers, psychologists, other support specialists, coaches and directors are likely to be represented in an ideal planning group.

Pre-performance planning

It is beneficial to have a structure against which to organize planning and Taylor (1995) identifies four elements: physical, technical, logistical and psychological (also sometimes referred to as technical tactical, physical and mental (TTPM)) that can be used as the basis for analysing performance needs in planning. Consider the example in Figure 23.1, taken from athletics (thanks to Dave Collins for the idea and ace logisticians David Dix and Simon Nathan for the refined model). It is possible to see the basis of this framework but with extended detail to separate medical and physical from physiological (dominated by plans for eating and drinking!). This example also emphasizes the need for planning to be time-phased and to contain key information (dates, locations, availability of personnel, contacts and resources). It is important that this information is made available for a planning session to be effective and efficient and that plans are updated as details, change, evolve and emerge.

The example shown in Figure 23.1 is a general plan and one that should be individualized and added to by each performer to provide the level of detail necessary. The plan makes allowance for an individual's psychological content; however, it is the psychological impact of reducing uncertainty and avoiding practical and logistical errors that is the primary reason for advocating its use.

The specific psychological needs of performers can be further addressed through individual plans such as the one suggested by Rushall & Potgieter (1987), who utilize a strategy planning sheet with three categories of information:

- **Primary behaviours**: functional activities that are almost inevitably going to happen, such as getting changed
- **Coping behaviours**: planned responses or actions to be completed at certain times (despite the term, Rushall & Potgieter include activities such as mental rehearsal not in response to another thought or action but just because it is part of the plan, so this category is not just 'coping')
- **Outcomes**: identify what the performer wants to achieve following the two categories of behaviour, such as feeling energetic, lively and powerful after a warm-up.

An excerpt from a modified version of the planning sheet is shown in Table 23.1 for a swimmer. In this

29th European Athletics Indoor Championships – Birmingham 2007 www.hotelwebaddress.com

Personal Coach ____________ **Performance Manager** ____________

Athlete ____________ **Event** ____________ **Team coach** ____________

PHASE 1: Arrival in Birmingham (Wednesday 28 February – between 14:00 – 17:00)
Team Hotel (tbc) Hotel Birmingham, Main Street, Birmingham B1 1AB
www.cpbhamcity.com 0870 2001 189

		Physiological	Mental/organizational	Technical/tactical	Physical/medical
DAY 1 (Wednesday 28 February 2007)	Depart UK home base to Birmingham Team Hotel (notify anti – doping)	**Hydration Strategy:** • Which drink? • How much? • Bottled water provided • Red Bull provided	**What to pack:** • GB kit check (new issue) • Passport (for accreditation)	**GBR Coaching team** <<coach names here>>	**GBR Medical Team:** Drs Baker/ Wilson John Sharp, Karen Elsworth, Nigel Redwood
		Nutrition Strategy: • Own food if required • What and when to eat	**Mental Preparation Plan:** • Distraction techniques (eg good book, DVD, cards)	**Training Load** • Danger of over-training prior to championships Dimension of spikes • Spikes should not exceed 6mm in length and 4mm in diameter	**Medical Plan pre champs:** • Anti-doping whereabouts to be kept up to date from selection • Complete uk:a medical form • TUE check • Forward medical plan from current EIS staff to BH
		Acclimatization: • Humidity in NIA • Air conditioning in hotel	**Accreditation:** • Hotel • 27/02 – 4/03 • 09:00 – 21:00	**Comp Regulations** • Athlete and coach aware of timetable, qualifying and final requirements?	**Anti-doping** • Importance of maintaining UK Sports whereabouts forms • IAAF "competition" doping regulations in force, before and during competition
		Recovery from Travel: • Check AA or BBC road watch to try to avoid rush hour and motorway congestion www.bbc.co.uk/birmingham	**Technical Plan:** • How much training? • Track training only at B'ham HPC not at NIA	**Accreditation Access:** • LOC rule presently states only athletes who are about to compete in that champ session will have access to warm up	**Medical Plan at champs:** • Athlete to confirm Physiotherapy and Massage programme with medical team
			Sharing a room with a team mate (unavoidable!) • Simple rules of sharing • Healthy living	**Personal Coach strategy** • See policy sheet	**Recovery:** • Ice Baths only at team hotel

Fig. 23.1 • Example planning format for athletics competition. From an original idea by Dave Collins carefully refined and applied by ace logisticians David Dix and Simon Nathan.

(Continued)

case activities were separated simply between mental and physical and the concept of 'Outcomes' was illustrated through bold, italicized statements in the mental activity column. Note that these statements were performer-generated, so helped with self-talk content (see later in this chapter). Using a systematic approach to planning ensures that the performer is absolutely clear in their own mind what it is they want to achieve and are able to determine if it has been achieved, or if additional action/coping is required if it hasn't.

Timelines and segmentation

One approach that can be used for an individualized plan is to consider various time phases in the period prior to a performance event and plan specific activities for each of the periods with increasing detail as the time to performance decreases (Fig. 23.2, p. 339).

Constructing timelines for planning is a useful exercise because it enables performer and practitioner to create and develop an overview and as a result answer the key question of what needs to be

PHASE 2: Pre-Championship Day Thursday 1 March
Stadium (NIA) viewing time 11:00 – 13:00 *note EAA/LOC rule on when athletes will be able to access warm up (HR/MW)
Meal timings Breakfast 06:00 – 10:00 Lunch 12:00 – 15:00 Dinner 18:00 – 22:00 (accreditation and room key required)

		Physiological	Mental/organizational	Technical/tactical	Physical/medical
DAY 2 (Thursday 1 March)	National Indoor Arena / Team Hotel / Birmingham HPC	**Hydration Strategy:** As above • Humid • Living with air-conditioning	**Refinement of Mental Preparation:** Plan B's Boredom	**Technical Plan:** • IAAF Indoor Competition Rules – check rules for qualification and lane draws or jumping order	**Medical Plan:** • Physiotherapy • Massage
		Nutrition Strategy: • Maintaining or adapting normal diet to meet Championship conditions • Danger of over-eating? • Confirming Nutritional Pack for competition day? **Essential Behaviour** • Drink bottle fluid • Caution with uncooked food, cold food and salads	**Timetable for day** • Team Leaders' stadium visit 11:00 • Official Training at NIA 11:00 – 13:00 • Training with starters 11:30 – 12:30 • Final Entry Confirmation 12:00 • GB Media Conference 14:00 • Technical Meeting 16:00 • 17:00 estimated release of start lists! • Team Meeting 18:00 • LOC Medical Meeting 18:00		• Pee Test • Check daily weight at same time • Sleep • Mood
			Training Times Birmingham HPC Wed 28/02 09:00 – 18:00 Thurs 01/03 08:30 – 16:00 Fri 02/03 08:30 – 16:00 Sat 03/03 08:30 – 16:00 Sun 04/03 10:00 – 12:00	• Team Leaders' stadium visit 11:00 • Technical Meeting 16:00	**Medical – General Health** • Gastroenteritis – take sensible precautions – wash hands regularly! • Cold/Flu – wash hands!
		Recovery / Cooling Strategy: • At competition site	**Communication plan for significant others!!** • Personal coach • Family members		
			Managing increased GB media interest with home champs		**Warm Up:** • Awareness of NIA procedures and systems • Entry point for NIA community hall for warm up

Fig. 23.1—Cont'd

(Continued)

planned for. The idea of increasing detail towards the performance itself is nicely demonstrated by the idea of performance segmentation recommended by Rushall & Potgieter (1987). They emphasize the benefits of segmentation for complicated and extended events such as endurance running. However, even short events such as a long jump run-up are effectively segmented in terms both of technical issues in training and also of the psychological benefits of orientating attention to what needs to be done in performance. An example of a segmented performance plan is shown below for a 200 m butterfly swimmer in a long course event (50 m pool) (Fig. 23.3, p. 340). Each segment in the plan is linked to key instructional information, including technical (long stroke), tactical (hold back), mental (relaxed) and physical (breathe) components. The instructional information is also grouped under mnemonic terms (eagle, dolphin, wind-up, etc.), some of which utilize evocative content to convey the essence of

Phase 3: Competition Day

Meal timings Breakfast 06:00 – 10:00 Lunch 12:00 – 15:00 Dinner 18:00 – 22:00
(accreditation card and room key card will be required)
Competition Sessions Friday 09:30 – 14:15 & 15:45 – 19:00 Saturday 09:30 – 11:45 & 13:15 – 16:30
Sunday 9:15 – 10:30 12:45 – 17:00
Opening Ceremony Friday 2 March at 14:50 (GB athletes required as host nation?)

	Physiological	Mental/organizational	Technical/tactical	Physical/medical
? add per individual Days to Event	**Hydration Strategy for Competition Day:** LOC will provide water and soft drinks **Nutrition Strategy for Competition Day**	**Athlete's individual competition organization** • Use official transport from team hotel (5mins transfer time) or walk? • Endurance runners w/up indoors or outdoors?	**Review qualifying requirements on publication** • When will I know my heats? Estimated as 17:00 01/03/07 but could be an optimistic estimate! • Tactics?	**Physio /Massage?** • As normal? • What is normal?
	Recovery / Cooling Strategy: • At track side • In team hotel	**Preparing for day(s) of competition (bringing it all together on a repeated basis):**	• Travel / Timing Arrangements to Venue: • Timing for call rooms (note difference between qualification and final) • Track (Q+F) 30mins / Infield 10mins • LJ/TJ/SP (Q) 55 / Infield 35 • LJ/TJ/SP (F) 40 / Infield 25 • HJ (Q/F) 70/50 / Infield 50/35 • PV (Q/F) 95/75 / Infield 75/55	**Warm Up:** Timing & content
	Environmental: Competing indoors in a full arena	**When to rehearse?** • Schedule / timing **When to relax?**	**Infield practice?** Field event athletes allowed two practices **Trials in-field events** LJ/TJ/SP in qualification 3 trials, final 6 trials	**Protests** In the first instant, protest must be made orally to the referee by the athlete OR by a responsible official acting on his/her behalf

Phase 4
Closing Ceremony Sunday 4th March at conclusion of last event – as host nation will be expected to have a good presence
Closing Banquet Sunday 4th March at 19:45 in International Convention Centre (again as host nation a good British attendance expected)
(Entry to closing banquet either with accreditation card and / or invitation card)
Medal Ceremony for 4 x 400 will take place during Closing Banquet (assume requirement for team kit not required)
Departure from Birmingham Monday 5 March (Check out before 11:00)

Fig. 23.1—Cont'd

performance in each segment. The mnemonic terms help recall, contribute to the information and provide a means of running through the race plan in short burst form. This could be usefully employed, for example, after a false start.

This plan, represented here just as the athlete drew it, shows the largest segment towards the start of the race and progressively smaller segments as the race concludes. The plan is also consistent with the idea of intensification (Rushall & Potgieter 1987) designed to offset fatigue and in this instance pain/discomfort. In essence, the intensification principle suggests that performers work mentally harder, utilizing more instructional and motivational self-talk, mood words and images and with more frequent changes between these, as fatigue and other factors detrimental to performance increase.

A segmented performance plan is likely to assist performers in several ways. First, it gives them a clear sense of control about what they should be doing at any stage. It enables them to attend to task-relevant instruction but phrased in such a way as to avoid the issue of exerting too much control that was outlined in the preceding chapter on attention and later in the section of this chapter on Self-talk. Developing a performance plan directly feeds into

Table 23.1 Planning sheet for swimmer day of race holding room

Time	Physical activity	Mental activity
6:00 am	Wake-up call, phone	
	Short walk and stretch	Loosen off from sleep
	Get up, shave, dry off, keep hydrated (0.5 L)	
	Check kit and add water bottle	Use checklist to ensure I've got everything I need. ***Preparation is complete***
	Breakfast (4 × OJ, cereals, toast/rolls + 0.25 L water)	
	Sit @ table (or outside), read paper if available + 0.25 L	Entertain self with easy chat or read
	Sit at 'meeting point'	
	Full plan included detailed warm-up and stretching sessions, plus diversion activities, at this point	
	Watch swimming with the rest. Keep hydrated and loose	Feel ***loose*** and ***ready***
	Take a walk (outside?) keep water bottle with me	Feel ***calm***
	Pick up kit go to change into race kit. Hat + goggles in pocket	
	Go back and put bag down. Speak to coach	***'Got everything I need to race'***

the development of the content of self-talk. While a performance plan helps to direct attention, it simultaneously helps to avoid the potential for a performer to become overly anxious. Keeping performers mentally busy and in control is fundamental to avoiding anxiety in performance situations. The performance plan also offers one further benefit, which we will return to later in this chapter: a focused, preplanned structure for evaluating performance.

In summary, planning is an essential component of performance. For most performers there is too much effort and investment at stake to risk getting it wrong on the day. Good planning not only reduces mistakes, it assists in creating the best opportunity for ideal mental and physical set-up. But even a realistic ideal will not match reality and performers must be prepared for quick adaptation of a plan to get the critical elements addressed and get to the *ready to perform* stage in as good a state as possible. To this end spending some time on contingency planning – what-ifs – helps performers make good decisions about how to react to the need for change. Often those charged with preparing performers will see advantages in extending this so that performers are presented with unexpected difficulties to overcome so that they learn directly how to react in such a way as to minimize any disadvantage to preparation. It is important that performers do not become seduced by the goal of getting or, worse, needing everything to be perfect in order to be able to perform. Frequently, delays occur in performance and these can be countered partly by using filler activities (e.g. stretching, mental rehearsal, music, puzzles) that can be easily deployed to occupy these time periods. Filler activities need to be combined with rapid refocusing of attention. The race plan above could be used for a global mental rehearsal and performance routines discussed in the following sections provide a sequenced

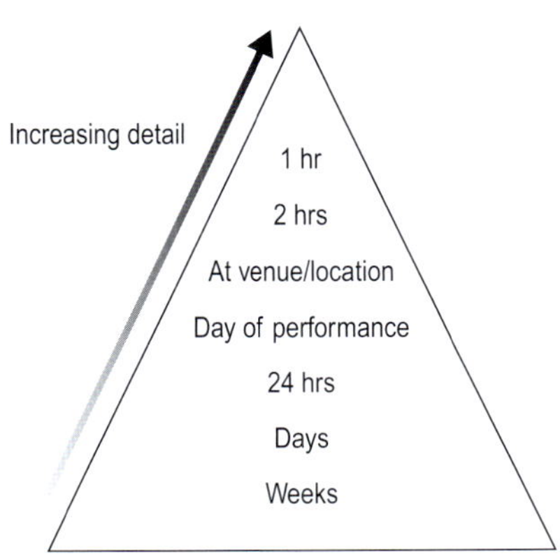

Fig. 23.2 • Planning activity can use time phases prior to performance as a structure.

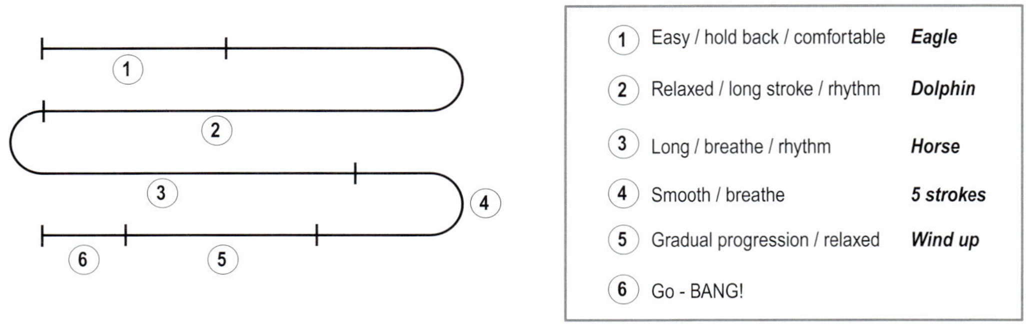

Fig. 23.3 • Segmented race plan for 200 m butterfly.

approach to focusing attention to a specific skill or performance component. Identifying filler activities with quick refocusing strategies and using these in practice, and in low level performance situations, is necessary for performers to help keep their heads under pressure.

Performance routines

Having considered planning and preparation strategies for performers to adopt in the build-up to an important event, we are now going to focus on a technique that can be used immediately prior to, and during, performance. The primary aim of a performance routine is to help the performer attain an optimal internal state in order to realize maximal potential. To meet this goal, a routine may encompass a number of specific techniques designed to self-regulate arousal, thoughts, performance expectancy and attentional focus. A routine can therefore act as a cocoon against the adverse effects of pressure, as, by concentrating on each step of the routine, performers learn to focus only on what they can control. The concept of 'control' is absolutely critical to what we are trying to achieve and we examine various ways to maintain control throughout this chapter.

Performance routines have been mainly linked with self-paced tasks, where performers tend to employ a systematic, routinized sequence of behaviours and movements prior to execution of the skill. In this way they are often termed *pre*-performance routines, and are a key component of a psychological skills intervention in such tasks (e.g. Boutcher & Rotella 1987). However, while performance routines are generally discussed in relation to self-paced tasks, any performer interested in achieving an optimal performance state can benefit from such a strategy. First, it is important to start with the 'end in mind'. How does the performer want to feel just before and during performance? This requires some detective work to determine exactly what the optimal internal state consists of before developing strategies to help achieve it. The detective work is based on getting answers to key questions such as: What is going through the performer's mind (thoughts and images) and how do they feel (arousal level and emotions), when performing at their best? This can be considered as an extension to the approach adopted by Hanin to determine an individual's zone of optimal functioning, discussed in Chapter 22.

As a demonstration, consider a dancer who has determined that a relaxed, confident state underpins her best performances. She can either (a) hope that on the day she feels confident and relaxed, and if not, she can reflect that it just 'didn't happen for her today' or (b) take control and develop a series of self-statements, images and arousal regulation techniques, fine-tuned during practice and directed at helping her feel confident and relaxed. This example also highlights the importance of the performer taking responsibility for the aspects of performance that they can control, including their pre-performance state. There may be occasions when an optimal state seems to just happen, and on other occasions it may be difficult to achieve (particularly if the pressure is intense). However, to establish an optimal performance state on a consistent basis, a performance routine is a likely prerequisite.

A five-step strategy to an optimal performance state

Although other similar routines are discussed in the literature (e.g. the Nebraska 3Rs: Ready, Respond, Refocus (Ravizza & Osborne 1991)), we are going to adopt Singer's Five Step Strategy (Singer 1988, 2000) as the basis for a flexible performance routine that can be applied across performance domains. The five-step strategy has been shown to facilitate learning and performance in a number of laboratory and field studies (Singer 2000, 2002), and focuses on creating the conditions for a 'just do it' performance state. The five steps are:

1. **Readying**: Obtain an optimal physical and mental set
2. **Imaging**: Mentally picture a successful technique and outcome
3. **Focusing**: Concentrate on one relevant external cue
4. **Executing**: 'Just do it'
5. **Evaluating**: Review effectiveness and adjust next time if necessary.

The first step is 'readying' and implies obtaining not only an optimal positioning of the body for the task but also an optimal mental state (attitudes and emotions). This may include using self-talk and arousal adjustment techniques to maintain emotional control and high confidence (see relevant sections in this chapter). This step sets the foundation for the rest of the routine and basically helps the performer ensure that they are physically and mentally in the right 'place'. The second step, 'imaging', reflects the importance of providing a picture and feeling of what successful completion of the task would be like. The third step, 'focusing attention', reminds the performer to focus on a relevant external cue or thought, while the fourth step, 'executing', reflects the importance of quieting the mind so that you can 'just do it'. Singer proposes that a final step, 'evaluation', allows the performer to evaluate the quality of execution, outcome achieved and the previous four steps of the routine, if time permits.

Singer's strategy was initially developed to help the learning of motor skills, as opposed to helping maintain performance in pressure settings. The five steps were intended as an instructional approach to distract learners from their own movements so that they could more quickly achieve the 'non-conscious' performance state associated with expert performance. However, as Masters (1992; Ch. 13 of this book) has suggested that a focus on the control of movement may also underlie choking under pressure, we argue that the five-step strategy may also provide a useful structure for skill execution in the performance environment. In order to be more flexible to the needs of expert performers, we suggest that the rigid, sequential structure may be modified slightly to allow a performer to (1) prepare an optimal performance set, (2) execute in a non-conscious manner and (3) review and evaluate performance to provide feedback for subsequent attempts. A modified performance routine for pressure situations is illustrated in Figure 23.4.

Figure 23.4 highlights three main phases of a performance routine: preparation, performance and review. The 'preparation' phase includes both the readying and imaging steps of Singer's strategy and reflects the fact that imaging may be used alongside other techniques to assist with mental 'readying'. The order in which these steps are incorporated into the routine can be flexible, so long as they help the performer feel ready to commit to entering the 'performance' phase. As the focusing step impacts directly on performance (see the discussion below) and can help create the 'quiet mind' associated with unconscious execution, we have linked steps 3 and 4 together as a 'quiet' period where detailed technical or strategic thoughts should be minimized. Performance (step 4) should occur non-consciously and as instinctively as possible, so, if a performer has any doubts, the time to 'pull out' and 're-prepare' should be at step 3, rather than reflecting on the error in step 5. Evaluating performance (the 'review' phase; step 5) is a critical element of continued improvement (see below). However, in-event it is important that this postperformance element of the routine helps the performer refocus and not dwell on any errors made (i.e. 'draw a line' under past performance).

Consistency is key: but consistency in what?

A key principle of performance routines is that, if the performer is consistent in thoughts and behaviours during performance, the performance itself will also be more consistent. However, it is important to note that it is the mental state just prior to and during performance that should be consistent, not specifically the behaviours linked to the routine. The behaviours and associated mental activity may need to be used flexibly depending on the initial mental state of the performer and the degree to which this differs from the ideal performance state. If a performer is already on a hot streak, he may not need to do much to get into an ideal state, but following a few mistakes doubts will occur and so obtaining an ideal state may be more difficult.

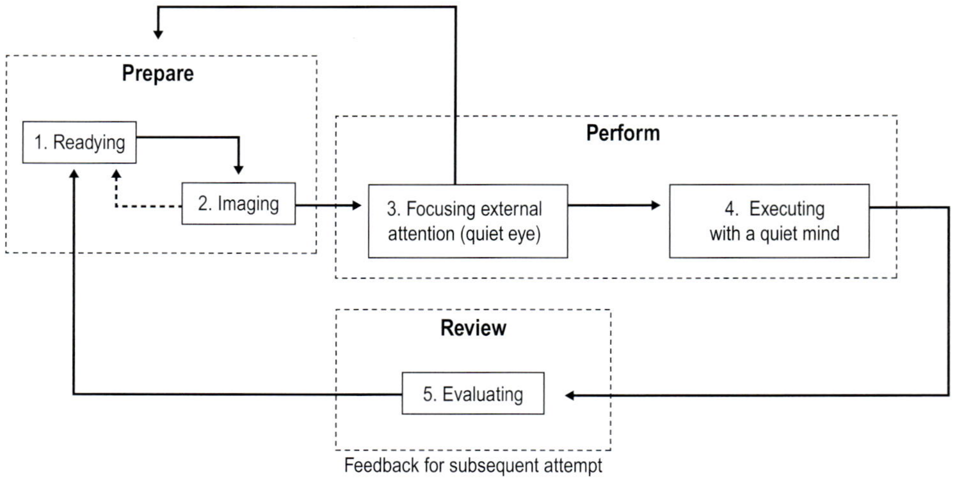

Fig. 23.4 • A flexible performance routine. Adapted, with permission, from R.N. Singer, 2002, Preperformance states, routines and automacity: What does it take to realize expertise in self-paced events? *Journal of Sport and Exercise Psychology* 24(4): 368.

For example, consider a golfer who usually 'waggles' his club three times prior to each shot (physical readying). He may use the cue words 'relax' (emotional readying), 'smooth' (a specific swing thought) and 'focus' (to direct focus to back of ball only) on each waggle. If, because of the demands of the situation, he still has doubts before he initiates his swing, it makes little sense to make the shot anyway, just because that is what the routine 'demands' should happen. The purpose of using a routine is to maintain control under pressure and so it would be more constructive to take one more waggle with a re-affirming thought or image, or perhaps even step back and repeat the whole routine (Fig. 23.4). The ability to consistently control our performance mental state is the goal we are seeking, not the ability to 'blindly' follow a set routine, or to run through a physically well choreographed set of movements while the brain races uncontrollably.

This flexible application may seem a little counterintuitive if performance routines are meant to be the same in different settings and help to make high-pressure performance 'feel' the same as a training environment. In reality, it is difficult to isolate the behaviour of the performer from the environment and context and even elite performers appear to adjust their routines slightly depending on the situation. As Aidan Moran highlighted in Chapter 22, the case study by Jackson & Baker (2001) investigating the consistency of the pre-kick routine of Neil Jenkins (at the time the world's leading point scorer in international rugby) demonstrated that he took longer on more difficult or more pressurized kicks. (These differences actually parallel similar patterns in physiological concomitants, such as heart rate deceleration.) Performers need to develop a consistent routine but also to recognize when a degree of flexibility is required to reach an optimal performance state.

Having discussed why a performance routine might be useful, we will now discuss the various techniques that might be adopted to help a performer maintain control of their performance state, starting with self-talk.

Self-talk

We spend a lot of time talking to ourselves, yet much of the time we are not aware of the existence of this internal dialogue, let alone its content. However, as there are strong links between our thoughts, our emotions and ultimately our actions, it is important that we regulate the information we provide to ourselves in the performance arena, via our self-talk. A colleague refers to this process as 'TEA-time' (Thoughts – Emotions – Actions; Moore 2000) and uses the phrase as a reminder to performers to check that their self-talk is constructive and likely to lead to an optimal performance state. Negative intrusions related to performance pressures may not feel voluntary, but performers *can* voluntarily do something to control these intrusions. It is necessary to learn to take control of thought processes and use self-talk appropriately to maximize the chance of achieving consistent and optimal performance; in short, performers need to take responsibility for TEA-time.

Self-talk has been defined as the 'internal dialogue in which individuals interpret feelings and perceptions, regulate and change evaluations and cognitions, and give themselves instruction and reinforcement' (Hackfort & Schwenkmezger 1993, p. 355). It has been called the key to cognitive control, and indeed the promotion of appropriate self-talk is commonly employed as a cognitive intervention in applied performance psychology (e.g. Zinsser et al 2006). However, there has been little systematic research in the area, and relatively little is known about the content of performers' self-talk (what they say), let alone where, when and why they use it (The '4Ws' of self-talk; Hardy et al 2005). As we are going to focus on the use of self-talk as part of a performance routine (where) in pressure settings (when), we will begin by exploring 'what' the content of self-talk might be and 'why' performers use it.

'What were they thinking?' – the content of self-talk

By far the most studied aspect of self-talk is the nature of the content; specifically, whether it is positive or negative (Hardy 2006). The general consensus amongst psychology consultants is that performers should adopt positive as opposed to negative self-talk (e.g. Zinsser et al 2006). This view stems, at least in part, from cognitive–behavioural therapy and the assumption that emotional problems result from maladaptive (negative) thought patterns (e.g. Beck 1976).The belief that positive, rather than negative, self-talk enhances performance has led to the implementation of a number of cognitive–behavioural techniques in the performance domain, namely thought stopping, cognitive restructuring and countering (see Zinsser et al 2006 for a detailed discussion of the use of cognitive–behavioural techniques in peak performance psychology).

So why should positive rather than negative self-talk assist performance? Positive self-talk may enhance performance through increases in confidence and anxiety control, whereas negative self-talk has been considered as being inappropriate, anxiety producing and counterproductive (Hatzigeorgiadis et al 2004). When examining the research findings relating to the content of self-talk, however, a more complex picture develops, with positive and negative self-talk both associated with both good and poor performance. For example, a recent study by Hamilton et al (2007) investigated the effect of positive and negative self-talk on performance in a cycling ergometer task. The results indicated that both forms of self-talk led to improved performance, in terms of total work completed in 20 minutes, compared to baseline conditions. Furthermore, in a study examining the self-talk of high-board divers, Highlen & Bennett (1983) found that elite divers actually reported using less positive self-talk than their non-elite counterparts.

Although it must be acknowledged that reviewing research into self-talk raises methodological concerns relating to different experimental designs and the susceptibility of performers to have biased or inaccurate recall, a number of reasons for these equivocal findings can be proposed. First, negative self-talk may only be harmful to the performance of certain individuals, since self-talk is a uniquely personal experience. The second reason is related to the function of self-talk and requires us to examine our second 'W', namely 'why' performers use self-talk.

Why do performers use self-talk?

Hackfort & Schwenkmezger's definition of self-talk highlights two main reasons why it might be used: instructional and motivational functions. Instructional self-talk is used by performers to help them both learn and execute individual skills and strategies. Instructional self-talk has long been proposed as a useful strategy in performance settings to focus attention on key aspects of performance (see Ch. 22). Self-talk helps athletes stay focused, not dwell on past errors, and remain in the present. Motivational self-talk, on the other hand, can be used in a general sense to maintain or increase drive and effort, to regulate arousal or to set an ideal mental set (in terms of mental toughness, confidence and focus).

The type of performance being undertaken will obviously have an influence on which type of self-talk is likely to be of most benefit. For example, research by Hatzigeorgiadis et al (2004) and Theodorakis et al (2000) found that the performance of motor tasks, requiring skill, timing and accuracy was enhanced to a greater extent by instructional self-talk (focusing on technical aspects of performance), than motivational self-talk. A purely endurance task, for example, may benefit more from motivational self-talk designed to maintain effort under extreme physiological demands. However, practitioners should be aware that it is an oversimplification to suggest that performers would not use both forms of self-talk, especially in competition or performance settings where both an ideal mental set (through motivational self-talk) and attention to suitable targets or strategies (through instructional self-talk) are required. Below is an example of such combination self-talk use, provided by an elite wrestler.

> With everything that I'm thinking before the match – instead of thinking about everything else negative – I'm saying 'OK, what you gotta do is go out, you gotta move, you gotta get to the "corner", you gotta stay on this guy for six minutes, go hard', telling myself, 'I win' out loud so my subconscious gets it. Tell myself to win at all costs.
>
> Eklund et al 1993, p. 44

Negative self-talk, negative performance?

While performance psychologists generally suggest that self-talk should be worded positively (e.g. Hardy et al 1996), this may depend very much on the purpose of the self-talk. Perhaps instructional self-talk should be worded in a positive manner in order to direct the performer's attention to the important cues and to avoid the potential for negative, ironic processing effects (Janelle 1999 and Ch. 22). Therefore, a golfer should phrase his pre-shot self-talk as 'Hit it down the middle', as opposed to 'Don't hit it in the water'. However, as discussed by Hamilton et al (2007), if the self-talk has a motivational purpose, it may not matter whether the phrasing is positive or negative. What is more important is the individual's preference for the type of self-statement they want to use and their interpretation of the content. For example, an endurance runner may find it more motivational to say 'Don't give up!' than 'Keep going! Stick at it!'

Although we will examine the practicalities of self-talk interventions in more detail later, it is worth taking stock of the discussion to date from a performer and practitioner viewpoint. It would appear from the research presented that positive content is generally productive in nature, so it is the safe option to ensure that self-talk has a positive impact. If a performer feels that negative self-talk is more motivational to them personally, then it is appropriate to use it. If instructional self-talk is required, be aware of the risks (e.g. ironic processing effects) of

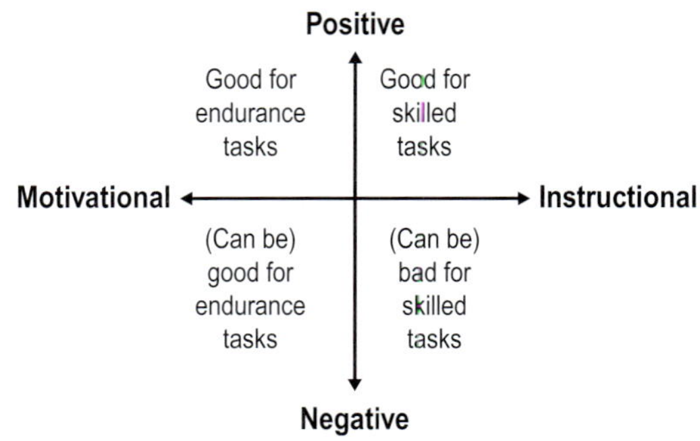

Fig. 23.5 • Types of self-talk: The vertical axis represents the 'what' and the vertical axis the 'why' of self-talk use.

adopting negatively phrased self-statements. We can summarize our discussion of the 'what' and 'why' of self-talk in Figure 23.5.

Prevention, cure or enhancement?

Much of the advice from performance psychologists with relation to self-talk interventions follows a similar theme, based on cognitive behavioural techniques (e.g. Zinsser et al 2006). First, it is important to identify self-defeating or irrational self-talk, then try and rationalize the thought processes, before finally replacing the negative thoughts with more productive ones. In this way, performers learn to take control of their thoughts with the positive impact this is likely to have on subsequent emotions and actions.

While this is a useful technique to apply in performance settings, it reflects a 'cure' as opposed to 'prevention' (or even 'enhancement') strategy. In the performance arena, the aim is not just to limit the negative influence of self-defeating thoughts but to attempt to create optimal mental and emotional states (TEA-time). Performers should therefore develop and fine-tune suitably motivating or instructional 'trigger' words or phrases in advance of performance in pressure environments. Because anxiety can make performers focus on what might go wrong (possible negative consequences) rather on what they should do right now, suitable cues can help performers focus on specific actions that can be performed in the moment – the processes underlying performance.

Hardy et al (1996) report an excellent example of how this focus on process in competition conditions might operate. When skier Tommy Moe was asked by the media prior to his Olympic gold medal performance whether he was thinking about winning, he indicated that he certainly wanted to win but had found in the past that when he thought about winning while racing he tightened up and did not perform well. He commented that he skied at his best when he focused on 'letting his outside ski run' and keeping his 'hands out in front' of himself. This example highlights the importance of focusing on what has to be done (the present moment), not on the desired outcome.

A focus on process

The benefits of using self-talk to provide a task-specific (process) focus in pressure environments are that self-talk is under the performer's control, can be very flexible and can be applied to any performance setting. In self-paced skills especially, self-talk may take the form of a cue-word or brief phrase directing the performer to attend to a specific aspect of the environment (e.g. 'Watch the ball'), their technique (e.g. 'Follow through'), or their mental set in terms of energy or mood (e.g. 'Blast', 'Easy', 'Hold on to it').

In more complex environments (fast-moving team sports, for example), process goals can still be useful, without having to be overly complex or numerous (i.e. you don't need one for every eventuality). For example, a useful way to continue to maintain focus even when anxious is to continually ask oneself 'What's my next job?' or to focus on the 'next 3 seconds'. Performers sometimes find it difficult to think about trying to maintain an appropriate focus over a full performance, which might last hours in some cases. However, this sort of process goal allows a performer to break performance down into manageable chunks and keep focused in the present. (See above on segmenting performances.)

There are potentially two concerns with adopting process-oriented self-talk, both of which can be refuted to a degree. The first concern is related to the predictions of the conscious processing hypothesis (Masters 1992), which suggests that skilled performance will deteriorate if performers try to exert conscious control over movements that were previously under automatic control. The mechanism behind this deterioration is the reinvestment in explicit rules about the way in which the skill should be performed (see Ch.13). Explicit rules are a form of verbalizable process goal, so it could be argued that the use of process goals may be counterproductive in pressured environments (e.g. Jackson et al 2006).

However, while a series of instructional cues during the completion of a skill may cause a performer to focus on the step-by-step mechanics of its performance, the use of one holistic cue should actually prevent such reinvestment occurring. For example, while a single holistic instructional cue (e.g. 'Smooth') might reflect a focus on the movement pattern being carried out, the focus is not on the step-by-step mechanics of the movement (e.g. head down; left arm straight; weight on back foot; etc.). Under pressure, therefore, a holistic cue may protect the performer from the potentially debilitating effects of reinvestment, as opposed to a situation where reinvestment may occur if no organized self-talk is in place. Again, the use of appropriate, proactive self-talk reflects a strategy of prevention, as opposed to thinking about having to deal with the consequences of reinvestment (cure). (These ideas are also examined by MacPherson et al 2009 and discussed in Ch. 13.)

The second concern refers to the fact that performers reliably report that peak performance states (e.g. flow; Jackson 2000), are characterized by a lack of conscious thought processes. Why, therefore, try to 'force' performers to actively think about what they are doing? Well, unfortunately, peak performance states are extremely rare, and individuals *do* tend to think when performing, especially in pressure settings. For this reason it is important to have a 'Plan B' if 'Plan A' (peak performance) doesn't work out. It is better to have some strategies planned to help direct attention and mental set in a productive way than discover that you have allowed the situation to affect your performance. The concept of TEA-time is useful here, in that it can act as a reminder that our thought processes are not automatically determined by the situation but that we can have control over them. By proactively managing our self-talk we can influence our emotional state and attentional set, which in turn will impact upon our subsequent performance (i.e. performance enhancement).

However, when performers are on a hot streak or having an amazing performance, it is probably not the time to try and 'force' self-talk interventions into the mix – they are not needed. There is no point trying to build confidence through self-talk if a performer is already experiencing peak performance or forcefully directing attention if it is already appropriate. However, helping performers be more consistent is often just as important for psychology support as helping performers improve their level of performance. If performers tend to be inconsistent and let the environment impact on their performance levels, then appropriate self-talk may assist in achieving a more consistent starting point for performance. Also, as described by Singer (2002), appropriate self-talk as part of a routine just prior to performance creates the environment by which an optimal performance state (e.g. flow) is more likely to occur subsequently.

Imagery

The use of motor imagery and observation for enhancing performance through mental practice has been discussed in detail in Chapter 16. However, in this section we want to briefly discuss the way in which performers can use imagery during performance as part of a flexible performance routine (Fig. 23.4). Singer (2002) explicitly included imagery as the second step of his five-step performance routine with the purpose of seeing and feeling the desired result prior to performing. Anecdotal support comes from golfer Tiger Woods, who proclaimed that 'You have to see the shots and feel them through your hands' before addressing the ball (Pitt 1998, p. 5).

In a similar fashion to self-talk, performers tend to use imagery for both instructional and motivational purposes. From an instructional viewpoint, imagery can be thought of as mental rehearsal and task-relevant focusing, allowing a performer to get a sense of what the performance might look and feel like (as described by Tiger Woods). From a motivational viewpoint, imagery can be used for arousal regulation (see next section) and also to set an ideal mental set (attention and confidence). As with self-talk, performers are likely to use imagery for both purposes in pressured settings. For example, attaching a positive outcome image to technical mental rehearsal will not only allow the performer to plan the actions to be carried out (instructional) but will create a confident and appropriately focused state (motivational). As Holmes & Calmels commented in Chapter 16, imagining an event has a similar effect on the brain's structures to performing the event in reality. As well as drilling the body, imagery during a routine can also 'trick' us into believing that we have performed successfully once and can therefore do it again, thus increasing confidence and reducing anxiety.

Arousal control

Arousal control is another key element of a peak performance state, and the aim of any performance routine is to try and ensure that an appropriate level of arousal is attained during performance. For this reason we are not going to consider activities that may be useful for regulating arousal in the build-up to performance (e.g. listening to music, progressive muscular relaxation scripts), as it is possible that a painstakingly created ideal state might be 'blown away' because of the changing demands of the situation during performance. Also, we would suggest that techniques designed to achieve deep relaxation are not appropriate close in time to performance itself, as deep, relaxed states are unlikely to be achievable (or appropriate for successful physical performance). We are therefore going to focus on a particular technique that can be applied briefly (as part of a routine) to help performers (re)control their arousal at the 'point of pressure'.

Reducing arousal – maintaining composure, regaining control

The ability to relax in pressure environments is often considered to be a key psychological skill for top-level performers, so that they may control their emotional response to these demands (e.g. Hardy et al 1996). While the principle behind this ideal (i.e. controlling responses to stress) may be appropriate, the idea that performers are relaxed during pressure events is unrealistic. In Chapter 22, Moran highlighted the example of Ronan O'Gara, who reflected that his heart rate might be 115 beats a minute in a game compared to the (more relaxed) 90–100 in training. Jonny Wilkinson (2003; England out-half) has been even more graphic in his description of his state of 'relaxation': 'You can actually see your shirt moving over your heart, the way your heart is beating. There's no way I stand there and kick in a game and I am perfectly relaxed. My heart is beating like mad.' As both these individuals have performed at the highest level, it can't be their inability to 'relax' under pressure that is holding them back. Neither Jonny nor Ronan may have been able to achieve a relaxed state when performing but they both maintain their *composure* and sense of *control*, and this is what the following technique seeks to achieve.

Breathing and breath control

'Breathing' may not be a revolutionary psychological technique but the control of breathing depth and rate is an effective (and simple) strategy for dealing with pressure. Again, we are back to that word 'control', and that is what makes a focus on breathing such a useful intervention for athletes who might be feeling that the demands of a stressful situation are getting to them. A performer who takes a moment 'out' to focus on breathing, ensuring it is deep and slow, is one who is regaining control of themselves and their composure. As experienced sport psychologist Ken Ravizza (2002, p. 10) comments, 'You have to be in control of yourself before you can control your performance... self-control leads to body control, which leads to skill control'. This is why breath control as a means of self-regulation is often a useful first intervention to explore with performers – it allows them to 'win back' some control.

Williams & Harris (2006) state that performers who are feeling stressed tend to find their breathing affected in one of two ways: either they hold their breath or they breathe rapidly and shallowly from the upper chest. These changes to the breathing pattern can create even more tension and impairment in performance. Learning to take a deep, slow, complete breath is relatively simple and can even be choreographed into pre-performance routines or the performance of certain skills. There are a variety of breathing exercises and techniques, many taken from Eastern martial arts practices, and some of these are outlined by Williams & Harris. However, the underlying principle is the concept of a *complete breath,* with the inhalation starting with the downward movement of the diaphragm. This pushes the abdomen out and creates a vacuum in the lungs, ensuring that the lungs fill up from the bottom.

To practise a deep complete breath, imagine that your lungs are divided into three parts. First fill up the bottom third with air by pushing the diaphragm down and your abdomen out; fill up the middle third by expanding the chest cavity and raising the rib cage; and finally fill the upper portion by raising the chest and shoulders slightly. The entire breath should progress smoothly and continuously before a pause is taken for several seconds at the end of the inhalation. Then exhale by pulling the abdomen in and lowering the shoulders and chest until all air is forced from the lungs. You should imagine that the lungs are emptying out the bottom, with the upper part emptying first, then the middle, then the bottom third. This point, at the end of the exhalation and before the next inhalation is the quietest moment of the breath and the point where it can be useful to reaffirm the feelings of composure you are trying to achieve ('centering'). In this way, appropriate, individually developed self-statements and imagery can be used to reinforce the feelings of composure gained from breath control. The performance routine is simply a means of ordering and coordinating these processes to achieve the optimal performance state.

Gaze control

The third step of Singer's routine relates to focus and, as Moran emphasized in Chapter 22, focused attention is best achieved by selecting one appropriate external cue. Maintaining attention on an external target helps prevent attentional disruption from non-productive (internal) thoughts and emotions. In addition, Vickers (Ch. 14) discussed how emerging research from cognitive and neural science shows a strong relationship between shifts of gaze and shifts of attentional focus, thus helping to provide an explanation for how focus and concentration contributes to physical performance.

Optimal visual attention: the quiet eye

Vickers (1996) identified a critical aspect of performers' visual attention, the 'quiet eye', defined as the final fixation on a target before the initiation of final movement. Theoretically, longer quiet eye periods allow performers an extended duration of processing of target information while minimizing distraction from other environmental cues. Vickers (2007) summarizes a number of studies that show that the quiet eye of elite performers is both earlier and longer than that of non-elite performers and is also longer during successful compared to non-successful performance. For example, during the preparation of an accurate basketball free throw, gaze is directed to a single location on the hoop (usually the front) and the fixation is maintained on that location for an optimal duration (approximately 1 second for this task). While this may seem like a rather obvious strategy to adopt, performers don't always control their gaze appropriately. Vickers (2007) reported that highly skilled basketball players tend to use fewer fixations during shots than less skilled performers, and fewer fixations on accurate shots than on inaccurate shots. The area over which the gaze is controlled on the target is also smaller for elite performers. To summarize; when performing successfully, experts focus on one key target and don't let their gaze 'wander' around a number of locations in the vicinity of the target.

While it is one thing to be able to highlight differences in gaze strategy between successful and unsuccessful performance, it is another to demonstrate that gaze control can be improved through appropriate training. Vickers and colleagues have previously demonstrated that the quiet eye can indeed be trained and that such training can contribute to large improvements in performance in a number of sports. For example, Harle & Vickers (2001) trained members of an elite basketball team to improve their gaze control during task execution of the free throw, through quiet eye training. Performers were guided to orient their gaze to the hoop as soon as possible and maintain this fixation for about 1 second (by saying 'Sight. . .focus'). They were instructed that the stability of the quiet eye on one location was crucial and used self-talk ('Nothing but net') and imagery (ball going in to the basket) to assist in the development of a positive mental state.

Effects of pressure

The scientific evidence confirms that pressure can influence attention (see Ch. 22), so this impact should also be reflected in changes in gaze behaviour, such as the quiet eye. Recent research (e.g. Behan & Wilson 2008, Vickers & Williams 2007, Wilson et al 2009) has demonstrated that the quiet eye period can be negatively impacted by increased pressure (i.e. made shorter), and this is associated with reduced performance. Performers tend to react to increased pressure by shortening their quiet eye period and moving their gaze around the target vicinity, rather than keeping it stable. Such a finding might be explained by Eysenck and colleagues' (2007) attentional control theory, which suggests that anxiety impairs a performer's ability to maintain goal-directed attention and inhibit distractions (see Wilson 2008).

Behan & Wilson (2008) argued that performance routines should therefore incorporate quiet eye control components to enhance attentional capabilities in stressful environments. By maintaining an effective visual orientation, through controlling the quiet eye, the negative effects of anxiety on performance may be alleviated. First, longer quiet eye periods extend subconscious processing of target information related to optimal performance (Vickers 2007). Second, by focusing externally on a target, rather than on the step-by-step mechanics of the performance, choking due to reinvestment should be prevented (Masters 1992). Third, the work of Wulf and colleagues (e.g. Wulf 2007) suggests that superior performance is linked with an external focus, which, in the case of quiet eye control, is achieved through vision. Finally, Singer (2002) suggests that a longer target fixation period serves primarily as a means of self-regulation to enter and sustain an optimal attentional state for performing. Whichever the mechanism, it is evident that performers should seek to create a quiet focus on a single external target to maintain optimal control and create the conditions for consistent, non-conscious, 'just do it' performance execution (step 4 of Singer's strategy).

Evaluating performance

The final phase of our routine and step 5 of Singer's strategy (Fig. 23.4) reflects a review process and the evaluation of performance. For performers to learn and develop they need to get accurate feedback on their performances. It is important that this is done relatively soon after performance to (1) maximize the benefits (the association between feedback and the event are more powerful the closer in time they are – an idea referred to by behavioural psychologists as *temporal contiguity*!) and (2) minimize any detrimental effects where performance outcomes have not been positive. Minimizing detrimental effects can be achieved by identifying positive subcomponents of performance, understanding what can be focused on to enhance future performances and ensuring the time spent reviewing performance is organized and limited so performers can 'move on' and prevent too much self-damning introspection. However, evaluation can quickly become resented and avoided by performers if it is perceived as a lengthy, burdensome chore; as time when they will receive negative comments and feel slighted, belittled or embarrassed; or as an unfocused waste of time. To counter these problems, Table 23.2 offers some principles to govern performance evaluation.

Table 23.2 Principles for evaluating performance

Performer-centred	Performers must be instrumentally involved and central to the process by providing and obtaining informative feedback, contributing to decisions about what the focus should be *For example, in rugby teams key players may be asked to review specific aspects of the game and isolate examples of good versus bad and relate back to fellow players and coaches key points and training implications*
Learning and development	Emphasis must be continually on learning how to improve. It is easy to focus on working out what went wrong and then to fall into the trap of blaming performers for mistakes. This will result in performers feeling defensive, learning less and concentrating on avoiding mistakes in the next performance
Cultural norm	Evaluations should follow every performance, good or bad. All performers and key staff must be expected and encouraged to offer and invite constructive criticism *For example, recent involvement with an elite military air display team revealed how central evaluation was to their performance culture. Rank, age and experience presented no barriers and comments were matter-of-fact, carefully considered by the team and remained focused on learning and development without threat of personal rancour*
Practical	Evaluation sessions should be time-efficient (too long and concentration will decrease), easy to complete, focused and well conducted
Process, not results	Evaluations should not be overly influenced by the outcome of performance and should identify what was done well and badly to reinforce the former and change the latter. An overall successful performance could have just as many learning points as an unsuccessful one but it frequently happens that good outcomes are followed by celebrations rather than by evaluation that will help learn how to do it again!
Confidential	Good evaluation is most likely to occur in an environment of trust where performers know that what is discussed does not become public knowledge and is not noted and recorded for other purposes (e.g. selection or contract renewal). Having people sit in on sessions may weaken this confidentiality so only those actively involved as participants in the evaluation process should be present

A key part of the evaluation involves an audit of both preparation and performance plans. This audit can be based on identifying answers to the following questions:

- Did the plan cover everything?
- What was planned but not done? Change required?
- What was done but not planned? Changes required?
- What factors caused main disruption to the plan?

Written plans can be efficiently used in the style of a checklist to complete this audit. While this can be done by a performer independently, evaluation is more effective when completed with, or at least reported back to, a psychologist, performance manager or equivalent to provide the necessary level of challenge and to control over- or underanalysis. In performances involving a large number of performers (corps, team or group) a buddy system or senior players can be used to ensure this takes place across all of the performers involved.

Performance data

Objective performance data, when available, can play a key role in evaluating performance, but the principle 'Process not results' must be kept in mind. Performance data are common in the sports domain but comparatively rare (and hard to establish) in other performance arenas such as dance or mountaineering. Times, distances, weight are simple performance data that avoid outcome focus through comparison with others, but these can be applied more effectively by zoning performance achievements in relation to preplanned targets. For example, increasing percentages towards a specified level, such as personal best, can offer performers graded levels of evaluation (Satisfactory, Good, Excellent) rather than simply success or failure (Collins & MacPherson 2007). The percentages can be adjusted to reflect other factors such as physical training status or return from injury and this would help performers avoid making unrealistic comparisons with ideals.

Performance data can also be analysed to examine performance aspects such as consistency and variation. The example in Figure 23.6, developed by former world champion codriver Robert Reid, shows performance data from a 3-day rally and uses the number of seconds per kilometre behind the winner of each stage as the variable of interest. The graph shows the times of the performer (who neither expected nor planned to challenge for a podium place), the average of a target group (selected from the field by performer and manager) and the overall winner of the rally. Using these data, the performer was able to identify six specific stages (circled on graph) where his speed deviated from the trend of the comparison group. The absolute speeds were not critical but stages where times were slower while the average speed of the target group was faster became the focus for more in-depth review. The graph also easily illustrates stages where speeds were closest to the stage winners (stages 8, 12 and 13), prompting evaluation of what was done well here. In this case, analysis of the overall winner was also instructive as it showed a progressive easing into performance in the first few stages, perhaps enabling acclimatization to conditions and changes in the car setup.

This graph demonstrates how performance data can be utilized with a high focus on process rather than outcome and with the capacity to identify specific components of performance to focus on. Furthermore, the simple presentation enables this element of evaluation to be completed quickly and easily. The graph also illustrates how it is possible to set targets to develop greater consistency so that, for example, achieving speeds less than 1.2 s/km slower than the stage winner would provide a meaningful goal for the performer. In this rally, five of 14 stages (36%) fell outside this target, so setting graded levels better than this (e.g. as above: Satisfactory, Good, Excellent) could be used to evaluate future performances.

Many performers and teams generate performance data from video analysis completed with stylized software to present potentially large numbers of statistics on performance. Two critical issues with this practice are to ensure that the information provided to performers is (1) *limited*, to avoid overload, and (2) *focused*, to ensure that the aspects selected are critical to performance, reflect current training aims and are appropriate to the performer (s) in the specific context. For example a performer required for a given performance to fulfil a specific,

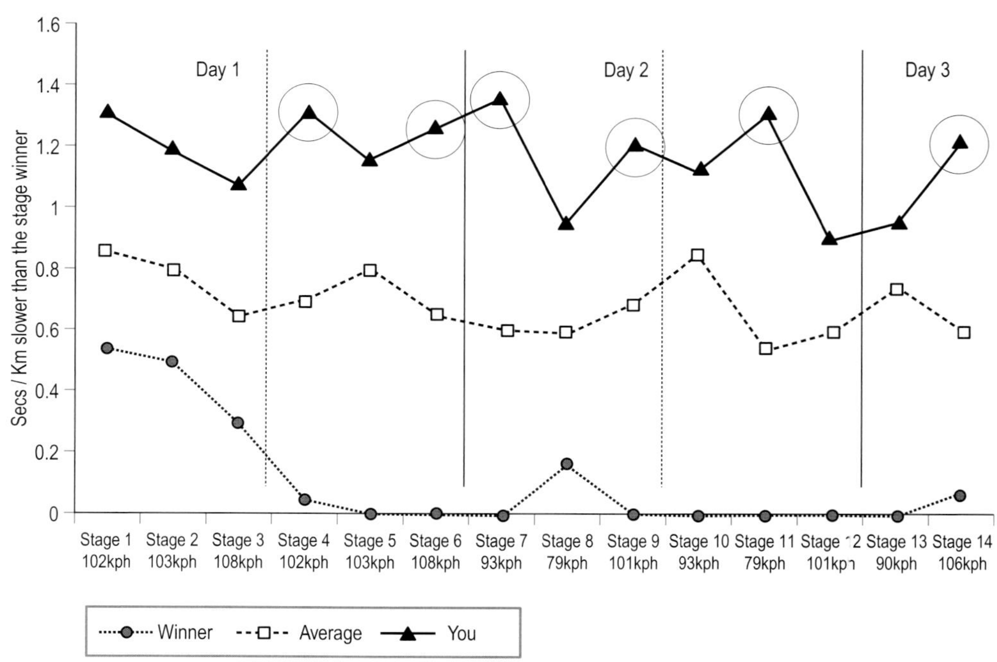

Fig. 23.6 • Analysis of performance data for a rally driver.

unusual role should not be judged on how well they performed other roles that might have demands conflicting with the ones they were assigned to. It is salient to note that some aspects of performance and high-visibility roles are naturally considered more desirable than others and contain inherent reinforcement for success. Performance evaluation can help to redress the balance by focusing on essential but less desirable roles and providing subsequent reward for good performance. For example, in team sport, scoring inevitably attracts attention so a professional rugby team made sure evaluation included a focus on defensive tackling to raise the perceived importance and esteem attributed to this crucial task (Richards & Richards 2002).

Performance criteria

In many physical performance domains performance data may not be available, or collecting information may be too costly in time, labour and equipment. Furthermore, data may not show the performance factors of primary concern to a performer on the basis of their current level, training or performance goals. A simple, practical solution to this is to use performance criteria, an idea developed and introduced to me by Richard L. Cox (personal communication, 2000) to evaluate performance. In this technique criteria are identified, in advance, that are representative of essential behaviours for optimal performance.

All criteria must be clear, observable behaviours that could realistically be assessed by a knowledgeable observer. This means terms like 'effective', 'quickly', 'confidently', which are open to interpretation and/or are hard to judge, must not be included. Selected criteria are not intended to provide an exhaustive list of performance factors but to be representative of key facets of performance. Consequently, it is highly likely that if all criteria are performed well then the overall performance will be good too. Selection may also reflect factors specifically targeted in current training or development plans. Criteria selected should reflect the breadth of performance demands, but avoid selecting too many and causing the subsequent evaluation process to become too cumbersome or lose focus.

Identifying representative performance criteria needs to be completed by the performer, under guidance, in order to ensure that they have ownership of the system and the criteria. As a guide, about eight to 10 criteria should be sufficient to address key facets of performance. Being able to establish what essential features of performance characterize good performances is a self-regulatory activity (see Ch. 20) and so learning how to do this under guidance can be construed as one way of achieving this aspect of self-regulation. Guidance also needs to focus on training the performer to describe behavioural rather than cognitive elements of performance so that they can realistically be evaluated by others too. Cognitive aspects can be evaluated more effectively by other means such as a think-aloud protocol using a video replay of performance. Typically, the process of identifying criteria is achieved through a repeated series of revisions (iterations) to achieve unambiguous, observable and representative criteria. Table 23.3 shows the development through an iterative process of a criterion for a badminton player.

Following performance, with sufficient time lapse to think clearly but not so much as to forget, the performer can rate themselves on how well each criterion was achieved (e.g. scale 1–10). This activity helps to increase self-monitoring and awareness of performance. Ratings can also be obtained from another who observed or could reasonably evaluate the performer. This could be another performer, manager, director or coach. Discussing discrepancies can help to identify future training and performance goals and when used with fellow performers the technique can aid the development of shared understanding (coherence), necessary for interactive performance teams. Performance criteria can be modified as performers develop, and be made appropriate to changing performance situations. In this way they can act as a form of goal setting and, for a team of performers, enhance task cohesion (see Chs 7, 8 and 24). Finally, performance criteria can provide the basis for the content of self-talk (see above), identifying specific task-relevant behaviours for performers to remind themselves of during performance and to maintain or regain attention (see the feedback loop element of Fig 23.4).

Table 23.3 The process of refining performance criteria through several stages

Initial criteria	Second attempt	Final criteria
Effective use of overhead shots; not predictable; challenge opponent	Variety of shots from overhead	Overhead shot placement on at least three different zones per match

Video-based evaluation

While performance criteria retain a strong behavioural basis to allow rating by others, it is clear that, for psychologists especially, mental activity is also important to review. One technique that can be employed to achieve this is video-based, stimulated recall (Gilbert et al 1994). Video footage can prompt thorough and detailed recall of mental activity prior to and during critical performance episodes. Being able to pause the playback enables the performer to explain decision making that might occur too rapidly to explain in real time. This process can be used to evaluate the accuracy of planned pre-performance routines, discussed earlier in this chapter, and to make necessary modifications or suggest additional practice and training requirements.

It is not uncommon for videos of performance to be given to performers without structure for analysis or any specific guidance. This can be a waste, as Bandura (1986, p. 51) noted that 'people cannot learn much by observation unless they attend to accurately perceive relevant aspects'. Unless the performer is very capable and knows what to look out for (can self-analyse and self-coach), providing video footage may be less effective than simply reminding performers of basic cues for a skill or movement. Unpublished preliminary investigative work by Adams (2006) showed that the flip-turn of experienced freestyle swimmers consistently improved when evaluation combined video replay with coach-identified attentional cues for future turns. Less effective was coach-identified attentional cues without video, and least effective was the performer just watching the video of their performance. The implication is that video alone has potentially the least benefit for enhancing performance yet may represent the biggest cost in time (to make and watch) and in technology. Although it may seem to provide a tempting feedback solution to those working with performers (especially larger groups and teams), using video alone needs to be considered very carefully in terms of both effectiveness and efficiency.

Cycle of performance development

Whatever option is chosen to evaluate performance, it should be stressed that evaluation is critical for performers to learn, develop and progress. Plans, performance data, performance criteria and video-based evaluations have all been outlined within this section. In addition to this, verbal debriefs and checklists can be used to good effect and easily conform to the principles outlined. Evaluation provides the essential link between performance and training/practice. Similarly planning and preparation occur as an output of good evaluations and in preparation for performance. These combine into a cycle of learning, development and enhanced performance (Fig. 23.7).

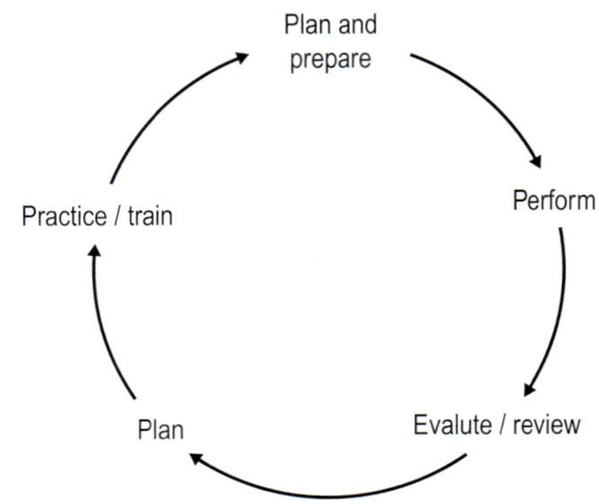

Fig. 23.7 • Cycle of performance development.

Bringing it all together: be 'safe' under pressure

Throughout this chapter, various approaches and mental skills have been described to help set an environment for the consistent attainment of optimal performance. There is very clear overlap in many of these areas: evaluation through performance criteria assists in the construction of self-talk; self-talk is a component of performance routines and routines may use focusing through gaze control. This overlap is understandable and to be expected because the single purpose of these skills is to maintain and enhance performance and so they converge towards this aim. This is particularly well illustrated in the case of performance routines, where a combination of techniques (breath control, self-talk and imagery) may be integrated into the 'Prepare' phase of the routine (steps 1 and 2 of Singer's strategy) in a manner that 'works' best for the individual concerned.

While the content is individual-specific it might be useful to consider the mnemonic SAFE as a reminder of the key elements of using a routine to maintain control under pressure:

- S: **Set** an optimal performance state (through breath control, self-talk and imaging techniques)
- A: **Adjust** routine if necessary (if optimal state has not been reached by 'standard' routine)

- **F: Focus** with a quiet eye (direct attention to key external target)
- **E: Execute** with a quiet mind (let conscious control go – 'just do it!')

Ultimately, the skills and approaches are tools that can be used in various ways and combinations to help performers meet the demands and pressures of achieving optimal performances.

Individual specificity: one size does not fit all

One further important message is to emphasize the need to ensure that psychological tools are applied appropriately to individuals. By way of an example: if a performer has a non-verbal cognitive preference, the practitioner's time would be better spent constructing an intervention strategy with an emphasis on imagery, as opposed to self-talk. Similarly, if the performer struggles to produce vivid and controllable images, then verbalized cue words may be more appropriate. This point reflects the importance of working with a performer to develop the most appropriate intervention to deal with the specific concerns and preferences they may have, not rehashing something that worked well previously with another performer.

The importance of a focus on individualized development was also raised in our discussion of negatively phrased motivational self-talk. We highlighted how the interpretation of the content of self-talk may be more important than the content itself (i.e. is it positive or negative?). It may be that, for some individuals, negative self-talk is not self-defeating but is instead interpreted as being challenging and motivational in nature. It is therefore important to consider exactly what the performer is trying to gain from their use of self-talk (the why), rather than simply focusing on the content (the what). By trying to force a performer to adopt positively worded self-statements, because that is what 'the research says', you may limit the motivational impact of the technique. This may not only limit performance but will also reduce the performer's trust in your understanding of their individualized needs.

We will finish this section with a final example (and warning) of why performance psychologists need to be careful not to try and force a specific psychological technique upon a performer simply because other psychologists or performers have found it to be useful. A news item in *The Psychologist* (Anonymous 2003) discussed the case of a seven-times world bowling champion and twice Commonwealth gold medallist who refused to attend national squad relaxation sessions run by the team psychologist. She was subsequently dropped from the team for failing to attend scheduled training sessions. This sorry story provides a few lessons for all performance consultants in terms of individualizing psychological techniques. Should we not be learning from such performers who have achieved success at the highest levels, not alienating them? Why should we think that group relaxation sessions are going to be relevant and effective for everyone in a squad? As the (female) bowler pithily commented, 'If I am going to lie on my back for an hour, I expect to be enjoying myself!' (Fig. 23.8).

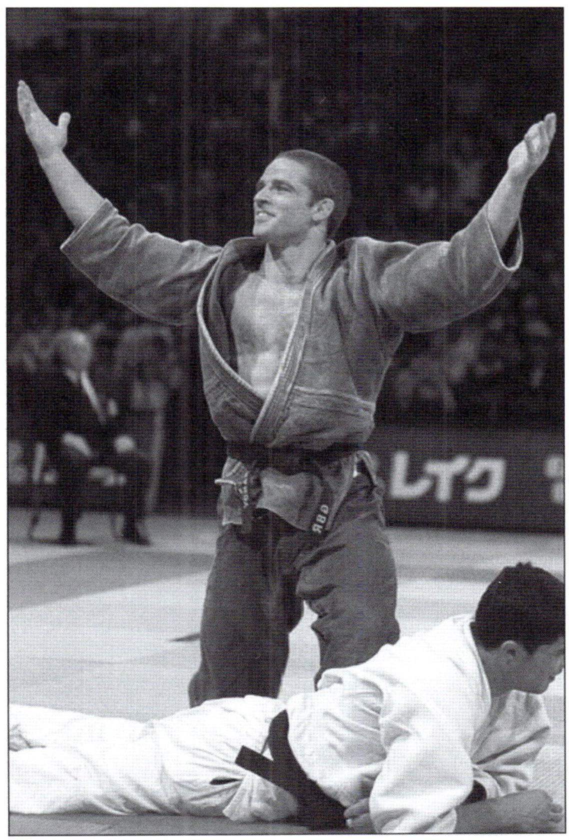

Fig. 23.8 • It's great when everything works. Graeme Randall celebrates winning Gold at the 1999 World Championships. © judosports.com and David Finch Photographs, with thanks.

Conclusion

All the techniques discussed in this chapter require practice in training before being unleashed in the pressure environment where the skills *must* be available if, and when, required (Fig. 23.9). Performers would not try out a new technical skill on the day of their most important performance without having drilled it in practice first. The same is true for mental skills, so, for example, a performance routine requires similar attention and fine-tuning in the practice arena and in lower-level performance opportunities. In this way, minor adjustments and improvements can be made to the techniques adopted, as well as the flow between these individual techniques making up the performance routine. Such practice will also lead to a level of automaticity, whereby the routine is automatically 'switched on' each time the performer is in a pressure situation. As we discussed earlier in the chapter, however, we need to leave some room for adjustments to the routine, to account for occasions when the optimal performance mental state does not occur following the 'standard' routine. 'What if?' planning may be a useful strategy to prepare for what steps should be taken when this situation does arise, so that the best chance for optimal performance is provided. In this way, the performer attempts to maintain control of the situation, even when external events may be raging out of control.

One final point, which may seem trite but is important in terms of our mantra of control being critical, is that it is important to maintain perspective in the face of pressure. Most performers choose to be there and enjoy the buzz of performing. By putting yourself out there for evaluation it is always possible that your performance does not match your aspirations. However, after a disappointing performance, you can control how you respond to that disappointment. Michael Johnson reflects the importance of perspective, having just failed to qualify for the 1992 Olympic 200 m final when he was favourite to win: 'Sure it was important to me, but to who else? The sun will be out tomorrow and the stars and the moon will be out tonight. It was only a race.' Guess what happened in 1996?

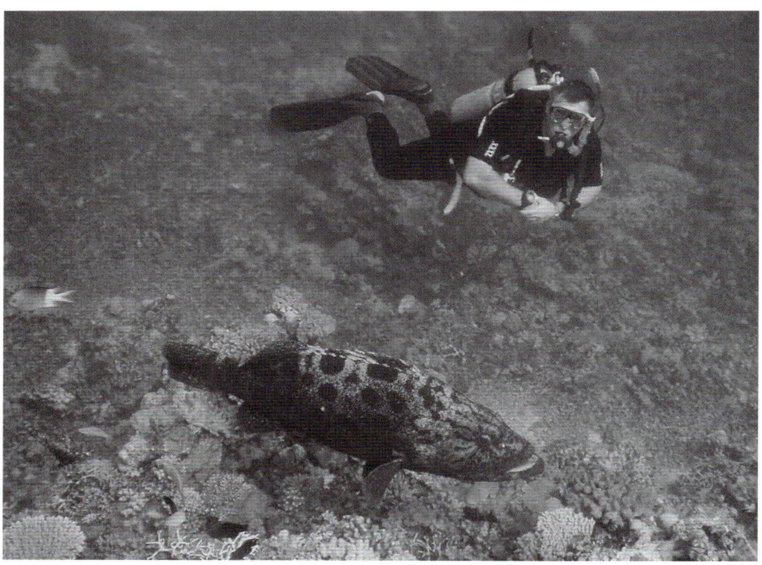

Fig. 23.9 • Low pressure. . .until it all goes wrong! Many outdoor adventure sports carry low risk so long as it is under control. So with Dave Collins underwater (he's the one with the tank).

References

Adams, D., 2006. Videotape replay as a method of feedback in the enhancement of the freestyle flip-turn. MSc thesis, University of Edinburgh.

Anonymous, 2003. Not bowled over by sport psychology. Psychologist 16, 117.

Bandura, A., 1986. Social foundations of thought and action: a social cognitive theory. Prentice Hall, Englewood Cliffs, NJ.

Beck, A.T., 1976. Cognitive therapy and emotional disorders. International Universities Press, New York.

Behan, M., Wilson, M., 2008. State anxiety and visual attention: the role of the quiet eye period in aiming to a far target. J. Sports Sci. 26, 207–215.

Boutcher, S.H., Rotella, R.J., 1987. A psychological skills educational program for closed-skill performance enhancement. Sport Psychologist 1, 127–137.

Collins, D., MacPherson, A., 2007. Psychological factors of physical preparation. In: Blumestein, B., Lidor, R., Tenenbaum, G. (Eds.), Psychology of sport training. Myer & Myer Sport, Oxford, pp. 40–55.

Eklund, R.C., Gould, D., Jackson, S.A., 1993. Psychological foundations of Olympic wrestling excellence: reconciling individual differences and nomothetic characterization. J. Appl. Sport Psychol. 5, 35–47.

Eysenck, M.W., Derakshan, N., Santos, R., et al., 2007. Anxiety and cognitive performance: attentional control theory. Emotion 7, 336–353.

Gilbert, W., Trudel, P., Bloom, G., 1994. Stimulated recall interviews as a data collection technique, Paper presented at the Association for the Advancement of Applied Sport Psychology, Lake Tahoe, CA.

Hackfort, D., Schwenkmezger, P., 1993. Anxiety. In: Singer, R.N., Murphy, M., Tennant, L.K. (Eds.), Handbook of research on sport psychology. Macmillan, New York, pp. 328–364.

Hamilton, R.A., Scott, D., MacDougall, M.P., 2007. Assessing the effectiveness of self-talk interventions on endurance performance. J. Appl. Sport Psychol. 19, 226–239.

Hardy, J., 2006. Speaking clearly: a critical review of the self-talk literature. Psychol. Sport and Exerc. 7, 81–97.

Hardy, L., Jones, G., Gould, D., 1996. Understanding psychological preparation for sport. Wiley, Chichester, West Sussex.

Hardy, J., Hall, C.R., Hardy, L., 2005. Quantifying athlete self-talk. J. Sports Sci. 23, 905–917.

Harle, S., Vickers, J.N., 2001. Training quiet eye improves accuracy in the basketball free-throw. Sport Psychologist 15, 289–305.

Hatzigeorgiadis, A., Theodorakis, Y., Zourbanos, N., 2004. Self-talk in the swimming pool: the effects of self-talk on thought content and performance on water-polo tasks. J. Appl. Sport Psychol. 16, 138–150.

Highlen, P.S., Bennett, B.B., 1983. Elite divers and wrestlers: a comparison between open- and closed-skill athletes. J. Sport Psychol. 5, 390–409.

Jackson, S.A., 2000. Joy, fun and flow state in sport. In: Hanin, Y. (Ed.), Emotions in sport. Human Kinetics, Champaign, IL, pp. 135–156.

Jackson, R.C., Baker, J.S., 2001. Routines, rituals, and rugby: case study of a world class goal kicker. Sport Psychologist 15, 48–65.

Jackson, R.C., Ashford, K.J., Norsworthy, G., 2006. Attentional focus, dispositional reinvestment and skilled motor performance under pressure. J. Sport and Exerc. Psychol. 28, 49–68.

Janelle, C.M., 1999. Ironic mental processes in sport: implications for sport psychologists. Sport Psychologist 13, 201–220.

Johnson, M., 1996. Slaying the dragon: how to turn your small steps into great feats. Harper Collins, New York.

Jones, G., Swain, A., Cale, A., 1990. Antecedents of multidimensional competitive state anxiety and self-confidence in elite intercollegiate middle distance runners. Sport Psychologist 4, 107–118.

Kipling, R., 1924. Rewards and fairies. Macmillan & Co., London.

MacPherson, A.C., Collins, D., Obhi, S.S., 2009. The importance of temporal structure and rhythm for the optimum performance of motor skills: A new focus for practitioners of sport psychology. J. Appl. Sport Psychol. 21, S48–S61.

Masters, R.S.W., 1992. Knowledge, 'knerves' and know-how: the role of explicit versus implicit knowledge in the breakdown of complex motor skill under pressure. Br. J. Psychol. 83, 343–358.

Moore, P.M., 2000. Preparation of an Olympic Team, Invited presentation to the BASES Annual Conference, Liverpool.

Pitt, N., 1998. Out of the woods. Sunday Times (Sport) 19 July, p. 5.

Ravizza, K.H., 2002. A philosophical construct: a framework for performance enhancement. Int. J. Sport Psychol. 33, 4–18.

Ravizza, K., Osborne, T., 1991. Nebraska's 3 R's: one play at a time pre-performance routine for collegiate football. Sport Psychologist 5, 256–265.

Richards, H., Richards, D., 2002. Tough defense. In: Hale, B., Collins, D. (Eds.), Rugby tough. Human Kinetics, Champaign, IL, pp. 179–203.

Rushall, B.S., Potgieter, J.R., 1987. The psychology of successful competing in endurance events. South African Association for Sport Science, Physical and Recreation, Pretoria.

Singer, R.N., 1988. Strategies and metastrategies in learning and performing self-paced athletic skills. Sport Psychologist 2, 49–68.

Singer, R.N., 2000. Performance and human factors considerations about cognition and attention for self-paced and externally-paced events. Ergonomics 43, 1661–1680.

Singer, R.N., 2002. Preperformance state, routines, and automaticity: what does it take to realize expertise in self-paced tasks? J. Sport and Exerc. Psychol. 24, 359–375.

Taylor, J., 1995. A conceptual model for integrating athlete's needs and sport demands in the development of competitive mental preparation strategies. Sport Psychologist 9, 339–357.

Theodorakis, Y., Weinberg, R., Natsis, P., et al., 2000. The effects of motivational and instructional selftalk on improving motor performance. Sport Psychologist 14, 253–271.

Vickers, J.N., 1996. Visual control when aiming at a far target. J. Exp. Psychol. Hum. Percept. Perform. 2, 324–354.

Vickers, J.N., 2007. Perception, cognition and decision training: the quiet eye in action. Human Kinetics, Champaign, IL.

Vickers, J.N., Williams, A.M., 2007. Performing under pressure: the effects of physiological arousal, cognitive anxiety, and gaze control in biathlon. J. Mot. Behav. 39, 381–394.

Wilkinson, J., 2003. The perfect ten (directed by Souster M, Kelly M). Video Collection International, London.

Williams, J.M., Harris, D.V., 2006. Relaxation and energizing techniques for regulation of arousal. In:

Williams, J.M. (Ed.), Applied sport psychology: personal growth to peak performance, fifth ed. Mayfield, Mountain View, CA, pp. 285–305.

Wilson, M., 2008. From processing efficiency to attentional control: a mechanistic account of the anxiety-performance relationship. Int. Rev. Sport and Exerc. Psychol. 1, 184–201.

Wilson, M.R., Vine, S.J., Wood, G., 2009. The influence of anxiety on visual attentional control in basketball free-throw shooting. J. Sport and Exerc. Psychol. 31, 152–168.

Wulf, G., 2007. Attention and motor skill learning. Human Kinetics, Champaign, IL.

Zinsser, N., Bunker, L.K., Williams, J.M., 2006. Cognitive techniques for improving performance and building confidence. In: Williams, J.M. (Ed.), Applied sport psychology: personal growth to peak performance, fifth ed. Mayfield, Mountain View, CA, pp. 349–381.

Putting them together: skill packages to optimize team/group performance

24

Dave Collins* Judy Collins†

*Grey Matters/UCLan; †University of Leicester, Leicester, UK

CHAPTER CONTENTS

Introduction

Working as a team is essential to all the performance environments that are the focus of this book. For individual performers, effective interaction is needed with a coach, director or teacher at the very least. In genuine teams or groups, where the outcome depends on effective collaboration, the interactions are even more central to effective performance. Team games are the best example of this, although extreme sports and dance settings increasingly offer environments that require equally team-like efforts. As a result, social elements become as important as cognitive ones in the setup, conduct and development of the environment. Reflecting this, our chapter focuses more on structure and interactions than on mental skills per se. We offer ideas, together with some techniques to implement them, that should underpin an effective performance group. The chapter should obviously be contextualized, indeed critiqued, using pertinent content from the others, particularly those in Section 2.

In the next section, we examine team preparation, focusing on the planning, design and style of methods that work best. The third section considers aspects for team performance, ranging from technical/tactical issues such as decision making through to confidence and cohesion. Finally, in the last section, we look at ways to optimize the contribution of the increasingly common 'team within a team': the support staff.

Preparing as a team

Deciding the agenda and optimum 'shape'

Whatever the team setting, two-headed with just coach and performer or multiple-personality such as a professional sports team or dance company, the first step is to decide on a strengths and weaknesses profile for each individual. There are many ways to make this evaluation, and psychologists have most commonly used some variant of the Performance Profile, based on personal construct theory (Kelly 1965) and developed in sport by Butler & Hardy (1992), which realizes a picture of strengths and weaknesses based on the individual's perceptions. In more structured situations however, and elite performance demands such structure, a more explicit and consistent method is often required. Figure 24.1 presents the format in use (at the time of writing)

DOI: 10.1016/B978-0-443-06734-1.00024-9

Name of Athlete: **Event:**

Coach:

	Factor	Rationale	Score
Outcome	**Consistency** High scores reflect consistent performances at, or close to, PB. Score is based on 4 best performances that season		Score 1 to 10 **Actual score:**
	Progression Provides a points score, reflecting the SB against the average performances of Gold/Bronze/Eighth athlete in the last three age specific majors (OG or World Juniors).		Score 1 to 10 **Actual score:**
	Technical/tactical ability Related to technical models developed by UKA and/or by independent evaluation by an SPC or other authority.		Score 1 to 10 **Actual score:**
	Competition placing Based on place in the major competition that year as agreed with the PM; 1st scores 16, 2nd 15 and so on.		Score 1 to 16 as a reverse item **Actual score:**
Process	**Professional attitude** The athlete's manner, especially in interaction with support professionals and fellow competitors in training and events.		Score 1 to 10 **Actual score:**
	Programme commitment Rate the athlete's willingness and commitment to involvement in relevant programmes, including testing, squads, etc.		Score 1 to 10 **Actual score:**
	Training commitment Rate the athletes work ethic in training. Score should be substantiated by exemplars and third party evidence.		Score 1 to 10 **Actual score:**
	Sport commitment Rate the athlete's commitment to progress in Athletics, as opposed to other areas of endeavour, including academics and other sports/activities.		Score 1 to 10 **Actual score:**
	Physical resilience Reflects the fragility or 'injury proneness' of the athlete. Remember past weaknesses may explain lack of progress rather than predict it!		Score 1 to 20 **Actual score:**

Fig. 24.1 • An exemplar athlete performance/potential template.

(Continued)

Process	**Mental toughness** Reflects the athlete's ability to 'produce the goods' in major championships and other pressure situations. Use data and exemplars to justify score.		Score 1 to 10 **Actual score:**
	Lifestyle Reflects the athlete's commitment to, and execution of, an appropriate lifestyle. An important but hard to define construct. Justifications for ratings need to be particularly clear here.		Score 1 to 10 **Actual score:**
	Environment Closely linked to lifestyle. Relates to the level of support enjoyed by the athlete across various areas such as finance, emotional support, facilities, etc.		Score –5 to +5 **Actual score:**
	Coaching quality Based on observation, quality of coach's planning/peaking and technical input, and commitment to this athlete.		Score 1 to 20 **Actual score:**
	Coaching development Reflects the coach's willingness and commitment to personal development, especially as pertaining to increasing their capacity to improve this athlete		Score 1 to 10 **Actual score:**
Athlete	**Physical suitability** Reflects the athlete's suitability for the current event, based on an estimation of his/her fully mature body shape/size.		Score 1 to 10 **Actual score:**
	Potential for this year's major event		Score 1 to 20 **Actual score:**
	Potential for next world level event		Score 1 to 20 **Actual score:**

Fig. 24.1—Cont'd

by British track and field athletes and coaches, a structured report form called the Athlete Performance Potential Template.

The approach can be modified for different environments by changing the headings and items, although the overall structure and many of the factors are generic. Repeated appraisals, season on season, provide a series of dynamic profiles from which a developmental work programmes can be designed, deployed, tested and refined, so keeping the team (however many are involved) always focused on improvement.

Further benefits can result from adjusting how the template is completed. In the planned athletics setting, based largely on professional athletes, coaches and performance managers, coach and athlete fill out the first draft and offer evidence for the scores they award. Subsequently, these scores are 'audited' by an independent other (in our case, the Performance Manager), who offers a critical questioning of the scores while also examining the action plans to address them. This 'external audit' is an important step if genuine development is to result. Whether the focus is on individuals, or key dyads such as coach–athlete or athlete–agent pairs, discussion must get into the 'Zone of Uncomfortable Debate' (see Ch. 8) so that weaknesses are genuinely considered and realistically addressed.

Finally, a word of caution. Whichever evaluation tool you use, they are usually best built around some form of self-scoring. In this regard, it is worth remembering that such scores have no 'special' value just because they are quantitative. These scores should be considered to be formative rather than summative, like the scores obtained from '360 feedback,' the current favourite in business circles. In other words, the values are used to show areas of relative strength against areas for development rather than as a formal pass/fail evaluation (McLean 1996). The need for informed interpretation of the relative values is further supported, as many of the constructs will inevitably be related. For example, work on strength will often restrict flexibility. Attention to one facet of performance may well impact on other factors just because, in the mind of the performer, one is emphasized over others! Accordingly, designing a development programme must focus on evolving towards the optimum balance of characteristics for the particular performance environment and, especially important in the team setting, each individual's particular role. All concerned must acknowledge the *yin–yang* balance of any characteristic (Lombardo & Eichinger 1996), that each one will carry both strengths and weaknesses.

Once a systematic analysis of the team has been completed, the initial decision facing the planner/coach/leader is how best to exploit the balance of strengths and weaknesses offered by the team members. Variously termed the shape, style or philosophy of the team, effectiveness often depends on how well the individuals fit the master plan, their degree of commitment to it and how flexible the plan is.

In simple terms, the decision has two extreme solutions and one compromise solution, which is probably the most practical and common answer. The two extreme solutions are:

- Design a system that fits perfectly with the performers available
- Go out into the market place and 'buy' different individuals who fit the exact specification.

There are examples of both these extremes in almost every performance environment. Unfortunately, for every success story, there are many failures. The first option requires extremely good knowledge and skills; the second your own captive multimillionaire! However, in both cases the absence of flexibility is a crucial drawback, making performances unidimensional and predictable. In the absence of the necessary conditions for either of the extreme solutions and to retain the competitive edge by developing new wrinkles ahead of the opposition, the midpoint compromise offers the most commonly effective option. In short, recruit as well as you can but always make sure that the style or shape of your team is making the optimum use of what you have. Many a coach has developed a strategy that 'would be great if we had…'.

The method relies on the ability to change each individual's natural inclinations, usually reflected by the strengths shown in their profiles, to a sufficient extent that all can fit into a 'best compromise' shape Specific ways to accomplish this compromise through developing individuals' commitment, understanding and skills to perform to the team's shape are offered in the final section of this chapter. For our present purpose, the message sent to team members must be carefully developed and evolved with both understanding and buy-in from team members, especially the leaders. The essential additional skill, which is based on the activity itself (e.g. rugby, ballet, mountain climbing) and not in the realm of performance psychology, lies in the design of the 'best fit' system.

Developing a 'cooperative' training environment

So an accurate analysis of strength and weaknesses is completed, well based plans have been made that offer the best fit for the skills-blend within the team and the ideas have been sold to and through team leaders. Now the final step in training your team lies in developing a cooperative training environment. This is the sort of collaborative environment in which team members are able to work with and for each other. Despite the competitive drives that underpin almost all the activities that are the focus for this book, there is a surprising amount of cooperation apparent between the most 'deadly' rivals. In fact, collaboration usually offers elite performers the best training opportunities. Thus, tennis players will 'hit' rallies against each other, judo players will attend international training camps and practise with future opponents, and dancers will 'take a class' with other companies, groups or choreographers; world-class performance requires world-class practice and world-class training partners.

This approach must be the norm, even among members of the same teams or training groups. Runners will talk about the need for group members to share the training load, to 'pull the laps'. Combat sports benefit from individuals who will 'role-play' different types of opponent (in fact, it helps the impersonator as well by developing their own vocabulary of techniques). Dancers need to take classes with others of equal or, preferably, higher skills (in fact, both seniors and juniors can benefit from this as well). Accordingly, setting a collaborative atmosphere is essential to the team's or training group's long-term health.

The key to this atmosphere and adoption by members of a 'quid pro quo' approach is balance. The sensible coach/teacher/leader will offer structure to training, making sure that each individual's specific needs are met through formally organized practices. Regular liaison with team leaders will help to 'check the temperature' and ensure that team members perceive that they are getting what they need and that others are pulling their weight. In fact, this sort of approach benefits everyone. In individual sports, performers get the chance to broaden their repertoire and understanding. For dancers, new moves and new approaches are developed in tandem with the extra boost to motivation. For team players, not only does the group get better and confidence in each other increase (see the discussion on mutual confidence/collective efficacy below) but better understanding of how moves are best countered just adds to the skill set to make them work.

Performing as a team

At first sight, performing as a team suggests a high level of acute or short-term interdependence where excellent performances occur when the team members are perfectly in tune with one another. Invasion games such as soccer or rugby and group performances in dance represent good examples of where this is the case. Even in these situations, however, it is important to acknowledge the need to ensure that the wider 'performance team' surrounding individual performers is operating with optimum effectiveness. We will consider the effective integration of support teams in a later section. Meanwhile, back to the interactive performance challenge.

The first thing to notice is that all the constructs elsewhere in this book apply to each individual involved in performance, whether they be performers or staff such as managers, coaches and directors. However, the interactions between these individuals represent an additional, and often awkward, complicating factor. The pioneering social psychologist Burt Carron (Carron et al 2002) put it very nicely when he observed that sport psychology work with a team required attention to each individual and to the team *and that these were separate concerns*. To put it another way, anyone working with the simplest rugby team in the world will end up with 17 clients: 15 individual players, one coach and a 16-headed monster called 'the team'. Bear this in mind as we work through the constructs that impact on team performance. Treat the group and the individual as distinct issues, linked but requiring separate evaluation and (almost always) distinct intervention plans.

There is obviously an immense amount of research that can be brought to bear on team performance but, for simplicity, we will consider all these factors under the three broad headings of Self-confidence, Decision making and Roles and reward.

Confidence and cohesion

Other chapters, particularly Chapter 23, touched on the important role of self-confidence and its situation-specific variant, self-efficacy (Bandura 1986). As we come to the group/team situation, recognize that all that's been said will apply to each individual. Thus, the four main techniques for improving self-efficacy, namely performance accomplishment, vicarious experience, verbal persuasion and arousal control, can all be used to good effect. For the present purposes, looking at the multi-headed monster that is the team, collective efficacy (CE) is an important additional idea. Put simply, CE relates to the extent to which members of any team or group believe that they and their fellow members will be effective in meeting a specific challenge. It is 'a sense of collective competence shared among individuals when allocating, coordinating, and integrating their resources in a successful concerted response to specific situational demands' (Zaccaro et al 1995, p. 309). This construct obviously applies very broadly. Thus, members of a dance company will have high CE and perform well so long as they are happy with the components that contribute to their performance. In short, 'I can do my bits' plus 'I know that the others can do theirs' is the simple recipe for high CE, high confidence and high performance! Exactly the same principles will apply to any sports or expedition team. So perceived competence of team members to meet the challenge, satisfaction with the preparation and strategies to be deployed, plus an 'X factor' that the team can handle whatever is thrown at it are all contributors to this important and desirable characteristic of most effective teams.

While CE has received a reasonable amount of research attention (e.g. Bandura 1993; Bray 2004) results have sometimes been equivocal. This may be due to the obvious cyclic relationship between CE and performance (note that the most important source of self-efficacy is 'performance accomplishment'). In short, performing well begets greater feelings of CE, which begets...! Nonetheless, most applied performance psychologists, coaches and managers would support the idea that boosting CE ahead of challenge is a good idea. Table 24.1 shows an example of a common way of achieving this by asking each performer to identify strengths of the other performers in the team. This example is taken from work with a curling team (five in the team, so four statements each – names changed!) prior to a major international event. The lists of strengths are then collected, collated and each player receives positive affirmations from his/her colleagues. The feedback was an effective reminder/reassurance to the individuals, who were able to focus on emphasizing these strengths throughout the tournament.

A similar principle should sensibly be applied to the preparation. Those involved in leading training and preparation need to be aware of the team's perceptions, of the team as a whole, of each individual and of themselves. Practice can be carefully structured to 'demonstrate' skill levels to all concerned (cf. ideas on feedback and performance evaluation in Ch. 23). So, if the group view is that performer *X* has a weakness, the sensible coach will arrange for practices that counter this view, although well in advance of the performance. If the perceptions are right, and player *X* is indeed weak in a certain area, demonstrating this to one and all in the final stages of preparation is potentially lethal! Not only would this impact on the CE of the team/group ('I told you he couldn't...what will we do if...'), it also detrimentally affects the individual through the construct of impression management (Leary 1992) mentioned later in this chapter. In simple terms, designing the practice and preparation schedule has psychological considerations, in particular ensuring CE is high before performance, that are every bit as important as the physiological concerns of peaking and periodization, which have traditionally underpinned this planning.

Cohesion can also play a part in promoting confidence, especially task cohesion. Those interested in exploring this important social psychological construct should read the work of Bert Carron (e.g. Carron et al 2002). For the present purpose, however, note that this approach divides team or group cohesion by two criteria. The first is a task or social and the second is the extent to which individuals are attracted to the group or perceive the

Table 24.1 Other team members' positive statements about specific performers

Name	Two strengths that he brings to the team are...	Name	Two strengths that he brings to the team are...
Fred	• Level headed input/attitude during heated/pressure situations • Great team member/player	Barney	• Judgement and power of sweeping • Good shot maker, particularly on clearing up
	• Deep thinker • Anticipates situations • Level head in tight situations		• Great sweeper • Good when it really counts
	• Level of tactical experience and additional voice to bounce problem situations off • Good shot making ability under pressure		• A great performer under pressure • World class sweeper and judge of a running stone
	• Easy going • Great lead		• Easy going – very approachable • Great team man

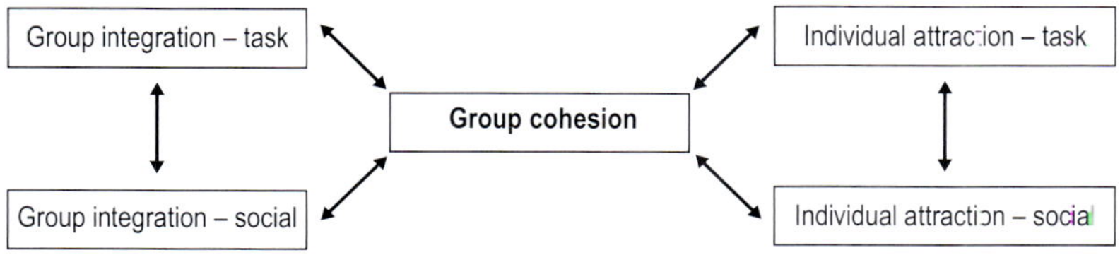

Fig. 24.2 • The structure of group cohesion according to Carron et al (1985). Adapted, with permission, from A.V. Carron, W.N. Widmeyer, and L.R. Brawley, 1985, The development of an instrument to test cohesion in sport teams: The Group Environment Questionnaire. *Journal of Sport and Exercise Psychology* 7(3): 248.

group to be well integrated. Figure 24.2 shows how the two criteria produce four factors associated with cohesion.

This structure has been supported by a large number of studies, most using the Group Environment Questionnaire (Carron et al 1985). Typical questions from each of the four factors are the easiest way to get a quick handle of these distinct but related constructs. Exemplars are as follows:

- **GI-Task**: 'Our team is united in trying to reach its goal'
- **GI-Social**: 'The team enjoy getting together socially'
- **ATG-Task**: 'I do not approve of the performance goals for this team' (*reverse item*)
- **ATG-Social**: 'I enjoy group/team parties'.

In recent research Carron et al (2002) has focused primarily on examining only the task-related cohesion factors suggesting, in line with our own views, that only 'task' factors have a strong link with group performance. The lack of unequivocal results from research on cohesion and performance leave a question mark over the impact of social factors on performance (the balance seems slightly in favour of the view that social factors do not have much impact) and also over the important issue of causality. The answer to whether cohesion causes enhanced performance or good performance causes enhanced cohesion is not easy to give from the current research and, indeed, the same points made on CE above may also apply here. As groups develop and establish a genuine identity (see the classic study on the life-cycle of groups by Tuckman & Jensen 1977), group attractiveness, traditions and adherence all increase. However, it seems most likely that there is a cyclic relationship between the overall cohesion construct and performance, in a rather similar fashion to CE (see Williams & Hacker 1982).

Three practical points emerge from consideration of the cohesion literature. The first, that success breeds good cohesion and this will probably lead to more success, is somewhat true but also somewhat lacking in utility! The second, that making the team socially cohesive is not really useful for performance, is also not much help; although it may stop people spending so much money on social bonding outings! The third is both important and practically applicable, however; it is *always* worth working on task components with any group.

Accordingly, team leaders/coaches/instructors should employ a range of team meetings, small group discussions and planning exercises to promote agreement, acceptance and commitment to the goals, methods, makeup and systems of the group from all members. As shown in Chapter 7, organizational effectiveness is always enhanced by closer agreement on these key characteristics (see also Zander 1982 for an 'aide memoire' of common-sense, but not necessarily commonly used, ways of promoting team identity and CE). In fact, such meetings act as a form of 'team coherence' (see below and concepts of shared mental models in Ch. 17), which contributes to the establishment, development and maintenance of a performance environment for the team, whatever its aims. Encouraging and facilitating open discussion between members is one of the best ways to build the mutual confidence, trust, spirit and commitment that typify effective teams.

Decision making

Almost all team games and many adventure sports group activities have a crucial 'decision-making' dimension, which is often the factor that determines the eventual outcome. Thus, as a time when physical preparation and practice of technique produce many good performers with skill and fitness, truly great performance teams are often distinguishable by being the ones capable of making the best decisions. Consideration of any three-stage model of motor control suggests that, in simple terms, making the right decision (stage 2 in the model shown in Fig. 24.3)

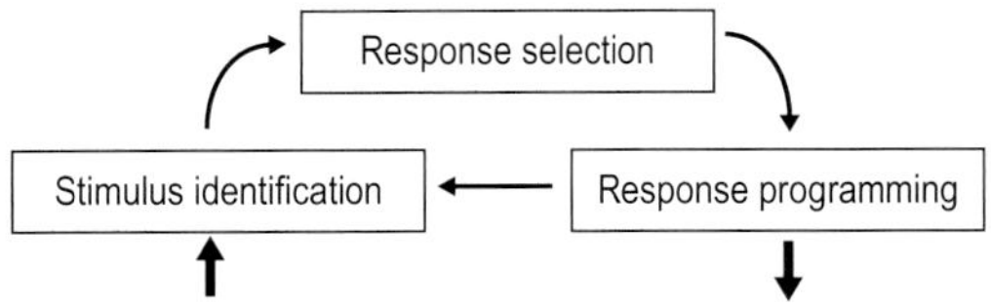

Fig. 24.3 • The simplistic three-stage model of motor control (not realistic but a good schematic for planning and understanding).

is highly dependent on appreciating and processing the right information (the perceptual stage). However, things are not quite as simple as they seem. For example, the decision that any team member makes will also have to take appreciation of the physical capabilities of his/her team mates and infer their decision making too. We will come back to this later. Meanwhile we will use the decision-making styles model outlined in Chapter 17, which identifies three types of decision making, namely Command, Standard Operational Procedures (SOP) and the highest order, Shared Mental Model (SMM) approach.

Command

Even at the highest level, there is a surprising amount of command decision making. One only has to watch the signals passing between ball carrier and team in basketball, catcher and pitcher in baseball, lead and belayer in climbing and skip and team in curling to see these systems in action. When decisions are made like this, in theory things should be easier since the decision is made by one performer, reducing the information processing load for everyone else (Eysenck & Calvo 1992). There are still a number of challenges however. First of all, the instructions need to be completely understood and, preferably, completely agreed with by the recipient. In some situations, curling and baseball for example, calling a time out for discussion can help to achieve understanding and acceptance. However, doing this too often carries a considerable cost. So, team meetings prior to performances need to clearly establish a general understanding and support for the often quite complex series of actions that follow the simple command. Even a basic call like rugby's 'Kit-Kat' (for those unfamiliar with the chocolate bar advert from which this comes, the command tells the player to feign injury and 'Have a break') has to have a series of steps associated with it if the whole thing isn't to become too obvious and the benefits lost. So, a team command, whether given verbally or visually, has to be simple and quick, with well rehearsed consequences. This makes it imperative that sufficient training time is provided for meetings to establish clear instructions for all aspects of the response and complete commitment from all the performers. A lack of confidence will limit buy-in to the action, increase potentially negative worry and provide a 'crack' in the team's performance that may be wedged and widened as the pressure builds. It should be obvious that even commands require the shared appreciation and buy-in that typify the SMM (Cannon-Bowers et al 1993).

It is also worth thinking about the ways in which the team's confidence in using commands can be optimized by applying SMM techniques. Thus, for example, consider the instructions of the curling skip to his/her player about to take a shot or the captain who sets a field in cricket. Previous discussion/team meetings/effective training and instruction must provide the commander (skip/catcher/captain) with sufficient knowledge about each team member so that they can adjust the decision based on understanding the characteristics of each team member as well as variable situation-specific issues such as state of the game or potential risk and individual fatigue. These factors must be overt, known and mutually agreed, not only by commander and recipients but also by the rest of the team. The constructs of self- and collective efficacy discussed earlier really apply here. Confidence and CE will be a lot higher if everyone knows and agrees with why the command is being issued. Finally, we need to recognize that, just as in military settings, the power/status of who gives the command will determine its impact. As such, it may be useful to limit the number of options/commands which a trainee commander may give, only releasing more complex command/lead routines as the players gain confidence in the individual.

In any case, once the commands have been established, they need to be practised in progressively pressured training situations and – a much neglected must – lower-pressure but real performance situations. Good feedback such as systematic expert observation, video feedback including notational analysis, and well organized performer input will enable the processes in response to the command to be evaluated. Follow-up discussion, practice and ongoing refinement are required to establish continual improvement. In our support work, we have developed the term *combination training* to describe the juxtaposition of highly technical skill practice with simple, physically fatiguing exercises to ensure performers can produce correct skills when fatigued (see Chs 20, 22 and 25 for details and exemplars). This approach can be equally well used to provide a means of training command-based decision making under progressive pressure. Thus, rugby players may be required to run command-initiated set plays at high speed while being progressively challenged by the drills being interspersed with high-intensity physical intervals.

This sort of work is increasingly common, with positive benefits accruing in team games, extreme sports and even some aesthetic activities. The real missing link, however, is the real performance-based practice that helps everybody to be completely confident that things will work in the 'heat of battle'. The recent (2007) rugby World Cup represents a perfect example. The New Zealand All Blacks were red hot favourites to win, having enjoyed a pre-eminent dominance in the world game for the previous 2–3 years. Unfortunately, this very dominance often carries a genuine risk in that players are unused to practising command-initiated, 'emergency' drills under pressure. The message is clear: for successful teams, performances where positive outcomes are fairly assured (or low-risk) represent crucial opportunities to practise emergency routines. In American team sport these are often called '2-minute team drills'. Once the command has been issued that the team is going for a drop goal, field goal, 3-pointer or possession-keeping strategy, all players should have a clear, predetermined and well rehearsed set of actions and follow-up decision options to fit.

Standard operational procedures

In simple terms, SOPs are just commands that either don't need to be said (everyone recognizes the need to do *X*) or have a longer or more comprehensive impact. The obvious example of SOP use is in response to emergencies such as the procedure a helicopter crew learns and adopts for ditching at sea or the response of medical staff to a patient's heart stopping. In team sport, SOP may be used for a 2-minute 'raise your game and play it tight' commitment from all members in the risky period following a score, either theirs or yours! Although traditional SOPs are quite stable, systematic and often based on minimizing risk and error, routinely in high-level sport SOPs are established on a weekly basis, based on scouting reports about future opposition. Such instructions are usefully summarized on a briefing sheet, which offers an aide-memoire of the moves practised in the weeks preceding and the circumstances in which they will be used (see Fig. 24.4 for an example). The 'if they..... then we'll....' nature of the SOPs is subject to the same concerns and constraints as the command. Also, as with commands, SOPs need to be evolved through broad-ranging discussion often initiated and guided by well prepared video of your own performances and video of the type of performance situations or opponents you are likely to encounter. To paraphrase a saying, 'Time spent in discussion is seldom wasted'. It might seem as if the SOP is clear and everyone is in agreement but, building on the ideas of procedural, declarative and tacit knowledge (see Ch. 15), the 'why' is more important than the 'what'. Establishing complete buy-in and common understanding makes the SOP a good deal more likely to work.

Consideration of Figure 24.4 will demonstrate many of the key features of such sheets. Common vocabulary, with simple terms used to summarize complex and well practised moves, is an essential feature. Note also the 'overall aims' section, which comes first, setting the context and establishing the mind-set for the team. This sort of overview, common practice in the best team settings, can also provide the basis for mental preparation at all levels.

There are a couple of government health warnings, however. First, overuse of SOPs can result in almost 'choreographed' styles of performance, which is disadvantageous if innovation, creativity and unexpected performances are valued. This is as true for a sports team that does not want to have predictable moves for which opponents will plan defences as for a dance company that seeks to develop new and exciting productions. Of course, many of the great dominant teams of the past have had a style (what soccer players call 'shape') that is apparent to even the most irregular observer. If you're dominant and it's working then change would seem illogical ('If it ain't broke, don't fix it!'). Nevertheless, there is a real need to develop and even deploy a few alternatives, which will give your team a longer shelf-life, however apparently dominant it is at present. Teams constantly need to reinvent themselves just as any other performer does (see later comments from the PP in Ch. 25).

The second point about SOPs is the need to build practice under increasingly pressured conditions. The combination training idea mentioned in the Command section above will cater for this in the early stages. The SOPs also need to be tried and tested in lower-pressure performance situations and, most crucially, the evaluation has to extend

XXXXX Vs YYYY

Team Objectives:

• Territory	- Play in their half
• Gain line advantage	- Attack 10 channel & outside 13 - Direct and physical
• Phase play	- Backs at 1st & 2nd receiver - Inside & outside runners needed off 10 - Early calls to organize support runners - Put appropriate numbers into breakdown
• Tempo of game	- Move forwards around - Minimise mistakes
• 1st Up tackles	- Line speed - Communication

Attack:

1. Play "Rap" rugby to start mixing with "Horse" runs and wide plays.
   - Inside & Outside support runners for 10 during phase play (especially slow ball)
   - 10 & 12 will race in defence – outside channels poorly defended

2. Counter attack

i. 2 passes wide or 1 pass and then back down short side

(4/5 players stay back – don't push up on outside)

3. Kicking

i. Back 3 are very good counter attackers, therefore

- Ball goes off field or
- Well behind wingers for them to chase back. OUR CHASE VITAL

4. Opportunities on restarts to move the ball wide. Poor chase from backs (4/5 stay back for kick)

Moves

Attacking '10' channel:

L/O's	6 & 7 man Diet 12 or 13 (All through 10's hands)			
	5 man Express Green			
Scrums	(LHS)	SKP		
	Hollywood 11			
	ACT 1			
	Fairy			
	(RHS)	Echo short & ACT 1		

Attacking wide:

L/O's	Ice Coke (6 & 7 man)			
	Double Lemonade (6 & 7 man)			
	Express White (5 man)			
Scrums	(LHS)	Hollywood T	CF Scrums	Liquid Y
		ACT 2		
	Hollywood Coke			
	(RHS)	Random		
		ACT 2		

Fig. 24.4 • Exemplar briefing sheet for a rugby team.

to every component of the SOP and every performer, not just to be based on whether it worked or not! Good use of video, subunit evaluations ('How well do you think we did...?') and team discussions should all be used to achieve effective evaluations.

Shared mental models

The SMM concept was introduced earlier. This represents the 'highest' order of team decision making, in which individual members take actions, without communication, that cater for and support the needs of other team members and the overall plan. SMMs were developed within the theoretical approach of naturalistic decision making (see Ch. 17) and are therefore optimally applied in high-pressure, time-urgent, short-duration situations. We have already suggested that the idea of SMM may also be relevant for effective teams for 'slower and more deliberate DM', related to the development of team procedures and goals. Thus, while we initially concentrate here on the development of SMMs in the direct performance environment (e.g. choosing who to pass to or whether to adjust timing in a group dance), we also suggest that similar principles may hold for the development of team ethos, spirit and goals.

At the simplest level, SMMs may emerge almost spontaneously from the juxtaposition of three key factors:

- Motivated and communicative team members
- Common knowledge (and ideally, common vocabulary) about the goals and methods of the performance environment)
- Encouragement for, and facilitation of, team problem solving.

Two contrasting but similar examples may help demonstrate this. Consider either a representative hockey team or a newly formed dance company getting ready for a tour...some contrast! Not so different, however, given that team members are knowledgeable and willing to talk about their particular discipline, an 'open to discussion' environment exists and team leaders (both formal and informal) encourage general discussion around clearly framed components of the challenge. In such an environment, it is more likely than not that team members will interact to address often self-identified and -defined issues, resulting in a genuine 'quality circle' approach and a consequent upward spiral in performance (we will elaborate more on the 'quality circle' idea later in this chapter).

So all can be sweetness and light? Unfortunately, 'it ain't necessarily so', and many blocks can derail this very effective self-development process. The role of the performance psychologist in this case is to assist in overcoming or avoiding these blocks. One such block is the personality of the performers. Incorporate a few big egos ('Why should I help him look better?') and our two touring teams may well never get past first base in terms of producing co-ordinated performances. Another key issue is the team vocabulary (the way problems are described and dissected) and goals (e.g. general agreement about the style of play or impression/motif to be followed). If these are not common across the team, different factions with low cooperation/communication will result. In fact, this can often be a problem when individuals from different systems come together with too little time given to 'setup'; assembling a national team from different club sides, for example. A third issue is that team members have to be sufficiently skilled to engage in this sort of team. The skills here are independent of the physical techniques of the activity and represent the elusive 'effective team member' characteristics likely to be found in performers with maturity/self-confidence, social competence and previous positive experience of working in this way. Finally, an autocratic, 'Mother knows best' leadership style can often stifle team members' almost natural inclinations to get things sorted. All these issues, and other threats to the self-perpetuating cycle of intrateam development, need to be addressed in the setup period. Well organized and well conducted team meetings on topics ranging from the most general (e.g. style, selection philosophy) to the specific (e.g. how will we cope with missed entrances, poor timing or a man-to-man defence?) are the primary means of addressing the SMM development without becoming blocked or derailed by the personality, vocabulary, individual competence in team situations or leadership style.

Opportunities to develop SMMs in this way do not exist only in the early stages of a team setup, but the sense of 'starting again' that is usually necessary does require some manipulation. So, to awaken a sleeping team one needs to initiate sufficient change to shake the current situation out of its rut. In this respect, the complex systems approach described in Chapter 9 offers an excellent mental model. Creating the necessary force for change, 'perturbing the system' in the language of dynamical systems, depends on how deeply etched and resistant the current system is. In simple terms, the deeper the rut, the greater the shake-up required. Perturbation can include introducing new team members, getting new leaders, rebranding or renaming, major successes or major failures; but all have to be carefully managed to create the right opportunity, then exploited in a timely fashion (see Ch. 9 for some examples of these ideas in action). Changing team leaders (new coach/ artistic director) or lead performers is a common approach, for example, but nature abhors a vacuum and too much delay in replacing a recently vacated leadership role or a lack of structure in the early stages and other, perhaps dysfunctional, leaders and systems may emerge. The next section will consider the roles that team members may play, and ways in which this situation may be manipulated to maximum advantage.

To finish this section, let's return to basics and consider the way in which practice can be structured to promote SMM development. Although the underlying principles are fairly simple, applying these effectively with a team does require some skilful handling. The simple principle is to expose the key question and encourage debate that moves towards solutions. Once again, a rugby example: the 2 versus 1 situation that underpins almost all team games (Fig. 24.5).

The progressions in Figure 24.5 are based on increasingly complex SOPs. By this means, performers gain an understanding of the goals, basic ideas (e.g. create then exploit 'space') and movements involved. In II, the players are forced to consider which sources of information offer the best indication of what the defender intends to do. As a result, the SMM benefits from common vocabulary (covering each possible position) and a 'weighting scale' is developed to offer common understanding for the relative importance of each factor. In III, the attackers are elaborating their SMM to develop a shared understanding of what each is trying to do in any given circumstance. This enables them to anticipate and support each others' actions.

We hope that this simple example will offer coaches, teachers and psychologists a starting point for practice design. A simple precis runs as follows:

1. Establish key ideas and goals. Make sure performers have the necessary moves to answer the questions set by the situation
2. Establish and refine a shared understanding and prioritization for the key variables. Encourage use of the 'Why this option' and 'What would have to change for you to...' questions to tease out, expose and internalize the 'limits' for each response
3. Ongoing elaboration of SMMs. Careful debrief and discussion (often best achieved informally) after performances. Video feedback is very useful here.

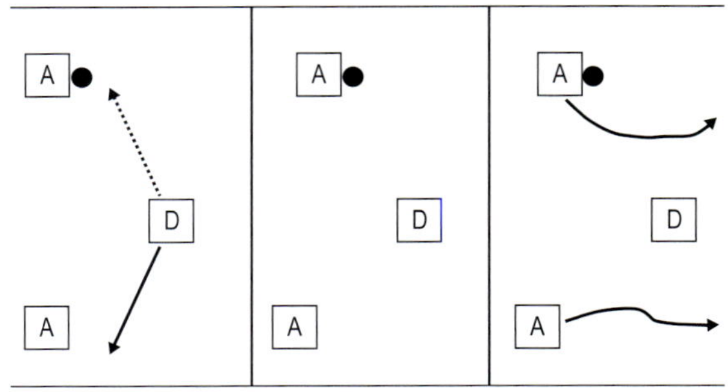

Fig. 24.5 • Exploring the complexities of a situation to expose the basics and develop SMMs (numbered I, II and III, left to right). I. Simple 2 v. 1. Depending on the defender (D) movement, the attacking player (A) with the ball must choose to draw the defender and pass or dummy the pass and go on to score. II. More advanced. Same setup as drill I but the defender is placed by the attackers in the most ambiguous/hardest to read position (in this case, obviously the middle!). Defender can choose a body position (e.g. left foot forwards). The two attacking players must agree a SMM covering each position/movement so that both know what they are going to do in any situation. This extends from drill I by emphasizing the information perception and processing for the two attackers, i.e. what do we look at and what does it mean for our actions. III. SMMs to take control. Attackers work to 'take control' of the defender. Debrief, review and repetition develop a mutual awareness which improves SMM and effectiveness. Thus, by setting off in different directions (termed running lines) the attacker influences the defender's position.

Best of luck! Remember that, so long as the groundwork is done correctly, you can afford to be innovative. Once the environment is established, the upward spiral is easy to keep spinning.

Roles and reward

Team performance is crucially dependent on all team members knowing and keeping to the correct role. This is true whether the team is a group of performers whose outcome depends on how well they interact or a group of professionals supporting one performer. We will cover the issue of support professionals in the next section. For now we will consider roles in performance teams and how buy-in can be optimized. The practical ideas should be considered against the more theoretical treatment of role clarity provided in Chapter 8.

Leadership roles and status

Many characteristics of effective teams can be driven by good leadership. Indeed, however much the social setting is 'engineered', two or three powerful personalities can confirm or eliminate the best laid and most logical plans. Other approaches (e.g. the Myers–Briggs Type Indicator (Briggs & Myers 1980)) offer insights into the optimum make up of teams, with detailed breakdowns of which types fit with which. In our experience, while useful as research instruments, these inventories offer comparatively little practical insight; despite the attractiveness of using psychometrics to determine the optimum make up of a team, the questionnaires offer more 'guidance as to tendencies' than a completely accurate and comprehensive picture. In simple terms, the complexities of team interaction in real life are only broadly described by such instruments, making them good for guidance but not for design.

There are simple steps that can be taken, however. Firstly, it is effective and efficient to make use of the 'natural' leaders within the group. Such individuals may just emerge, have an acknowledged leadership status because of their role within the team or just have the leader mentality within their make up. Exploring what makes a 'natural leader' is outside the scope of this chapter, although most will spot such individuals fairly easily – the real skill lies in making the best use of their charisma, determination and drive. Whatever the genesis of the leadership, however, getting these performers aligned with and accepting of the plan, structures and systems at the earliest opportunity is a good investment of time. This can be effectively achieved by developing features of the plan in association with this central subgroup.

Leadership, or at least some aspects of it, may not have to rely just on those with explicit formal leadership roles such as captains. The Scandinavian sport psychologist, Willi Railo, coined the term 'cultural architect' to describe those influential individuals within a team who, if on board with the direction of change, could subtly influence others towards the new way. Railo has used this idea effectively in several high-performance, culture-change projects, most famously (in the UK at any rate) while working with Sven-Göran Eriksson and the English football team.

Whether the culture change uses natural or emergent leaders, there are three basic principles, which must be employed in parallel. These emerge from consideration of behavioural approaches to psychology and are as follows:

- Team members must have high-status role models who are exhibiting most, or preferably all, of the 'new and desired' behaviours
- Rewards must be used systematically to reinforce changes towards the new and desired behaviours
- Leadership, both overt and covert, must be used to encourage change by challenging the status quo, suggesting/facilitating change in the desired direction, and supporting the desired behaviour.

Rewards and perceived equity

The previous section focused on the role of leaders to enhance the performance of a team and to support such change through systematic reward structures. Of course, many high-performance environments now involve more 'quantitative' rewards, many of which are linked to outcomes. Sound behavioural psychology principles must be applied to such rewards; put simply, make sure that you reward the behaviours you want because the rewarded behaviour is likely to persist! It is all too easy to reward the obvious, 'high-status' behaviour (e.g. scoring) rather than the less obvious 'hard graft' that may facilitate it. Furthermore, since most interactive teams are made up of a number of different roles, reward systems must be sophisticated enough to reinforce the appropriate behaviours for each of these roles. Attention to these 'crucial details' is essential, as effective reward underpins the likelihood of effective behaviour, whether this be tackling, dancing or changing tyres effectively!

These concerns are largely intra-individual; in other words, the leader/coach needs to make sure that each performer is rewarded for doing what they need to do for the whole team to work effectively. Just as crucial, however, are the social perceptions associated with the reward. Problems will occur if performer *A* thinks performer *B* is getting more than is fair. This 'perceived fairness' is the key factor here; it isn't just a case of giving everyone the same reward, be it money, recognition, praise or other markers of status. The key issue is to establish 'perceived equity', not equality, within the team (e.g. Bretz & Thomas 1991). In simple terms, most of us are sufficiently reasonable to recognize that different roles carry the potential for different levels of reward. Thus, quarterbacks get more than linemen, principal dancers more than supporting performers, and drivers get more than mechanics. What counts is not the difference, rather it's the size of the difference. Ensuring that the group perceives rewards as 'proportionate' is important and requires a two-pronged educational process. First, each team member must be informed and accepting of others' roles and their importance for the overall performance (coincidentally, this also helps with group integration and the task elements of cohesion). Secondly, team members must have a SMM (that term again!) that includes a similar and performance-appropriate weighting scale for the relative contributions of each role.

While the first paragraph above is very much an executive concern (although the leader will sensibly make use of team-generated/endorsed statistics in determining reward), the second concern cries out for good use of team meetings, a well established, open communication style and application of transparent policies for decisions associated with valued rewards. Both aspects need to be addressed since, by definition, rewards can generate envy and green-eyed team members rarely if ever perform effectively!

Quality circles

Changing the behaviour of team members so that they individually and thus collectively become more effective can be achieved by building on the theory of impression management (IM; Leary 1992). In essence, IM proposes that individuals are not so worried about what they think of themselves but are often more worried about what they think others think of them. These self-presentational concerns are often a major source of stress (James & Collins 1997), as performers worry that they aren't looking good, doing well enough or doing the right thing. As Leary (1992, p. 347) observes, performance is a perfect arena for IM: 'Whenever people compete, they run the risk of conveying negative images of themselves – that they are unskilled, incompetent, unfit, unable to handle pressure, or whatever – to observers, team-mates, coaches, opposing team members, and, often, the world at large'.

The good news is, however, that countering this source of stress is often an equally effective means of raising performance by ensuring that team members stay focused on their roles. The idea is very close to a comparatively recent innovation in business termed 'quality circles'. The team is split into small groups of four or five; these can be intact units (e.g. defence, corps de ballet) but ideally are individuals who have similar or even interdependent roles within the team. In each performance, one individual is 'scored' by the rest of their subgroup, then debriefed on the key positives and points to work on (strictly in that order!). This may sound like a recipe for conflict but, once educated into the positive and critically constructive emphasis that the approach requires, the subgroups become really supportive in their 'firm but fair' feedback.

Additional benefits include a counter to IM as a source of stress as individuals become very aware of what they need to demonstrate to gain approval from the most important social group – their own peers. So long as these expectations are realistic (and contextualized to the particular challenge), the 'What are they thinking of me?' pressures are reduced. Furthermore, SMMs are reinforced by the increasingly common understanding that accrues from discussion and feedback in the quality circle. Finally, members of the subgroup learn to offer task-relevant feedback and encouragement during the performance itself. Since task-relevant cognitions represent one of the best foci during the event (see Chs 20, 21 and 23), encouraging in-team communication patterns built on this can only be good.

The one issue in all this is that the tasks and roles that are encouraged are the right ones! IM concerns lead many to concentrate on a more 'public' but, for overall performance, dysfunctional set of behaviours. For example, team members may tend to avoid hard but comparatively invisible tasks in favour of more obvious, high-reward attempts; goal hanging at the expense of defence is an obvious example. Accordingly, the wise coach/teacher/leader/performance psychologist will listen carefully to the subgroup feedback and watch/listen to see which aspects of performance lead individuals to express pride. Subtle adjustment can often be effectively achieved by changing the group feedback to off-track individuals. After all, seeking approval from your peer group is human nature.

Performance versus commercial concerns

One further key factor worthy of consideration is the tension that will almost always occur in professional performance organizations (PPOs). Examples include professional sports teams (e.g. Manchester United or New York Yankees), major dance companies such as the Royal Ballet or 'X' sports franchises. In all cases, the PPO's reputation was established, and is maintained, by performance. However, many such organizations have shareholders or other similar structures, which require financial success. Therein lies the potential tension; performance can be inconsistent and very difficult to control, so much so that, even if winning occurs, positive marketplace outcomes do not result (Gilson et al 2001, Gladden & Milne 1999). As a result, the two management structures that are almost inevitably involved (performance management (PM) and business management (BM)) can end up in competition if roles and required rewards are not carefully set and adhered to.

The potential clash between the BM and PM subunits is further highlighted by how much structure they optimally require. The PM will usually suffer under too much structure. Too much structure renders a sport PPO subunit predictable, handing the opposition a big advantage. In similar fashion, all but the most secure performing arts environment must offer innovative and alternative approaches to the traditional portfolio. By contrast, the BM subunit may require a longer period of structure within which to consolidate business strategies, revenue generating initiatives and cost reduction strategies. Finally, unless roles are clear and primacy consistent, much effort will be wasted in civil wars! As an example, consider the arguments that might have occurred between the PM and BM units at Manchester United when David Beckham was sold. Sir Alex obviously won, but think of the loss in 'other income' to the franchise when such a marketable commodity was lost.

The bottom line for all these factors is to have strong and commonly understood team structures with good communication. These apparently simple characteristics take effort and skill to develop and cannot be left to chance.

Supporting as a team

All but the most individualistic of performers in the most individual of sports make use of support from a team of specialists. Even climbers, who invariably trust only their buddy on the other end of the rope, will make use of medics and a range of '-ologists' to realize their best performance. What is not often recognized, however, is the fact that the organization of these teams also needs careful consideration to ensure they operate to maximum effect.

The way in which these teams work has evolved over the last few years through three distinct types of support. It's worth noting that different performance environments are at different stages of development, employing different types of support. For example, at the time of writing, we can think of high-level performers in the UK whose support structures exemplify each of the three types. The first is *unidisciplinary* support, which, as the name suggests, involves the performer getting support from one discipline. Typically, professional boxers will make use of a trainer (a.k.a. the strength and conditioning specialist) in addition to the boxing coach. The logical progression of this is to use a number of different specialists from a variety of disciplines, resulting in *multidisciplinary* support. At present this is probably the most common form of support across performance environments in the UK. Generally, the input from the various specialists is moderated/controlled by one individual, normally the coach, manager or artistic director. Both these approaches possess obvious weaknesses. In the first, only one component of performance is being addressed. In the second, the moderating/controlling individual has to know, understand and correctly spot all the potentially important and often subtle interactions between different performance components. Added to this potential limitation is the fact that in this support structure the various specialists miss out on the chance to build on each others, advice.

Consider one common performance challenge: recovery from injury. Generally the realm of the physiotherapist, optimum recovery and return to performance will clearly involve medical, psychological, nutritional and mechanical issues as follows.

- Doctors, e.g. diagnosing the injury!
- Psychologists, e.g. the mental challenges of rehab and return to performance
- Nutritionists, e.g. adjusting intake while workload is lower
- Biomechanists, e.g. checking for injurious patterns of movement so preventing further problems.

Our point here is simple: it takes a very knowledgeable and adroit individual to effectively moderate and control all the input effectively and harmoniously. Not many coaches, managers and artistic directors will have had the training, nor possess the knowledge or be able to devote the time, to keep this complex process on track.

This brings us to the third and highest order of support, which is the ideal for effective support for a high-level performer. In an *interdisciplinary* support structure, specialists work in various combinations to bring the full weight of their expertise to bear at any one time. This sounds great but it does take time and concerted effort if it is to work optimally. Two concerns exist: management and role clarity.

Firstly, let us briefly consider the management of the interdisciplinary team. The person responsible for coordinating and managing the support has a number of functions to perform. With so much specialist input (and egos!) involved, there is a real risk that the performer can get swamped with support or confused by potential contradictions as each expert weighs in with their important contribution! This is best avoided by making sure that one individual knows exactly what is happening in all the areas at long-term (macro), intermediate (meso) and day-to-day (micro) level. In most performance environments this is best achieved by use of another specialist, the performance manager (PM), whose training and oversight keeps things in balance. In a sports setting the PM can make sure that things are working well, leaving the coach to focus on the technical development and preparation of the performer. Figure 24.6 shows this diagrammatically and represents the system developed for use in British track and field athletics.

The most important function that the PM can serve is to maintain and ensure good communication between all members of the team. Thus, in Figure 24.6, support specialists communicate freely and often about issues that have been identified by the coach/athlete pair. Individual specialists or subsets of the full team address previously identified specific issues with the coach/athlete client, keeping the PM informed. Useful tools for the PM process include full team 'case conferences' at which all can discuss a particular project (e.g. increasing power) or issue (e.g. injury rehabilitation). This sort of model also enables optimum allocation of resources to make the maximum difference to performance. All support participants are oriented to a 'performance benefit' focus by peer pressure *and* line management.

Another tool, especially when support teams are working with more than one client, is a regular progress chart that keeps everybody on track. Figure 24.7 provides an example, once again designed initially for use in British track and field. The third tool is the simplest, although actually the most powerful. Coffee conversations between various members of the team should be regular, facilitated by close working proximity and enabled by sufficient observation and interaction to ensure that everyone in the team has a real sense of both the performance environment and the individual's strengths and weaknesses.

Use of all these tools is accompanied by the golden rule of 'not in front of the client'! Effectively managed conflict, open disagreement and vigorous debate are essential in a high-performance environment to keep the cutting edge sharp. However, the crucial role of confidence highlighted earlier means that all must be careful to resolve disagreements and reach consensus away from the performer, presenting a positive and united front on the agreed plan. All these components mean that support systems must be thought of as performance teams in their own rights with all the factors addressed elsewhere in this book taken into consideration.

A final and particular role for the PM is to avoid the spectre of dependency, which can so often frustrate the benefits of the increasingly complex support teams that typify professional performance environments. Such developments can be quite insidious and develop so subtly and quietly that they

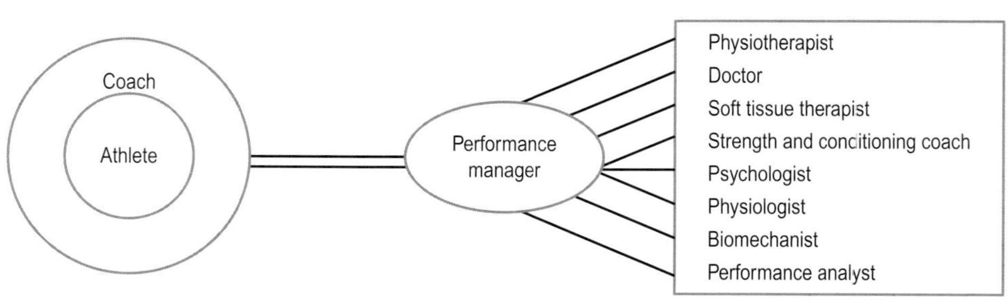

Fig. 24.6 • Schematic of performance management with an interdisciplinary support team.

Athlete	2007/8 Point of contact	Medicine	Physio	S&C	Massage	Physiology	Nutrition	Psychology	Biomechanics	Comments / Actions
Athlete A	Coach 1		F							Olympic A qualifier in France this past weekend
Athlete B	Coach 2		M							Programme in place for shoulder stability. Making good S&C progress. Review by on 06/02/2008
Athlete C	Coach 3		F							Spending little time in here at present - limited practitioner input and programme visibility. Meeting scheduled during w/c 18/02/2008
Athlete D	Coach 4		I							Meeting with Specialist on 08/02/08. Case Conference with key people to be arranged a.s.a.p, possibly 14/02/08?
Athlete E	Coach 5		M							Rescheduled nutrition appointment for next week
Athlete F	Coach 6		I							Continuing to improve
Athlete G	Coach 7		F							Nutrition appointment on 05/02/08 - trialling competition nutrition strategy for this weekend
Athlete H	Coach 8		F							Intensive coaching input from foreign coach - based in Leeds at the moment
Athlete I	Coach 9		F							Referred to nutrition - arranging to meet next week

F = Full Training
M = Modified Training
I = Injured

- Outside target with no improvement or deteriorating trend
- Inside target but with deteriorating trend or outside target with improving trend
- Inside target with improving or level trend

Fig. 24.7 • Exemplar weekly update form for use within an interdisciplinary support team.

only cause the performer to crash and burn in the highest-pressure circumstances. The problem is, in no small part, human nature. Most members of the support team like to support! In short, they feel fulfilled and good about themselves when the performer acknowledges and even seeks out their input. Add to this that the most effective support personnel generally have good personal skills and you have a potential recipe for disaster. Performer and specialist work closely together and form an increasingly tight relationship; in fact, doing this in a professional way is an essential precursor for optimum interaction. From here, however, it is a short step to seeking the specialist's opinion on all sorts of matters outside their speciality. The effective management of an interdisciplinary support team must work to 'keep it real and honest' between the specialists, making sure that conflicts or differences of opinion are exposed and solved away from the performer while also avoiding the green-eyed favourites trap. In many support structures, rotating specialists is a good way to keep things fresh and professionally appropriate. For example, it does no harm for a performer to get used to being seen by a different physiotherapist: a fresh pair of eyes and an informal audit of work completed is almost always positive for the long-term enhancement of performance of the support team.

The other concern that faces the use of an interdisciplinary support structure is the need for establishing role clarity within the support team. In this regard, all the considerations raised earlier in this chapter also apply. As described, there is nothing more destructive to the close working relationships that are essential to interdisciplinary support than one specialist trespassing on the role of another. Whether this trespass is genuine or perceived is almost irrelevant to the impact! Thus, even for the support team, role clarity is key.

Most of these problems can be avoided, and the interdisciplinary process enhanced, with careful setup and open discussion. We want to emphasize that a focus on establishing and promoting smooth running in support systems is every bit as much a performance enhancer as the most esoteric mental strategy! Unfortunately, however, optimizing the efficacy of support systems has not traditionally been a major focus for performance psychology to date. The detail and exemplars presented in this section demonstrate that it is a crucial part of performance and one that requires specific and careful attention to get right.

This level of attention is nicely shown in the following two examples, showing dynamic roles and interaction of specialists over time, which were developed by Dr Bruce Hamilton and Neil Black, at that time respectively Chief Medical Officer and Chief Physiotherapist at UK Athletics, in response to real life issues of role clash. Without role clarity it is perfectly conceivable that, in the scenario of an injured athlete, doctors might be suggesting treatment while physios might be booking in athletes for scans. In both cases each professional is straying into the other's area of professional expertise. Quite apart from the interpersonal issues between practitioners that might occur in this scenario, the confused message to the athlete is likely to decrease confidence and slow the whole process. The delineation shown in Figure 24.8, developed through discussion of both general philosophy and specific case studies (see our earlier ideas about developing SMMs), keeps everyone on track, helps to ensure that a consistent message is given to the athlete/client, maintaining their confidence and adherence to the programme, and optimizes the benefits of the interdisciplinary interaction.

The second example (Fig. 24.9) takes the rehab process through to its logical conclusion, delineating the respective roles of physio and strength and conditioning specialist. An important, value-added

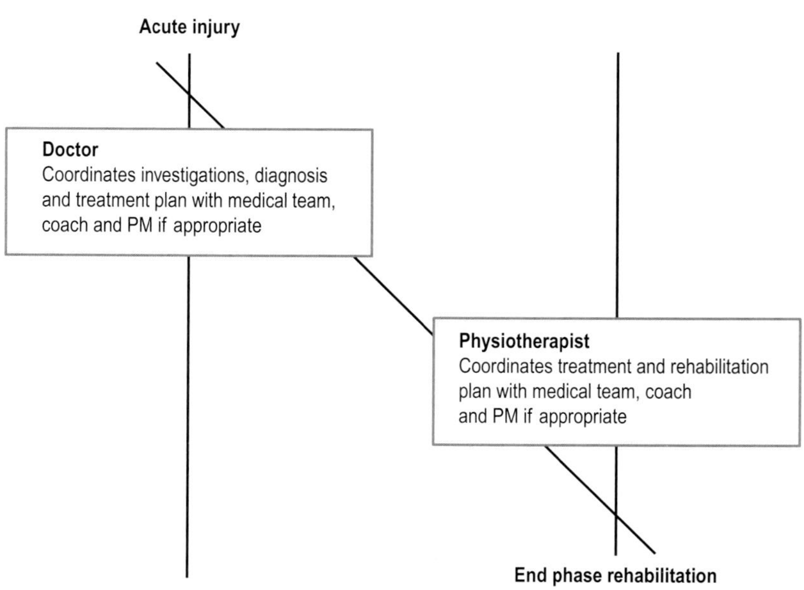

Fig. 24.8 • Role responsibility between doctor and physiotherapist from injury to rehab completion.

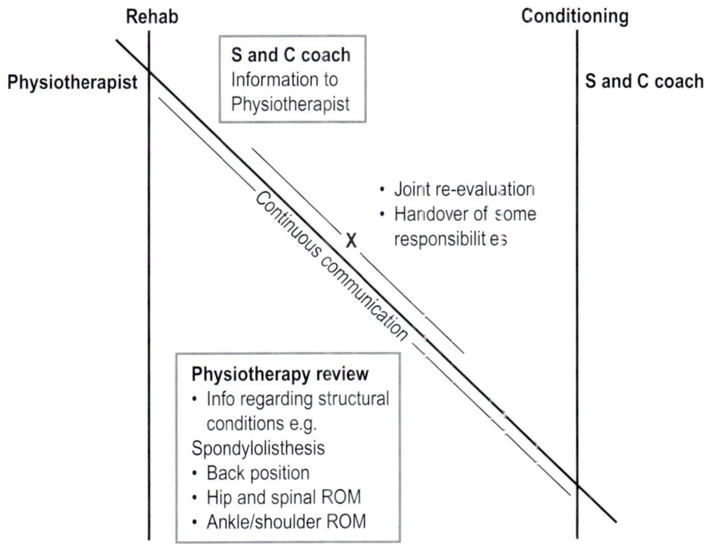

Fig. 24.9 • Roles and handover between physiotherapist and strength and conditioning coach.

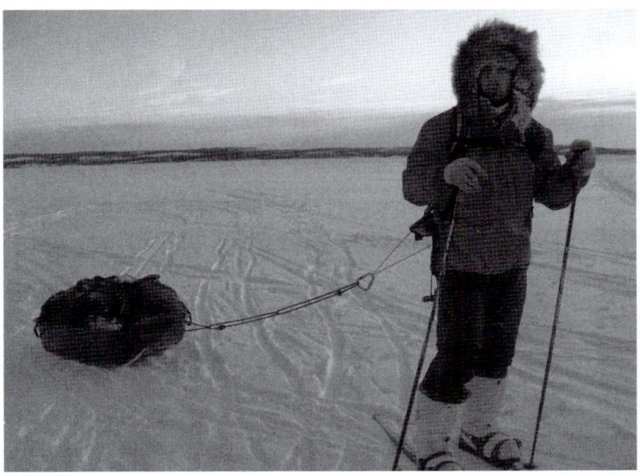

Expedition work places a particular emphasis on teamwork. High consequences of failure and unremitting pressure, both physical and mental. Photo with thanks to Pat Falvey © www.patfalvey.com

benefit is that prophylactic 'prehab' is also facilitated. Nothing beats identifying such important activities into a clear role specification.

Conclusion

In this chapter, we have firmly identified the need for careful attention to the detail of working systems within the team. The practical advice within this chapter should be compared and contrasted with the more theoretical, organizational psychology perspective offered in Chapter 8. Concentration on the working systems of any group is a worthwhile focus that will enhance the output of your performance and support teams more than any expensive team building trips!

References

Bandura, A., 1986. The explanatory and predictive scope of self-efficacy theory. J. Clin. and Social Psychol. 4, 359–373.

Bandura, A., 1993. Perceived self-efficacy in cognitive development and functioning. Educational Psychologist 28, 117–148.

Bray, S.R., 2004. Collective efficacy, group goals, and group performance of a muscular endurance task. Small Group Research 35, 230–238.

Bretz, R.D., Thomas, S.L., 1991. Perceived equity, motivation and final offer arbitration in major league baseball. CAHRS Working Paper Series. Center for Advanced Human Resource Studies, Ithaca, NY.

Briggs, I., Myers, P.B., 1980. Gifts differing: understanding personality type. Consulting Psychologists Press, Palo Alto, CA.

Butler, R.J., Hardy, L., 1992. The performance profile: theory and application. Sport Psychologist 6, 253–264.

Cannon-Bowers, J.A., Salas, E., Converse, S.A., 1993. Shared mental models in expert team decision-making. In: Castellan, N.J. (Ed.), Individual and group decision-making. Lawrence Erlbaum Associates, Hillsdale, NJ, pp. 221–246.

Carron, A.V., Bray, S.R., Eys, M.A., 2002. Team cohesion and team success sport. J. Sports Sci. 20, 119–126.

Carron, A.V., Widmeyer, N.W., Brawley, L.R., 1985. The development of an instrument to assess cohesion in sports teams: the group environment questionnaire. J. Sport Psychol. 7, 244–266.

Eysenck, M.W., Calvo, M.G., 1992. Anxiety and performance: the processing efficiency theory. Cognition and Emotion 6, 409–434.

Gilson, C., Pratt, M., Roberts, K., Weymes, E., 2001. Peak performance. Business lessons from the world's top sports organisations. Harper Collins, London.

Gladden, J.M., Milne, G.R., 1999. Examining the importance of brand equity in professional sports. Sport Marketing Quarterly 8, 21–29.

James, B., Collins, D., 1997. Self-presentational causes of competitive stress during performance. J. Sport and Exerc. Psychol. 19, 17–35.

Kelly, G.A., 1965. The psychology of personal constructs. Norton, New York.

Leary, M.R., 1992. Self-presentational processes in exercise and sport. J. Sport and Exerc. Psychol. 14, 339–351.

Lombardo, M.M., Eichinger, R.W., 1996. FYI for your improvement: a development and coaching guide. Lominger, Minneapolis, MN.

McLean, G.N., '360-degree feedback: Does it belong in the practitioner's toolkit'. Paper presented at the 1996 American Society for Training and Development Internal Conference and Exposition, June 1996.

Tuckman, B.W., Jensen, M.A., 1977. Stages of small-group development revisited. Group and Organisation Studies 2, 419–427.

Williams, J.M., Hacker, C.M., 1982. Causal relationships among cohesion, satisfaction, and performance in women's intercollegiate field hockey teams. J. Sport and Exerc. Psychol. 4, 324–337.

Zaccaro, S.J., Blair, V., Peterson, C., Zazanis, M., 1995. Collective efficacy. In: Maddux, J.E. (Ed.), Self-efficacy, adaptation, and adjustment: theory, research, and application. Plenum Press, New York, pp. 305–328.

Zander, A., 1982. Making groups effective. Jossey-Bass, San Francisco, CA.

Practical dimensions of realizing your peak performance

25

Dave Collins

Grey Matters/UCLan

CHAPTER CONTENTS

Introduction

As I stressed in the opening chapter, this Section covers the 'sharp end stuff' which for many is the core of performance psychology. Although work on the actual performance is the most common subspecies of our subject, it would be a mistake to pay most attention to this phase. Indeed, if the other three sections have been attended to properly, problems in the performance itself may be few and far between. Things still go wrong though, that is the joy of the challenge after all, so avoiding these pitfalls and having some cunning plans practised and in the pipeline is always going to be an important area for attention.

Key practical issues

Something to acknowledge right up front is how comparatively easy it is for performers to commit performance suicide or, at least, tie a metaphorical ball and chain to their own ankle. The commonness of 'self-defeating strategies' is not down to anything complexly 'Freudian' or to some hidden unconscious need to avoid success. Rather it's just that we find it so easy to think the wrong things. RR talks about the big rock in the middle of a white water rapid that 'seems to become magnetic' the more paddlers are told not to hit it. As Aidan highlights in Chapter 22, the structure and function of the human brain includes some characteristics that are often dysfunctional for performance environments. To repeat a key quote, 'the intention to concentrate creates conditions under which mental load enhances monitoring of irrelevancies' (Wegner 1994, p. 7). In other words, many performers become distracted because they try not to. So does this mean they shouldn't try?! No... the answer is to change the method, not the intention. Aidan's chapter offers a number of very practical ideas in this respect, so there isn't too much to add.

DOI: 10.1016/B978-0-443-06734-1.00025-0

Combination training

One extra idea, though, which actually addresses the specific issue raised in Chapter 22 by the Irish rugby kicker Ronan O'Gara, is the need to be physically aroused to an equivalent level in practice as in the event itself. My approach to this, which I have called 'combination training', is to combine practice of very technical, challenging skills with hard physical work. The approach is not particularly innovative, maybe even common-sense but, like many similar ideas, not particularly common! So in Ronan's case, kicks would be taken in short blocks of two or three, in the middle of the full team session or interspersed with fitness work such as interval training. In similar fashion, SB used to complete technical timing drills for the final three strides of his javelin throw interspersed with 200 m strides. A motocross rider, to address his weakness of work on sand, would complete a 5-minute technical circuit on his motorbike followed immediately by a mile's mountain bike ride in full kit, then the circuit, and so on (Collins et al 1993). Such a combination of physical work and technical task is often more similar to what is required in the event itself. The approach also works psychologically, however; so golfers can beneficially combine challenging putts with sprints or press-ups because they learn to overcome a physical distraction (fatigue) that acts in a similar fashion to the more mental challenge (e.g. fear of failure) they will face in the event. In Chapter 20, Hugh illustrates how such combination training can meet the important requirements of learning and pressure-testing coping skills, helping to bridge the training gap from practice and training to high-intensity performance.

This approach can be used with mental practice as well. So, in preparation for fighting specific opponents, judo players can mentally rehearse their strategy against a particular individual during the walk-back recoveries of an extremely hard, 'puke-creating' interval session. Not only does this ingrain the plan, it also adheres to the PETTLEP (Holmes & Collins 2001) precepts in that the arousal is matched to the context in which the tasks will be used.

Finally, the same idea can be employed with different kinds of 'pressure'. KB reports that, as Welsh coach, he would stop team practice mid-session and 'invite' Neil Jenkins, his world-class kicker, to 'win the game' with a challenging penalty kick while the rest of the team tried to distract him. When finding it difficult to 'get mentally up' for qualification, SB would invent a new reality in which the final was cancelled so his practice was focused on a one-time throw to win ('Your focus determines your reality' (Master Yoda, 2005)). Whatever pressure you apply, you can get very creative with these ideas, so give them a go.

The behaviour–cognition–emotion triad

The other key issue to emerge from Section 4 relates to the idiosyncratic and ever-evolving interaction between emotions, thoughts (cognition) and behaviour. Indeed, this 'unholy trinity' underpins almost all the advice included in the section, albeit each of the components, in an attempt to clarify an extremely complex picture, is often considered, if not in isolation, as the prime factor. Despite this, however, the interaction between the factors, and therefore the need to consider the full picture, should be clear to the thoughtful and informed reader. As an example, consider some possible interactions between coping, emotions and attention (Chs 20, 21 and 22, respectively). As Hugh highlights in Chapter 20, the decision to engage in coping is driven by a combination of thoughts and emotions surrounding the challenge (e.g. Can I cope with it? Can I control what it is doing to me?), coupled with the allocation of attention to the various components of the challenge and the mental reactions it is generating. Certainly the practical methods presented throughout the section are optimally effective when they address two or even all of the emotion–cognition–behaviour triad. One important implication here is that any attempt by the athlete or practitioner to control challenges/enhance performance by attention to only one of these components is likely to be doomed.

Another facet of this triad is its idiosyncratic and context specific nature. In simple terms, the interactive pattern of reaction will not only vary from individual to individual but also intraindividually from context to context. Thus, for example, Dave might be completely confident getting shot at or jumping out of planes but is a bag of nerves at a Saturday-night disco (it's true I'm afraid!). Interestingly, this individual/context-specific reaction is also vulnerable to sudden 'chaotic' change. In other words, one small change in a component of the triad can generate an almost complete flip-flop in attitude and behaviour. Complex systems theories seem to offer the best explanation for this, although some field-specific approaches such as reversal theory also get close. The latter seems an overly complicated approach, however, at least to my mind, with practical implications difficult to derive mechanistically from the theory itself. The interested reader is referred to Kerr (1999) if you fancy taking on this challenge (see also Ch. 9).

The main implication of this bifurcating variation (it changes a lot and very suddenly) is the need for highly individualized, constantly refined and multi-layered plans. Self/performer knowledge, evolved and refined over a long period of careful observation, coupled with carefully thought through and well rehearsed plans that address the problem through all three components, will be the best way forwards. Built-in flexibility and 'Plan Bs' to cope with unexpected changes in demand or perception/reaction will help to make the action plan bomb proof. It is perhaps for these reasons that we rather 'nail our colours to the mast' in Chapters 20 and 21, presenting cognitive behavioural therapy as the most efficacious tool for the performance practitioner, given that appropriate training is completed. Certainly, the degree of control and flexibility inherent in the approach, coupled with its 'head-on' tackling of the cognition–behaviour–emotion triad, makes it a very attractive tool for the performance environment.

Things to think about

Developing a 'mindless' performance – in several brains at once

The astute reader will be led to 'compare and contrast' the advice included in this book, and the PP were well up to this challenge. As one very important example, compare and contrast the advice offered by Aidan in Chapter 22. His emphasis on skilled performers' use of an external focus (i.e. on the outcome of the action rather than the action itself) echoes many of the points made in Section 3; wherever possible, skilled execution should be almost 'mindless', allowing the performer's mind–body system to get on with doing what it has been prepared to, and what it knows it can, do. The idea certainly isn't new; *mushin-no mushin* or 'mind – no mind' is a traditional principle of martial arts that still resonates today. Sixteenth-century advice, 'Take as your thought the thought of no thought', transfers directly from *The Seven Samurai* to the Olympic final. In similar fashion, SM highlighted that:

> in dance we talk about technique not being the end goal, it's what you say with your technique, so the interpretation becomes the focus in performance, the specific technique has become automatic. But the process which gets you to that point through rehearsal goes from learning the steps to intense focus on technique and technical challenges to then analysis and development of artistic interpretation including musicality and characterization. So by the time the performance comes you trust your body to perform the technique, which frees you up to focus on others on stage or the audience.

Furthermore, the mindlessness idea is (yet) another of the possibly counterintuitive ideas that permeate the book; it certainly contrasts starkly with the screams to 'concentrate' and 'think about it' that characterize so many coaching episodes. All members of the PP commented on this. RR stressed the need for such automatic, apparently calm action, especially when in the middle of a white-water rapid that has the capacity to kill you... not a good CV entry! With typical Irish loquaciousness, RR also highlighted the planning ahead/Plan B thinking highlighted in the previous block. Stressing the need to be 'more reactive than a block of Semtex in a sauna', he highlights the need for mindlessness, actually multiple mindlessness, in descending a high grade rapid.

> the good guys have the knack of letting the boat run, not doing too much, creating time and space in the midst of overwhelming pressure that acts on the boat, on the mind and on the body. Maybe you can see in this the different levels of attention at work. The river runner has to be more than a man in a barrel falling downstream. Steering, following a preselected line means working your radar. Getting part of your head up in front, preparing the ground, long before the leading edge of the boat touches it isn't just desirable – it's crucial. It's a completely different level of attention from the guiding, correcting, accelerating and side-slipping that makes up the boat control. Throw in some glacier meltwater temperature, as well as looking out for your mates, and you've got an air-traffic control issue for sure!

In such a varied, high degrees of freedom environment, it is almost impossible to generate and remember the required number of Plan Bs. Accordingly, it might be best to think about the plans as principles, ways to think and priorities to address rather than hard and fast 'do this' statements (cf. NDM in Ch. 17).

My best example of this multiple mindlessness is running down a slope. You move smoothly, quickly and safely, so long as you maintain an 'open' focus and keep a steady rhythm; your attention is 'out front', about 4–5 m ahead of your feet, while your body movements and balance are accounted for by a separate system. Focus, usually all of a sudden, on one rock or on a stagger, and the consciousness kicks in with an accompanying burst of trepidation. This sort of split focus, controlling movement while getting your attention out front, should be familiar to all high-speed sports performers, especially perhaps downhill skiing/biking and motor sports. In fact, in some sports a third brain can be incorporated to offer even more 'out-front-ness'. Thus, the expert rally driver will use his bottom and inner ear to know where the car is, his eyes to set the next corner and the pace notes to set up for what is coming next. Unfortunately, most speed sports don't cater for codrivers. So, in events like skeleton bobsleigh, downhill skiing and slalom, the performer must provide their own internal pace notes. Developing and internalizing these plans is a major part of the preparation to perform, a skill that makes combined use of mental practice and sensory reintegration to develop a 'feel-drive plan' for execution.

The chapters offer a variety of ways to accomplish this educated mindlessness; assuming, of course, that the right training and preparation has been completed to ensure that the performer has a strong and consistent internalized programme for the skill or skills required. Many of the ideas presented by Mark and Hugh in Chapter 23 suggest ways in which this 'automatization and trust' ('I can do it automatically and know I can and can let my body get on with it') can be developed. For coacting groups, this auto-trust has an added dimension in that what you are letting your body get on with must fit to the team's or group's agreed system. If not, everyone regresses to their 'natural' or best established style and the team, quite literally, falls apart.

Being ready for when it goes wrong

Of course, this won't always be easy to do, and all accept the pressures that pull the performer(s) towards dysfunctional styles of thinking, movement control and execution. Accordingly, much of the section is about what you can do to cure, if the prevention hasn't worked. It's important to practise this as well, using whatever means to disrupt or challenge performance, so that effective strategies for getting back on track are also internalized and trusted. Concepts of progressive exposure, simulation, combination training and mirroring performance states to enhance the transfer of practice receive a comprehensive discussion in Chapter 20. Without this practice, however, performers must fatalistically learn to accept that 'today isn't the day' and get off the pitch/stage/arena/river as soon as possible with as much psychologically and physically intact as can be salvaged. This 'Oh well' approach is more common than one would think, and there are certainly individual and group performers who don't see their brain as controllable but rather prey to a group of unidentifiable gremlins. Fine if you can pack it in and try your challenge (e.g. a first ascent) tomorrow. Unfortunately, most Olympics or first nights are arranged in advance and tickets sold, so 'I'll be fine tomorrow' doesn't help. In this case, techniques from counselling (see Ch. 21) can be used to very good effect, getting performers to challenge and reconceptualize their views of what they can and cannot control. Certainly, for those domains where opting out is not an option, good coaches will prepare Plan B options in advance. Solutions may sometimes have to be somewhat ad hoc, however. For example, SM recalled a dancer dislocating his knee on stage, so the group danced closely around him as he crawled off!

The points made in Chapter 24 on impression management are also important here. Many athletes learn early to 'talk the talk' but can go a whole career with little or no confidence in their ability to live up to the levels of control that they proclaim so confidently. PP members recognized this and spoke of the need to get these issues in the open at an early stage. KB stressed the need for a grasp of psychology as an essential part of the coach's toolbox. The acknowledgement that directors, instructors and coaches need a T-shaped knowledge (depth in a few topics, breadth in many) was considered in Section 3. The performance environment offers just one of many applications where the breadth, and an understanding of how the various factors interact, is an essential component for those working closely with performers. Too often, a lack of knowledge and confidence in the dark art of performance psychology leave such issues undiscussed – often termed 'the elephant in the room' (although how you could ignore one I'm not sure!). In fact, try to expose them and many will try to hush up the conversation in case it pollutes minds and leads to the very breakdowns it is supposed to prevent. Such 'only accentuate the positive' coaches do have one point; you don't usually start examining someone's doubts and concerns the night before a final. Leaving it unaddressed at other times, however, is just plain negligent. As with so many behaviour change exercises, recognition and acceptance of the problem is an important first step (see the Transtheoretical or 'Stages of Change' Model (Prochaska & DiClemente 1984)). Coaches who demonstrate a performer's weakness, at the right time, with the right intentions and with the tools to solve it, are doing exactly what they should. The models of behaviour change clearly emphasize that generating a readiness, even an eagerness, to change is crucial. A variety of data will help do this effectively, so practitioners may usefully employ performance videos, notational analysis, external reports and the performer's own diary/logs in combination. The only caveats are, as already pointed out, timing, starting with some solutions in mind and plans ready, and the recognition that the change process will take time, so allowing for the slump and rebuild that will often be associated with the change process. SM highlights the need for close one-to-one support through this process, to reassure and maintain the motivation of the performer so they accept and work through the inevitable slump.

Using counselling but not playing at it

The need for communication and support from practitioner to performer is a clear implication of this section, indeed of the whole book. The good news is that techniques from the science of counselling psychology can be used whatever your level of training. So, reading through some basic 'How to' books to improve your awareness of your own communication styles, or to develop some alternatives, is time well spent whether you have a formal training in psychology or not.

However...

this isn't an invitation to consider yourself qualified to probe into the mental 'nooks and crannies' of your performer, looking for problems to solve with your new-found skills. Professionally qualified psychologists and counsellors complete long periods of training for a reason and specialist skills are likely to be needed just to spot some of the potential risks as you dig down. In this regard, it is both irritating and worrying to see the number of 'short but expensive' courses that confer 'Grand Wizard' or 'Master Practitioner' status after a 2-week learning experience. It simply isn't possible to gain the necessary skills that quickly. Of course, some individuals only want to 'go deep' with one or two of their performers. The relationships between performer and coach are often very deep, and there are temptations for both parties to explore, both widely and deeply, the psyche of the other. There should be clear boundaries to this exploration but the problem is that the lines can get very fuzzy and hard to set.

Drawing these lines and sticking to them is important for anyone in the people business, and the frequent power imbalances make establishing boundaries all the more important. So how can you draw the line without constant access to a consultant's input? The most sensible approach I have seen comes from Derek Milne, a clinical psychologist and educator who also works in sport. His ideas are paraphrased in Figure 25.1. Along the bottom, from left to right, is a continuum of increasingly serious interpersonal discussions. It should be very clear that, while everyone should be happy to take part in the left-hand exemplar, only clinical psychologists or psychiatrists who happen to be reading should be willing to take part in the one on the right! The trick is where to place the cutoff between these two extremes. This is very open to debate but the thick black vertical line may represent a common-sense splitting point which delineates things you can help with and topics that should be referred to someone with specialist training.

The bottom line is to help, and improve your capacity to help but, as Clint Eastwood says, 'a man's got to know his limitations .

So what should you do?

As I said at the start of this chapter, there is an understandable tendency to pay more attention to the 'on the day' challenges, if only because they so clearly impact on the performances that are the aim of the whole process covered by this book. This is an all too common mistake but, as you are reading this book, I know that it is a mistake you will avoid!

Seriously, though, there are a couple of other common pitfalls that need attention, together with a synthesis of the key messages from the chapters. For a start, you might consider the focus of attention for the different phases of preparation.

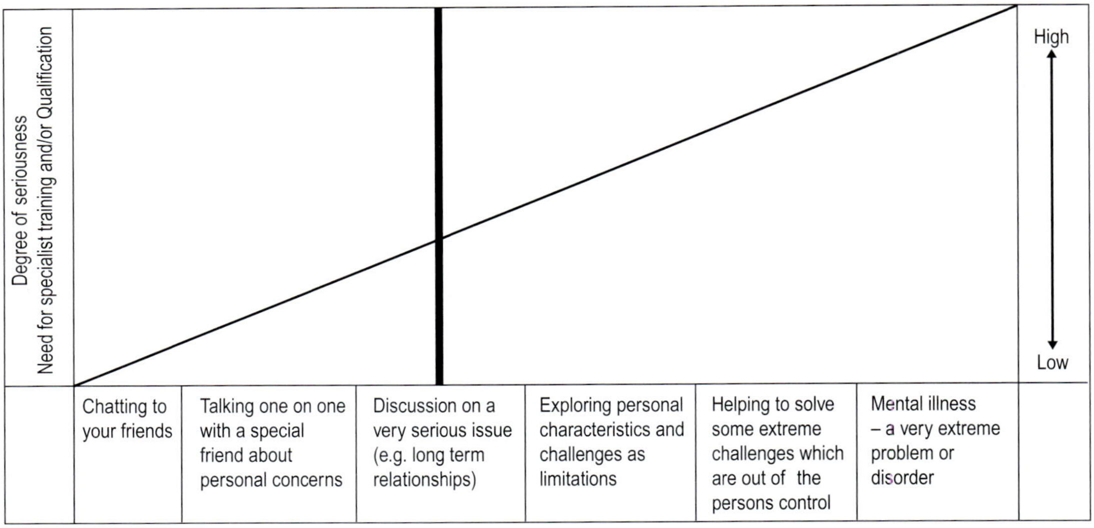

Fig. 25.1 • Seriousness/need for training in 'interpersonal discussion' situations. With kind permission of Derek Milne.

Preparation strategies should include at least two psychological cycles

Chapter 10 has already offered some important ideas about planning and periodization – some may have read this as solely concerned with physical preparation. Not so, of course, as skill acquisition and tactical development will also be big parts of the picture. Mental development should also play a part, though, and the arrangement of training preparation phases before performance phase should allow for at least two cycles. The reason for this is presented graphically in Figure 25.2 and uses as an example a comparison between former World Heavyweight Champion Lennox Lewis and one of his many challengers, the comparatively unknown 20/1 outsider Hasim Rahman.

Now Lennox was a lot better than Hasim, a fact shown on the graph by his higher 'real potential'. When it came to the bout, however, Lennox underperformed. A combination of limited preparation, poor climatic and time-zone adjustment, taking part in a movie (*Ocean's Eleven*) just before the bout, and perhaps not taking his opponent seriously enough, meant that, on the day, he performed well below his real potential while Hasim, seizing the day, performed at his absolute best. As a result, Hasim stole the bout on points. Lennox prepared better the second time around and won the rematch but I hope the lesson is clear.

For the present purpose, consider the focus for most coaches. They spend all their efforts teaching new skills, developing new methods and recruiting the best talent (for teams and companies) to make the Actual Potential column as big as possible. For some, however, comparatively little time is spent avoiding the pitfalls that limit 'on the day' achievement. My point is that there is a switch point, after which further work on actual potential is actually less impactful on the day than making sure that limitations are kept to a minimum. In short, the preparation to perform should include at least two cycles, one of building up and the other of consolidation to avoid things breaking down. Some actual data from performers may help to show this; consider Figure 25.3.

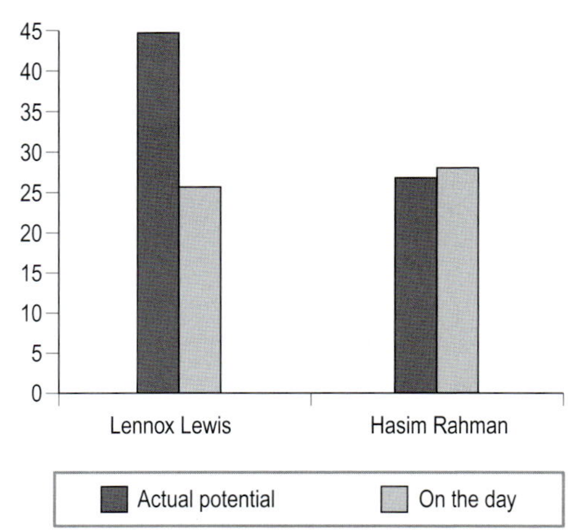

Fig. 25.2 • Actual potential versus 'on the day' performance.

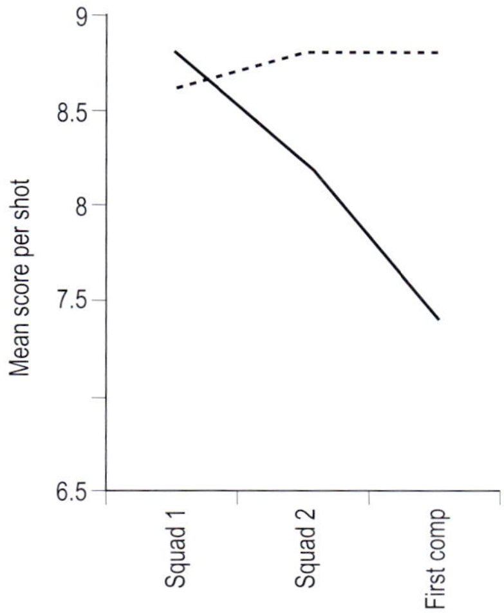

Fig. 25.3 • Mean scores per shot for two international target sports athletes in the run-up to the season.

At the first squad weekend in February, both performers were working on technical issues. Their performance levels were very close, a situation that had characterized their records the previous year. By the second squad, in early April, the first performer (shown as the solid line) had 'put this technical evolution away' for that season, making the decision with his coach to go with what he had and focusing his efforts on completion simulations. In contrast, the second performer (shown as the dashed line) continued to seek the 'perfect technique'. By the start of the season, in mid May, the first athlete was maintaining a good level of consistency; the second was (pardon the pun) shot!

Performers who actually give a performance, specifically aesthetic sports and dance, should consider how close to the 'opening night' they leave it before considering the second-phase work of minimizing limitations. SM explained that, unfortunately, it is common practice to get your costumes the day before the performance, despite efforts to practise in performance-like kit through rehearsal. As an aesthetic philistine but performance aficionado (look them up in the dictionary – I had to!) this strikes me as asking for problems. Perhaps some culture change is essential; I don't think Manchester United would be presented with their brand new strip on the first day of the season!

So, shifting from build to consolidate at the notional split point in your preparation is an important feature of getting the optimum performance out of performers. This shift should be explicitly discussed and advertised to ensure buy-in from all parts of your performance team (see the next section). After the split point is reached, concentrate on making the most of what you have rather than trying to add further to your repertoire.

Work on understanding the exact components of peak performance in the potential building phase

A short, succinct but crucial point. When considering your training phase, take the time and trouble to ensure a deep and shared understanding of what each component is and why it is important. Some practices have an almost traditional place in training and others are included for reasons of political or personal preference. This is particularly an issue when support teams are used; it is entirely possible for one or more of the support professional/coaching/specialist staff to get a bee in their bonnet about one particular facet or issue of preparation. This then gets included without question, or even takes on a disproportionate status in the total programme. Such biases towards performance components are particularly common when the support professional/coach is a former performer: everyone ends up working on the particular strength (or weakness) from that individual's history. So rather than the whole judo team working on one throw because it is a favourite of the coach, each should be addressing his or her individual needs. Rather than including preventative drills against ankle problems (the injury that finished the teacher's career), each has a personalized schedule. Think it unlikely? Well both happened, so please make sure you evaluate all practice and development activity for its contribution to performance and avoid wasted effort.

Use combination training and simulations to test/confirm in the run-up to performance

Chapter 22 has already offered some useful ideas about training attention, and the combination approach discussed in this chapter, plus Chs 21, 23 and 20, provides a practical system for preparing performers to reproduce skilled performances under pressure. Concentration on this sort of training has been a common feature of good performance psychology for a number of years. Brent Rushall was one of the leaders in the field, but has unfortunately been neglected by some practitioners. I present two suggestions based on his work, which may help maximize the return.

First of all, attentional training drills can offer a useful but all too rare opportunity to objectively evaluate mental skills in reasonable isolation. The idea is that, if an attentional focus is any good, this should show up in outcome. In a typical application of these ideas, Rushall & Shewchuck (1989) contrasted the performance differences of three different attentional sets in swimming. One was superior and resulted in a performance improvement over the other two. Now if the same idea is applied to combination training, then performance measures on the relevant task (the kick or technical bike ride, as considered earlier) will be maintained across sets, even as the performer gets more fatigued. The performance measures in this case can be outcome (keeping up a good time or scoring rate) or process (holding form, stride/stroke length or aesthetic quality). The point is that mental focus, or at least the effect of it, can be evaluated: important for motivation, for monitoring and, if it works, for confidence!

The second point concerns what performers should be attending to during performance and has already received some attention in Chapter 3 and specifically in the section on self-talk in Chapter 23. In his classic *Psyching in Sports*, Rushall (1979) makes some excellent suggestions about the combinations of mood words, positive self-talk and task-relevant cognitions that should be used to combat the mental impacts of stress and fatigue. Mood words are those that sum up the action; 'Smooth' or 'Glide' for skaters are good examples. Mood words should be personally meaningful and, as identified in Chapter 13, offer either an 'analogy' or 'rhythm' cue (Poolton et al 2006 and MacPherson et al 2009, respectively), as opposed to a more complex set of 'explicit' verbal instructions. The take-home message here is to avoid long-winded wordy attentional sets, meaningless noise ('Faster', 'Tackle' or 'Concentrate') and to apply the KISS principle (Keep It Simple, Stupid!). Rushall also talked about the intensification principle as physical challenge progresses, thereby increasingly taxing attention. Reflecting and anticipating this, the cycle between self-talk, mood words, etc. should increase in frequency and become more emotive (swearing too) so that the changing content can help to maintain focus.

One exception to this rule relates to more complex situations. In this case, providing a set of short, sharp aide-memoires through which the performer can shift is often a good idea. Let me offer an example from our own work in motocross (Collins et al 1993), which is shown in Figure 25.4.

This plan represents the biker's 'mental model' of the course (cf. our earlier discussion on internal pace notes). In the run-up to the event, he dusts off the plan from last year, using it as a stimulus for practical (e.g. combination) and mental (e.g. mental rehearsal) training. On arrival at the site, he makes adjustments to refine towards a specific plan (this year's course, this year's climate, this year's bike and this year's body), then uses that as the basis for development through formal practice and qualification.

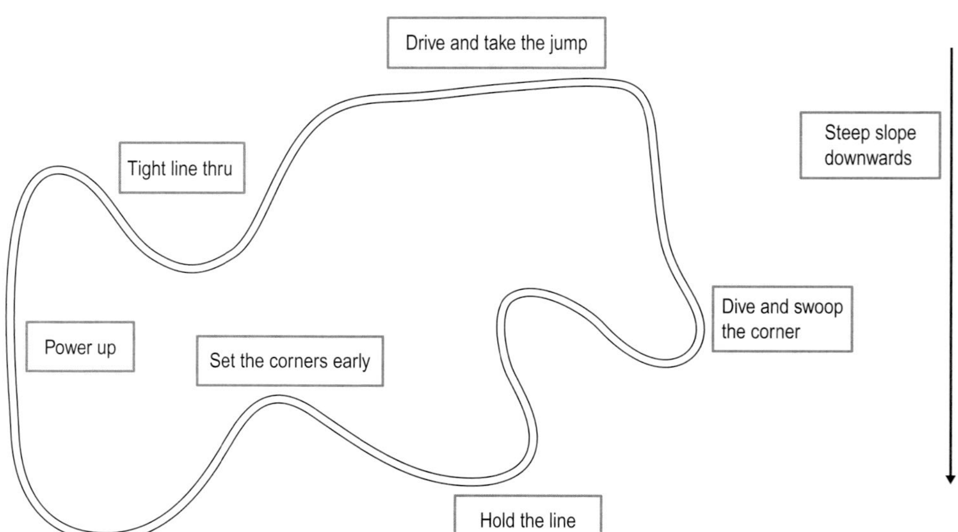

Fig. 25.4 • A 'key focus' plan for a motocross course (kept simple for illustrative purposes!).

'Fred Bloggs'

Event ______________________

Date ______________________

Completed by ______________________

Poor Average Excellent

	1	2	3	4	5	6	7	8	9	10
Pre-event										
Equipment check										
Right training										
Diet and fluids										
Resting										
Sleep										
Self belief										
In event										
Pre-race preparation										
Race plans										
Pre-race focus										
Post-race debrief										
Confidence										
Diet and fluids										
In race										
Starts										
Aggression										
Awareness										
Racing to plan										
Decisive										
Endurance										
Explosion										
Flow										
Position in blend										
Reaction										

Fig. 25.5 • Exemplar post-event checklist used with short-track athletes. With kind permission of Alan Luke.

The plan is longer-winded (more explicit) than some of the earlier recommendations (in Chapter 13 for example) may suggest. Recognize, however, that the performer is going to be constantly switching from one to the next to the next as he races around the course. As such, the level of detail represents a 'shorthand' for the technical and tactical foci necessary. A similar approach can also be seen in the swimmer's race plan in Chapter 23 and can also be used for phases of any longer-duration event, to break it down into manageable chunks. Thus, invasion games can have sets of principles for different parts of the pitch (see Fig. 24.4), downriver runs can be planned rapid by rapid, climbs pitch by pitch or dance performances act by act. Layer on some emotional cues as well (see Ch. 21) and your preparation, simulation/rehearsal and performance should be optimized.

Make sure everyone knows what they need to do

Highlighted for teams by Chapter 24 and in Chapter 9, role clarity is always crucial, whether the team are performers, support staff or both combined. Confidence in each other and, for the performer(s), that the level of performance will meet their goal is a key benefit that cannot help but accrue if you ensure this through a variety of means (for example, the application of performance criteria from Chapter 23 with groups of performers). The methods suggested in the chapter, together with many of the ideas from Section 2, should provide you with a number of different tools. Figure 25.5 offers another example of using such criteria to strengthen common understanding.

In this application, developed with the then national coach for short-track speed skating, Alan Luke, both skater and coach completed a personalized post-event checklist (PEC), rating self/skater on a number of key behaviours. The PEC added clarity in three ways. Firstly, as the criteria were developed, the whole support team evolved a common understanding of the concepts and methods needed for each skater. Secondly, comparisons in score between skater and coach provided for 'healthy debate' on future action plans to evolve performance. Finally, more detailed debrief of each criteria, specifically why the score was what it was, identified areas of concern that specialists could get to work on. In this example, at the pre-Olympic event, sleep was identified as an issue and addressed in time for the event itself.

As per the advice throughout this book, using different approaches to promote and 'triangulate' the constructs and characteristics required is a key function for coaches and/or performance managers.

Conclusion

The aim of this section was to offer you a variety of tools and the reasons underpinning them. I hope this chapter has offered some hints on how creative you can get in developing original and innovative combinations, all with the consistent and well understood aim of performance enhancement.

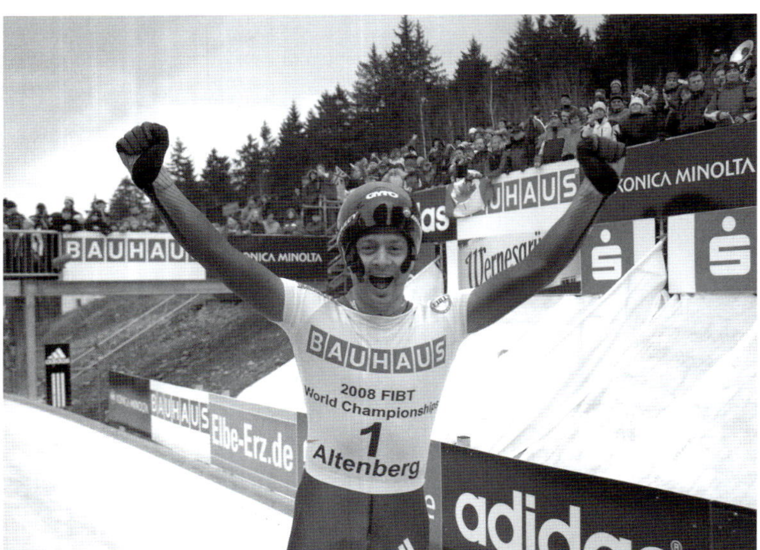

Even better when it works all season! Kristan Bromley celebrates the 'triple crown' of European, World Cup and World Championship Gold in Skeleton Bobsleigh. With thanks to Kristan Bromley.

References

Collins, D., Doherty, M., Talbot, S., 1993. Performance enhancement in Moto Cross: a case study of the sport science team in action. Sport Psychologist 7, 290–297.

Holmes, P.S., Collins, D., 2001. The PETTLEP approach to motor imagery: a functional equivalence model for sport psychologists. Journal of Applied Sport Psychology 13, 83–106.

Kerr, J.H., 1999. Reversal theory: motivation and emotion in sport. Psychology Press, London.

MacPherson, A., Collins, D., Obhi, S., 2009. The importance of temporal structure and rhythm for the optimum performance of motor skills: a new focus for practitioners of sport psychology. Journal of Applied Sport Psychology 21, S48–S61.

Poolton, J.M., Masters, R.S.W., Maxwell, J.P., 2006. The influence of analogy learning on decision-making in table tennis: evidence from behavioural data. Psychology of Sport and Exercise 7, 677–688.

Prochaska, J.O., DiClemente, C.C., 1984. The transtheoretical approach: crossing traditional boundaries of therapy. Dow Jones–Irwin, Homewood, IL.

Rushall, B.S., 1979. Psyching in sports. Pelham Books, London.

Rushall, B.S., Shewchuck, M.L., 1989. Effects of thought content instructions on swimming performance. Journal of Medicine and Physical Fitness 29, 326–334.

Wegner, D.M., 1994. Ironic processes of mental control. Psychol. Rev. 101, 34–52.

Conclusion: Where next? Getting help in your pursuit of excellence

Amanda Martindale* Dave Collins†
*University of Edinburgh, Edinburgh UK; †Grey Matters/UCLan

CHAPTER CONTENTS

Where next?

This chapter aims to provide direction on how to get help in your pursuit of excellence. The sections on the four Ps (Preparation, Provision, Practice and Performance) have hopefully heightened your awareness of the psychological underpinning of peak physical performance. This understanding, along with your own experience, may well have stimulated further questions, ideas or directions that you wish to pursue. Consequently, the first part of this chapter provides information for the athlete or coach wishing to secure professional assistance from a qualified sport or performance psychologist. This includes: developing aims and objectives; what to look for; where to look; and a guide to accreditation systems. Alternatively, for the coach or practitioner seeking to implement some of the applied concepts discussed in this book, the second part of this chapter provides direction on putting theory into practice and how to maximize your professional autonomy and independent judgement in the decisions you formulate on the journey towards peak physical performance.

Securing performance psychology assistance

Developing your aims and objectives

Prior to seeking the services of a sport or performance psychologist, it is well worth considering your aims and objectives. For example, are you seeking performance enhancement or life development skills, intervention or education, a brief consultation or a more enduring consultation process? It is also worth bearing in mind that the focus of your support may dictate the type of relationship, approach and/or way of working with the psychologist. For example, performance enhancement may have an emphasis on change, challenge and possibly discomfort, while life development skills may have more of an emphasis on comfort and gentle questioning. It is likely that you will have an idea of some areas that you would like to work on or address and this can be the initial starting

DOI: 10.1016/B978-0-443-06734-1.00027-4

point for discussion with a potential provider. In taking this forward, there are a number of questions that you may wish to ask regarding the way in which the psychologist operates. Sometimes this process is agreed in collaboration, depending on the context, logistical and practical circumstances. The next section provides some background information on what to look for in a potential performance psychology service provider.

What to look for

One of the first lines of enquiry for sounding out a potential provider of psychological services is to establish their theoretical orientation (and most importantly to establish that they have one). The orientations or paradigms utilized in sport and performance psychology include cognitive–behavioural and variations of this (e.g. rational–emotive behavioural) and humanistic orientations (e.g. person-centred). Cognitive–behavioural orientations are more prevalent in performance psychology as they consider cognitions (thoughts) and behaviours (actions) and provide direction, skills, techniques and strategies to enhance these in training and performance arenas (see Ch. 21). This can involve leading and training athletes to perform outwith the bounds of their comfort zone and challenging them to overcome difficulties in pursuit of enhanced performance. In contrast, humanistic orientations are typically non-directive and involve low levels of resource provision. This type of practice may involve questioning to assist the performer in understanding and discovering where they want to go. You may already have an inclination about the type of support you are most likely to respond to; however, it's important to keep an open mind and discuss the implications of practice with the provider themselves as they will probably have a clear rationale for why they operate according to their chosen orientation (Fig. C.1).

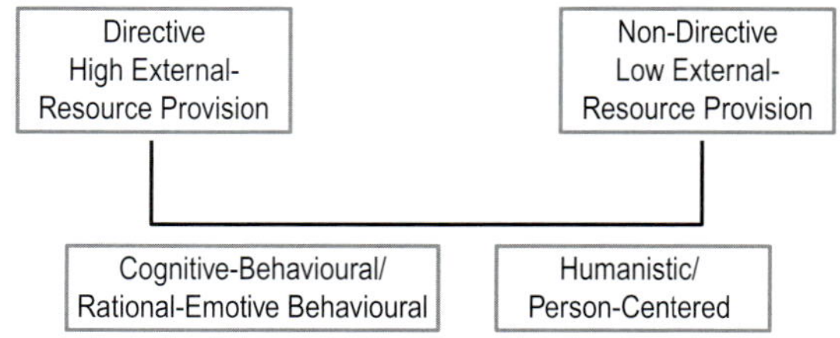

Fig. C.1 • Continuum of applied sport psychology theoretical orientations: direction and external resource provision.

A related, but distinct line of enquiry you may wish to pursue is to establish the provider's professional philosophy. The possible responses to this question can be vast and varied; however, it is promising if the provider includes fostering empowerment, independence and/or self-sufficiency in the performer (Kremer & Scully 1998). This would suggest that they recognize the process of skill development and may ultimately be seeking to make themselves redundant (i.e. to provide the performer with the ability to know when and how to utilize certain skills and strategies without the need for the provider to be present).

The psychologist should be able to talk you through their model of practice and /or intervention. This will help to clarify what you can expect and the necessary stages of the process. Typically, the cognitive–behavioural process (see Murphy 1995 for more detail) will begin with a phase of needs analysis to ensure that the practitioner has a sound understanding of the performer's situation, task demands, and current levels of operation and performance. Once the goals have been clearly identified, the psychologist will work in collaboration with the athlete and coach to develop skills, enhance techniques and design strategies for performance enhancement. It is important to clarify that these interventions are theoretically and scientifically underpinned and in accordance with the principles of best practice. Ideally, the provider will keep up to date with current developments in peer-reviewed journals, for example. You should feel free to discuss the scientific underpinning as to why the intervention is likely to be of assistance. This can sometimes aid buy-in and understanding as to what you may experience and the likely development process. As part of the process the psychologist should build in time-framed evaluation to gather and provide feedback on how well you are progressing towards your goals.

Sometimes refinement of the intervention is required or goals may need to be re-addressed if improvements are not progressing as quickly as hoped. It is important to be aware, however, that rarely are interventions of this kind a 'quick fix' process; more typically, they require a period of education, learning, development, maintenance and then a period of sustainability before the process of change can be said to have taken place (as per the stages of change model (Prochaska & DiClemente 1984)).

Another factor you may wish to consider before deciding on your helping professional is whether they have the human or people skills that you think will either complement or bring an added dimension to your existing support team. For example, superior communication skills are necessary in order to be able to express understanding, scientific rationale in laymen's terms, and sometimes to convince less than enthusiastic members of the team that certain directions are worth pursuing. If you are hoping that the practitioner will operate as an 'agent of change' then these communication skills should be accompanied by sound empathy and an ability to challenge in a manner that is acceptable and appreciated by the athlete.

You might even think about the 'consumer resistance' to the idea of working with a psychologist; might it be too great for an immediate implementation? Gould & Damarjian (1998) identify several barriers, which can often be automatically erected at the first use/appearance of the 'psycho':

- Performer's stereotype of psychologists – 'I'm not mental'
- A perceived/actual lack of knowledge about performance
- Lack of knowledge/unaware of organizational politics (see Section 2)
- Coming in 'too heavy' or 'all-knowing' – as a result poor first impressions/expectations hamstring subsequent efforts
- Hero worship – the psychologist is quite literally 'starstruck' and gives certain performers far too much fawning respect
- Failure to be practical – too 'ivory tower' and theoretical.

These barriers are based on stereotypes but are all too often true or self-fulfilling. Any psychologist worth the name will be aware of these challenges and will take care to embed themselves carefully and with consideration. The coach can help by addressing these concerns head on, but it may well be that the performance environment, its traditions and mores mean that the introduction must be handled with particular care and at a particularly slow pace.

Finally, it is worth considering whether the provider has the ability to organize and to develop support systems and networks, and displays an awareness or willingness to learn about other support sciences and methods. Be wary of practitioners who appear to know all the answers (see Ch. 10), use broad-brush generic interventions or work in isolation from the coach and other support providers. Performance psychology is not an exact science and, as a result, providers of this service may need to operate with a 'test and adjust' approach whereby interventions are tailored over time to the individual requirements of the performer and their setting. A skilled practitioner will be creative in their design of interventions and remain open to the feedback and ideas of the athletes and coaches. The most successful interventions are often those that have evolved through collaboration between athlete, coach and psychologist as each provides input about their own area of expertise (as an example relating to technical change, see Collins et al 1999).

Where to look

The professional bodies that govern sport and performance psychology in the UK are the British Psychological Society (BPS, Division of Sport and Exercise Psychology) and the British Association of Sport and Exercise Sciences (BASES). In the USA the recognized bodies are the American Psychological Association (APA; Division 47) and the American Association for the Advancement of Applied Sport Psychology (AAASP). Each of these bodies has a website through which you can navigate to find contact details of registered consultants. A list of web addresses is provided at the end of this chapter. Not all providers choose to be listed in this way, however, and there are various other ways of locating a suitable specialist. For example, institutes of sport commonly employ sport psychologists to work with athletes and teams, although they may have restrictions on providing support to athletes outside these systems. Many performance psychologists employed by universities consult in addition to their teaching and research activities and these individuals are typically up to date with current literature and research. It is also well worth keeping your ear to the ground, as word of mouth can often be a valuable source of information as to how well a particular individual has been received by other athletes, coaches and service providers. Of course, different styles suit different individuals; however, it may save you valuable time if you receive insight on their knowledge, professional conduct and interpersonal style from a trusted contact. However you find a potential practitioner, it is important to clarify their professional status to ensure that you will be receiving the highest level of service. The following section on accreditation systems explains more about what to look out for.

Accreditation systems

You should seek to establish whether the potential provider is a member of one or more of the bodies mentioned above and their stage of development within that group's particular pathway. For example, a Probationary Sport and Exercise Psychologist is a member of BASES who is going through the process of Supervised Experience. If a provider has undergone the full training cycle required then they will have accredited (e.g. BASES) or chartered status (e.g. BPS) of the relevant professional body. This means they have gone through a period of supervision and have been recognized as able to practise independently. This status also ensures that the practitioner is adhering to a code of conduct, is following recognized standards of professional ethics and is regularly undertaking continuing professional development activity. By choosing a provider who is recognized by a professional body of psychology or sports science you are ensuring professional accountability and a quality level of service; make sure you ask for a copy, or at least a reference to, the code of conduct to which they work.

Be aware that there are practitioners operating with minimal qualifications in the field who do not follow an accreditation system. In fact, at the time of writing, anyone in the UK can call themselves a psychologist. It may be worth checking out why this is the case; it can be a painstaking and long process to become qualified, which demonstrates diligence, commitment and dedication on the part of the provider.

As a final note, psychologists may well (indeed should) utilize peer supervision; this is where they anonymously discuss cases with another fully qualified psychologist to ensure that their conceptualization and intervention strategies are well founded. This is typically an indicator of quality practice and is becoming increasingly common following the lead of some of the more traditional branches of psychology (e.g. clinical and counselling psychology). Such discussion is within the bounds of confidentiality in most codes of conduct. Even so, it is considered good practice for the psychologist to advise you of such activity.

If you want to read further, Kate Hays (2006) has provided an excellent overview of some of the professional issues in performance psychology. Read and think about what characteristics you really need for effective, safe and evidence-based support in your particular performance domain.

Implementing psychology for physical performance

How to make the most of this book

One of the five principal criteria of professionalism identified by Carr (1999) is that a high degree of individual autonomy and independence of judgement is required for effective practice. Physical performance situations present novel problems, often with no clearcut or 'correct' answer. As such, solutions may be 'advisory' and ultimately dependent on the quality of deliberation and reflection by the practitioner. Thus, practice must be informed by science and theory, while still applied creatively to meet the specific demands and requirements of each unique situation.

This autonomy and independence of judgement is where we believe the skill and quality of the practitioner predominantly lie (i.e. Why are they doing what they are doing? How have they arrived at that suggested course of action?). Consequently, the emphasis of this section on implementing psychology for physical performance is placed on maximizing coaches' and/or psychologists' decision-making capabilities.

A central facet underpinning sound professional judgement and decision making is scientific knowledge. Indeed, Sibeon (1991, p. 7) suggests that 'one of the recognized hallmarks of a profession is an underlying knowledge base, a body of specialized knowledge which acts as the basis of professional expertise'. We hope that this text will assist you in using knowledge to enhance your practice, whether as a performer, psychologist or coach. This concept of necessary knowledge is captured by Thompson's (2000) 'Thinking and Doing Model', which describes how 'thinking' provides us with opportunities to use theory to enhance practice while 'doing' provides us with opportunities to learn from experience, which in turn may enhance the 'thinking' element of practice.

We are inclined to take this concept a step further and suggest that critical thinking is an essential aspect of professional practice (i.e. Why is this likely to create an impact? Why has that period of training/intervention not produced the desired outcome?). Furthermore, we suggest that critical thinking can be enhanced through the development of professional judgement and decision-making skills.

A professional exemplar: coach decision making

In examining the knowledge bases and decision-making processes required for effective coaching, Abraham et al (2006) carried out the validation of a coaching schematic based on expert coach consensus. This schematic is suggested to illustrate the coaching process, at a conceptual level, through referral to the required knowledge, concepts, decision making and resulting behavioural/observable output of coaches (see Ch. 15, Figure 15.1).

The expert consensus revealed that coaches use a 'hierarchy' to make decisions in an integrated fashion (i.e. a hierarchical set of rules helps to organize coaches' decision making). This approach enables coaches to utilize a broad range of information when identifying areas for development and generating potential directions. This complex approach to achieving outlined goals is termed the 'breadth-first approach' to problem solving (Abraham & Collins 1998). As part of this approach, expert coaches are accessing several knowledge bases (sometimes with competing or conflicting rationales) to make a 'best-fit' decision.

In exploring this broad range of knowledge sources used by expert coaches to underpin their decision making, Abraham et al (2006) identified the two most important sources of knowledge to be sport-specific and pedagogic in nature. In addition, expert coaches identified the importance of what were termed the '-ologies' (e.g. physiology, psychology, biomechanics, motor control, etc.) as a source of information about the ways in which decisions must be tweaked to meet the needs of each individual. As such, there is a growing consensus that knowledge of psychological factors influencing performance (along with other scientific disciplines) helps to underpin informed decision making in coaches of pre-elite and elite athletes.

Such awareness, namely what knowledge bases are informing decision making, can allow coaches to gain an enhanced conceptual understanding of the process they are going through to guide the development of their athletes. The quest for interdisciplinary knowledge is predominantly self-driven and, while there are numerous opportunities for continued professional development (e.g. coaching qualifications, courses, experience, higher education courses, own reading, etc.), Abraham et al (2006) suggest that expert coaches may be more akin to 'knowledge magpies' than 'filing cabinets'. Understanding and exploring the complexity of coach decision making is still at an early stage; however, it is clearly a worthy research endeavour. Some further clarity and understanding may be gleaned from considering the professional judgement and decision-making processes undertaken in other parallel professions and, in particular, from recent research in the provision of applied sport psychology practice.

A more detailed treatment of these issues can be found in Section 3; specifically, Chapters 22 and 25.

A more pertinent application for this book – PJDM in action

In parallel to the developments in coach education, the importance of professional judgement and decision making (PJDM) has become increasingly recognized within the applied sport psychology literature (e.g. Gardner & Moore 2005, Martindale & Collins 2005, Poczwardowski et al 1998). This reflects the importance credited to decision-making processes in parallel professions such as teaching and medicine, and in other branches of psychology, such as clinical and counselling (e.g. Curtner-Smith 1999, Hill 1992, Patel & Ramoni 1997).

One rationale for this deserved attention is based on the suggestion that 'issue conceptualization' has been previously been neglected in applied sport psychology practice and research (Poczwardowski et al 1998). Issue conceptualization refers to the phase between the needs analysis and the associated intervention/s (i.e. where the issues surrounding the situation are established and an appropriate course of action has been formulated). Martindale & Collins (2005) have suggested that issue conceptualization represents a dynamic and multilayered process in which the practitioner may consider issues across various timescales (e.g. short, medium and long) and levels of support (e.g. session, intervention and programme). For example, the practitioner may consider how they intend to impact on the performer's behaviour, cognitions or emotions across these various layers throughout the process of change (Greenberg 1986).

This focus on issue conceptualization is due to the engagement in decision making that is required at this time; although decision making is integral throughout the process of support provision, intuitively it is especially important during this phase.

The skilled practitioner will reflect on a broad range of information and knowledge bases (e.g. needs analysis results; psychological, interdisciplinary, personal, and situational knowledge) alongside their theoretical orientation, professional philosophy and past experience to arrive at a considered and informed course of action.

This combination of factors can have considerable consequences for the nature of the goal and the nature of the relationship established between practitioner and client. For example, if a practitioner has adopted a cognitive–behavioural orientation and is operating as an agent of change (i.e. with performance enhancement as the goal) then they may relate to the client in a challenging manner, questioning the logic of certain thoughts, beliefs and behaviours. In contrast, a humanistic practitioner working towards life development as the agreed goal may operate in a much less directive manner, encouraging the client to discover their own solutions. Of course, both approaches are entirely valid, so long as method matches objective. The point is that both positions should hopefully have been arrived at through a series of conscious decisions if practice is to be delivered in a coherent manner.

These decisions are manifest in the practitioner's 'intentions for impact', which represent 'the cognitive component that mediates the choice of intervention' (i.e. why the practitioner has chosen a certain intervention rather than what the intervention is (Hill & O'Grady 1985)). These intentions offer insight into how the practitioner is thinking about and planning for the intervention with the performer.

In order to demonstrate these decision making processes 'in action', a case study of an international judo athlete rehabilitating from a serious and potentially career-ending injury to her knee (ruptured anterior cruciate ligament) is provided in Figure C.2 to illustrate the multilayered and 'nested' characteristics of issue conceptualization and intentions for impact.

The uppermost section of Figure C.2 represents the overall 'programme' of support, which in this case was longitudinal and spanned several years. The practitioner is likely to have over-riding intentions for work with each client; in this case to foster empowerment, independence and self-sufficiency, and to prepare the client for career transition (retirement). These intentions may be strongly influenced by the provider's theoretical orientation and professional philosophy.

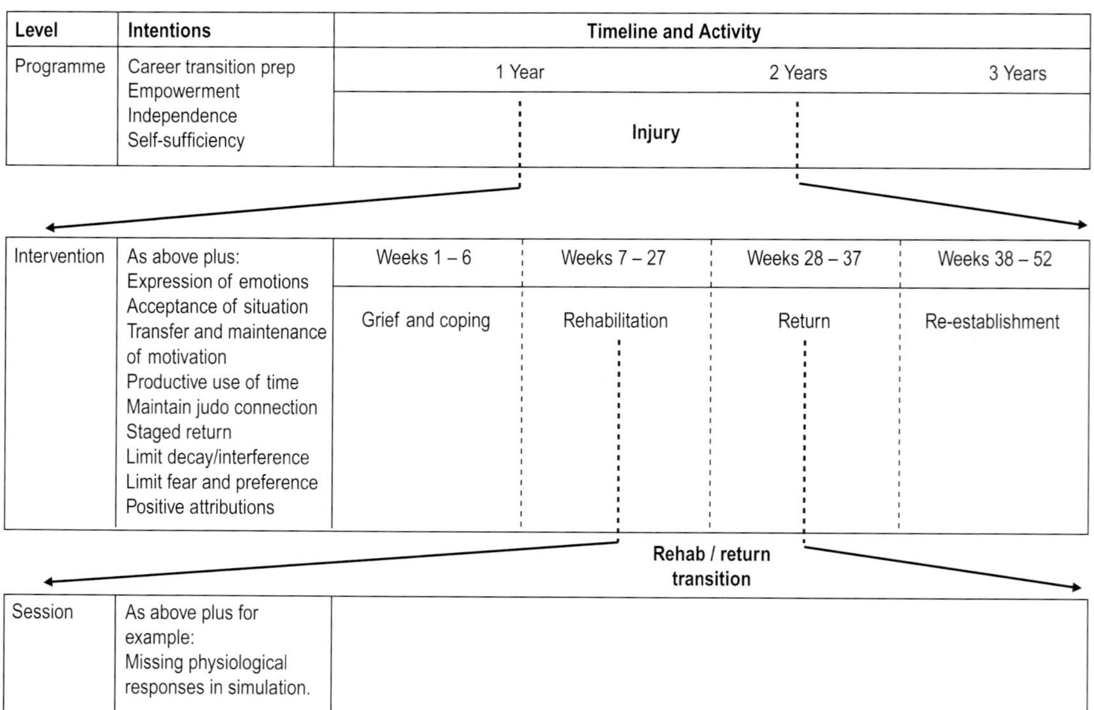

Fig. C.2 • Multilayered nature of client issues/practitioner intentions for impact across programme, intervention and session levels of support.

The middle section of Figure C.2 represents one block of 'intervention' carried out as part of the support; in this case the phase of intervention lasted approximately 1 year. A further layer of 'intentions' may be formed for each new phase of intervention based on a continued needs analysis. The formation of these intentions will be led by the specific context and the client's presenting needs. However, despite this more elaborate layer of intentions, whatever its nature, the practitioner should still be working to meet the programme-level intentions previously established; thus the 'nested' approach to coherent support begins to emerge. In this case, the client was expected to move through a series of 'stages' in her recovery from injury (namely, grief and coping, rehabilitation, return and re-establishment). The intervention required during each phase will logically differ and, in the case of serious injury, require psychological, emotional, social, motor control and physiological elements.

A further layer of intentions can be exposed by considering that, throughout any given phase of intervention, the provider will conduct individual 'sessions' with the client. In our case study, for example, sessions during the rehabilitation and return phases of intervention included refinements to a performance simulation programme (such as countering the lack of physiological sensations). These short-term issues presented themselves in sessions with the client, and the provider was therefore required to formulate an intention for impact and design a suitable refinement. As part of this level of the intervention process, the practitioner should be mindful of intentions formed at the intervention and programme levels in order for the support to remain coherent and appropriately focused.

This exemplar case study illustrates some of the complexity and intricacy involved in issue conceptualization. Notably, but also typically, it is a 'multilayered' dynamic process manifested throughout the support with intentions for impact 'nested' within each layer to maintain a coherent approach. We suggest that this depth of consideration and analysis is beneficial for the provider in the planning, implementing and evaluation of support.

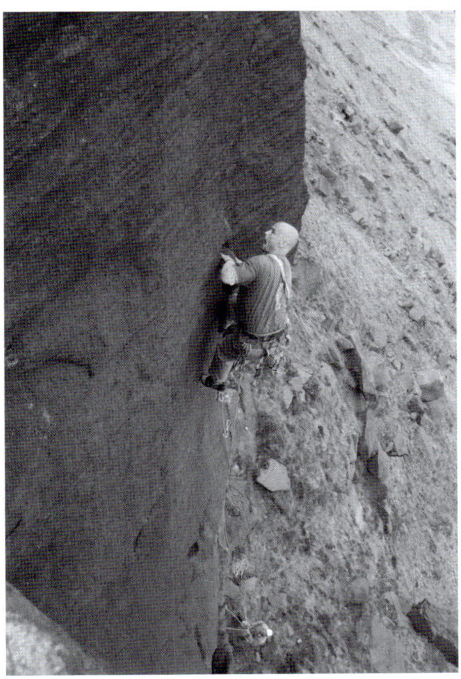

Ace biomechanist Dr John Buckley applies his mechanical skills to a practical task.

A summary, special circumstances and future directions

Evaluating psychology for physical performance

In evaluating the application of psychology for the enhancement of physical performance it is important to consider both outcome and process. The most important outcome is the improvement in performance; however, it can be difficult to pinpoint just what factor or combination of factors is responsible for such gains. Nevertheless, outcome can be evaluated at session, intervention and programme levels of support (e.g. by using session impact scales, gauging the level of experiencing/adherence and conducting behaviour change interviews – see Martindale & Collins 2007).

A further level of evaluation can be gleaned by considering the process of support. For example, clients may be unsure if psychology support has stimulated a quantifiable difference in terms of performance outcome, but perceive themselves to be in a better 'mental state' before and during performance. This enhanced 'state of being' may in itself be considered a success and more likely to allow the individual to produce performances to their full capability.

The provider too, can evaluate the process of their support through undertaking peer supervision and reflective practice. In particular, we suggest that focus should centre on the critical reflection of professional judgement and decision-making processes (see Martindale & Collins 2007 for a fuller explanation).

A key issue – when to pass it on?

One big issue, already addressed but still worthy of careful consideration, is the need for and timing of referral. This chapter, indeed the whole book, espouses a level of detail that is, we feel, not only essential but also the natural expectation of the performer. In short, if they can be bothered to put in the time and commitment necessary for peak performance, then so should we as performance enhancers! The need to refer is implicit to this detailed consideration of a client/performer's needs, and such a step should be an obvious decision when one is motivated by the client's needs. Chapters 21 and 25 explore this issue, so detailed consideration is available elsewhere. At this juncture, however, we should emphasize the need to ask for input, not just when you think things are going wrong but in anticipation of that fact. In short, audit your decisions wherever possible (see our earlier comments on 'peer-supervision') and always place the client/performer's needs as the first priority.

Pursuit of knowledge and professional practice

Ultimately, we hope this book and this chapter have stimulated your pursuit of knowledge, psychological and otherwise, to support your current practices in physical performance. In addition, we hope to have stimulated your desire to seek and/or implement the provision of professional applied performance psychology practice to ensure our performers receive the highest level of service and support that they so deserve.

References

Abraham, A., Collins, D., 1998. Examining and extending research in coach development. Quest 50, 59–79.

Abraham, A., Collins, D., Martindale, R., 2006. The coaching schematic: validation through expert coach consensus. J. Sports Sci. 24, 549–564.

Carr, D., 1999. Professional education and professional ethics. J. Appl. Philos. 16, 33–46.

Collins, D.J., Morriss, C., Trower, J., 1999. Getting it back: a case study of skill recovery in an elite athlete. Sport Psychologist 13, 288–298.

Curtner-Smith, M.D., 1999. The more things change the more they stay the same: influencing teachers' interpretations and delivery of national curriculum physical education. Sport, Education and Society 4, 75–97.

Gardner, F.L., Moore, Z.E., 2005. Using a case formulation approach in sport psychology consulting. Sport Psychologist 19, 430–445.

Gould, D., Damarjian, N., 1998. Insights into effective sport psychology consulting. In: Hays, K.F. (Ed.), Integrating exercise, sports, movement and mind: therapeutic unity. Haworth, Binghampton, NY, pp. 111–130.

Greenberg, L.S., 1986. Change process research. J. Consult. Clin. Psychol. 54, 4–9.

Hays, K.F., 2006. Being fit: the ethics of practice diversification in performance psychology. Professional Psychology: Research and Practice 37, 223–232.

Hill, C.E., 1992. An overview of four measures developed to test the hill process model: therapist intentions, therapist response modes, client reactions, and client behaviours. Journal of Counseling and Development 70, 728–739.

Hill, C.E., O'Grady, K.E., 1985. List of therapist intentions illustrated in a case study and with therapists of varying theoretical orientations. Journal of Counseling Psychology 32, 3–22.

Kremer, J., Scully, D., 1998. What applied sport psychologists often don't do: on empowerment and independence. In: What sport psychologists do. British Psychological Society, London, pp. 21–27.

Martindale, A., Collins, D., 2005. Professional judgment and decision making: the role of intention for impact. Sport Psychologist 19, 303–317.

Martindale, A., Collins, D., 2005. Enhancing the evaluation of effectiveness with professional judgement and decision making. Sport Psychologist 21, 458–474.

Murphy, S.M. (Ed.), 1995. Sport psychology interventions. Human Kinetics, Champaign, IL.

Patel, V.L., Ramoni, M.F., 1997. Cognitive models of directional inference in expert medical reasoning. In: Feltovich, P.J., Ford, K. M., Hoffman, R.R. (Eds.), Expertise in context. MIT Press, Cambridge, MA.

Poczwardowski, A., Sherman, C.P., Henschen, K.P., 1998. A sport psychology delivery heuristic: building on theory and practice. Sport Psychologist 12, 191–207.

Prochaska, J.O., DiClemente, C.C., 1984. The transtheoretical approach: crossing traditional boundaries of therapy. Dow Jones–Irwin, Homewood, IL.

Sibeon, R., 1991. Towards a new sociology of social work, Avebury, Aldershot, Hampshire.

Thompson, N., 2000. Theory and practice in human services. Open University Press, Buckingham.

Web resources

The British Psychological Society website:, www.bps.org.uk

The British Association of Sport & Exercise Sciences website: www.bases.org.uk

American Psychological Association website:, www.apa.org

The American Association for the advancement of Applied Sport Psychology website: www.appliedsportpsych.org

Index

Note: Page numbers followed by *b* indicate boxes, *f* indicate figures and *t* indicate tables.

Q

R

S

T